Dilemmas in Drug Therapy

HARRY BECKMAN, M.D.

*Houghton Fellow in Clinical Research and
Consulting Physician, Columbia Hospital,
Milwaukee; Consulting Physician, Milwaukee
County General Hospital; Honorary Physician,
Saint Mary's Hospital, Milwaukee; Editor,
Year Book of Drug Therapy; Professor (Emeritus)
of Pharmacology, Marquette University School
of Medicine.*

W. B. Saunders Company, Philadelphia and London, 1967

W. B. Saunders Company: West Washington Square
Philadelphia, Pa. 19105

12 Dyott Street
London W.C.1

Dilemmas in Drug Therapy

To the Staff of

COLUMBIA HOSPITAL

in gratitude and admiration

Preface

MANY YEARS AGO, having been asked to create a department of undergraduate pharmacology, I found it necessary to separate the experimental matter from actual therapeutics in order to present the subject acceptably to preclinical students. The therapeutic portion, as it sifted out, seemed almost automatically to form itself into a book, and so my "Treatment in General Practice" was launched upon a long career.

Now another occurrence has provoked somewhat similar action. A long-time consultant, official and unofficial, on the use of drugs in my area, I have recently been asked to come into one of the hospitals as full-time consultant in this field. And so once again the sorting-out process! And willy-nilly (mostly nilly this time, being now really too old for this sort of thing), another book has found itself being written.

"Here is the patient and these are the circumstances. This drug has failed and so has that. Who has used another unusual one instead and why? What are the risks? Is there something I should know and do not? What would you do?" These are the questions the consultant on drugs is asked. The book is an attempt to answer them for all physicians who may want the benefit of requested opinion. Mark you, please, I have said *opinion*, for the sort of temperament that can consider itself outside subjectivity is not mine. I try to consider all sides of a question objectively, and then offer the answer of a human being and not of a computer.

Should the book prove to be of service in a very confused field, I shall be pleased.

It is a pleasure and privilege to acknowledge the generous support of the great publishing house of W. B. Saunders Co. in this my rather tremulous swan-song, and to extend to Judith (Mrs. Thomas) Jones my thanks for her faithful secretarial assistance.

HARRY BECKMAN

Columbia Hospital
3321 N. Maryland Avenue
Milwaukee, Wisconsin 53211

Contents

(THERE ARE NUMEROUS ENTITIES IN THE INDEX THAT
DO NOT APPEAR IN THE TABLE OF CONTENTS.)

ABDOMINAL DISTENTION

"I do not know precisely what gaseousness is, but I do know that in some of my patients, after a complete work-up and treatment that is otherwise adequate, all that I have left is a persisting complaint of this trouble. And all I can do is rely upon what they tell me regarding the extent of relief I am able to give them, since I don't know how to measure the amount of gas in their gastrointestinal tracts either at the beginning or at the end of the treatment. I have heard there is a silicone preparation that is sometimes effective as a carminative in cases of this sort. What is the drug?"

Reply: Simethicone (Mylicon, Silain), which is methyl polysiloxane in a silica aerogel, is a physiologically inert preparation that is sometimes used for the purpose you have in mind. Milton Lieberthal and David Frank, at the Bridgeport, Conn., Hospital, carried out a double-blind study with an earlier but similar preparation in 108 patients. The tablet they used incorporated, in addition to the silicone as specific agent, some digestive enzymes which may have been useful; but the employment of the silicone certainly seems rational. Sixty-nine of the patients were "more than satisfactorily" relieved by the drug and not by the placebo, whereas 31 were not relieved by either agent.

Milton M. Leiberthal and H. David Frank. Silicone in Relief of Gaseousness: Double-Blind Study. Connecticut Med. 27:548, 1963. I. N. Marks, S. Bank and A. Groll. A Trial of Methyl Polysiloxane in the Treatment of Abdominal Distention. South African M. J. 39:476, 1965.

"It is popular nowadays to scoff at the carminatives, but as a matter of fact I believe that they are effective agents. But all of the members of the group, such as alcohol, capsicum, cardamom, cloves, ginger, mustard and the volatile oils generally are violently irritant to the gastrointestinal mucous membranes and provocative of excessive peristaltic activity unless they are much diluted and carefully 'blended' so that they only engender a warm and pungent feeling in the mouth and pharynx. However, I have not been able to devise an entirely satisfactory prescription to accomplish this—could you provide one?"

Reply: The following is a satisfactory combination:

Tincture of capsicum 2.0
Spirits of peppermint 8.0
Tincture of ginger............................. 60.0
Alcohol to make................................. 120.0
Label: 1 teaspoonful well diluted every half-hour until relieved.

It seems to me not unlikely that the carminatives in such a mixture may initiate reflexes promoting upward expulsion of gas and perhaps even its downward propulsion in the colon. Admittedly, however, animal experimentation cannot demonstrate these things. The bile salts have none of these pungent qualities and simply act directly to increase peristalsis. They seem to be effective in persons who suffer the sort of gaseous distention that wakes them in the night. One or 2 of the 240 mg. tablets of dehydrocholic acid (Decholin) are said often to bring quick relief.

ABORTION—PREMATURE LABOR

"I have been raised in the conservative tradition regarding missed abortion; i.e., to allow the patient to evacuate the uterus spontaneously, merely examining blood samples periodically to be certain that a coagulation defect is not developing. But now I understand that there is some stir of interest in more active measures employing drugs. Could you say a word about these?"

Reply: One method is to give a large intravenous dose of oxytocin (Pitocin or Syntocinon), but the risk of water intoxication associated with such therapy has deterred most men from using it. Another technique is to inject a hypertonic solution of either 50% dextrose or 20% saline transabdominally into the amniotic sac. Explanations of how such solutions may act are entirely speculative. It is said that there is usually a latent period of 24 hours before effective contractions begin and an additional 12 hours before the uterus is evacuated under this therapy.

Charles A. White. The Management of Missed Abortion. J. Iowa M. Soc. 55:461, 1965.

"I have heard that therapeutic abortion can be easily achieved through the intra-amniotic injection of hypertonic saline; can you describe this?"

Reply: The report I shall cite is that of Alexander Turnbull and Anne Anderson, at the University of Aberdeen, who used the method in 7 women in whom pregnancy had reached at least 19 weeks, the indications for termination being rubella in early pregnancy in 2 and psychiatric disturbances in 5. Transabdominal amniocentesis was performed under local anesthesia, a small bore polyethylene cannula was introduced and connected to apparatus through which uterine activity could be measured by the changes in amniotic pressure. Sodium chloride, 180–200 ml. of 22.5% solution, was injected into the amniotic sac through the polyethylene cannula, usually aspirating a similar amount of liquor beforehand. There was transient lower abdominal pain in only one of the cases. Most patients experienced fairly intense thirst within one hour of the saline injection, which persisted for some hours, but the extremely strong contractions induced by the injection were almost painless until a late stage. Starting from the beginning of dilatation of the cervix, usually about 6 hours before abortion, the contractions became increasingly painful, and analgesics were then required. The fetus was usually expelled when dilatation reached 3–5 cm., abortion being spontaneous in all instances and manual removal of the placenta necessary only in one. In the only case in which fetal heartbeats were audible before injection they became faint and irregular within 90 seconds of the injection and a few heartbeats were detected at intervals for a further 20 minutes. The abortion process required from 23 to 45 hours for completion despite the high-pressure contractions that were measured and that the uterus had been contracting with increasing force for from 40 to 80 minutes after the injection of the saline. There has been recent report of 2 cases in which it appeared that injections of this sort were responsible for widespread cerebral infarction.

Alexander C. Turnbull and Anne B. M. Anderson. Changes in Uterine Contractility Following Intra-Amniotic Injection of Hypertonic Saline to Induce Therapeutic Abortion. J. Obst. & Gynaec. Brit. Common. 72:755, 1965. J. M. Cameron and A. D. Dayan. Association of Brain Damage with Therapeutic Abortion Induced by Amniotic-Fluid Replacement: Report of 2 Cases. Brit. M. J. 1:1010, Apr. 23, 1966.

"In using such progestational agents as norethindrone (Norlutin) and medroxyprogesterone acetate (Provera) in threatened abortion, is there likelihood that masculinization of the female fetus may occur even though evidences of virilization in the mother are not provoked?"

Reply: Yes, according to Jacobson (St. Peter's General Hospital, New Brunswick, N.J.), fetal masculinization may result from doses too small to be androgenic in treated mothers. In his series some virilization occurred in 10 of 182 pregnant women given 10–40 mg. daily of the drug you mentioned for 4–35 weeks, and masculinization was seen in 15 of 82 female infants born to treated mothers (18.3%). I think one should add, however, that labioscrotal fusion will not be effected if the drugs are not used until after completion of the first trimester.

Benjamin D. Jacobson. Hazards of Norethindrone (Norlutin) Therapy During Pregnancy. Am. J. Obst. & Gynec. 84:962, Oct. 1, 1962.

"Although some of my associates claim fair success with progesterone preparations in threatened abortion, my own record is a very poor one. What has been the general experience?"

Reply: In the matter of spontaneous abortion, many competent observers consider that it is extremely difficult to dislodge the fetus if a pregnancy is normal. In their opinion the fetus that is spontaneously aborted is defective and an attempt to prevent its loss is not desirable. The question is rather academic it seems, at least from the pharmacologic standpoint, because it is not a matter of record that the use of drugs is of much value in stopping the process. In fact, there are observers who feel that the therapy must be begun before conception if it is to be effective; a few years ago, Tyler and Olson, experienced investigators in this field, stated their belief that, all routine studies having been made and correctable defects treated, one should begin progesterone therapy as soon as possible after ovulation if anything is to be expected of it. There are, however, some minority reports, such as that of Benjamin Jacobson, in New Brunswick, who has studied the matter extensively and says that abortions closely related to endocrine (progesterone) deficiency, as manifested by arborization in cervical smears (and not related primarily to pathologic, anatomic or mechanical factors) are preventable by maintaining adequate progestational therapy. There have been some reports of the use of the contraceptive pill but they have not been impressive.

Benjamin D. Jacobson. Abortion: Its Prediction and Management. Fertil. & Steril. 16:604, 1965. Edward T. Tyler and Henry J. Olson. (University of Calif., L. A.) Fertility Promoting and Inhibiting Effects of New Steroid Hormonal Substances. J.A.M.A. 169:1843, Apr. 18, 1959. R. R. Macdonald. Norethynodrel and Mestranol (Enovid) in the Prevention of Recurrent Abortion. Lancet 2:362, Sept. 21, 1965.

"As the only obstetrician in our small community, I am unable to compare my results with the isoxsuprine (Vasodilan) treatment of premature labor with others. Is an increased fetal heart rate generally a frequent finding?"

Reply: Yes, it appears to be. In the experience of Lewis Shenker, in Flushing, New York, an increased fetal heart rate was noted in 25 of 40 instances but there were no effects on the fetal ECG. However, there are some interesting effects on the woman in labor, in addition to the significant suppression of uterine activity that is sometimes achieved. Have you observed a fall in blood pressure and increased blood flow into the extremities, or increases in both heart rate and contractile force? Occasionally there is also a small amount of bronchodilatation and intestinal inhibition; and psychic stimulation has been reported.

Lewis Shenker. Effect of Isoxsuprine on Fetal Heart Rate and Fetal Electrocardiogram. Obst. & Gynec. 26:104, 1965.

"Has any study been made of the effect of prophylactic thiazides on the prematurity rate in pregnant juveniles?"

Reply: Yes, at the District of Columbia General Hospital, Frank Finnerty and Frank Bepko studied the effect of prophylactic thiazides on both perinatal mortality and prematurity rate in patients of this sort. Their population comprised 3083 entirely normal Negro patients 17 years of age and under. Using the alternate case technique, 1541 patients were treated with thiazide diuretics and 1542 remained untreated. Chlorothiazide (Diuril) in dosage of 500 mg. twice daily was used in 936 individuals, and chlorthalidone (Hygroton) in 50 mg. dosage daily in 404 individuals. An infant was considered premature when its birth weight was 5 pounds 8 ounces (2.5 kg.) regardless of the period of gestation. Seventy-three of the thiazide-treated patients were delivered of premature infants, whereas 223 of the nontreated patients were delivered of prematures. While it seemed likely that there were several factors other than thiazide therapy that may have affected the result in this study, it appears nevertheless that the difference in the result in the two groups is possibly significant.

Frank A. Finnerty, Jr., and Frank J. Bepko, Jr. Lowering the Perinatal Mortality and the Prematurity Rate: The Value of Prophylactic Thiazides in Juveniles. J.A.M.A. 195:429, Feb. 7, 1966.

ACANTHOSIS NIGRICANS

"I have a case of 'benign' acanthosis nigricans that developed in early childhood and has now flared up severely at puberty, though it seems to be becoming stationary. Has the disease ever responded to drug therapy of any sort?"

Reply: Usually it has not, and in the malignant cases that develop in later life in association with a malignant tumor that is usually an adenocarcinoma, there is always progression until the primary tumor has been removed, after which there is remission or complete disappearance of the lesions but reappearance if metastasis occurs. However, I have seen report of a case treated by Dige-Petersen, in Denmark, that had all the earmarks of the malignant form though during 20 years or more no malignant lesion was ever found. Progress was as follows under corticosteroid therapy: after 5 months there was some subjective but no objective improvement; after 9 months objective improvement began; and after 3 years the skin disease had subsided so much that it was much less a problem than the patient's rheumatoid arthritis.

Harriet Dige-Petersen. A Case of Acanthosis Nigricans Treated with a Steroid. Acta Dermat.-Venereol. 44:431, 1964.

ACNE

"I have heard that Enovid has been used effectively in acne. Is this correct?"

Reply: Bernard Wansker (Charlotte, N.C.) has reported the effective treatment of 40 females, aged 14–39, who had had acne for an average of 7 years. The drug was used just as it is in contraceptive practice, and the results were said to have been excellent in 32 patients. But I should certainly be hesitant to institute this therapy in most young girls in the age group in which this malady is most often annoying.

Bernard A. Wansker. Norethynodrel with Mestranol (Enovid) in Treatment of Acne. South. M. J. 57:917, 1964.

"It seems to me that, in my general practice, the best thing I can do for my adolescents with acne is protect them against infection and thus prevent scarring. So I put them on oral sulfonamides with a high fluid intake and do not at all experience the dire results that some men associate with the use of these drugs. Is there an explanation?"

Reply: Of course there is Lady Luck. But I should say that the greatest danger is from the prolonged use of a sulfonamide with regularity, followed by a fairly long period of abstinence, and then a return to the therapy. This is the sort of thing that induces the hypersensitization type of reaction, and once an individual has experienced a reaction he is extremely likely to experience it again, more quickly and more violently, on readministration of the drug after a lapse of time. Since you may count on most of your patients being quite erratic in their use of the drugs you prescribe for them, it would seem to me that your safest procedure would be to provide only a week's supply of the drug at any one time. Courses of a week may be frequently repeated without fear of establishment of hypersensitization. Some of the fear of serious adverse reactions to the sulfonamides is undoubtedly a residual from the earlier period when topical, highly sensitizing applications of the drugs were made.

"There has been report of effective use of tetracycline in treatment of acne vulgaris, and it has seemed to have some value in my own practice. How would one explain this, since acne is certainly not an infectious disorder?"

Reply: At Harvard Medical School, Freinkel's group felt that their studies supported the concept that free fatty acids in sebum have a major role in the pathogenesis of acne, and that since these fatty acids are probably largely produced by lipolytic action of the normal bacterial flora of the skin, this might serve as a rational basis for the therapeutic efficacy of antibiotics in this disorder.

Ruth K. Freinkel, John S. Strauss, Shing Yiu Yip and Peter E. Pochi. Effect of Tetracycline on the Composition of Sebum in Acne Vulgaris. New England J. Med. 273:850, Oct. 14, 1965.

"If the systemic use of antibiotics in acne is as good as some observers are claiming, why do we still have the acne problem with us?"

Reply: The answer is that it really is not as good as it has appeared to some observers, for there are adequately controlled studies showing such therapy not to be significantly superior to that with a placebo. The most recent such study to come to my attention was that of Robert Crounse, University of Miami, who found placebo to be just as good as either tetracycline or demethylchlortetracycline (Declomycin).

Robert G. Crounse. The Response of Acne to Placebos and Antibiotics. J.A.M.A. 193:906, Sept. 13, 1965.

"I recently had a patient being treated for premenstrual tension with hydrochlorothiazide (Esidrix) who lost her acne while on the therapy. Unfortunately she moved out of the city and I have not been able to follow up to learn the result of more or less continuous diuretic therapy. Would such a thing be rational and has anybody done it?"

Reply: Some years ago Cooper and Gant (George Washington University) reported a result of precisely this sort in 16 females and 2 males whose severe facial acne, with lesions over the chest and back in some instances, cleared rapidly under 3 or 4 Esidrix tablets daily. Of course there was striking diuresis and weight loss for the first few days in all patients. I have been waiting to see or to hear of confirming studies, which do not seem to have been forthcoming.

C. David Cooper and James Q. Gant, Jr. Treatment of Acne Vulgaris with Esidrix-KCl: Preliminary Report. M. Ann. District of Columbia 29:75, 1960.

ACROMEGALY

"Is there any drug therapy that is specifically helpful in acromegaly?"

Reply: None.

ADDICTION

"Recent experience has indicated to me that drug abuse and addiction is much more common in the population than the records indicate. Just how much drug abuse and addiction is seen in the hospitals and recognized as such?"

Reply: In a careful study at the Boston City Hospital, John Schremly and Philip Solomon learned that the incidence is actually much higher than is recognized when a search for it is not made. During an 8 month period in which approximately 100,000 patients were admitted to the emergency floor of this large hospital, which deals primarily with patients in the lower socioeconomic group, a total of 82 drug abusers and addicts was uncovered. The drugs and the number of instances in which they were involved were the following: heroin, 32; terpin hydrate with codeine, 5; paregoric, 3; morphine sulfate, 2; dihydrohydroxycodeinone (Percodan), 1; codeine, 1; barbiturates, 17 (1 of these also abused meperidine [Demerol]); meprobamate (Miltown, Equanil), 5; dextroamphetamine (Dexedrine), 4; both barbiturates and dextroamphetamine, 3; glutethimide (Doriden), 2; bromides, 2; an inhaler (Valo) containing 150 mg. of 2-amino heptane carbonate, 150 mg. of d-1 desoxyephedrine carbonate, 50 mg. of phenylpropanolamine carbonate, menthol and aromatics, 2; chlordiazepoxide (Librium), 1; ethchlorvynol (Placidyl), 1; propoxyphene (Darvon), 1. Among the heroin addicts, 2 also abused marijuana; 1, lysergamide (LSD-25) and 1, propoxyphene.

John A. Schremly and Philip Solomon. Drug Abuse and Addiction. J.A.M.A. 189:512, Aug. 10, 1964.

"Having become convinced that there is much more barbiturate addiction in this country than is commonly recognized, I am now closely questioning all patients in whom there is suspicion of this. However, I do not recognize all of the barbiturate preparations by name. Could you supply a list?"

Reply: The AMA Committee on Alcoholism and Addiction has supplied the following list of barbiturates available on the U.S. market:
Barbital (Veronal)
Mephobarbital (Mebaral)
Metharbital (Gemonil)
Phenobarbital (Luminal)
Amobarbital (Amytal)
Aprobarbital (Alurate)
Butabarbital (Butisol)
Diallylbarbituric acid (Dial)
Probarbital (Ipral)
Talbutal (Lotusate)
Vinbarbital (Delvinal)
Cyclobarbital (Phanodorn)
Heptabarbital (Medomin)
Hexethal (Ortal)
Pentobarbital (Nembutal)
Secobarbital (Seconal)
Hexobarbital (Cyclonal, Evipal, Sombulex)

Methitural (Neraval)
Methohexital (Brevital)
Thiamylal (Surital)
Thiopental (Pentothal)
Allylbarbituric acid (Sandoptal)
Butethal (Neonal)
Cyclopentenyl allylbarbituric acid (Cyclopal, Cyclopen)
Butallylonal (Pernocton)

Of course the number of preparations in which barbiturates are combined with other agents is legion.

AMA Committee on Alcoholism and Addiction. Dependence on Barbiturates and Other Sedative Drugs. J.A.M.A. 193; 673, Aug. 23, 1965.

"I have a 21-year-old male patient who had visual and auditory hallucinations and was caught in the act of exhibitionism; but there has been no evidence of thought disorder, and psychometric studies have shown no evidence of schizophrenia. When hospitalized for a short period all of the symptoms disappeared. Could any sort of drug addiction account for such a picture?"

Reply: Indeed, yes. This fits precisely the picture of the psychotic manifestation of amphetamine addiction. Was your patient also paranoid during his episode? In Australia, D. S. Bell has reported 14 cases quite similar to yours and pointed out that amphetamine intoxication can precipitate the onset of this schizophrenic episode.

D. S. Bell. Comparison of Amphetamine Psychosis and Schizophrenia. Brit. J. Psychiat. 111, 701, 1965. Philip H. Connell. Clinical Manifestations and Treatment of Amphetamine Type of Dependence. J.A.M.A. 196:718, May 23, 1966.

"The family of a patient of mine, who had had barbiturates withheld from her after a long period of addiction to them, called me because she had developed convulsions. It was touch-and-go for awhile but she pulled out of it all right. What is the full symptomatology of barbiturate withdrawal?"

Reply: Sudden withdrawal of barbiturate, or even reduction to 50% of the accustomed dose, may be more dangerous to life than sudden withdrawal of morphine. There is improvement during the first 12–16 hours, and signs of cerebellar dysfunction disappear, but the patient then becomes apprehensive and so weak that he can hardly stand. Fasciculation appears, there is coarse tremor of the hands and face, and the deep reflexes are hyperactive. The patient is sleepless, nauseated, has abdominal cramps and frequently vomits; blood pressure and pulse rate are elevated, and there is fever. There may be a 12 pound weight loss in 36 hours. Nonprotein nitrogen is elevated and there are hyperglycemia and hemoconcentration. The patient often develops difficulties in making cardiovascular adjustments on standing, but no clinical or electrocardiographic evidences of myocardial damage appear. The most serious aspect of this withdrawal is the appearance of typical grand mal convulsions, usually at about the thirtieth hour. The development of a psychosis, which is not unusual, may delay recovery beyond the usual 2 or 3 weeks.

"In the discussions preceding the legislation against the 'pep-pill' traffic there has been frequent mention of the amphetamines as addicting drugs. I had always thought of them as merely drugs of habituation and not true addiction; am I wrong?"

Reply: It is only recently, as the result of such reports as that of Oswald and Thacore, in Scotland, that we have felt justified in accepting drugs of this group as truly addicting rather than merely habituating agents. Definitions: habituation is emotional or psychologic dependence on a drug; addiction is habituation plus the development of tolerance that necessitates increasing the dose in order to obtain the original effect when the drug is taken repeatedly, coupled with the necessity, called physical dependence, to continue use of the drug to prevent appearance of the characteristic illness from the "abstinence syndrome."

I. Oswald and V. R. Thacore. Amphetamine and Phenmetrazine Addiction. Brit. M. J. 2:427, 1963.

"In our city, addiction to paregoric, which contains 130 mg. of opium per ounce, is becoming a matter of major importance. What complications of this addiction are to be anticipated? The drug is usually concentrated by boiling before intravenous injection."

Reply: This matter has been thoroughly studied by Frederick Oerther and associates, in Detroit, who find that users often mix paregoric with the amphetamines, secobarbital (Seconal), glutethimide (Doriden) or tripelennamine (Pyribenzamine). It is said that the talcum filler of tripelennamine has been associated with diffuse pulmonary granuloma and subsequent pulmonary hypertension. Paregoric contains benzoic acid, camphor and anise, and these irritants lead to occlusive sclerosis after intravenous injection. The veins used are the median cubital, femoral, popliteal, axillary, saphenous and even the external jugular; indeed the latter is the most frequent site of injection, and it is therefore said that a scar at the base of the neck just above the clavicle is pathognomonic of paregoric addiction. Endocarditis, sepsis, abscess at injection site, cerebral abscess, purulent meningitis and septic arthritis have been seen in paregoric users with bacterial infections. Oerther's group also observed homologous serum hepatitis. Tetanus, mycotic endocarditis and malaria, which have occurred in heroin addicts, can be expected to be seen ultimately in these paregoric addicts.

Frederick J. Oerther, Joseph L. Goodman and A. Martin Lerner. J.A.M.A. 190:683, Nov. 16, 1964.

"There is much agitation in our metropolitan center for bringing about a radical change in the therapy of opiate addiction. The reasons given are the following: 1. The opiate addict is treated as a criminal, though alcoholism is a larger and more dangerous problem, and the alcoholic is not so treated. 2. Present treatment is a failure, as proved by the high proportion of patients who relapse quickly. 3. If the addict were supplied with drugs legally, the results would be: (a) his criminality would cease and he would accept withdrawal, psychotherapy and rehabilitation more willingly; (b) illicit traffic in drugs would cease because no longer profitable; (c) recruitment of new addicts would stop and the number would be reduced by treatment and death.

"Somehow I feel in my bones that this is all wrong, but I am unable really to formulate my reasons. Would you care to state your position in the matter?"

Reply: I can only say to you that many close students of the subject object to the proposed change and type of approach to the addiction problem for the following reasons:

1. Character defects and socioeconomic handicaps would not be changed by supplying the addict with drugs. 2. Few addicts could be persuaded to undergo withdrawal and accept psychotherapy while being supplied with drugs at the same time; indeed, many of these people feel that in the drug they have the answer to their problem and do not regard themselves as psychiatrically abnormal. 3. The best controlled studies contradict the view that most addiction is due to peddler contact rather than to association with addicts or potential addicts. 4. Supplying drugs to addicts might only serve to spread addiction. It is pointed out that the legal availability of alcohol does not decrease the inordinate interest of youths of weak character in this drug. 5. Since the present market for illicit narcotics is greater than can be supplied by smuggled drugs there is no great underworld interest in enlarging it, but if some of this were lost there might be a considerable upsurge in proselytizing activity. 6. The addict continues to take his drug not only to avoid the abstinence syndrome but because he wants to be jolted by a great and rapid alteration in physiologic status. If given just enough drug to avoid withdrawal symptoms he would be likely to supplement the supply with purchases from illicit sources. 7. Addicts would be required under the proposed plan to register at special clinics, and it is unlikely that many would desire to do this, either because of unwillingness to be stigmatized as an addict or through fear of identification by the police. 8. It is very probable that the plan would be self-defeating because of the expenses incurred not only in operating the clinics but in maintaining the amount of surveillance necessary to prevent diversion of much of the drug supply into illegal channels. Addicts, furthermore, would tolerate this surveillance very badly.

"Is codeine really a drug of addiction?"

Reply: Yes it is undoubtedly, but the incidence is so low that I have never felt that one has to take the likelihood seriously when using the drug under ordinary circumstances, i.e., to relieve pain with it in average dosage for a limited period of time. However, its addicting potentiality has been recently accentuated in most interesting fashion through report of withdrawal symptoms in an infant born to a mother who had been taking 6 to 8 grains of the drug daily for 2 months for relief of pain associated with metastatic malignancy.

G. Van Leeuwen, R. Gutherie and F. Stange. Narcotic Withdrawal Reaction in a Newborn Infant Due to Codeine. Pediatrics 36:635, 1965.

"For the first time in my experience I have a pregnant heroin addict. What shall I expect?"

Reply: Some unpleasantness certainly. Of the 66 such cases reported from the Metropolitan Hospital in New York by Roy Stern, 27 showed obstetrical complications (toxemia, abruptio placentae, retained placenta, postpartum hemorrhage, ruptured marginal sinus, cephalopelvic disproportion and breech presentation). The incidence of 15.1% of toxemia of pregnancy was highly significant as compared with 5.2% of all obstetrical patients in the hospital; the incidence of abruptio placentae (9%) and postpartum hemorrhage (9%) was also significantly high. There was an 18.5% of premature infants, which was significantly high. Practically all of the women continued to use heroin up to the time of delivery, and 20% of them signed out of the hospital against advice, 5 of them within 24 hours of admission and generally within 2 days. Stern pointed out that not only is the physical condition of the pregnant addict poor because of the conditions under which she obtains and uses the drug, but the conditions of her addiction also make her liable to hepatitis, multiple abscesses, thrombophlebitis and emboli. Furthermore, she is uninterested in improving her condition so long as she can obtain enough heroin for her needs. Obviously, such a person may be expected to be less concerned with prenatal care than with the effect this will have on her obtaining money enough to buy her drug. Stern did not find labor prolonged in the addict. You should be warned, however, that within 24 hours after delivery at the most, the mother may be expected to begin to show withdrawal symptoms. It is likely that the best treatment for these withdrawal symptoms is through the use of methadone, as described elsewhere in these Replies.

Roy Stern. The Pregnant Addict. Am. J. Obst. & Gynec. 94:253, 1966.

"It seems to me that I am seeing considerably more paralytic ileus and atony of the urinary bladder in my surgical practice than formerly. Could this be ascribable in any way to the large number of drugs in use nowadays?"

Reply: I should say it is due to the deprivation of accustomed drugs rather than to their administration. Specifically I have in mind the current addiction to sedatives and hypnotics. For example, I recall a patient in our hospital who developed unaccountably severe postoperative ileus and urinary bladder atony which was only explainable when other manifestations of the glutethimide (Doriden) withdrawal syndrome appeared. Numerous somewhat bizarre occurrences in hospitalized patients could easily be explained on the basis of withdrawal symptoms if careful examination were made into drug habituations of patients when they are admitted.

ADDISON'S DISEASE

"At long last I have diagnosed a case of Addison's disease in my own practice. With proper use of the corticosteroids, sodium chloride and supplementary use of desoxycorticosterone if needed, what is the prognosis in an average case?

Reply: With luck, i.e., a nice balance of these things you list, your patient is likely to live out a life of normal length unless he has complicating tuberculosis. Even the latter disease does not necessarily mean an earlier death, but it unquestionably complicates the picture through introducing the possibility of effecting spread of the tuberculous process through use of the corticosteroids (please note that I said *possible* and not *probable*).

AGAMMAGLOBULINEMIA

"I have a patient with agammaglobulinemia who of course requires high dosage of antibiotics for the least little infection. What amount of gamma globulin would be effectively protective?"

Reply: Initial dosage of 0.6 ml./pound with maintenance dosage of 0.3 ml./pound intramuscularly at monthly intervals for children and 2 week intervals for adults.

AGRANULOCYTOSIS

"Since agranulocytosis is the commonest adverse hematologic reaction to drugs, with a mortality rate of 20 to 50% if infection develops, even though treatment is early and appropriate, I am wondering whether you could supply a list of the drugs most frequently associated with this unfortunate reaction?"

Reply: If one is to apply the strictest definition of agranulocytosis, i.e., that it is a malady characterized by great diminution in leukocytes in the peripheral blood, neutropenia and the clinical manifestations of fever, prostration, buccal ulcerations, then perhaps not all of the drugs herewith listed truly qualify; since, however, they have all been associated with at least granulocytopenia, they may be considered to be potential if not actual causative agents in this syndrome. Aminopyrine (Pyramidon, etc.), dipyrone (Novaldin, etc.), amithiozone (Tibione, Panrone), antithyroid drugs (propylthiouracil, methimazole [Tapazole], methylthiouracil [Methiacil, Thimecil]), arsenicals, busulfan (Myleran), carbonic anhydrase inhibitors, colchicine, sodium colistimethate (Coly-Mycin Injectable), ethosuximide (Zarontin), fluorouracil, gold salts, lincomycin (Lincocin), nitrogen mustards, novobiocin (Cathomycin, etc.), organomercurials (Neohydrin, Meralluride, Dicurin, etc.), PAS, phenacemide (Phenurone), phenothiazines (Thorazine, etc.), phenylbutazone (Butazolidin), primaquine, primidone (Mysoline), quinine, ristocetin (Spontin), sulfonamides, suramin (Bayer 205, etc.), trimethadione (Tridione), mephenytoin (Mesantoin), 6-mercaptopurine (Purinethol), methyldopa (Aldomet), vinblastine (Velban), vincristine (Oncovin), imipramine (Tofranil), oxyphenbutazone (Tandearil), chloramphenicol (Chloromycetin), indandione anticoagulants (Danilone, Eridione, Hedulin), tolbutamide (Orinase), chlordiazepoxide (Librium).

"In what time relationship with regard to administration is a patient likely to develop agranulocytosis when given one of the drugs most prone to cause that type of reaction?"

Reply: Agranulocytosis is most likely to occur in a patient who has been continuously treated for from 2 to 8 weeks or indeed for many months, but it may occur after one dose of a drug to a patient who has had occasional doses of that drug for months or even years.

"We have just had a case of agranulocytosis definitely attributable to aminopyrine (Pyramidon), prescribed elsewhere. Are all cases of agranulocytosis drug-induced?"

Reply: No, but it has been possible to incriminate drugs in about half of the recorded instances. At the University of Montreal, Pretty's group summarized 30 cases of acute agranulocytosis seen between 1946 and 1964. In 14 cases the agents incriminated were aminopyrine, phenylbutazone, sulfonamides and chlorpromazine. Aminopyrine alone was responsible for 8 of the cases. In the remaining 16 cases no definite etiology was established. These observers emphasized, however, the possibility that drugs are involved in many more cases than can be definitely proved since patients are often admitted to hospital in a helpless state and questions about previous drug ingestion are either ignored by the patient's family, or (this I add myself) the family may be ignorant of the drug-taking habits of the patient or refuse to recognize a familiar preparation that has been used for a long time as a "real" drug. Elsewhere in these Replies there are listed most of the drugs whose causative role in the malady has been established.

Harry M. Pretty, Gilles Gosselin, Guy Colpion and L. -A. Long. Agranulocytosis: A Report of 30 Cases. Canad. M. A. J. 93:1058, Nov. 13, 1965.

ALCAPTONURIA

"Are there any drugs that are helpful in the treatment of alcaptonuria or for the ochronosis associated with it?"

Reply: Certainly nothing of specific value, but administration of vitamin C (ascorbic acid) may delay darkening of the urine in alcaptonuria through its reducing properties. There is, as you know, an associated arthritis in this disease, but it is not responsive to the drugs used in treating rheumatoid arthritis.

ALCOHOLISM

"I have heard of the intravenous administration in acute alcoholism of $100-200$ μg. of triiodothyronine. Would this be rational and safe therapy?"

Reply: If one recalls that an excess of thyroid hormone in the circulation can detrimentally affect cardiac function, it would seem a risky thing to do. Actually, there have been contradictory reports regarding the efficacy of this therapy. At St. Vincent's Hospital, Worcester, Massachusetts, Marshall Goldberg and associates concluded that triiodothyronine is useful in conjunction with such measures as parenteral infusion of fluids, vitamins and tranquilizers, but not as a means unto itself. But in Toronto, Kalant's group concluded that the drug had no effect on the rate of recovery from an alcoholic episode. Elsewhere I have remarked that the world would probably not lose a great deal if many of its alcoholics were to be projected into fatal myocardial infarctions, but since not all of these people are total bums, one faces again the old euthanasia question: Who is to choose the candidates for promotion?

Marshall Goldberg, Robert Hehir and Marc Hurowitz. Intravenous Triiodothyronine (Cytomel) in Acute Alcoholic Intoxication: Preliminary Report. New England J. Med. 263:1336, Dec. 29, 1960. H. Kalant, G. Sereny and Rita Charlebois. Evaluation of Triiodothyronine in Treatment of Acute Alcoholic Intoxication. New England J. Med. 267:1, July 5, 1962.

"I have only recently begun exploring the usefulness of disulfiram (Antabuse) in some of my alcoholics but have found it extremely difficult to use. Have you any suggestions?"

Reply: Disulfiram's usefulness in combating alcoholism lies in the fact that the presence of the drug in the body makes alcohol ingestion an extremely unpleasant experience, and this is precisely the reason for its failure more often than not. The difficulty is a three-faceted one. If the patient is hospitalized for the indoctrination, as he should properly be, he may be so frightened by the reaction he gets when given a test dose of alcohol that he will have nothing to do with disulfiram thereafter, reasoning that no one is going to catch *him* going around with that poison in his system. Or the physician, being aware of the risk involved in the test procedure, settles for merely describing to the patient the reaction he will experience if he takes even a small amount of alcohol while on the drug; and then, when the patient does drink and does have his reaction, he is not unlikely to claim that he was not adequately warned of the severity of the thing. And finally (and probably the most frequent occurrence militating against use of disulfiram) the patient is very likely to feel superior to the use of the drug, arguing that he can really stop drinking any time he wants without taking any sort of "poison" to help him do it.

"I know what I can accomplish in alcoholism with disulfiram (Antabuse), which indeed is very little; has citrated calcium carbimide (Temposil) in the main been any more serviceable?"

Reply: From hearsay and from the two reports cited below, I have gained the impression that Temposil sensitizes to alcohol in only a few hours rather than the few days required by Antabuse to accomplish the same thing;

however, the effect is milder and appears to wear off more quickly. It seems, too, that in some individuals there is an increased craving for alcohol in the beginning of the treatment. However, the drug is newer than Antabuse and the true status of the one vis-à-vis the other is not yet fully established.

Alfred Minto and F. J. Roberts. Temposil: New Drug in Treatment of Alcoholism. J. Ment. Sc. 106:288, 1960. T. Wada, Z. Tanaka, T. Sakurada, K. Shirmada, K. Sato and S. Horigome (Hirosaki University). Citrated Calcium Carbimide (Temposil) in Treatment of Alcoholism. Postgrad. Med. 28:188, 1960.

"In our municipal hospital we have latterly been injecting a central nervous system stimulant intravenously into Saturday-night drunks in order to awaken them sufficiently in the emergency room to gain some responsiveness and cooperation. The thing works pretty well, but how much risk are we running?"

Reply: Considerable, I should say. Presumably most of these patients are unknowns who are necessarily handled somewhat hurriedly under circumstances in which careful cardiovascular studies are not easily accomplished. So there is a risk. And what of preexisting psychoses; are you not accentuating some of these?

"In the case of a patient who is admitted with the 'delirium tremens'-like syndrome associated with alcohol withdrawal, but in whom it is impossible to elicit a history of alcoholism, sudden withdrawal of what other agents may be considered as possibly responsible for production of the picture?"

Reply: Hypnotic and tranquilizing drugs of quite diverse chemical structure have been associated with withdrawal symptoms of the sort you indicate; the following list is probably not complete: barbiturates, chloral hydrate, paraldehyde, glutethimide (Doriden), methyprylon (Noludar), ethchlorvynol (Placidyl), meprobamate (Miltown, Equanil), promazine (Sparine), reserpine (Serpasil), imipramine (Tofranil).

"Is there any difference in the efficacy of the potent drugs used in the treatment of the psychoses and the true tranquilizing agents in treatment of the alcohol-withdrawal syndrome?"

Reply: In a study in Toronto, Sereny and Kalant made a double-blind comparative evaluation of promazine (Sparine), chlordiazepoxide (Librium) and placebo in 58 male alcoholics admitted to the hospital within 24 hours of their last drink. Promazine was given in daily dosage of 400 and 800 mg., and chlordiazepoxide in daily dosage of 200 and 400 mg. It was found that both promazine and chlordiazepoxide were more effective than placebo in promoting sleep and diminishing sweating, but tolerance quickly developed to promazine though not to chlordiazepoxide. Tremor was reduced significantly by promazine but not by chlordiazepoxide; indeed the latter even increased it. Promazine rapidly produced striking postural hypotension and compensatory tachycardia, while the onset of hypotension under chlordiazepoxide was more gradual. Neither drug improved the appetite compared with the placebo. Grand-mal seizures or delirium tremens occurred in 5 patients on promazine, 1 on placebo, and none on chlordiazepoxide. These investigators concluded that chlordiazepoxide appeared to be superior to promazine but that the total benefit produced by it constituted a relatively small addition to the placebo effect.

G. Sereny and H. Kalant. Comparative Clinical Evaluation of Chlordiazepoxide and Promazine in Treatment of Alcohol-Withdrawal Syndrome. Brit. M. J. 1:792, 1965.

"I have a case of severe alcoholism in a 55-year-old patient who is also diabetic and has had one coronary occlusion and one cerebral vascular accident. He is still at work, when not off on an alcoholic bout, and now and then tries to prove (always unsuccessfully) that he can take just one drink and then leave it alone. He refuses to try disulfiram (Antabuse) because a friend of his had a severe reaction with it, and feels himself superior to participation in Alcoholics Anonymous. What might I try?"

Reply: Very interesting report of the use of metronidazole (Flagyl) in 53 patients has been made by J. A. T. Taylor, in Los Angeles. The effect of this drug on drinking was stumbled upon during its use for other purposes. Metronidazole in this study caused a favorable physical response in acute alcohol withdrawal, a decreased compulsion to obtain alcohol, decreased tolerance for quantity of alcohol, changes in the central nervous system and psychic effects of alcohol, objective physical improvement and the development of an aversion to alcohol. It does, however, cause an Antabuse-type reaction upon the ingestion of alcohol, and therefore of course may be unsuited to use in your patient who appears to be very uncooperative.

Jo Ann T. Taylor. Metronidazole—A New Agent for Combined Somatic and Psychic Therapy of Alcoholism. Bul. Los Angeles Neurol. Soc. 29:158, 1964.

"When a patient is admitted in a mild to severe state of alcoholic intoxication, has it really been shown that anything is accomplished by placing him under the influence of tranquilizing drugs during the withdrawal period?"

Reply: Yes, several investigators have shown this to be the case. With adequate tranquilization the course of recovery is usually more rapid and smoother, the period of restlessness and depression not being nearly so long or pronounced. Sometimes, through becoming more rapidly comfortable and able to eat and sleep, the patient is enabled through the drug to build up what Martin Kissen at St. Luke's Hospital, Philadelphia, has well termed "his sadly depleted psychic and physiologic resources." And once in a blue moon during this period he may even gain the strength to attempt the course that is his only salvation, i.e., total abstinence for the rest of his life.

Martin D. Kissen. Management of Psychomotor Agitation in Acute Alcoholism: Double-Blind Study Using Chlordiazepoxide (Librium). Dis. Nerv. System 26:364, 1965.

"Do we have a drug as effective as Alcoholics Anonymous?"

Reply: An impertinent question, my friend, and the answer is no.

"One of my associates recently had a case of Wernicke-Korsakoff syndrome in a chronic alcoholic that fortunately had been diagnosed early so that daily intramuscular injection of 100 mg. of thiamine supplemented with oral vitamin B complex was able to effect rapid improvement. But when the dehydration, a prominent feature of the episode, was treated by intravenous glucose solution, the symptoms rapidly returned and the patient quickly deteriorated. How could this be explained?"

Reply: Parenterally administered glucose, as in your case, will rapidly wash out the body stores of glucose in these patients who have become nutritionally deficient through practically living on alcohol to the exclusion of real food. Had your associate added 100 mg. of thiamine to each of his glucose infusions the debacle would almost certainly have been avoided.

ALLERGIC MALADIES

"My patient was admitted vomiting dark red blood and passing bright red blood rectally; no other symptoms. X-ray studies caused gastric carcinoma to be considered, but at a second study in 48 hours there were no longer signs of deformity. Later gastroscopy showed evidence of both old and fresh bleeding areas and a projecting hyperemic mass; after 2 weeks there were no longer any signs of inflammation or hyperemia. The whole episode was strongly suggestive of a reaction to ingestion of a foreign substance, but this was denied. Could a drug have done this nevertheless?"

Reply: This was certainly an unusual experience, but I have actually seen the report of a practically identical happening which followed the ingestion of a single oral penicillin tablet by a patient known to be allergic to penicillin. Patients, of course, have their own notions regarding what is and is not a potentially toxic foreign substance. Many individuals, as you know, no longer look upon aspirin as a "real" drug, and it appears that penicillin is rapidly entering the same lay classification.

S. P. Bralow and L. S. Girsh (Temple University). Urticaria of Gastric Mucosa with Massive Hemorrhage Following Oral Penicillin Anaphylaxis. Ann. Int. Med. 51:384, 1959.

"I do not believe that the manufacturers are promoting antiserotonin compounds for treatment of allergic maladies, but one of my associates claims to be getting good effects with them. Have any good studies been performed?"

Reply: I have seen a few reports in which cyproheptadine (Periactin) and methysergide (Sansert) were used on the assumption that there is a serotonin factor in the pathogenesis of the allergic state. None of the findings provided more than very qualified support for use of the drugs in any of the variety of allergic disorders.

Egon Bruun and Henning Letman (Copenhagen). Clinical Results of Treatment with Antiserotonin (Periactin) in Allergic Patients. Acta allergol. 17:343, 1962. Hugh Smellie and Lionel Fry (King's College Hospital, London). Comparison of an Antiserotonin, Cyproheptadine (Periactin), and a Pure Antihistamine, Chlorpheniramine (Chlor-Trimeton), in Hay Fever, Acta allergol. 17:352, 1962. Walter Pinsker and Kent H. Thayer (VA Hosp., Long Beach, Calif.) Treatment of Allergic Conditions with Methysergide (Sansert) (1-Methyl-D-Lysergic Acid Butanolamide Bimaleate), a New Antiserotonin Drug: Pilot Study. Ann. Allergy 21:200, 1963. William C. Grater (Dallas). Serotonin and Antiserotonins in Allergy. South. M. J. 56:1287, 1963.

"We are all nowadays of course quite apprehensive regarding hypersensitization to drugs but do not have to hand much information of a safeguarding nature. What, for example, are the influences of size and spacing of doses, heredity, sex, age, etc., in the matter?"

Reply: If we could always know that a dose of a certain size is required in the case of a certain drug, either to hypersensitize or to elicit the hypersensitivity (allergic) reaction in most individuals, the safety with which numerous potent drugs could be used would certainly be greatly enhanced. But we do not know this. Scratch and intradermal tests for hypersensitivity, in which minute amounts of the drug are used, are unreliable diagnostic tools in allergic practice and may occasionally provoke reactions of utmost severity. The patch test is more reliable, but it also may set off severe systemic responses. Thus experience with diagnostic tests teaches that in highly sensitized individuals very little of the drug is needed to initiate the reaction. Clinical therapeutic experience confirms this, since almost absurdly small doses administered in treatment have at times been responsible for reactions. Fortunately, however, many hypersensitized individuals can take reasonably adequate therapeutic dosage of a necessary drug and experience the reaction only when that dosage is exceeded. The effect of the route of administration on the incidence of reactions in already hypersensitized individuals is not fully elucidated. Other factors enter to confuse the picture considerably in clinical studies, and results of animal experimentation in this field cannot be extrapolated into human affairs with impunity. It is probably safe to say, however, that in the case of many drugs oral administration is by and large safer than any type of parenteral administration. Whether there is any direct relationship between the incidence of allergic maladies and the likelihood of becoming hypersensitized to administered drugs in human families or in the individual person is an undecided question. I do not find clinical evidence that is of more than suggestive value to indicate that age plays an important part in the likelihood of developing hypersensitization to drugs. However, young laboratory animals are poor producers of antibodies, and time may reveal significant differences between reaction incidences in man at the extremes of age and during the middle period. The sex differences in susceptibility that have been observed are possibly for the most part attributable to extraneous circumstances. For example, woman's greater use of analgesics may explain the higher incidence in her of angioneurotic edema and, in the aminopyrine era, of agranulocytosis. There is no established relationship between sex and the incidence of clinical allergies as a whole or the incidence of anaphylaxis in protein-sensitized guinea pigs. In rather rare instances a state of hypersensitivity will diminish or disappear while use of the incitant drug is continued. But certainly it is dangerous to gamble on such an occurrence in a clinical situation unless the reaction is not of a serious type and more especially unless the drug in point has never been reported in association with serious reactions of hypersensitivity. I know of no findings that would justify the glib pronouncement that drug allergies wear themselves out. Rather it seems that disappearance may be expected in only slightly over half the cases in a variable number of years. Furthermore, the severity of the potential reaction will probably have increased in about 1 of every 12 patients. I take this to mean that the physician who readministers at any time a drug to which there has been an overt

hypersensitivity reaction does so at considerable risk.

"We hear much today about drug allergy and 'hypersensitivity' and are warned that it is dangerous to incur such reactions, but no one tells us just which reactions are of an allergic nature. Can you list them?"

Reply: The principal systemic reactions are the blood dyscrasias, comprising agranulocytosis, thrombocytopenic purpura and hemolytic and aplastic anemia; the serum-sickness type of reaction, in which there is fever, urticaria, arthralgia, lymphadenopathy, etc.; bronchial asthmatic attacks; periarteritis nodosa; hepatitis; allergic conjunctivitis and rhinitis; angioneurotic edema; drug fever without other accompanying manifestations; and anaphylactic shock. The last of these is the most frequently fatal.

Actually, most of the allergic reactions to drugs occur as skin eruptions, which are seen in the following forms: (a) eczematous dermatitis of both contact and internally disseminated types, the essential lesion being edema with vesicles situated within the epidermis; (b) urticaria (hives), a lesion whose primary focus lies within the deeper blood vessels of the skin, which dilate and become permeable to plasma constituents; (c) exanthematic eruptions, which are erythematous, scarlatiniform, macular, papular or morbilliform; (d) exfoliative dermatitis, which is shedding of the superficial skin to reveal inflammatory layers beneath, usually being associated with serious systemic manifestations; (e) erythema multiforme–like eruptions; (f) purpura simplex; (g) fixed eruptions, which reappear at the same sites each time a drug is taken.

"Will the use of iodides in the treatment of an asthmatic interfere with allergic skin test reactions?"

Reply: The drugs have not been found to diminish either immediate or delayed skin test reactions.

"In our hospital recently a life was lost because full facilities for coping with an anaphylactic drug reaction were not immediately available in the area where they were needed. Could you suggest a 'set' of the various emergency medications that might be ready in some central station in mobile form or else placed in duplicate in the principal stations in the hospital in which these potentially fatal reactions are most likely to occur?"

Reply: Here is the "anaphylaxis set" that is always available in numerous areas at the Mayo clinic.

ANAPHYLAXIS SET

Materials	How Supplied
Medications:	
Epinephrine hydrochloride, 1:1000	Two 1 cc. ampules for ordinary hypodermic syringes or two 1 cc. Tubex ampules
Aminophylline, 7½ gr.	Two ampules, 3¾ gr. each, for intravenous use
Ephedrine sulfate, 25 mg. (⅜ gr.)	One ampule suitable for subcutaneous, intramuscular or intravenous use
Diphenhydramine hydrochloride solution: 10 mg./cc.	Benadryl hydrochloride Steri-Vial, 10 cc., for intravenous use
Corticosteroid	Soluble prednisolone, 50 mg., for intravenous use or Solu-Cortef (hydrocortisone sodium succinate), 290 mg., for intravenous use
Penicillinase, 800,000 units	Neutrapen, single-dose vial, for intramuscular or intravenous use
Metaraminol bitartrate, 10 mg./cc.	Aramine, 10 cc. vials for intramuscular, subcutaneous or intravenous use
Levarterenol bitartrate 0.2% solution	Levophed bitartrate, two 4 cc. ampules, for intravenous infusion
Dextrose, 5% solution	1000 cc. for intravenous use
Water, sterile and triple distilled	Two 5 cc. ampules (for dissolving dry medications for injection)
Materials to facilitate injections:	
Hypodermic syringes	Two 1 cc. disposable syringes with needles and one Tubex syringe, one 20 cc. syringe
Hypodermic needles	Two with disposable syringes; one 1 inch needle for intramuscular injections; and one 4 inch needle for intracardiac injections
Administration set for intravenous solution	Type to fit enclosed bottle of dextrose solution
Tourniquet	Length of rubber tubing, 16–20 in.
Isopropyl alcohol sponges	Tubex individual packets
Surgical Supplies:	
Scalpel	One with attached blade
Hemostat	One, small
Suture material	Plain surgical catgut (00) with attached needle
Sterile gauze sponges	
Resuscitative devices:	
Plastic airways adaptable to mouth-to-mouth breathing	Resuscitube airways, adult and pediatric sizes

Louis E. Prickman. Prevention and Management of Anaphylactic Reactions. Minnesota Med. 45:905, 1962.

"I find in my allergic patients who need steroids that I can control the medication much more readily by injection than by prescribing the drugs for oral ingestion. But many of the individuals complain bitterly of pain and soreness at the injection site, and in a few instances I have had subcutaneous fat necrosis there. What can be done about this?"

Reply: That is real pain and 1 out of 4 or 5 patients is going to object to it pretty strenuously. The only thing I know to do, if you do not want to have the drugs taken orally, is to review the situation thoroughly and assure yourself that all of the patients in whom you are using corticosteroids really require this therapy. Have you fully exhausted the possibilities of the antispasmodics, sympathomimetic amines, theophylline and tranquilizers in all cases?

"I have an allergic patient under treatment with cyproheptadine (Periactin) and another under methysergide (Sansert). There has been a moderately impressive response in both instances, but both patients are gaining considerably in weight. Is this due solely to increased appetite or is it one of the early evidences of Cushing's syndrome?"

Reply: William Grater (Dallas), reporting his experience in more than $3\frac{1}{2}$ years with these drugs in ambulatory patients with allergies of various sorts, said that probably the most important single side action was the increased appetite and weight gain. Increased linear growth was also evident in many asthmatic children who had had subnormal growth patterns. In discussing Grater's paper, T. E. Van Metre, Jr., of Johns Hopkins, said that his own experience made the weight gain ascribable solely to the increased food intake and not to the Cushing manifestation.

William C. Grater. Serotonin and Antiserotonins in Allergy. South. M. J. 56:1287, 1963.

"In the prophylaxis against reactions in repository pollen therapy, is the addition of an antihistamine to a corticosteroid worthwhile?"

Reply: Mayer Green (University of Pittsburgh) had no immediate or delayed systemic reactions to his 922 injections with either corticosteroid alone or corticosteroid combined with an antihistaminic compound; but he had about twice as many local reactions when corticosteroid alone was used than when corticosteroid plus an antihistaminic was used. His steroid capsule was 4 mg. 6-alpha-methylprednisolone, and the antihistaminic was 12 mg. chlorpheniramine maleate (Teldrin); 1 capsule of each was taken the evening before injection, another 1 hour before, and another the evening after injection.

Mayer A. Green. Repository Pollen Therapy: Placebo-Controlled Comparison of Corticosteroid Prophylaxis with and Without Antihistamine. Ann. Allergy 22:187, 1964.

"Has the intranasal application of corticosteroids been used effectively in the treatment of hay fever?"

Reply: Yes, there have been several reports of satisfactory employment of this therapy. The most recent to come to my attention was that of Philip Norman and Walter Winkenwerder, at Johns Hopkins Hospital. They used the cartridge of dexamethasone aerosol for intranasal application (Turbinaire), the dose being two inhalations in each nostril three times daily for a total daily dose (at the nozzle) of about 1.0 mg. of dexamethasone. The patient was instructed to shake the unit vigorously, insert the nozzle into the nostril with vial upside down, and to sniff in when the aerosol was delivered. Two of the 40 patients selected for study were unable to use the aerosol because of irritation immediately after spraying. Adequate data for evaluation were obtained from 36 patients, and the study was thoroughly controlled. On the basis of their physician interview and examination, 29 of 35 patients were improved; according to the patient's subjective opinions of the severity of their symptoms, 28 of 37 were improved; and according to a daily symptom diary, 24 of 32 were improved. Overall, it therefore appeared that about three-fourths of the patients were favorably affected by the therapy. But in 2 patients among those who were not improved the symptoms seemed actually to be intensified.

Philip S. Norman, Walter L. Winkenwerder. Suppression of Hay Fever Symptoms with Intranasal Dexamethasone Aerosol. J. Allergy 36:284, 1965.

"I have a patient who experiences a secretory otitis media each year in late winter and early spring in association with a tree pollen allergy. Surprisingly, the corticosteroids have not been effective, but as a matter of fact all other types of treatment have failed also. Can you suggest anything?"

Reply: You have probably prescribed the corticosteroids for oral use. Try the long-acting intramuscular methylprednisolone (Depo-Medrol), as used very effectively by John Heisse, at the University of Vermont. He gave a dose of 80 mg. in adults and older children and 1 mg./lb. in children weighing less than 80 lb. It was found incidentally that the drug does not obliterate the skin sensitivity reactions, thus enabling an allergic investigation to proceed in a patient whose symptoms have been remitted by the therapy.

John W. Heisse, Jr. Secretory Otitis Media: Treatment with Depo-Methyl-Prednisolone (Depo-Medrol). Laryngoscope 73:54, 1963.

"We are all aware that the outstanding evidences of overaction of the antihistaminics are usually drowsiness, dizziness, dryness of the mouth and gastrointestinal disturbances; also that less frequently occurring reactions are faintness, headache, blurring of vision, apprehension, confusion, tremulousness, paresthesia, urinary frequency, difficulty of micturition and insomnia. But what are the rarer reactions?"

Reply: Some of the rarer reactions, usually following grossly excessive dosage: muscular incoordination, convulsions, jerky speech, Ménière-like symptoms, hallucinations, hysteria, impotence, toxic psychosis, substernal pain, shock, agranulocytosis, hematuria, hemolytic anemia and pancytopenia. Among the severe reactions, a preliminary period of excitement and convulsions is most likely to occur in children, and central nervous system depression from the beginning in adults. These drugs must be used with care in patients with convulsive disorders, since at least some members of the series have been found capable of inducing seizures in such persons even in ordinary dosage.

There is evidence that the antihistaminics are important as the cause of chronic recurrent dermatoses in industrial workers, these drugs being widely used in industrial plants in the attempt to control the common cold. Cross sensitization to chemicals, whose possession of a common immunochemical grouping with the antihistaminics is unsuspected, appears to be responsible for these reactions. The antihistaminics should not be administered when skin testing with tuberculin is being done because they lessen the intensity of the reaction.

Intravenous diphenhydramine (Benadryl) elevates systolic and diastolic blood pressures, which would probably contraindicate this administration in hypertension. The contraindication should probably apply also to heart disease because the drug given intravenously causes some cardiac acceleration, shortening of diastole, evidence of atrial tachycardia and changes in the T and P waves that point to a possible myocardial effect.

In experiments on both human and rabbit eyes it has been found that 0.5% antazoline (Antistine) is not toxic to the cornea and does not affect the pupil or accommodation. However, 1%, and especially 2%, strengths are definitely toxic.

Chronic toxicity of any sort in individuals taking these drugs during long periods has not been demonstrated. Paradoxically, the antihistaminics sometimes are reacted to allergically themselves and they may also aggravate allergic manifestations.

"The great number of available antihistaminics has become quite confusing. Could you perhaps mention some features that distinguish individual members of the group?"

Reply: The following listing is probably not complete but it certainly includes the principal antihistaminics:

ANTAZOLINE PHOSPHATE (ANTISTINE). This compound, used topically in the eye, though milder and less irritating than others of the group, is weaker in its antihistaminic action than most of them. Some side actions in about 20% of patients, most frequently drowsiness and nausea.

Dosage: 1 or 2 drops of the 0.5% solution in each eye every 3 or 4 hours.

BROMPHENIRAMINE MALEATE (DIMETANE). Much resembles chlorpheniramine (see below) in action and uses.

Dosage: 4 mg. orally three to six times daily, or sustained-action tablet every 8–12 hours; children under 6 years, 2 mg. three times daily, over 6, half adult dosage. Subcutaneously, intramuscularly or intravenously, 5–20 mg., or may be added to transfusion blood.

CARBINOXAMINE MALEATE (CLISTIN). As potent as any and as few side effects. Atropine-like or even ganglionic-blockade action like that of hexamethonium is possible but very unlikely to occur. The action of epinephrine is not potentiated, and the drug does not have local anesthetic action.

Dosage: 4 mg. three or four times daily, up to 8 mg. if needed; children over 6 years, 2 mg.

CHLORCYCLIZINE HYDROCHLORIDE (DI-PARALENE, PERAZIL). There is nothing particularly distinctive about this drug except that it has prolonged action and a low incidence of toxic effects.

Dosage: 50 mg. two or three times daily.

CHLOROTHEN CITRATE (TAGATHEN). No particular advantages or disadvantages are notable for this drug.

Dosage: 25 mg. three times daily.

CHLORPHENIRAMINE MALEATE (CHLOR-TRIMETON, TELDRIN SPANSULES). Good efficacy and a low incidence of side effects characterize this drug. Note should be taken when giving parenterally of incompatibility with allergenic substances and with preparations that contain oil; avoid use in the same syringe.

Dosage: Oral, 2–4 mg., or a sustained-action tablet every 8–10 hours and at bedtime. Subcutaneous, intramuscular or intravenous dosage, or to be added to transfusion blood, 5–20 mg.

CLEMIZOLE HYDROCHLORIDE (ALLERCUR). There seems to be nothing very distinctive about this one. Daily adult dosage is 80–160 mg., given in divided amounts.

CYCLIZINE HYDROCHLORIDE (MAREZINE). Principally used in treatment of motion sickness in 50 mg. adult dosage, one-half this for children 6–10, one-fourth for others.

CYPROHEPTADINE HYDROCHLORIDE (PERIACTIN). Principally used in treatment of pruritus. Adult daily dosage from 4 to 20 mg. in divided doses.

DEXBROMPHENIRAMINE MALEATE (DISOMER). This drug differs from brompheniramine only in being the dextro isomer, the older drug being the racemic mixture. Appears to be just as good with possibly lower incidence of side actions.
Dosage: 2 mg. four times daily.

DEXCHLORPHENIRAMINE MALEATE (POLARAMINE). Dextro isomer of racemic chlorpheniramine, which it appears to resemble in efficacy with possibly lower incidence of side actions. Adult dosage 2 mg. three or four times daily or a sustained-action tablet morning and evening.

DIMENHYDRINATE (DRAMAMINE). Principally used in treatment of motion sickness in adult dosage of 50 mg.

DIMETHINDENE MALEATE (FORHISTAL). Apparently useful for all antihistaminic purposes, including the therapy of pruritus. Usual adult dosage is 1 mg. three times daily.

DIPHENYLPYRALINE HYDROCHLORIDE (DIAFEN). A satisfactory drug with a low incidence of side actions.
Dosage: 2 mg. every 4 hours.

DOXYLAMINE SUCCINATE (DECAPRYN). The only distinctive thing about this drug appears to be that the incidence of sedation in association with the use of full therapeutic dosage is high.
Dosage: 12.5–25 mg. three or four times daily.

MECLIZINE HYDROCHLORIDE (BONAMINE). Used principally in the treatment of motion sickness in adult dosage of 25–50 mg.

METHAPHENILENE HYDROCHLORIDE (DIATRINE). There is some tendency for gastrointestinal irritation with this drug, but otherwise the incidence of side actions appears low.

METHAPYRILENE HYDROCHLORIDE (HISTADYL, SEMIKON, THENYLENE AND NUMEROUS OTHERS). The incidence of sedation in association with use of this drug appears to be exceptionally low.
Dosage: 50–100 mg. three or four times daily; 20 mg. may be added to transfusion blood.

METHDILAZINE (TACARYL). A phenothiazine derivative compound used for general antihistaminic purposes, and possibly has greater antipruritic efficacy than some of the other agents. Usual adult dosage is 8 mg. twice daily but may be given three or four times a day.

PHENINDAMINE TARTRATE (THEPHORIN). Rather than sedation, this drug may cause stimulation, and it has been effectively employed in combination with some of the other drugs of the group to offset their sedative action; but it may cause palpitation, nausea and insomnia.

PHENIRAMINE MALEATE (TRIMETON). There is nothing distinctive in the report on this drug. Usual adult dosage is 25 mg. three times daily.

PROMETHAZINE HYDROCHLORIDE (PHENERGAN). This is one of the most potent antihistaminics; it also has use in combating motion sickness, as an antiemetic, as a sedative and in dentistry to prevent or reduce swelling, pain and trismus. Nausea and vomiting of several types may be favorably affected, including that associated with pregnancy and surgical procedures. Alone, or to potentiate other central nervous system depressants, the drug is used in both surgical and obstetric cases. Barbiturates should be eliminated or at least very much reduced when used with this drug, and the use of morphine and all other depressant analgesics should be reduced in dosage by one-quarter to one-half. Since the incidence of drowsiness or dizziness varies with individuals, patients should be warned against getting into potentially dangerous situations. Jaundice, excessive hypotension or hematopoietic damage have not been reported to my knowledge.
Dosage: Antihistaminic, 12.5 mg. before meals and on retiring, but less may be adequate; rectal, intramuscular or intravenous administration also feasible; nausea and vomiting, prophylaxis or therapy, 25 mg. every 4–6 hours; surgical sedation, 25 mg.; obstetric sedation, 25–75 mg.

PYRATHIAZINE HYDROCHLORIDE (PYRROLAZOTE). This phenothiazine derivative, related to promethazine (see above), is an effective antihistaminic, sometimes causing slight nausea. Agranulocytosis has been reported when the drug was used in excessive dosage for a prolonged period.
Dosage: 25–50 mg. three or four times daily.

PYRILAMINE MALEATE (COPSAMINE, NEOANTERGAN, PARAMINYL, PYRA-MALEATE, PYRAMAL, PYRILAMINE, STAMINE, STANGEN, STATOMIN, THYLOGEN). The distinctive feature of this drug is the low incidence of sedation in association with its use.
Dosage: 25–50 mg. three or four times daily.

PYRROBUTAMINE PHOSPHATE (PYRONIL). Distinguished by a low incidence of side actions, including sedation.
Dosage: 15 mg. three or four times daily.

THONZYLAMINE HYDROCHLORIDE (ANAHIST, NEOHETRAMINE). In order to obtain effect with this drug the dosage must be higher than with most of the others, but the incidence and degree of side actions are less, particularly that of sedation.

Dosage: 50–100 mg. three or four times daily.

TRIMEPRAZINE TARTRATE (TEMARIL). A phenothiazine derivative compound that is principally used in treating pruritus. Usual adult dosage is 2.5 mg. four times daily or 5 mg. of the sustained-release preparation every 12 hours.

TRIPELENNAMINE HYDROCHLORIDE (PYRI-BENZAMINE). This effective antihistaminic may be given parenterally as well as orally, and the solution for injection may be mixed with allergens for their subcutaneous injection. Gastrointestinal irritation occurs rather frequently but it is not severe, and sedation is moderate; occasionally there is stimulation of the central nervous system.

Dosage: 50–100 or even 150 mg. daily will usually be tolerated orally in divided doses; 25 mg. may be added to transfusion blood every 4–6 hours. There is also a citrate salt for more pleasant oral administration in liquid form.

TRIPROLIDINE HYDROCHLORIDE (ACTIDIL). Some drowsiness may occur with this drug, but the overall incidence of side actions has not been high.

Dosage: 2.5 mg. three times daily.

"Can one obtain falsely negative skin wheal reactions in a patient on corticosteroids?"

Reply: Some observers have doubted this, but in what appeared to be a careful study of the matter in Oslo, Hauge and Vale showed an inhibitory effect of triamcinolone (Aristocort, Kenacort) of some importance. Thirty-three positive intradermal tests in 10 untreated asthmatics were repeated during oral administration of triamcinolone, 4 mg. three times daily; 8 of the 33 reactions turned negative, apparently as a consequence of the corticosteroid therapy.

H. E. Hauge and J. R. Vale. The Influence of Triamcinolone on the Allergic Skin Wheal Reaction. Acta Allerg. 20: 496, 1965.

ALOPECIA

"In a case of alopecia areata I have tried all the usual remedial measures with complete failure of results. My patient is willing to try anything, even though a bit 'off beat,' provided no danger is involved. Do you know of anything fitting this description?"

Reply: I have seen a Letter to the Editor describing the disappearance of these lesions upon use of the oral contraceptive pill by a woman in whom pregnancy had always also effected clearance.

M. G. T. Fisher. Oral Contraceptives and Alopecia Areata. Brit. M. J. 2:1246, 1965.

"I have heard that the long-term corticosteroid therapy of alopecia universalis is sometimes effective in restoring hair growth. Shall I risk it?"

Reply: It is true that 2 successfully treated cases have been reported from separate practices, and probably a good many other patients have been more or less effectively treated. I should think that your risk would be not so much in provoking cushingoid symptoms as in perhaps having a very difficult person to deal with when you stop the corticosteroids and the hair all falls out again. You would have of course to stop it at some time, and wouldn't this be a severely traumatic experience?

Walter B. Shelley, Joseph S. Harun and Joseph M. Lehman (Univ. of Pennsylvania) Long-Term Triamcinolone Therapy of Alopecia Universalis: Case Report. Arch. Dermat. 80:433, 1959. I. I. Lubowe Arch. Dermat. 79: 665, 1959.

AMEBIASIS

"At our large general hospital we are in need of a plan for long-term institutional prophylaxis and therapy of amebiasis and shigellosis. Kindly advise."

Reply: The most extensive recent study in this field was that of Gholz and Arons, at the Sonoma State Hospital, Eldridge, California, who thoroughly endorsed iodochlorhydroxyquin (Vioform) for both prophylactic and therapeutic use in both diseases. After establishment of an endemic prevalence rate for *Entamoeba histolytica* of 40%, their patients were placed on a dosage regimen of 250 mg. Vioform with each of the three meals. At the time of their report, 4000 patients and 50,000 patient-months of treatment had been covered, with 1200 patients having been continually on the drug for more than 3.5 years. Not a single positive stool had been found during this time. For treatment of patients with the active disease, the same dosage was used with isolation for 10–14 days and medication being continued for at least 1 year; negative stools were achieved in all of the 142 individuals. Among the 4000 patients on the prophylactic treatment, 9 cases of subclinical shigellosis appeared during the first year of the study. In patients with clinical infection with *Shigella sonnei* and *S. flexneri*, Vioform in the same dosage used throughout the study caused clinical remission within 48–72 hours. Incidentally, the drug was completely ineffective against *Salmonella typhimurium, S. enteritidis, S. infantis, Giardia lamblia, Trichuris trichiura, Strongyloides stercoralis* and *Enterobius vermicularis.*

Lawrence M. Gholz and Walter L. Arons. Prophylaxis and Therapy of Amebiasis and Shigellosis with Iodochlorhydroxyquin (Vioform). Am. J. Trop. Med. & Hyg. 13:396, 1964.

"In our large general hospital we have been using iodochlorhydroxyquin (Vioform) prophylactically against amebiasis after an outbreak of amebic colitis two years ago. The results have been excellent, and the lack of serious toxic reactions has been astonishing. May we have to pay dearly very suddenly for our feeling of security with this regimen?"

Reply: No, I think not; the drug is surprisingly innocuous. In its long-term administration in 4000 patients, Gholz and Arons did observe an unusual gait change in 20 individuals, 18 of whom recovered completely. Thirteen of the latter were rechallenged with the drug for many months without return of symptoms, and it was the belief of these investigators that Vioform was actually not the etiologic agent in this reaction.

Lawrence M. Gholz and Walter L. Arons. Prophylaxis and Therapy of Amebiasis and Shigellosis with Iodochlorhydroxyquin (Vioform). Am. J. Trop. Med. & Hyg. 13:396. 1964.

"In the follow-up examination of patients treated for intestinal amebiasis, what is the most satisfactory diagnostic method?"

Reply: In Egypt, A. Z. Shafei, in a large follow-up study, found the examination of mucus collected during sigmoidoscopy superior to stool examination.

Aly Z. Shafei (Alexandria University). Treatment of Amebiasis with Resotren Compound. J. Trop. Med. & Hyg. 64: 282, 1961.

"In our practice we do not often see a case of amebic dysentery nowadays. What is the present position of the antibiotics in this therapy?"

Reply: Elsdon-Dew's group at the University of Natal found tetracycline, chlortetracycline (Aureomycin) and oxytetracycline (Terramycin) equally effective in dosage of 1 gm. daily, but the main disadvantages of this therapy were expense, failure to prevent hepatic involvement, and a significant relapse rate. Best results were achieved in patients who were given tetracycline combined with diiodohydroxyquinoline (Diodoquin) and chloroquine (Aralen). *Dosages:* Tetracycline, 50 mg. three times daily for 10 days; diiodohydroxyquinoline, 600 mg. three times daily for 20 days; chloroquine, 800 mg. immediately, followed by 400 mg. 6 hours later and then 200 mg. twice daily for 14 days.

S. J. Powell, A. J. Wilmot and R. Elsdon-Dew. Potentiating Effect of Quinolines on Action of Tetracycline in Amebic Dysentery. Lancet 1:76, Jan. 9, 1960.

"Am I correct in believing that chloroquine (Aralen) has replaced emetine in the treatment of amebic liver abscess?"

Reply: Not entirely, I believe. Chloroquine alone is certainly the drug of choice between these two when there is complicating cardiovascular disease, but otherwise, at least in the experience of Wilmot and associates (University of Natal), a course of emetine combined with a standard dose of chloroquine reduces the minimal tendency to relapse. *Dosages:* Chloroquine (Aralen) 600 mg. followed by 300 mg. 6 hours later and then 150 mg. twice daily for 29 days; this to be coupled with 60 mg. emetine hydrochloride intramuscularly daily for 10 days.

A. J. Wilmot, S. J. Powell and E. B. Adams. Chloroquine Compared with Chloroquine and Emetine Combined in Amebic Liver Abscess. Am. J. Trop. Med. & Hyg. 8:623, 1959.

"What is presently the accepted therapy for amebiasis?"

Reply: At the U.S. Naval Hospital in Philadelphia, Jones and Nielsen recommend that in cases with minimal or mild bowel symptoms and signs, carbarsone be given orally in dosage of 250 mg. two, three or four times daily for 10 days, to be followed by iodochlorhydroxyquin (Vioform), 250 mg. three or four times daily for 10 days, or by diiodohydroxyquin (Diodoquin), 630 mg. three times daily for 14–20 days. If there is accompanying dysentery the drugs are to be repeated in one or more courses, and in the presence of obvious secondary infection, cultures are to be taken (preferably from purulent exudate of ulcers) and oxytetracycline (Terramycin) is to be given orally (subcutaneously if indicated) in doses of 500 mg. every 6 hours for 7–10 days pending more definitive study of the cultures, blood cultures and sensitivity studies. Emetine hydrochloride is to be considered in dosage of 60 mg. daily for 4–6 days deeply subcutaneously only in the severest forms, especially if associated with extraintestinal lesions other than hepatic, and if there are no cardiac contraindications.

H. Leonard Jones, Jr., and Orville F. Nielsen. Colitis: Management Based on Pathogenic Mechanisms. M. Clin. North America 49:1271, 1965.

AMYLOIDOSIS

"By coincidence, we have simultaneously in our small hospital a case of amyloidosis complicating an old resistant suppurating wound and one of primary systemic amyloidosis in which the congestive heart failure appears intractable. Can you suggest any drugs other than the obvious ones that might be indicated in these two situations?"

Reply: None.

AMYOTROPHIC LATERAL SCLEROSIS

"Are there drugs that are specifically helpful in amyotrophic lateral sclerosis?"

Reply: No.

ANEMIAS

"We are all aware that any of the iron preparations suitable for oral administration will, if given in proper dosage, correct all of the iron deficiency anemias with the few exceptions in which the use of parenteral iron seems advisable, but what is the sequence of events that occurs in an individual during the development of iron deficiency?"

Reply: Iron is first mobilized from the reserve, which amounts to 1000–1500 mg. in the adult male and probably somewhat less in the female. When these stores are depleted, serum iron falls, and iron granules no longer appear in the cytoplasm of maturing normoblasts; hemoglobin synthesis is retarded, and an excess of protoporphyrin accumulates in the erythrocytes. Microcytosis and hypochromia, anisocytosis and poikilocytosis appear after several months, and the familiar physical signs occur after the process has become one of long standing. Erythrocytes are thought by most hematologists to be derived from primitive endothelium of the intersinusoidal capillaries of the bone marrow. Anoxia differentiates this endothelial cell into the earliest erythroid cell, the megaloblast. The next stage in production of the erythrocyte, the transformation of megaloblast into erythroblast, requires the action of the erythrocyte-maturation factor, cyanocobalamine (vitamin B_{12}). The only part—but an extremely important one—played by iron in the process is in the formation of the hemoglobin that is to be stored in the erythrocyte.

"Will an injection of iron-dextran complex (Imferon), given neonatally, prevent the anemia of prematurity without the necessity for further therapy?"

Reply: Yes, according to W. D. Elliott (Manchester, England), but only if mixed feeding is provided in the fourth month. Elliott studied 57 premature infants who received an intramuscular injection of 50–250 mg. of elemental iron in the form of Imferon neonatally, 75 who received oral iron during the first 6 months, and 70 who received no prophylactic iron. The oral iron preparation was a mixture containing 1 gr. of ferrous sulfate, and it was given three times daily starting before the 6-week period. He found that infants with birth weights of 2 to 3 pounds and 3 to under 4 pounds who received intramuscular iron responded better than those given oral iron or no treatment at all. In infants of 4 to under 5 pounds at birth, the results were similar with oral and intramuscular iron.

W. D. Elliott. Prevention of Anemia of Prematurity. Arch. Dis. Childhood 37:297, 1962.

"Iron preparations of the sustained-release type are being promoted for the treatment of anemia. Are they acceptable?"

Reply: To make the bold pronouncement that they are not acceptable would be unwarranted from the evidence, but I can tell you that several commercially available preparations of this sort were studied at the Canadian Department of National Health and Welfare by Middleton and associates and found not to have the sustained action that was claimed for them.

E. J. Middleton, E. Nagy and A. B. Morrison. Studies on the Absorption of Orally Administered Iron from Sustained-Release Preparations. New England J. Med. 274:136, Jan. 20, 1966.

"Preparations of iron with cobalt added are being promoted to us in our area. What precisely is the overall position of cobalt in the anemias?"

Reply: Under experimental conditions cobalt stimulates erythropoiesis in both children and adults and also protects animals from developing anemia during the course of induced sterile suppuration. Definite responses have been observed in a fair proportion of patients with moderate anemia associated with chronic infection, inoperable carcinoma of the stomach, chronic renal disease, Cooley's, sickle cell and some other refractory anemias. Responses have not been reported, to my knowledge, in the anemia associated with hepatic cirrhosis, and very little evidence of effect has been obtained in the lymphomatous diseases, i.e., lymphosarcoma, leukemia, etc. Claims have been made for the supplemental use of cobalt in the anemias of pregnancy and prematurity and the iron deficiency anemia of infants born at full term, but it seems to me that none of the studies was very critical.

There is definitely no indication for routine employment of the element as an adjuvant to cyanocobalamine or iron therapy in anemias of any sort. In fact, Bush's conclusion to his review of the subject is subscribed to by all conservative and disinterested observers; it remains to be determined whether the benefits of cobalt therapy outweigh the possible disadvantages. Certainly the use of the drug should be confined to anemias in which all other methods of treatment have failed, in other words to the refractory anemias. Considerable gastrointestinal disturbances are the most frequent occurrences when cobalt is taken, but other things have been reported also, such as precordial pain, skin rashes, renal injury, tinnitus and temporary deafness, thyroid hyperplasia with hypofunction, and thrombocytosis. Until something more is known about the mechanism of cobalt's action, I think that it should be looked upon as a potentially dangerous drug.

J. A. Bush. The Role of Trace Elements in Hemopoiesis and in the Therapy of Anemia. Pediatrics 17:586, 1956.

"The manufacturers of Simron, a preparation of ferrous gluconate with a potentiator, recommend a 30 mg. a day dosage, but I have not succeeded with this in cases in which there has been chronic gastrointestinal disturbance. Of course, I am aware that one must get the iron absorbed in an iron deficiency anemia, but with a preparation devised to accomplish precisely this, why have I failed?"

Reply: It appears that in their eagerness to accomplish the correction of iron deficiency anemia with a preparation containing less iron than would be likely to be disturbing, the manufacturers have somewhat undershot the mark in their recommended dosage. Charles Brown (Cleveland Clinic) obtained very satisfactory responses when he used a dosage of 40–60 mg. daily.

Charles H. Brown. Oral Iron Therapy in Patients with Acute and Chronic Gastrointestinal Diseases. Am. J. Gastroenterol. 40:634, 1963.

"I have never known precisely how much my patient has to pay for iron when I prescribe it for him in one or another of the numerous preparations that are available nowadays. Has any study of this matter been made?"

Reply: Yes, in Volume I of The Medical Letter, page 56, July 24, 1959, the statement appeared that the approximate cost of 100 mg. of iron was at that time as follows for the listed preparations: Exs. Ferrous Sulfate U.S.P. 1.5 cent; Feosol Tablets (SKF), 2.3 cents; Fergon (Winthrop), 3.8 cents; Mol-Iron (White), 3.8 cents; Roncovite (Lloyd), 6.8 cents; Chel-Iron (Kinney), 7.5 cents; Feosol Spansules (SKF), 18 cents. It has been alleged that the addition of ascorbic acid (vitamin C) acts as a reducing substance to convert ferric food iron into more easily assimilable ferrous forms and that it will delay the formation of ferric from ferrous iron that is administered as a drug, and this is true. But an additional truth is the fact that the amount of ascorbic acid necessary to accomplish these things is far beyond that which is incorporated in most of the iron-with-vitamins mixtures that are commercially available. I should certainly be unwilling to have my patient pay additional for his iron in order to obtain the ineffective amounts of vitamin C if one views it merely as an aid to absorption of iron.

"It has been generally accepted that iron stores once depleted cannot be replenished or at best can be replenished only with great difficulty. If this is the case, is it then true that women, whose pregnancies have greatly drained their iron stores, cannot ever again refill these stores?"

Reply: That has certainly been the consensus, but since the careful study of Jack Pritchard and Ruble Mason, in Dallas, we know the assumption to be unwarranted. In their observations on 3 men and 6 women who were studied a total of 12 times, there was clearly demonstrated an ability to store iron when the ingestion of ferrous gluconate was continued after the correction of their anemia. With the daily ingestion of 110 mg. of medicinal iron, the rate of accumulation of storage iron averaged about 4.5 mg. and ranged from 3 to 6 mg. per day. It is therefore predictable that the otherwise normal adult with depleted iron stores will accumulate 0.5 gm. or more of storage iron when taking one 0.3 Gm. ferrous gluconate tablet three times a day for 4 to 6 months, which iron is readily available for hemoglobin synthesis.

Jack A. Pritchard, Ruble A. Mason. Iron Stores of Normal Adults and Replenishment with Oral Iron Therapy. J.A.M.A. 190:897, Dec. 7, 1964.

"The impression is conveyed by innuendo that of the two preparations available for parenteral administration of iron, the newer one, Jectofer, is superior to the earlier Imferon because of fear that the latter may cause sarcoma. Is there any justification for this attitude?"

Reply: Certainly not. The contention that Imferon may be dangerous for the reason you mention has been thoroughly repudiated by the Food and Drug Administration.

"I recently placed an anemic woman on daily intramuscular injections of the iron–sorbitol–citric acid complex called Jectofer. Now the urine has become dark olive color and turns black upon standing. Is this a phenomenon of sinister significance?"

Reply: No, apparently not. Boyle's group (Royal Infirmary, Edinburgh) found that 5 specimens from 10 patients turned black within 24 hours and 4 of them within 4 days, the remaining 1 not turning black within 10 days. Probably bacterial action frees the iron from the sorbitol–citric acid complex, permitting the formation of some insoluble ferric compounds.

D. Boyle, A. W. Dellipiani, J. A. Owen, D. A. Seaton and R. W. Tonkin. Black Urine after Jectofer Injections. Brit. M. J. 1:285, Feb. 1, 1964.

"When is it advisable to use iron and vitamin B_{12} concomitantly?"

Reply: Addition to iron therapy of the agents used in the hyperchromic-macrocytic anemias – cyanocobalamine (vitamin B_{12}), folic acid, dried stomach preparations – is not ordinarily profitable except to the purveyors of the drugs; true dimorphic anemias are rare except in certain postgastrectomy and gastroenterostomy cases.

"When is it desirable to administer iron parenterally rather than orally?"

Reply: Since there are few things more sure than the response to orally administered iron in the hypochromic-microcytic anemias, the desirability of administering the drug parenterally will likely be recognized only in the following instances: first, in some cases of sprue in which there may be as poor absorption of iron as of other nutritive substances; second, in the occasional patient who has excessive gastrointestinal reactions to orally administered iron; third, in the rare patient who develops an allergic type of reaction (in one such reported case parenterally administered iron was tolerated though orally administered iron invariably caused angioneurotic edema and pruritus); fourth, after extensive bowel resection and in patients with ulcerative colitis or a functioning colostomy; fifth, in patients with a hemorrhagic diathesis or esophageal varices or severe peptic ulceration, in whom repeated bleeding episodes may be expected (orally administered iron will not reconstitute the iron stores, as needed in these individuals); sixth, in cases in which the requirement for iron is exceptionally high, this circumstance possibly explaining the response in some recorded instances of anemia in association with rheumatoid arthritis when the failure of oral therapy had been shown not to result from deficient absorption – in short, in cases of refractoriness to iron, if such a

state truly exists; seventh, in instances in which it seems imperatively necessary to recoup the hemoglobin loss more rapidly than is usually possible with oral iron administration.

"We are taught that iron is absorbed from the intestinal tract in only very minute amounts and as needed, and yet one occasionally hears of a case of severe poisoning in an infant who has chewed large numbers of ferrous sulfate tablets. How would you explain this, and what is the best treatment in such a case?"

Reply: Necropsy findings have indicated that the barrier to absorption of iron through the intestinal wall is abolished by the escharotic effect of large amounts of the drug. Severe hemorrhagic gastritis and enteritis occur in these cases and also hemorrhagic periportal hepatic necrosis unless death takes place very early. The patients go into shock, presumably because of the fluid loss through vomiting, diarrhea and enteric hemorrhage, though direct vasodepressor action of the iron has not been excluded in the causation of this collapse. Methemoglobinemia occurs, and there is also evidence of disturbance in the blood clotting mechanism.

Entirely satisfactory therapy for cases of acute ferrous sulfate poisoning has not been developed, but it seems advisable to get raw eggs and milk into the child quickly to promote absorption of the iron. Gastric lavage with sodium bicarbonate solution would convert corrosive ferrous sulfate to the less irritant ferrous carbonate. BAL has not been beneficial and might even enhance the toxicity of the iron. Whole blood transfusion, or better still exchange transfusion, is definitely indicated, and it is rational to use methylene blue to combat methemoglobinemia.

"Is the use of calcium disodium versenate, commonly known as EDTA, justified in the treatment of ferrous sulfate poisoning?"

Reply: Its use is rational at least, for it will exchange its calcium for iron and in this way remove the latter from circulation. At Cook County Hospital, Thomas Covey, who observed 20 instances of iron poisoning among 1427 children who ingested potentially poisonous substances during one year, treated his cases by inducing emesis and initiating gastric lavage with sodium bicarbonate, at the end leaving a solution of sodium bicarbonate and a saline cathartic in the stomach. He then began intravenous fluids, containing 50–75 mg./kg. daily of EDTA divided into 2 doses, as soon as possible. After the first phase in a severe case of ferrous sulfate poisoning, in which there is hemorrhagic gastroenteritis, shock, acidosis, coagulation defects and possibly coma, there is a second phase of delayed, profound shock; during this second phase the agent is given intramuscularly for a total of 4 or 5 days. Covey would have it used even in the absence of symptoms if the history of ingestion of 1 gm. of ferrous sulfate or more is well documented. Peritoneal or hemodialysis are also considered if the urine flow is greatly reduced or absent; intravenous and oral vitamins to help prevent liver damage, and oxygen as indicated. Unfortunately, EDTA's usefulness is severely limited if there is greatly reduced urinary volume.

Thomas J. Covey. Ferrous Sulfate Poisoning: Review, Case Summaries and Therapeutic Regimen. J. Pediat. 64:218, Feb., 1964.

"Is it a fact that administration by stomach tube of the new antidotal compound, desferrioxamine (Desferal) in cases of ferrous sulphate poisoning will bind iron remaining in the gastrointestinal tract to prevent its absorption?"

Reply: I believe this is the case, but Henderson and associates have recorded an instance in a 14½-months child in which, after giving an initial oral dose of 5 Gm., they gave 92 mg./kg. intravenously on three occasions at 12 hour intervals. The serum iron fell rapidly in this case to normal levels and there was an excretion of about 25 mg. iron in the urine. Of course, as is the case with EDTA, a severely diminished urinary volume would limit the usefulness of this drug.

F. Henderson (St. Louis Children's Hosp.), T. J. Vietti and Elmer B. Brown (Washington Univ.). Desferrioxamine (Desferal) in Treatment of Acute Toxic Reaction to Ferrous Gluconate. J.A.M.A. 186:1139, Dec. 28, 1963.

"Would you kindly provide a brief statement of the various ways in which cyanocobalamine (vitamin B_{12}) can be administered to a patient with addisonian pernicious anemia?"

Reply: When the drug is used parenterally, which is the preferable method, it is advisable in order to restore the vitamin B_{12} concentration of depleted tissues to give an injection of 100 μg. twice weekly until hemoglobin levels have been returned to normal. Thereafter, a single 100 μg. injection monthly suffices in most individuals indefinitely, though it is advisable to raise the dosage during infections. And if there are neurologic complications at the time therapy is begun it is well to double the dosage until remission is achieved. Then the same maintenance dosage is used as in cases without complications.

Intravenous administration of cyanocobalamine has been found feasible, but it is difficult to see what advantages this route of injection would have.

It has also been shown that if the drug is given orally in extremely high dosage, of the order of 300 μg. daily, full hematopoietic effects can be obtained in pernicious anemia, since it appears that the difference between a patient with this malady and a normal individual is only quantitative in the matter of cyanocobalamine intestinal absorption. However, such oral therapy is expensive, the patient may frequently omit a dose, and it is not always successful.

A preparation of cyanocobalamine with added intrinsic factor obtained from hog stomach was formerly official in the U.S.P. Such preparations as Bifacton, Extralin F, etc., are still available. They will effect remissions quite satisfactorily, but increasing experience shows that the results of their use are disappointing in the long run; i.e., after varying periods of from 6 months to 2 years the blood count begins to fall and macrocytosis reappears. Increasing dosage at that time does not remedy the situation, or at most only temporarily. Except in instances in which there is rebellion against continued monthly injections, or when oral administration may be imperatively necessary for a short period for some other reason, it does not seem that the use of these cyanocobalamine–intrinsic factor preparations should be the preferred type of therapy. The tablets or capsules contain ¼ and ½ unit as defined in former editions of the U.S.P. (15 μg. of cyanocobalamine and 300 mg. of the intrinsic factor concentrate). Two other trade-named preparations containing both cyanocobalamine and intrinsic factor are Ventriculin, which is the dried and defatted wall of hog's stomach, and Extralin, which is obtained by incubating liver with minced hog's stomach. They contain both intrinsic and extrinsic (cyanocobalamine) factors, the former because it is a gastric secretory product and the latter because stomach muscle and liver contain cyanocobalamine. In giving them, one therefore provides not only the vitamin but also the factor necessary to accomplish its absorption. Unfortunately the amounts of both present in Ventriculin are small, and it is necessary to use this material in large quantities. About 40 Gm. (4 heaping teaspoonfuls) must be taken in divided dosage throughout the day in water, milk or fruit juice to obtain hematopoietic responses equivalent to the requirements for 1 former U.S.P. oral unit. This is an expensive and not very popular preparation. The daily dosage of Extralin is 12 large capsules; this too is an expensive and not much used preparation.

"What is the longest interval between vitamin B_{12} injections that has satisfactorily held pernicious anemia patients in remission?"

Reply: Until the report of Collins and Jackson (Bluffton, Indiana) appeared, who held their 8 patients in satisfactory condition with 1000 μg. doses of the vitamin intramuscularly every 6 months, the longest interval I have ever seen was 3 months: 87 of Kinloch's 100 patients were effectively held at that interval with doses of 1000 μg. intramuscularly.

Jack T. Collins and Charles E. Jackson (Caylor-Nickel Clinic). Twice Yearly Vitamin B_{12} Therapy in Pernicious Anemia. Am. J. M. Sc. 243:27, 1962. J. D. Kinloch (Royal Infirm. Glasgow). Maintenance Treatment of Pernicious Anemia by Massive Parenteral Doses of Vitamin B_{12} at Intervals of 12 Weeks. Brit. M. J. 1:99, Jan. 9, 1960.

"What is the position of folic acid vis-à-vis cyano-cobalamine (vitamin B_{12}) in the macrocytic anemias?"

Reply: The neurologic complications of addisonian pernicious anemia are not prevented by folic acid and indeed may be worsened unless cyanocobalamine dosage is concomitantly increased. The megaloblastic anemia of infancy usually responds to folic acid but not always to cyanocobalamine. In the megaloblastic anemia in pregnancy, folic acid is regularly effective and cyanocobalamine rarely, if at all. There is good response in the nutritional megaloblastic anemia syndrome to the combined use of cyanocobalamine, folic acid and large doses of thiamine. The following are best treated by the combined use of cyanocobalamine and folic acid: anemias of sprue, fish tapeworm infestation, gastrointestinal disease and surgery (when they are of the macrocytic type), and celiac disease.

"I have a pernicious anemia patient who rebels against further vitamin B_{12} injections. What is the status of liver extract nowadays?"

Reply: I do not believe that there is any longer a place for raw liver, crude liver extract or refined liver preparations in the therapy of addisonian pernicious anemia, because the fact is adequately established that vitamin B_{12} is the sole factor necessary to effect symptomatic reversal. Why not treat her (?) with 300 μg. daily of an oral cyanocobalamine preparation such as Rubrafolin until you can lead her back again into acceptance of the injections?

"Has the minimum daily adult requirement for vitamin B_{12} been established?"

Reply: Yes, Louis Sullivan and Victor Herbert have done so at the Boston City Hospital, Thorndike Memorial Laboratory. In their study the minimal effective daily dose of vitamin B_{12} was defined as the quantity that, administered daily to patients with uncomplicated pernicious anemia, would result in slight but distinct reticulocytosis and a rise in erythrocyte count, hemoglobin and hematocrit, without the significant changes in bone-marrow morphology, serum iron or serum vitamin B_{12} levels that attend therapy with larger doses. By this definition, the minimal effective daily dose of vitamin B_{12} was demonstrated to be in the range of 0.1 μg.

Louis W. Sullivan and Victor Herbert. Studies on the Minimum Daily Requirement for Vitamin B_{12}. New England J. Med. 272:340, Feb. 18, 1965.

"Nowadays one very rarely sees a full-blown classical case of pernicious anemia. This is probably because in our affluent society people tend to have medical attention relatively early in most debilitating maladies, and also I think it not unlikely that some benefit may be derived from the overstuffing with complex vitamin mixtures in which so many individuals indulge. But the disappearance of the classical case is not an unmixed blessing since it fails to keep us fully in touch with all of the potentialities of the disease and also makes the patient lackadaisical in attention to his therapy through not having experienced a serious manifestation before coming in for diagnosis. Would you therefore kindly provide a statement of what is to be expected from therapy if one were to have the good luck to encounter a real textbook case?"

Reply: When cyanocobalamine (vitamin B_{12}) is given by injection in proper dosage in this malady, the marrow is converted from a megaloblastic to a normoblastic state in 48–72 hours, reticulocytes appear in the peripheral blood and rise within 5 to 6 days to a peak whose height, other things being equal, is inversely proportional to the level of the red cells. The soreness and burning associated with glossitis disappear in a few days and lingual papilla regeneration is usually complete in less than 6 weeks, though with advanced cord involvement the tongue lesions may persist. Usually within 6–8 weeks the count of mature erythrocytes is within normal limits, where it may be kept by maintenance dosage thereafter. The abnormalities in other cell systems such as gastric epithelial cells and cells in the sputum and oral and vaginal smears are also reversed. The skin begins to acquire color in the first week and later becomes healthy and moist in appearance. This improvement is shared by the mucous membranes. Murmurs, angina and spleen palpability disappear. The edema, too, usually disappears, but it may be accentuated as the patient becomes ambulant if there is much cord involvement. Some patients have polycythemia for awhile and consequently a very red appearance. Appetite, physical strength and sexual power return. Gastrointestinal symptoms disappear, possibly with bowel looseness for a short time. Dizziness, blurred vision, headache and dyspnea disappear.

Overall improvement in neurologic status is striking, even individuals with the most severe symptoms usually recovering except for minor evidences of involvement. Cerebral and mental symptoms appear to be completely curable, though 6–12 months may be required. Loss or perversion of the sense of smell is cured in 2–4 months, and muscular weakness and atrophy in a few weeks; impairment of superficial sensibilities clears unless there is actual cutaneous anesthesia, and even ataxia disappears except perhaps for some unsteadiness in the Romberg position. The returning tendon reflexes may be exaggerated. Poorest prognosis is in regard to involvement of the lateral columns of the cord, abnormal plantar and exaggerated tendon reflexes nearly always persisting permanently. Since neurologic residuals remaining after 10–12 months of intensive treatment probably represent irreversible degenerative changes, the importance of the earliest possible diagnosis cannot be exaggerated. In very rare instances the full cyanocobalamine effect may not be apparent because of concomitant folic acid or ascorbic acid deficiency; supplementary administration of these two agents will quickly correct the situation.

Pregnancy used to be considered a calamity for the pernicious anemia patient, but women are now carried through safely to the birth of healthy babies. Major surgical procedures probably tend to precipitate or increase neurologic symptoms, but patients receiving cyanocobalamine therapy are on the whole good surgical risks. Neither free hydrochloric acid nor intrinsic factor appear in the gastric juice during an induced remission.

"In a patient with pernicious anemia on vitamin B_{12} therapy, I was recently able to obtain gastric juice containing acid after I had placed the patient on a corticosteroid. Has such an experience been recorded?"

Reply: Yes, at Cornell University, Graham Jeffries obtained fasting and stimulated gastric juices containing both acid and intrinsic factor in a patient who, having been for a long time on vitamin B_{12} therapy, was given prednisolone (Meticortelone, etc.) for 4 months. Gastric biopsy specimens also contained normal glands with an abundance of parietal and chief cells between areas of relative atrophy. It has been shown that the corticosteroids sometimes enhance the absorption of cyano-

cobalamine through stimulation of the gastric secretion of intrinsic factor.

Graham H. Jeffries. Recovery of Gastric Mucosal Structure and Function in Pernicious Anemia During Prednisolone Therapy. Gastroenterology 48:371, 1965.

"I have recently placed a patient with pernicious anemia on vitamin B_{12} therapy and had a peripheral thrombosis to treat about 10 days later. Could there have been any connection between the drug and this occurrence?"

Reply: There have been reports of such cases. In the 4 patients of Klemetti, in Helsinki, the thrombosis occurred immediately after the reticulocyte peak had been reached in 1, 9 days after the peak in 1 and about 2 months after the peak in 2. This has been common to all reported cases, that have usually been in aged persons with a history of cardiovascular disease.

Lahja Klemetti. Is Vitamin B_{12} Treatment of Pernicious Anemia a Predisposing Factor for Thromboses in Aged Patients? Acta med. scandinav. 176:121, 1964.

"If cyanocobalamine (vitamin B_{12}) is to be used orally in treatment of pernicious anemia, what should be the dosage?"

Reply: In their 37 patients who were treated for 18–43 months, Thompson and associates found 100 μg. daily to be inadequate; normal hematologic values were accomplished without neurologic complications, but the serum levels of the vitamin fell progressively and at the end were not felt to be within the safe range. With such low dosage there is also great risk involved if the patient skips a dose. The studies of both Waife and associates (Indianapolis) and Withey and associates (Cardiff, Wales) established 300 μg. daily as the minimal fully effective dosage.

R. B. Thompson, D. W. Ashby and Edna Armstrong. Long-Term Trial of Oral Vitamin B_{12} in Pernicious Anemia. Lancet 2:577, 1962. S. O. Waife, C. J. Jansen, Jr., R. E. Crabtree, E. L. Grinnan and P. J. Fouts. Oral Vitamin B_{12} Without Intrinsic Factor in Treatment of Pernicious Anemia. Ann. Int. Med. 58:810, 1963. J. L. Withey, J. H. Jones and G. S. Kilpatrick. Long-Term Trial of Oral Treatment of Pernicious Anemia with Vitamin B_{12} Peptide. Brit. M. J. 1:1583, June 15, 1963.

"What drugs are effectively used in the megaloblastic anemias other than addisonian pernicious anemia?"

Reply: There are indications that the *megaloblastic anemia of infancy* may be a syndrome rather than a single entity, since it sometimes responds to crude liver extract and nearly always to folic acid, but now always to cyanocobalamine. The *megaloblastic anemia* *of pregnancy* frequently responds very slowly if at all to liver extract or cyanocobalamine, but folic acid is effective; blood transfusions may also be needed, however, in an occasional instance to carry the patient through. The *nutritional megaloblastic anemia syndrome*, of which tropical macrocytic anemia is a geographic type only, appears to result from failure to absorb cyanocobalamine, folic acid and possibly also such factors as choline and pantothenic acid. The claim has been made that these anemias do not respond well to refined liver extract but only to the crude form, but this position has been questioned. There is good response to the combined use of cyanocobalamine, folic acid and large doses of thiamine. The *anemias of sprue (both types), fish tapeworm infestation, gastrointestinal disease and surgery (when they are of the macrocytic type), and celiac disease* respond best to the combined use of cyanocobalamine and folic acid.

"One of my colleagues has a case of megaloblastic anemia in which he is beginning to think he has precipitated polycythemia vera by the use of folic acid. Is this likely?"

Reply: There have been a few reported instances of this sequence, which were thought to have been merely coincidental until Grönbaek and Larsen (Frederiksborg County Hospital, Hillerőd, Denmark) reported their case in which there was strong evidence of folic acid in the causative role. On 10 mg. folic acid three times daily polycythemia had developed, but it reverted after halving of the dosage for some months. Unfortunately, return to high dosage was not done, which would have been the true test.

Palle Grönbaek and Jörgen Vive Larsen. Polycythemia Vera Following Treatment of Megaloblastic Anemia with Folic Acid. Acta med. scandinav. 174:781, 1963.

"There have been several reports, differing in detail, of the use of small doses of folic acid as a differential procedure in megaloblastic anemia. Has anyone attempted to standardize the measure?"

Reply: Yes, Thirkettle's group (University of Bristol) has done so. All patients in their series who truly had megaloblastic anemia responded to small doses of folic acid except those with the malabsorption syndrome, who will not respond. After 8 days on a diet containing no red meat or offal and low in vegetables containing folic acid, their patients are given 200 µg. folic acid daily for 10 days. They considered that they had a positive diagnosis if a reticulocyte response (over 4%)

was obtained, and the folic acid treatment was continued in such cases.

J. L. Thirkettle, K. R. Gough and A. E. Read. Diagnostic Value of Small Doses of Folic Acid in Megaloblastic Anemia. Brit. M. J. 1:1286, May 16, 1964.

"After a considerable diagnostic hassle we have finally settled upon it that one of our patients does not have true addisonian pernicious anemia but rather has a megaloblastic anemia in association with diverticulosis of the small intestine, truly a rare entity. Tetracycline therapy has corrected the situation, at least temporarily, but we do not understand what is going on. Can you explain?"

Reply: I certainly do not feel that I can explain, but I can cite Paulk and Farrar's thorough study of a case in Atlanta in which they laid the blame for the malabsorption of vitamin B_{12}, that underlies the anemia, upon the presence of a flora in the stagnant areas that produces large amounts of a substance which interferes with absorption of the vitamin. The action of the antibiotic would then be explainable on the basis of its allowing the emergence of a resistant strain that does not produce significant quantities of the hypothetical toxin.

E. Alan Paulk, Jr. and W. Edmund Farrar, Jr. Diverticulosis of Small Intestine and Megaloblastic Anemia: Intestinal Microflora and Absorption Before and After Tetracycline Administration. Am. J. Med. 37:473, 1964.

"What is the status of the stimulation of erythropoiesis by androgenic hormones?"

Reply: In B. J. Kennedy's series at the University of Minnesota, there were 3 good responses in 8 cases of anemia in myelofibrosis; 1 in 9 cases of leukemia; 2 in 16 cases of renal disease; 3 in 3 cases of hypogonadism; 2 in 3 cases of refractory anemia; and 1 in 4 cases of aplastic anemia; making a total of 12 good responses in 43 cases. *Dosages:* intramuscularly, testosterone propionate, 50–100 mg. three times a week; stanolone, 100 mg. three times a week; testosterone enanthate, 400–800 mg. weekly or testosterone cyclopentylpropionate, 200 mg. weekly; and orally, fluoxymesterone, 20 mg. daily; methyltestosterone, 50 mg. daily or testosterone linguets, 20 mg. daily. The period of administration should be at least 2 months.

B. J. Kennedy. Stimulation of Erythropoiesis by Androgenic Hormones. Ann. Int. Med. 57:917, 1962.

"Testosterone has considerable erythropoietic action in addition to its androgenic action. Is this favorable effect on hemoglobin levels retained in the synthetic substitutes for testosterone that have been developed principally for their anabolic rather than androgenic activity?"

Reply: I am unable to give a categorical answer, but will cite the study of Mullin and DiPillo (Long Island College Hospital, Brooklyn), who obtained gratifying increases in hemoglobin level when using stanozolol (Winstrol) in individuals with mild to moderate anemias and also in a group of patients with terminal metastatic carcinoma in which all modalities of treatment, including radiotherapy and chemotherapy, had been exhausted.

William G. Mullin and Frank Di Pillo. Influence of Stanozolol (Winstrol) on Hemoglobin Levels. New York J. Med. 63:2795, Oct. 1, 1963.

"I have been using testosterone cautiously with good effect in a case of refractory anemia, but now some evidence of masculinization is beginning to appear. Is there a preparation with which I can retain the desired effect with less virilizing activity?"

Reply: Sanchez-Medal's group (Mexico City) used the anabolic hormone, oxymetholone (Adroyd; Anadrol) with fair satisfaction in 19 cases. During the first 2 months of the treatment, 5 of the patients died, 4 failed to respond to therapy, and the anemia improved in 10. *Dosage:* 0.6–3.7 mg./kg. body weight daily. All patients gained somewhat in weight, and hoarseness and hirsutism appeared in 8 of them.

L. Sanchez-Medal, J. Pizzuto, E. Torre-Lopez and R. Derbez (Mexico City). Effect of Oxymetholone (Adroyd; Anadrol) in Refractory Anemia. Arch. Int. Med. 113:721, 1964.

"Is there a case for cobalt therapy in the anemia of pregnancy?"

Reply: Claims have been made for the supplemental use of cobalt in the anemias of pregnancy and prematurity and the iron deficiency anemia of infants born at full term, but it does seem to me that none of the studies were very critical. Responses to this agent have sometimes been observed in patients with moderate anemia associated with chronic infection, inoperable carcinoma of the stomach, chronic renal disease, sickle cell and some other refractory anemias, but there is certainly no indication for *routine* employment of the element as an adjuvant to cyanocobalamine, iron or folic acid therapy in anemias of any sort. In situations in which help is often really badly needed, such as in anemias associated with hepatic cirrhosis and in the lymphomatous diseases, there has been very little evidence of effectiveness of cobalt. And the agent is quite toxic: gastrointestinal disturbances, precordial pain, skin rashes, renal injury, tinnitus and temporary

deafness, thyroid hyperplasia with hypofunction and thrombocytosis.

"I have a child with congenital (erythroid) hypoplastic anemia in whom I have had the good fortune to effect an arrest with corticosteroids. If I take this patient gradually off the drugs and she eventually relapses, may I expect again to succeed with the corticosteroids?"

Reply: Among the 12 of Donald Allen and Louis Diamond's (Harvard University) 22 corticosteroid-treated patients who showed a sustained remission while under treatment, none ever failed to respond when there was subsequent need for the drugs. They found that a level of 5–7.5 mg. prednisone daily was usually adequate to maintain a hemoglobin above 9–10 Gm./100 ml. In the beginning of the therapy, an average of 30 mg. daily was used, with response usually noted within 14 days.

Donald M. Allen and Louis K. Diamond. Congenital (Erythroid) Hypoplastic Anemia: Cortisone Treated. Am. J. Dis. Child. 102:416, 1962.

"We have in our practice a case of pyridoxine-responsive anemia in which the response to pyridoxine has been quite satisfactory. We are, however, uncertain how to proceed on the long-haul basis."

Reply: Perhaps the best criterion would be the experience of Beaupre and Growney (University of Pennsylvania) in their very severe case, which in fact was the first reported to have an associated peripheral neuropathy. The patient was given 100 mg. pyridoxine intramuscularly daily. On the fourth day there was a peak reticulocytosis of 7%, and after 2 weeks of therapy the hemoglobin had risen to 11.5 Gm./100 ml. The patient was then able to walk normally and was discharged on 5 mg. pyridoxine orally three times daily. After 3 months of this, all signs of the neuropathy had disappeared, but they returned after a year and a half. On increasing the dose to 40 mg. daily, they diminished, and disappeared on raising it to 60 mg. daily.

Eugene M. Beaupre and Patrick M. Growney. Pyridoxine-Responsive Anemia with Neuropathy. Ann. Int. Med. 59:724, 1963.

"In the painful crisis of sickle cell anemia one often has to resort to the use of narcotics to effect relief. But we do not like to do this of course for fear of addiction; in fact, it is sometimes difficult to evaluate this pain because the patient subject to frequent crises is likely to exaggerate his symptoms in order to receive a narcotic drug. Has any other agent been effectively used?"

Reply: The most interesting departure in therapy that has come to my attention was that of Diggs and Williams (Memphis, Tennessee), who used papaverine in 18 patients with sickle cell anemia and 4 with sickle cell hemoglobin disease with severe pain. In all, 32 crises were treated with initial dosage of 0.065 Gm. papaverine intramuscularly, repeating in 30–60 minutes if the pain continued. Further treatment with 0.032–0.065 Gm. intramuscularly or orally was given every 2–4 hours for the next 24 hours. In some patients, pain diminished dramatically within 1 hour; in others, it decreased temporarily and then recurred, after which it responded partially or completely to subsequent medication. However, the relief did not last as long as that provided by narcotics, and in 1 patient there was prompt relief on one occasion and none on another. This therapy was rationalized on the belief that pain in sickle cell disease is due to impediment in blood flow in capillaries and terminal blood vessels because of increased viscosity of the blood containing sickle cells, with subsequent tissue hypoxia and injury. If there is vasoconstriction of vessels adjacent to areas in which there is marked stasis of blood, the use of the vasodilator agent is rational. The shortcoming of papaverine, however, for use in such a situation is that it is quickly and actively bound to plasma proteins and thus has a very fleeting analgesic action. This limitation can be overcome by incorporating it in a rectal suppository to yield it at a fixed rate to the bloodstream during a prolonged period. I have heard also of the use of anticoagulants in the sickle cell crisis, but have seen only one report, that of Rodman and associates (VA Hospital, Philadelphia), who appeared to have been encouraged by the use of these drugs in their 1 patient. However, it was the experience of Salvaggio and associates (Charity Hospital, New Orleans) in their 12 patients that the complications of anticoagulant therapy outweighed the slight clinical improvement obtained.

L. W. Diggs and Dorothy L. Williams. Treatment of Painful Sickle Cell Crises with Papaverine: Preliminary Report. South. M. J. 56:472, 1963. Theodore Rodman, Ralph M. Myerson and Bernard H. Pastor. Prevention of Painful Crises of Sickle Cell Anemia with Prothrombinopenic Anticoagulants: Report of Case. Am. J. M. Sc. 242:707, 1961. John E. Salvaggio, Charles A. Arnold and Charles H. Banov. Long-Term Anticoagulation in Sickle Cell Disease: Clinical Study. New Eng. J. Med. 269:182, July 25, 1963.

"Since it has long been the clinical impression that infections predispose to sickling crises in individuals with sickle cell anemia, would it be worthwhile trying to reduce the incidence of these episodes through the prophylactic use of antibiotics or chemotherapeutic agents?"

Reply: In Uganda, where the commonest early childhood infections are malaria and respiratory infections and the mortality in sickle cell anemia is high, M. A. Warley and associates put this matter to the test. The prophylactic group were given 1,200,000 units of long-acting benzathine penicillin by injection and one 200 mg. tablet of chloroquine (Aralen) at the weekly attendance at the clinic and a similar chloroquine tablet to take on the intervening week between two attendances. The control group received 0.5 ml. of sterile water by injection. The groups were of equal size, 66 in one and 60 in the other, and about three-fourths of the children were under 6 years of age. Statistical studies and clinical impressions agreed that the treated group was at a definite advantage over the control group. It could only be determined with certainty, however, that the chloroquine was responsible for this advantage since protection against malaria eliminated the fall in hemoglobin value that had always occurred before; the role played by the long-acting penicillin could not be clearly determined.

M. A. Warley, P. J. S. Hamilton, P. D. Marsden, R. E. Brown, J. G. Merselis, and N. Wilks (Kampala, Uganda). Chemoprophylaxis of Homozygous Sicklers with Antimalarials and Long-Acting Penicillin. Brit. M. J. 1:86, July 10, 1965.

"I have a patient with idiopathic autoimmune hemolytic anemia. Are there any drugs that might be effective?"

Reply: The prognosis is grave in this malady and treatment frequently ineffective. When the usually recommended therapy— ACTH, corticosteroids and splenectomy— fails to induce a remission, antineoplastic agents have occasionally been effective, though the mechanism of their action is not understood. Robert Matthews, in California, has reported the case of an elderly woman with severe, idiopathic autoimmune hemolytic anemia that was initially controlled by splenectomy, but in whom a relapse associated with development of severe autoimmune thrombocytopenic purpura failed to respond to large doses of prednisone (Meticorten, etc.); these symptoms were controlled to a variable degree with azathioprine (Imuran).

Robert J. Matthews. Idiopathic Autoimmune Hemolytic Anemia and Idiopathic Thrombocytopenic Purpura Associated with Diffuse Hypergammaglobulinemia, Amyloidosis, Hypoalbuminemia and Plasmacytosis. Am. J. Med. 39:972, 1965.

"I have a patient with autoimmune hemolytic anemia, whom I am treating with corticosteroids. Is this therapy being superseded by the antineoplastic agents in the centers where specialized studies are being done?"

Reply: No. Robert Schwartz and William Dameshek (Tufts University) have authoritatively stated that, while the antineoplastic agents may be useful adjuncts to corticosteroid therapy, or alternatives when corticosteroids are contraindicated or ineffective, their toxicity precludes them from recommendation for routine treatment of the disease.

Robert Schwartz and William Dameshek. Treatment of Autoimmune Hemolytic Anemia with 6-Mercaptopurine (Purinethol) and Thioguanine (Thioguan). Blood 19:483, 1962.

"I have a patient with autoimmune hemolytic anemia in whom splenectomy has not been helpful and there has been no response to corticosteroids. I am very dubious of the advisability of using such potentially toxic agents as the antineoplastic drugs. Have you anything to suggest?"

Reply: At the Henry Ford Hospital in Detroit, Ten Pas and Monto have used heparin effectively in one case, giving 100 mg. subcutaneously every 8 hours and gradually reducing the dosage to 25 mg. twice daily.

Andrew Ten Pas and Raymond W. Monto. The Treatment of Autoimmune Hemolytic Anemia with Heparin. Am. J. M. Sc. 251:63, 1966.

"When there is reason to suspect a drug in the causative role of hemolytic anemia, what agents should one have in mind?"

Reply: Acetanilid, phenacetin, amithiozone (Tibione, Panrone), PAS, primaquine, quinine and quinidine, sulfonamides, sulfones (Promin, Diasone, Promizole, Avlosulfon, DDS), suramin (Antrypol, Germanin, Bayer 205), vitamin K, trimethadione (Tridione), nitrofurantoin (Furadantin), methyldopa (Aldomet). In the case of some of these drugs the occurrence of a hemolytic anemia has been recorded only a few times.

"Is there any drug therapy that is effective in the hemolytic anemias?"

Reply: In the hemolytic anemias resulting from abnormality intrinsic in the erythrocyte as it develops we have no very useful pharmacologic agents (see preceding Replies), but in some of the extracorpuscular hemolytic anemias there is much that we can do with corticotropin and the corticosteroids. The entities most often benefited, according to Lichtman, are the idiopathic acquired hemolytic anemias with and without demonstrable antibodies, the symptomatic hemolytic anemias (those associated with malignant lymphomas, chronic lymphocytic leukemia, collagen diseases and miscellaneous tumors) and the hemolytic states resulting from drug sensitivities.

H. C. Lichtman. Status of Therapy in Anemias. J.A.M.A. 167:735, 1958.

"I have recently had a patient who was discovered to have erythrocytes deficient in glucose-6-phosphate dehydrogenase when he developed a severe hemolytic anemia upon ingestion of primaquine together with chloroquine (Aralen) after returning from a malarious zone. I understand that it was the primaquine and not the chloroquine that caused the trouble, but should like to know what other drugs this individual should avoid. Could you supply a list?"

Reply: I believe that between 40 and 50 compounds have been identified in association with this reaction. The following, however, is a condensed list of the drugs most likely to be encountered: acetylsalicylic acid (aspirin), aminopyrine (Pyramidon, etc.) acetophenetidin (Phenacetin), furazolidone (Furoxone), nitrofurantoin (Furadantin), para-aminosalicylic acid (PAS), primaquine, probenecid (Benemid), salicylazosulfapyridine (Azulfidine), sulfacetamide (Sulamyd), sulfamethoxypyridazine (Kynex), sulfanilamide, sulfoxone (Diasone), thiazolsulfone (Promizole), quinacrine (Atabrine), sulfisoxazole (Gantrisin), diaminodiphenyl sulfone (D.D.S.), dimercaprol (BAL), phytona (Mephyton, Konakion), menadiol sodium diphosphate (Synkavite, Kappadione, Thylokay).

Walter J. Stuckey, Jr. Hemolytic Anemia and Erythrocyte Glucose-6-Phosphate Dehydrogenase Deficiency. Am. J. M. Sc. 251:104, 1966.

"I have recently had the misfortune to have a case of aplastic anemia that was ascribable with fair certainty to a self-administered drug. What are the chief drugs that have been associated in an etiologic role in aplastic anemia and what proportion of the total cases have they accounted for?"

Reply: A chemical substance taken as a drug or otherwise encountered is thought to be responsible for about half the reported cases of aplastic anemia. The compounds most importantly implicated have been listed by Allan Erslev (Jefferson Medical College): chloramphenicol (Chloromycetin), sulfonamides, sulfonamide derivatives such as acetazolamide (Diamox), the thiazide diuretics and the sulfonylurea antidiabetic compounds, phenylbutazone (Butazolidin), anticonvulsants such as mephenytoin (Mesantoin) and trimethadione (Tridione), benzene, other organic solvents, insecticides such as benzene hexachloride (Lindane), chlorophenothane (DDT), chlordane, gold salts. To this list of Erslev's, I would add acetaminophen (Apamide, Tylenol, etc.), arsenicals, colchicine, ethosuximide (Zarontin), hydralazine (Apresoline), phenacemide (Phenurone) and streptomycin. Since many of these are valuable drugs or organic chemicals, and aplastic anemia is a very rare complication, the mandate is not to abandon use of all of these agents but merely to be extremely cautious in their employment.

Allan J. Erslev (Jefferson Med. College). Drug-Induced Blood Dyscrasias. J.A.M.A. 188:531, May 11, 1964.

"There is much complaint in our area about the difficulty of getting infants to take ferrous sulfate in liquid form because of its alleged unpalatability. I have not had trouble of this sort myself, but most of my associates are turning to use of the new organic iron-carbohydrate complex, polyferose (Jefron Elixir). This preparation is said to contain approximately 50% iron by weight, but since three-fourths of it is in the ferric form, I am doubtful of its efficacy in comparison with the more readily absorbable ferrous preparation. What is the true state of affairs?"

Reply: I can only tell you that although this preparation has achieved considerable popularity among pediatricians, there have been adverse reports. The most recent to come to my attention was that of Jean Ross, at the Boston Floating Hospital, who reported 4 cases of iron-deficiency anemia of infancy that did not respond to the administration of this preparation. It is certainly legitimate to wonder whether palatability may not have been substituted for therapeutic reliability in the case of this item.

Jean D. Ross. Failure of Iron-Deficient Infants to Respond to an Orally Administered Iron-Carbohydrate Complex. New Eng. J. Med. 269:399, Aug. 22, 1963.

"Since it is the deoxygenation (reduction) of hemoglobin S molecules that brings about the distortion of the erythrocytic cell membrane that is ultimately responsible for the crises in sickle cell anemia, would it not be logical to administer a carbonic anhydrase inhibitor to a patient with this malady, as carbonic anhydrase is the enzyme responsible for the hemoglobin reduction?"

Reply: Quite logical, and it has been done, but with very little success. For example, there was no sustained improvement in the 7 patients treated with the potent carbonic anhydrase inhibitor, dichlorphenamide (Daranide, Oratrol) by Finney and Hatch, of Diggs's group in Memphis. These observers felt it likely that the inhibition of carbonic anhydrase tends to produce a hyperchloremic metabolic acidosis which increases intravascular sickling and hemolysis sufficiently to circumvent any benefit derived from blockage of erythrocytic carbonic anhydrase.

Raymond A. Finney, Jr., and Fred E. Hatch, Jr. Effect of a Carbonic Anhydrase Inhibitor, Dichlorphenamide, on Sickle Cell Anemia. Am. J. M. Sc. 250:154, 1965.

"Is anything to be gained from the use of hormonal therapy in aplastic anemia?"

Reply: The chances of success with either corticosteroids or androgens are certainly small but remissions have been recorded in both congenital and acquired cases when the drugs have been used for several months. McKenna and Erslev speak of androgen dosage in terms of 100–200 mg. of testosterone enanthate intramuscularly weekly, or oxandrolone (Anavar), 15 mg. daily by mouth, or methandrostenolone (Dianabol), 15–20 mg. daily. Corticosteroid dosage is often 40 mg. daily of prednisone (Meticorten, etc.) or other corticosteroid in equivalent dosage. Infection should be combated with the appropriate antibiotic.

Patrick J. McKenna and Allan J. Erslev. Treatment of Anemias. M. Clin. North America 49:1371, 1965.

"Is it possible for orally administered iron to cause severe rectal burning and no other gastrointestinal disturbance?"

Reply: Yes, it appears to be. Philip Nast and James Roth, in Philadelphia, have reported the case of a patient who had severe fulminating ulcerative colitis, in whom a capsule of Simron caused such burning within 6–8 hours in two separate trials, and also in a third trial when the contents of the capsule were added to her food without her knowledge. It is possible that any other iron salt and not merely Simron might have had this effect, but such trial was not made.

Philip R. Nast and James L. A. Roth. Use of Oral Iron in Anemia Associated with Gastrointestinal Disorders. Jour.-Lancet 86:69, 1966.

"What drugs have been found useful in treatment of autoimmune hemolytic anemia?"

Reply: In this malady the erythrocytes are destroyed prematurely by antibodies generated by the patient's own immune system. In many instances the condition is a complication of one of the lymphomas or of systemic lupus erythematosus, with a few cases being associated with other collagen disorders, myeloma, sarcoidosis, ulcerative colitis, ovarian cysts. Acute episodes have also occurred in primary atypical pneumonia and infectious mononucleosis. Of course blood transfusion is much employed, usually with packed cells because erythrocytes and hemoglobin are more needed than plasma; but difficulties in crossmatching often arise. Corticosteroids are highly valued in this therapy, being especially effective in the "warm" antibody type. Latterly, there has been some use of the immunosuppressive drugs, such as azathioprine (Imuran) and 6-mercaptopurine (Purinethol). In the so-called "cold" antibody type of the disease, penicillamine (Cuprimine) has been used with some effect. Splenectomy is sometimes resorted to in autoimmune hemolytic anemia when drug therapy has failed.

ANTHRAX

"What is the specifically effective antibiotic in the treatment of anthrax?"

Reply: One has to hedge a bit in answering this question because if the disease has advanced into the disseminated stage when diagnosed it is unlikely that any drug will be very helpful. Penicillin is the drug of choice with the tetracyclines probably in second place. But in these fulminating cases it is best to use a corticosteroid as supplemental therapy.

ANTIBIOTICS

"We are charged so frequently with 'abusing' the antibiotics that one grows a bit weary of hearing the thing. Just what are these heinous abuses?"

Reply: I suppose one must say that the worst one of them all is yielding to the demand of a patient who will have a certain antibiotic "or else." Then there is the failure to warn the patient strictly against self-administration of an antibiotic that may be "left over" after treatment of an acute episode is terminated; serious reactions may have become fully established in such a patient before he seeks help. Antibiotics should not be administered to a patient merely because he has a fever whose cause you cannot easily and quickly determine; the dire possible results of doing this have been dealt with elsewhere in this volume. And surely there is dubious justification for the prescription of an antibiotic over the phone without having examined the patient. There is absolutely no excuse for administration of these drugs in maladies which you know to be of viral origin, for the drugs have been fully determined to be worthless in these disorders. In the case of streptococcal pharyngitis it is an abuse to administer a single dose of an antibiotic for its quick "curative" effects unless it be one of the very long-acting ones, for the organism involved in this malady requires continuous exposure to penicillin for at least 10 days if the patient is to be fully protected against recurrences and the rheumatic fever which always hovers in the background. Continuing the use of an antibiotic when superinfection has appeared is also reprehensible because it perpetuates the circumstances under which the new organism has been able to establish a pathogenic hold. Failure to stop administration of a given antibiotic when certain types of reaction appear is also an abuse. Louis Weinstein lists the following as such reactions that should warn the physician of danger: an anaphylactoid reaction, thrombopenia, severe leukopenia, hemolytic anemia, disturbance of vestibular or auditory function, evidence of renal insufficiency, serum sickness, angioneurotic edema, exfoliative dermatitis, purpura. Failure to make searching inquiry into the possibility that the patient may have experienced a previous reaction to the drug that is to be used is certainly a dereliction of duty and therefore an abuse. And finally, the use of certain antibiotics without definite knowledge that the patient is free of renal disease; Weinstein says that the only ones that can be used safely in full dosage in an individual with severe renal failure are chloramphenicol, erythromycin, novobiocin and chlortetracycline. Even the dosage of penicillin must be reduced in a patient with renal insufficiency.

Louis Weinstein, *in* L. S. Goodman and A. Gilman. The Pharmacological Basis of Therapeutics, Third Edition. New York, The Macmillan Co., p. 1171, 1965.

"Some bacteria have developed resistance to the antimicrobial drugs and others have not. Could you supply a statement of the situation at present?"

Reply: Fred Gill and Edward Hook, at Cornell, have reviewed the matter thoroughly. The following may be gleaned from their publication. Penicillin is still the most effective agent for the prevention and treatment of group A streptococcal infections. Sulfonamides are effective in prophylaxis but they will not eradicate group A streptococci from the pharynx, regardless of the sensitivity of the organism, and therefore do not constitute adequate therapy for streptococcal pharyngitis. Erythromycin is the agent of choice in the patient who is allergic to penicillin. The tetracyclines can no longer be effectively used in streptococcal infections. The susceptibility of the pneumococci to antimicrobial agents has remained remarkably stable. Tetracyclines and erythromycin are excellent alternative drugs in patients who are allergic to penicillin, which is the drug of choice. However, it does appear that the usefulness of the tetracyclines is diminishing. Regarding the meningococcal infections, it is now evident that sulfonamide-resistant organisms are widely distributed throughout the United States and that the sulfonamides can no longer be relied upon for effective chemoprophylaxis or treatment of meningococcal infections; at the present time penicillin G constitutes the therapy of choice, and there is no advantage in the addition of a sulfonamide. Chloramphenicol may be effectively substituted in a patient who is sensitive to penicillin, but there is no evidence that the new penicillinase-resistant penicillins and cephalothin have established value either in prophylaxis or therapy of meningococcal infections. Decreased susceptibility of gonococci to penicillin has been confirmed in laboratories throughout the world. Penicillin is still the drug of choice in gonorrhea but must be used in much higher dosage now than formerly. Other effective agents against gonococci are the tetracyclines, erythromycin, streptomycin and chloramphenicol. However, since streptomycin-resistant strains of the organism have occurred when the drug is widely used in an area, it is best to use tetracycline or erythromycin if the patient is not responding to penicillin. At present, from one to two thirds of the strains of staphylococci isolated from clinical sources are resistant to penicillin G, streptomycin, tetracycline and erythromycin. But the new penicillinase-resistant penicillins—methicillin, oxacillin, cloxacillin and nafcillin—are all active against these organisms. Nevertheless, the position is not entirely secure here because we are beginning to learn that there are a few strains, which are apparently widespread, virulent and communicable, that are resistant to all of these agents. The present position regarding the enteric bacteria is that most strains of *E. coli* are sensitive to ampicillin, colistimethate (or polymyxin B), tetracycline and chloramphenicol, but strains acquired outside the hospital are more likely to be fully sensitive than are hospital-acquired strains. Ampicillin is the most active drug against *P. mirabilis* and kanamycin against indole-positive strains of *Proteus*. Most strains of *Klebsiella-Aerobacter* are sensitive to colistimethate or kanamycin, a smaller proportion to chloramphenicol or tetracycline. Nearly all strains of *P. aeruginosa* are sensitive to colistimethate (or polymyxin B) but resistant to other agents. Tetracycline is satisfactory in the treatment of most cases of shigellosis in the United States, and nearly all strains of salmonella are still susceptible to chloramphenicol.

Fred A. Gill and Edward W. Hook. Changing Patterns of Bacterial Resistance to Antimicrobial Drugs. Am. J. Med. 39:780, 1965.

"When a patient is seen with what appears to be a life-threatening infection and is placed on antibiotics and supportive measures as indicated, is there advantage to be expected from the routine use of corticosteroids in addition?"

Reply: This matter was studied by leading investigators in five university hospitals in this country, whose accumulated data provided no evidence of important benefit resulting from the use of hydrocortisone in patients under these circumstances.

Ivan L. Bennett, Jr., Maxwell Finland, Morton Hamburger, Edward H. Kass, Mark Lepper and Burton A. Waisbren.

Effectiveness of Hydrocortisone in Management of Severe Infections: Double-Blind Study. J.A.M.A. 183:462, Feb. 9, 1963.

"Which of the antibiotics in current use are bactericidal and which bacteriostatic?"

Reply: Those that are primarily bactericidal are penicillin, streptomycin, bacitracin, neomycin, polymyxin B (Aerosporin), colistin (Coly-Mycin), kanamycin (Kantrex), vancomycin (Vancocin), ristocetin (Spontin), methicillin (Staphcillin, Dimocillin-RT), nafcillin (Unipen), ampicillin (Penbritin, Polycillin), oxacillin (Prostaphlin, Resistopen), cephalothin (Keflin). Those that are primarily bacteriostatic are novobiocin (Albamycin, Cathomycin), erythromycin (Erythrocin, Ilosone, Ilotycin, Pediamycin, Erythromycin), oleandomycin (Cyclamycin, Matromycin) and lincomycin (Lincocin).

"When is one justified in using combinations of antibiotics?"

Reply: The authoritative review of this subject by Harry Dowling at the University of Illinois, provided the following replies to your question. (1) The only clear indications at present for combining antibiotics are in streptococcal bacterial endocarditis and tuberculosis. (2) In other cases, preliminary in vitro studies are desirable before antibiotics are given in combination, except when time is insufficient for laboratory tests. (3) When there is not time for such tests, it is advisable to combine antibiotics that are primarily bactericidal and to avoid combining a primarily bactericidal with a primarily bacteriostatic antibiotic for fear that antagonism may result. (4) If an antibiotic of a bacteriostatic and a bactericidal group must be combined, large doses of the primarily bactericidal antibiotic should be given.

Harry F. Dowling. Present Status of Therapy with Combinations of Antibiotics. Am. J. Med. 39:796, 1965.

"We habitually say that gram-negative organisms are not susceptible to the action of penicillin and let it go at that. But what if we were to give enormous dosage of penicillin in some of the gram-negative infections?"

Reply: In a thorough study of this matter in Boston, Louis Weinstein and associates divided gram-negative bacilli into the following three groups on the basis of in vitro studies: (1) "resistant," or those sensitive to 1250 units or more per ml. (this level is difficult to attain in blood); (2) "moderately sensitive," or those inhibited by 156–625 units per ml. (this concentration may be achieved by injecting 5,000,000–10,000,000 units of penicillin); (3) "sensitive," comprising strains susceptible to 2.5–78 units per ml. (serum levels of this order are attained when moderate amounts of penicillin are given). They then put the matter to the clinical test. Seventeen patients with various gram-negative bacilli infections were treated with 1 million–80 million units of penicillin daily in divided intravenous doses at 6 hour intervals. After 2-6 weeks of treatment there was complete control of the infection in 13 of the 17 patients; 2 patients did not respond, 2 others responded initially but did not do so upon relapse. The causative organism was *Aerobacter aerogenes* in 7, *E. coli* in 7, a proteus strain in 2 and klebsiella and *S. typhimurium* in 1 each. Mixed infection of proteus and *A. aerogenes* was present in 1 patient and of *E. coli* and proteus in another.

Louis Weinstein, Phillip I. Lerner and William H. Chew. Clinical and Bacteriologic Studies of Effect of "Massive" Doses of Penicillin G on Infections Caused by Gram-Negative Bacilli. New England J. Med. 271:525, Sept. 10, 1964.

"What modifications in antibiotic dosage should be made in a patient with known renal disease?"

Reply: The following is Sanford and Reinarz's compilation from several sources: chloramphenicol (Chloromycetin), normal or slight decrease in dosage (but follow reticulocyte counts and serum iron levels for evidence of toxicity); colistimethate (Coly-Mycin), 2 mg./kg./48–72 hr.; erythromycin (Erythrocin, Ilotycin), normal dosage; kanamycin (Kantrex), 1 Gm. loading dose, then 0.5 Gm./48–96 hr.; methicillin (Dimocillin, Staphcillin), 1 Gm. intravenously/8–12 hr.; oxacillin (Prostaphlin), 1 Gm. intravenously/4–6 hr.; penicillin G, aqueous penicillin every 4-12 hours; streptomycin 1 Gm. loading dose, then 0.5 Gm./48 hr.; tetracycline (Achromycin, etc.), 1 Gm. loading dose, then 0.5 Gm./48–96 hr.; chlortetracycline (Aureomycin), normal dosage (but metabolic effects of the drug inactivated in vivo are unknown; it may have toxicity); oxytetracycline (Terramycin, Terrabon), 1 Gm. loading dose, then 0.5 Gm./48–96 hr.; vancomycin (Vancocin), 0.5 Gm./48–72 hr.

Jay P. Sanford and James Allen Reinarz. Complications Associated with Antibiotic Therapy. Disease-A-Month, Nov., 1964.

"In the crowded wards of our large antiquated municipal hospital we treat ordinary pneumococcus pneumonia with penicillin with very satisfactory results. But I feel that, in order to insure maximum use of our beds, we are routinely giving higher dosage than necessary. Other than wastage of the drug, are we running any danger with this practice?"

Reply: At least a theoretic danger. At Cornell University, Louria and Brayton showed that the incidence of superinfection was much higher with excessive penicillin dosage than when just sufficient dosage was used; i.e., new microorganisms, including staphylococci and gram-negative enteric bacteria, appeared more often in the sputum. Often the bacteriologic evidence of superinfection disappeared spontaneously when administration of the antibiotic was stopped. But undoubtedly appearance of those organisms does introduce an added risk.

Donald B. Louria and Robert G. Brayton. Efficacy of Penicillin Regimens: With Observations on Frequency of Superinfection. J.A.M.A. 186:987, Dec. 14, 1963.

"I have a patient who has experienced a rather frightening acute psychotic reaction after the intramuscular injection of penicillin. Are sequelae to be feared?"

Reply: No, the psychiatric disturbances associated with penicillin administration have generally been free of serious sequelae, but I am obliged to point out that Sheldon Cohen (Emory University) did report the cases of two young adults who showed the classic picture of anaphylactic shock associated with penicillin hypersensitivity, and then later developed impairment in all phases of living as measured by their premorbid adjustments. And to compound the felony, it happened that one of the patients had an infection that was penicillin-resistant, and the other had self-administered the drug for treatment of a cold.

Sheldon B. Cohen. Brain Damage Due to Penicillin. J.A.M.A. 186:899, Dec. 7, 1963.

"Is it true that cases of nephropathy associated with penicillin and the newer semisynthetic penicillins are being seen?"

Reply: In Seattle, Robert Schrier and associates reported the ninth case of methicillin (Staphcillin, Dimocillin) nephritis and 3 additional cases of penicillin nephritis. However, they carefully made the point that all evidence relating penicillin allergy to renal disease must still be circumstantial because of the difficulty in establishing an unequivocal relationship between penicillin or any sensitizing agent and specific renal lesions, without adequate methods to establish the hypersensitive state.

Robert W. Schrier, Roger J. Bulger and Paul P. Van Arsdel, Jr. Nephropathy Associated with Penicillin and Homologues. Ann. Int. Med. 64:116, 1966.

"What proportion of individuals experience an allergic reaction to a first injection of penicillin?"

Reply: I think it impossible to answer this

question with accuracy. Prior to 1954, the incidence of reactions appeared to vary between 3 and 6%; this was during the period in which crystalline penicillin G and penicillin G in peanut oil and beeswax were being used. Subsequently, when procaine penicillin G became available, the rate was estimated to be 1–2%. And now, when so much benzathine penicillin G is being used, the rate is apparently slightly lower still. From the data accumulated by Bernstein and Hauser it appears that among 56,901 military personnel who volunteered symptoms of reactions following injection of 0.6 million units of benzathine penicillin G, the reaction rate ranged from 0.74 to 1.78, with a mean of 1.028%. And Frank and associates reported that among 76,130 Navy recruits receiving this drug only 0.83% volunteered symptoms of penicillin allergy. For the most part, the reactions in this latter group were of the primary serum-sickness type, which would suggest that these reactions represented initial sensitization to penicillin rather than immediate reactions due to prior sensitization; however, one can not be certain of this since Rytel and associates reported that 84% of 1022 Navy recruits arriving at Great Lakes expressed knowledge of previous penicillin treatment.

S. H. Bernstein and H. B. Hauser. Sensitivity Reactions to Intramuscular Injections of Benzathine Penicillin. New England J. Med. 260:747, Apr. 2, 1959.

Paul F. Frank, Gene H. Stollerman and Lloyd F. Miller. Protection of a Military Population from Rheumatic Fever. J.A.M.A. 193:775, Sept. 6, 1965.

M. W. Rytel, F. M. Klion, T. R. Arlander and Lloyd F. Miller. Detection of Penicillin Hypersensitivity with Penicilloyl-Polylysine. J.A.M.A. 186:894, Dec. 7, 1963.

"Now we hear that penicillin can cause hemolytic anemia, which is surely something new under the sun. Are we really to be in fear of this occurrence?"

Reply: No, I do not think so since the reported cases have so far been only a few. But if you are using penicillin in high dosage, as in a case of subacute bacterial endocarditis, I should be on the qui vive and watch the hematocrit.

"Am I properly open to criticism if I do not initially use a combination of penicillin and a sulfonamide in an infection in which it is later shown that this might have been an advantageous procedure?"

Reply: No, I do not think that you are, for it seems to me usually a quite defensible procedure to use one drug alone until evidence justifies inclusion of the other or a switch to the other. There are so many things to be taken into account in the treatment of an infectious disease with an antibiotic or a chemothera-

peutic agent: the amount of protein binding in the individual instance and of inhibiting substances in the body fluids; the amount of conjugating material available in the particular patient, and indeed the actual state of that patient's defensive mechanisms at the moment. Certainly one can routinely use a penicillin-sulfonamide combination when evidence of the true etiology of an infection is not immediately available, but this is certainly not very elegant therapy. Other reasons given by some men for always using this type of therapy (and not very cogent reasons in my opinion) are the hope of having one effective agent still operating if resistance develops to the other, and the desire to hit with full force if the organism is found to be sensitive to both of the drugs. In Boston, Louis Weinstein's group found that in 25–30% of the patients in their study the effectiveness of penicillin, and in 32–37% that of sulfadiazine, was reduced when both drugs were given simultaneously.

Louis Weinstein, Charles A. Samet and William H. Chew. Studies of Effects of Penicillin-Sulfonamide Combinations in Man. Am. J. M. Sc. 248:408, 1964.

"Are the new semisynthetic penicillins safe to use in a patient who is sensitive to penicillin G?"

Reply: I do not think it is possible as yet to give them blanket clearance, but at the University of Tennessee, Edgar Luton found 8 patients who had penicillin G anaphylaxis tolerant to methicillin (Dimocillin, Staphcillin). But he did some very careful testing before beginning use of the drug.

Edgar F. Luton. Methicillin (Dimocillin, Staphcillin) Tolerance after Penicillin G Anaphylaxis. J.A.M.A. 190:39, Oct. 5, 1964.

"Are there any practicable penicillin sensitivity tests available?"

Reply: No, this matter is still in an unsatisfactory state, although interesting observations have recently been reported by Howard Voss and associates in New York.

Howard E. Voss, Anthony P. Redmond and Bernard B. Levine. Clinical Detection of the Potential Allergic Reaction to Penicillin by Immunologic Tests. J.A.M.A. 196:679, May 23, 1966.

"We have just had a case in our hospital of respiratory arrest after the parenteral administration of neomycin. Fortunately, the quick administration of neostigmine saved the patient's life, but this was a very frightening experience. What other antibiotics have caused this sort of thing, and is neostigmine always effectively antidotal?"

Reply: Apnea has been associated in rare instances with the parenteral administration of streptomycin, neomycin, viomycin, kanamycin, colistin and polymyxin B. Neostigmine is an effective antidote to all of these except colistin and polymyxin B. These two drugs possibly prevent repolarization of the nerve endings, as does a skeletal muscle relaxant such as succinylcholine (Anectine), and are therefore not susceptible to the cholinesterase-inhibiting action of neostigmine. It is possible that any one of the following will increase the likelihood of occurrence of an apneic reaction to any one of the incriminated antibiotics: chronic debilitating disease, renal disease (or azotemia developing during the episode), hypoxic states, corticosteroids, narcotics, sedatives and, of course, muscle relaxant drugs.

Charles R. Ream (Saint Elizabeth Hosp., Elizabeth, N. J.). Respiratory and Cardiac Arrest after Intravenous Administration of Kanamycin with Reversal of Toxic Effects by Neostigmine. Ann. Int. Med. 59:384, 1963. Guenther Pohlmann. Respiratory Arrest Associated with Intravenous Administration of Polymyxin B. J.A.M.A. 196:181, Apr. 11, 1966. Eric W. Davidson, Jerome H. Modell, Frank Moya and Oscar Farmati. Respiratory Depression Following Use of Antibiotics in Pleural and Pseudocyst Cavities. J.A.M.A. 196:456, May 2, 1966. Gertie F. Marx, Edward J. Bennett, Louis R. Orkin. Oral Neomycin and Respiratory Failure. Canad. Anaes. Soc. J. 12:415, 1965.

"I have a patient whose onset of deafness seems suspiciously associated with her taking of neomycin by mouth. Is this a likely sequence?"

Reply: It is unlikely, but it has happened. Richard Fields (USAF Hospital, Washington, D.C.) spoke of 2 reported cases of deafness resulting from orally administered neomycin and 6 due to topical neomycin or its use as an aerosol or an irrigating solution. He then reported a case of his own of deafness associated with rectal and colonic irrigations with the drug.

Richard L. Fields. Neomycin Ototoxicity: Report of Case Due to Rectal and Colonic Irrigations. Arch. Otolaryng. 79:67, 1964.

"I have a patient who is claiming that her progressive deafness is due to neomycin that I prescribed for treatment of an enteric bacterial infection. Since the hearing disturbance did not begin until about 10 days after discontinuance of the neomycin, could the drug be held responsible?"

Reply: Yes, I believe that it could, since Lowell Greenberg and Hassen Momary (Los Angeles) reported an instance of both audiotoxicity and nephrotoxicity due to orally administered neomycin. But the occurrence is so rare that it cannot be construed as a contraindication to use of the drug. However, you are doubtless aware that parenteral administration of neomycin is much more likely to cause the serious side action.

Lowell H. Greenberg and Hassen Momary. Audiotoxicity and Nephrotoxicity Due to Orally Administered Neomycin. J.A.M.A. 194:827, Nov. 15, 1965.

"In our area a great deal of chloramphenicol (Chloromycetin) is prescribed, and we are not experiencing severe reactions, and yet there is constantly a great clamor on the part of medical educators against use of the drug except in a few specific infections; even the manufacturer's package insert carries a warning. How is one to reconcile these things?"

Reply: Relatively easily, in fact. In the first place, granting that a busy practitioner may prescribe the drug rather freely without ever experiencing a case of pancytopenia, it is nevertheless true that many such cases have occurred and that they have often been fatal. The second reason why the drug should not be freely used is simply that we now have other agents that are more effective and less toxic in the same situations. In upper respiratory tract infections and bacterial pharyngitis penicillin is usually perfectly satisfactory. For *E. coli* infections of the genitourinary tract there are the sulfonamides, nalidixic acid, nitrofurantoin (Furadantin) and furazolidone (Furoxone). In systemic infections with gram-negative organisms there are sodium colistimethate (Coly-Mycin Injectable) and kanamycin (Kantrex), which are actually more effective than chloramphenicol, though admittedly they have toxicities of their own and must be used with great care. And in the staphylococcal infections, for which so much chloramphenicol is prescribed, we now actually have better agents in oxacillin (Prostaphlin, Resistopen), methicillin (Dimocillin-RT, Staphcillin) and nafcillin (Unipen).

"I have a patient with hypoplastic anemia that appears attributable to the ingestion of chloramphenicol (Chloromycetin), but the drug was taken more than 2 months ago. How long after the taking of such a drug may a reaction occur in the blood?"

Reply: In 1962, Kurtides and Alt (Northwestern University) reported a case of hypoplastic anemia in an individual who had ingested chloramphenicol on two occasions, 9 and 17 months before onset of the illness, but just how long before the diagnosis was made this patient had actually begun to undergo a hematologic reaction is unknown. In Sharp's 1963 review of 40 cases of blood dyscrasias associated with the use of this drug, the most frequent interval after cessation of therapy was 1–3 months, but in 2 cases it was 9 months, and in 1 case 1 year.

Efstratios S. Kurtides and Howard L. Alt. Remission of Hypoplastic Anemia in an Adult Following Combined

Androgen and Corticosteroid Therapy. Quart. Bull. Northwestern Univ. M. School 36:325, 1962. A. A. Sharp. Brit. M. J. 1:735, 1963.

"One very astute observer in our area habitually uses much higher chloramphenicol (Chloromycetin) dosage than any of the rest of us, sometimes giving as much as 8–10, or occasionally I believe even as high as 18 Gm., daily. He says that since chloramphenicol-induced aplastic anemia is strictly on an allergic basis, and that it occurs very rarely and is as likely to be associated with low as high dosage, he sees no reason for not dosing heavily and getting full effect of the drug in as short time as possible. Is this good reasoning?"

Reply: Here in my own city, Burton Waisbren practices precisely this sort of thing and apparently with impunity since he presides over antibiotic therapy at the large general hospital and his record with high dosage of chloramphenicol is no worse than others with more conservative dosage. But many of us are hesitant, perhaps unreasonably, to use what is known hereabouts as "Waisbren dosage," and I think that the recently published study of James Scott and associates, in Los Angeles, tends to support our position. These observers presented findings strongly implying that chloramphenicol hematologic reactions are on a purely pharmacologic and not hypersensitivity basis. The implication from this would be of course that with increasing dosage the likelihood of such occurrences also increases. But this is only an implication, to be sure, and it is highly desirable that the subject be further investigated, for it is true that Waisbren often obtains fine results with his bold use of the drug.

James L. Scott, Sidney M. Firegold, Gerald A. Belkin and John S. Lawrence. Controlled Double-Blind Study of Hematologic Toxicity of Chloramphenicol. New Zealand M. J. 272:1137, June 3, 1964. Burton A. Waisbren, Clifford Simski and Poo-Liang Chang. Administration of Maximum Doses of Chloramphenicol (Chloromycetin). Am. J. M. Sc. 245:1, 1963.

"I have had considerable success with the new antibiotic, lincomycin (Lincocin), in dermatologic practice, but have had to abandon the use of the drug in all cases because it caused the patients to have numerous watery bowel movements. Has this been general experience?"

Reply: It has been a deterrent in use of the drug quite often, but Ben Kanee (Vancouver, B.C.) found that by reduction in dosage from an-initial 1000 mg. followed by 500 mg. every 6 hours, four times daily, to 500 mg. every 8 hours, three times daily, he could reduce the bowel disturbance to a tolerable degree. In his experience, however, pruritus ani required discontinuance of the therapy in 2 of the 14 patients with pyodermas.

Ben Kanee. Lincomycin in Dermatologic Practice. Canad. M. A. J. 93:220, July 31, 1965.

"From what I hear of the new antibiotic, cephalothin (Keflin), it begins to appear that it should be the 'first drug' of choice pending bacterial susceptibility studies. Is this a correct inference?"

Reply: This semisynthetic agent resembles the semisynthetic penicillins—ampicillin, methicillin, oxacillin and nafcillin—in not being inactivated by penicillinase, and there is suggestive evidence of effectiveness against staphylococci resistant to the penicillins, erythromycin, tetracyclines and chloramphenicol. Gram-negative organisms, too, are more susceptible to cephalothin than to any of the penicillins except ampicillin, though *Pseudomonas* is resistant. But the drug cannot be given orally because of poor absorption, and intramuscular injection may be painful and intravenous administration may cause thrombophlebitis. There have also been reports of a few allergic skin reactions, less often eosinophilia and neutropenia, and latterly evidence has been produced of the possibility in rare instances of cross-sensitivity between the penicillins and this new drug. So I should say that at the present time this does not seem to be the ideal "first drug," but increasing experience may advance it into that prized spot. I shall cite a few individual experiences.

At the King County Hospital, Seattle, Marvin Turck's group used the drug in treatment of 103 hospitalized patients with infections due to *Diplococcus pneumoniae*, penicillinase- and nonpenicillinase-producing staphylococci, streptococci, *Escherichia coli*, *Klebsiella-Aerobacter*, *Proteus mirabilis* and other gram-negative organisms. There was clinical and bacteriologic improvement in 76% of the patients. After cessation of treatment, relapse was common in patients with chronic urinary tract infections. A disadvantage of the drug was that it had to be administered parenterally at frequent intervals and the injections were usually accompanied by pain. No other untoward reactions were encountered, however, except for the development of rash in 3 patients. Nine patients with a history of previous penicillin allergy were given the new drug without incident.

At the Ohio State University Hospital, Robert Perkins and Samuel Saslaw treated 51 patients with various severe infections and obtained cures regularly in those in which staphylococci and pneumococci were involved but only occasional impressive responses in gram-negative bacillary infections; generally unfavorable treatment results were observed for mixed infections due to a staphylococcus plus a gram-negative bacillus, or two or more gram-negative bacilli. There was successful cephalothin treatment of serious infection in 10 of 12 penicillin-allergic patients. Comparable results were had by Stephen Merrill's group at the Wadsworth VA Hospital in Los Angeles, but the possibility that there may be cross-allergenicity between cephalothin and the penicillins arose in this study and caused the investigators to advise that suitable precautions be observed in the use of cephalothin in a patient who has had a life-threatening reaction to one of the penicillins.

Louis Weinstein, Kenneth Kaplan and Te-Wen Chang. Treatment of Infections in Man with Cephalothin (Keflin). J.A.M.A. 189:829, Sept. 14, 1964. Richard S. Griffith and Henry R. Black (Indiana Univ.). Cephalothin (Keflin)— A New Antibiotic: Preliminary and Laboratory Studies. J.A.M.A. 189:823, Sept. 14, 1964. Sherwin A. Kabins, Bernard Eisenstein and Sidney Cohen (Michael Reese Hosp.) Anaphylactoid Reaction to Initial Dose of Sodium Cephalothin. J.A.M.A. 193:165, July 12, 1965. Marvin Turck, Kenneth N. Anderson, Ronald H. Smith, James F. Wallace and Robert G. Petersdorf. Laboratory and Clinical Evaluation of a New Antibiotic—Cephalothin. Ann. Int. Med. 63:199, 1965. Robert L. Perkins and Samuel Saslaw. Experiences with Cephalothin. Ann. Int. Med. 64:13, 1966. Stephen L. Merrill, Alvin Davis, Bernard Smolens and Sydney M. Finegold. Cephalothin in Serious Bacterial Infection. Ann. Int. Med. 64:1, 1966.

"Word is going around that the concomitant administration of chymotrypsin and tetracycline will raise the blood level of the latter. Is there any basis for the rumor?"

Reply: At Columbia University, Seneca and Peer have been reporting such findings. They have found that a 20 mg. oral dose of chymotrypsin each time a dose of tetracycline is given will very considerably raise the titer of the antibiotic in both blood and urine. Clinical applications in the actual treatment of infectious diseases are not yet published.

Harry Seneca and Pat Peer. Enhancement of Blood and Urine Tetracycline Levels with a Chymotrypsin-Tetracycline Preparation. J. Am. Geriatrics Soc. 13:708, 1965.

"What is the position of lincomycin (Lincocin) among the antibiotics?"

Reply: At the New England Medical Center Hospitals, Louis Weinstein and associates have determined that the drug inhibits most strains of *Staphylococcus aureus* and *Streptococcus pyogenes* and *D. pneumoniae*, and that gram-negative bacilli and enterococci are highly resistant to it. Highest drug levels are achieved when the drug is taken in the fasting state, and it appears to be equally effective when given orally or parenterally: effective dosage in the experience of these observers appeared to be 50–100 mg./kg./day for children and 600 mg./6–8 hr. for adults.

So far very little toxicity has been reported, though diarrhea sometimes occurs. So in lincomycin we have another drug with which to combat infections with staphylococci, pneumococci and *Streptococcus pyogenes*, a list which includes the penicillins, cephalothin (Keflin), erythromycin (Erythrocin, etc.), vancomycin (Vancocin).

Kenneth Kaplan, William H. Chew and Louis Weinstein. Microbiological, Pharmacological and Clinical Studies of Lincomycin. Am. J. M. Sc. 250:137, 1965.

"I know that nephrotoxicity occurs frequently when amphotericin B is used, but has the drug ever been known to cause nephrocalcinosis?"

Reply: I have seen only the one case report of Finlayson's group (Duke University), in whose patient with sporotrichosis the drug did seem clearly to be responsible for the nephrocalcinosis that occurred.

G. Rolland Finlayson, Jose L. Miranda, Charles J. Mailman and J. Lamar Callaway. Sporotrichosis Treated with Amphotericin B: Nephrocalcinosis as a Therapeutic Complication. Arch. Dermat. 89:730, 1964.

"I have a patient with coccidioidomycosis, whom I am treating with amphotericin B. He has become very weak and developed a flaccid paralysis of the lower extremities. What do I do in this emergency?"

Reply: Stop the drug at once and give supplemental potassium orally, and intravenously if necessary, for the drug has probably damaged the kidney sufficiently to cause both a decreased tubular reabsorption and increased potassium excretion. Several cases of this sort have been reported.

John A. McChesney and John F. Marquardt. Hypokalemic Paralysis Induced by Amphotericin B. J.A.M.A. 189:1029, Sept. 28, 1964.

"I have recently had a patient on amphotericin B (Fungizone) who developed a sufficient degree of anemia to require discontinuance of the therapy. Is this not unusual?"

Reply: Yes, it is. In studying this matter at the National Institutes of Health, Brandriss's group, who were treating various mycoses with the drug, found a reduction in mean hematocrit volume from 41% before therapy to 27% during therapy in most of the patients, being nearly always normocytic and normochromic, with bone marrow aspiration revealing erythroid activity to be normal in most instances. And there is no change in the rate of hemolysis of erythrocytes during the therapy. So they concluded that the anemias are caused by depression of red cell production by amphotericin imposed on mild preexisting hemolysis due to systemic infection. These anemias do not often require discontinuance of amphotericin or blood transfusion, but they nevertheless constitute one of the reasons for using the drug only when the indications are absolute.

Michael W. Brandriss, Sheldon M. Wolff, Russell Moores and Frederick Stohlman, Jr. Anemia Induced by Amphotericin B (Fungizone). J.A.M.A. 189:663, Aug. 31, 1964.

"One hears that the tetracyclines will discolor the teeth in infancy. What is the extent of this problem?"

Reply: This discoloration occurs when these drugs are given during the formative period of the crowns of the teeth. In discussing the subject, Joan Weyman has said that for the deciduous anterior teeth this is from mid-pregnancy to about 4–6 months postnatal, and for the permanent anterior teeth from 6 months to about 5 years of age. Perhaps the least productive of this objectionable staining is oxytetracycline (Terramycin).

Joan Weyman. Tetracyclines and the Teeth. Practitioner 195:661, 1965.

"Can you give me some indication of acceptable antibiotic dosage in newborn and premature infants?"

Reply: At the University of Buffalo, Sumner Yaffe, a member of the Pediatrics Panel of the AMA Registry on Adverse Reactions, in an article invited by the Section of Adverse Reactions of the Council on Drugs, stated the following dosages: *Bacitracin*: 1000 units/kg. (900 units/kg. for premature infants)/day, in divided doses at 8–12 hour intervals: when diluted, the drug should be refrigerated at 4° C. and discarded after 24 hours. *Chloramphenicol*: 25 mg./kg./day may be therapeutically effective but also toxic; it is necessary to maintain blood levels of $10-20$ μg./ml. to obtain maximal therapeutic effect. *Colistin* and *Polymyxin B*: up to 1.5 mg./kg./day, intramuscularly for not longer than 7 days. *Erythromycin*: adequate serum levels, greater than 0.5 μg./ml., in premature infants have been reported following oral administration of erythromycin estolate in dosage of 10 mg./kg. every 6 hours; when given parenterally, 10 mg./kg./day suffices. *Kanamycin:* therapeutic serum levels of 15–20 μg./ml. have been produced in premature and newborn infants with parenteral administration of 15 mg./kg./day in two divided doses at 12 hours. *Neomycin*: dosages up to 100 mg./kg./day have been used extensively for as long as 3 weeks. *Novobiocin*: blood levels of 18–90 μg./ml. have been reported in the newborn infant following oral administration of a single dose of 12.5 mg./kg. *Penicillin*: it has been found that a single injection of 30,000 units of penicillin G in premature infants results in blood levels of 80–140 units/ml., with detectable activity present 24 hours later; satisfactory blood levels have been produced in the newborn by giving 40,000 units/kg. every 24 hours orally; the more resistant phenoxymethyl penicillin may be given in dosage of 30,000 units/kg. every 8 hours. Little information is available on the use of the newer penicillins in prematures and the newborn. Long-acting penicillin preparations should not be used because of the likelihood of producing sterile abscesses at the injection site in these very young individuals. *Streptomycin*: serum levels of 5 μg./ml. in 12 hours have been reported following a single dose of 6.6 mg./kg.; most physicians use 20 mg./kg./day for the newborn, although double this dosage has been employed without evidence of accumulation or renal or auditory damage. *Tetracyclines*: oral administration in the newborn of 100 mg./kg./day provides therapeutic serum levels, with some accumulation (levels of 10–18 μg./ml.) at the end of a week of therapy; much smaller doses (15 mg./kg.) can be given parenterally.

Sumner J. Yaffe. Antibiotic Dosage in Newborn and Premature Infants. J.A.M.A. 193:818, Sept. 6, 1965.

"The broad in vitro bactericidal spectrum for cephalothin (Keflin) suggests potential usefulness for treatment of infection due to mixed bacterial populations. Has this promise been fulfilled in clinical experience?"

Reply: Not very well, unfortunately. For example, in the study reported by Robert Perkins and Samuel Saslaw, in Columbus, Ohio, there were 6 patients who had mixed infections of the lower respiratory tract and 1 who had an infection of the skin due to a coagulase-positive staphylococcus plus one or more gram-negative bacilli; treatment failed in 5 of these patients, 2 of whom had flora including pseudomonas. Comparable results were had in 8 patients with infection of one site due to two or more gram-negative bacilli; treatment failed in 7 of the 8, and 4 of these had pseudomonas as part of the infecting flora. Possibly, however, these unfavorable responses were at least partially due to the type and stage of underlying disease, the nutritional status of the patients and the possible production of a cephalosporinase, particularly by pseudomonas organisms. In this same experience, comparably ill patients with similar underlying diseases and infection due to only a single gram-negative bacillus occasionally responded dramatically and there were higher infection cure rates; particularly impressive in this group were cures in 5 of 6 individuals with acute *Klebsiella* pneumonia, although 2 of the 5 had underlying myelogenous leukemia.

Robert L. Perkins and Samuel Saslaw. Experiences with Cephalothin. Ann. Int. Med. 64:13, 1966.

"Penicillin's potential for producing epileptiform convulsions has restricted its subarachnoid and intraventricular administration; may it not be that the extremely high intravenous dosage nowadays recommended for subacute bacterial endocarditis, and sometimes for gram-negative bacillary infections, may also provoke such convulsions?"

Reply: This is certainly a remote but definite possibility. Two patients who developed generalized seizures and other signs of nervous system dysfunction associated with high doses of penicillin were reported by Peter New and Charles Wells, at Vanderbilt University. Shortly after penicillin therapy was begun each patient developed muscular hyperirritability, myoclonic jerking movements and generalized convulsions; one individual developed visual and auditory hallucinations, the other became semicomatose. It should be remarked, however, that both of these patients had evidence of impaired renal tubular function and that both patients retained remarkably high penicillin levels for many hours after the drug was stopped. So it would appear that at least in a patient with renal dysfunction there is some potential hazard of cerebral toxicity with very high penicillin dosage.

Peter S. New and Charles E. Wells. Cerebral Toxicity Associated with Massive Intravenous Penicillin Therapy. Neurology 15:1053, 1965.

"May the tetracyclines be used safely in individuals with kidney impairment?"

Reply: Only very cautiously because these drugs increase the nonprotein nitrogen titer through interference with protein synthesis. Consider dosage readjustment if a patient develops anorexia, nausea and vomiting, and have the BUN level immediately re-evaluated. In fact, azotemia can occur under these drugs in the presence of normal renal function, because of the increased load of the products of amino acid metabolism that is presented to the kidneys for excretion when protein synthesis is interfered with. This may occur with dosage that is entirely within the accepted therapeutic range.

Aubrey J. Pothrer, Jr., and E. Everett Anderson. Tetracycline-Induced Azotemia. J. Urol. 95:16, 1966.

"Do effective amounts of ampicillin (Polycillin) pass the placental barrier?"

Reply: In Bristol, England, T. E. Blecher and associates gave 500 mg. of ampicillin orally at 6 hour intervals to 42 women, collecting amniotic fluid and maternal blood samples at the time of amniotomy or amniocentesis, between 3¼ and 5¾ hours after the third dose. Samples of maternal and cord blood were collected at the time of delivery from 23 women who received the drug in the same dose schedule by mouth during labor. The drug was recovered in every specimen of amniotic fluid and serum examined and the concentrations were felt to be sufficiently high to be effective against the high proportion of the bacteria likely to be encountered in intrapartum infection; but the concentrations in the cord serum were considered to have been probably ineffective against a significant proportion of these organisms.

T. E. Blecher, W. M. Edgar, H. A. H. Melville and K. R. Peel. Transplacental Passage of Ampicillin. Brit. M. J. 1:137, Jan. 15, 1966.

"Could you recommend oral antibiotic dosages for the newborn infant?"

Reply: Sumner Yaffe, at the State University of New York at Buffalo, proposes the following: chloramphenicol (Chloromycetin), 25 mg./kg. total per 24 hours in divided dosage at 12 hours; colistin sulfate (Coly-Mycin Sulfate), 5 mg./kg. divided at 6 hours; erythromycin propionyl lauryl sulfate (Ilosone Lauryl SO₄), 25–40 mg./kg. divided at 6 hours; neomycin sulfate, 50 mg./kg. divided at 6 hours; phenoxymethyl penicillin (Pen-Vee L-A, V-Cillin), 90,000 units/kg. divided at 8 hours; tetracycline, 100 mg./kg. divided at 6 hours.

Sumner J. Yaffe. Antibiotics for the Newborn Infant: A Discussion of Dosages. Clin. Pediat. 4:639, 1965.

"When it is impossible to administer an antibiotic orally to a newborn infant, what agents may be used and how?"

Reply: Sumner Yaffe, at the State University of New York at Buffalo, proposes the following: chloramphenicol (Chloromycetin), 25 mg./kg., divided at 12 hours and given intramuscularly; sodium colistimethate (Coly-Mycin), 1.5 mg./kg. or less, divided at 8–12 hours and given intramuscularly; kanamycin sulfate (Kantrex), 15 mg./kg., divided at 12 hours and given intramuscularly; potassium penicillin G, 20,000 units/kg., divided at 12 hours and given intramuscularly or intravenously; polymyxin B (Aerosporin), 1.5 mg./kg. or less, divided at 8–12 hours and given intramuscularly; streptomycin sulfate, 10–20 mg./kg., divided at 12 hours and given intramuscularly; tetracyclines, 15 mg./kg. divided at 12 hours and given intramuscularly.

Sumner J. Yaffe. Antibiotics for the Newborn Infant: A Discussion of Dosages. Clin. Pediat. 4:639, 1965.

APHTHOUS PHARYNGITIS

"What about the aphthous pharyngitis that those of us working in summer camps for children see so often; is there any specific drug therapy?"

Reply: No.

ARRHYTHMIAS

"In our hospital we have never used acetylcholine in the differential diagnosis of arrhythmias, but it is rumored that 'they' have found it useful elsewhere. Is this a fact, and what are the dangers?"

Reply: Schoolman and his group studied the matter at the University of Illinois and found that in tachycardias of known supraventricular origin the drug has differential diagnostic value through its ability to cause a transient block of A-V conduction, revealing the pattern of atrial activity previously obscured by overlying QRS complexes. They also found it valuable for clearly delineating the mechanism of atrial flutter, especially in the presence of bundle branch block simulating the ECG appearance of ventricular tachycardia. In an individual with a rapid heart, an ECG was recorded while carotid sinus pressure was applied. Then an intravenous infusion of 5% glucose was started to facilitate rapid administration of multiple acetylcholine doses. *Dosage:* 10–20 mg. acetylcholine hydrochloride dissolved in 1 ml. of saline solution were added to the glucose infusion at 3-5 minute intervals, the largest single dose being 220 mg.

Harold M. Schoolman, Lionel M. Bernstein, Armand Littman and Luke R. Pascale. Acetylcholine in Differential Diagnosis and Treatment of Paroxysmal Tachycardia. Am. Heart J. 60:526, 1960.

"In a refractory case of ventricular tachycardia would it be dangerous to add potassium to the quinidine regimen?"

Reply: At about the turn of the present century the ability of intravenously injected potassium chloride to terminate ventricular tachycardia and fibrillation was demonstrated in the dog, but because of the narrow margin of safety the compound was not used in man until Sampson and Anderson employed it orally with success in 1930. In ventricular tachycardia there is an intracellular loss of potassium, and its replacement is logical. At Vanderbilt University, Crawford Adams has described his successful use of potassium chloride together with quinidine in a case of the sort you have in mind. Potassium chloride, 120 mEq. daily, was initially administered in-travenously and then 1.0 Gm. was given orally with 0.4 Gm. of quinidine sulfate every 6 hours. During a succeeding period of many months, 4.0 Gm. of potassium chloride and 3.2 Gm. of quinidine sulfate were administered daily in divided doses without complication and without recurrence of the arrhythmia. You must be aware, however, that potassium excretion occurs mainly by way of the urinary system and that if there is impaired renal function there is real danger in using the drug. However, the alterations in intracellular potassium concentration can be successfully monitored by the electrocardiogram.

Crawford W. Adams. Treatment of Refractory Ventricular Tachycardia and Fibrillation by the Administration of Potassium and Quinidine. Dis. Chest 46:364, 1964.

"In a case of ventricular tachycardia unresponsive to cardiac depressants, might I hope to effect control through the use of a pressor amine?"

Reply: A sympathomimetic amine will sometimes do it through acceleration of the basic idioventricular pacemaker with resultant suppression of ectopic activity, or possibly even through increased coronary blood flow and improved myocardial stability, as suggested a few years ago by H. Gold and E. Corday. The case of William Underhill and John Tredway (Hamot Hospital, Erie, Pa.) is illustrative. Quinidine and procaine amide having failed to terminate the attacks, they were discontinued and intravenous infusion of isoproterenol (Isuprel, Aludrine, etc.), 0.4 mg. in 500 ml. of 5% dextrose in water, was begun. The attacks promptly ended, and after 2 days the infusion was replaced with sublingual Isuprel, 10 mg. every 4 hours. After 20 days of this, the Isuprel was discontinued, quinidine therapy was resumed, the attacks immediately recurred, and the patient died suddenly on the next day.

H. Gold and E. Corday. Vasopressor Therapy in the Cardiac Arrhythmias. New England J. Med. 260:1151, 1959. William L. Underhill and John Tredway. Treatment of Paroxysmal Ventricular Tachycardia with Isoproterenol. Ann. Int. Med. 60:680, 1964.

"When applying direct-current countershock for the treatment of cardiac arrhythmias does it matter whether the patient is under the influence of digitalis at the time?"

Reply: There is evidence that it does. At the New York Upstate Medical Center, Robert Gilbert and Richard Cuddy studied the records of 28 patients receiving digitalis and converted from atrial fibrillation or flutter to sinus rhythm with direct-current countershock. There were ECG signs suggesting digitalis intoxication following the conversion in 20 of these cases, and 2 of the patients died in ventricular fibrillation several hours after apparently successful conversion. No such ECG abnormalities occurred among 6 patients on digitalis treated with countershock but not converting and 5 patients converted with countershock who were not receiving digitalis or in whom digitalis had been discontinued for several days. These investigators recommended that digitalis be withheld for several days in subjects for whom a conversion attempt is planned. Stern recommended a digitalis suspension period of 7–12 days. But suppose such a course precipitated ventricular tachycardia as the digitalis effect wore off; that could be embarrassing, too.

Robert Gilbert, Richard P. Cuddy. Digitalis Intoxication Following Conversion to Sinus Rhythm. Circulation XXXII, 1965. Schlomo Stern. The Effect of Maintenance Doses of Digitalis on the Rate of Success of Cardioversion. Am. J. M. Sc. 250:509, 1965.

"I have recently had a patient who, 2 hours after electrical countershock for conversion of an arrhythmia, had five attacks of syncope within about 3 hours. She had been premedicated with quinidine sulfate 0.3 Gm. every 2 hours for four doses. Could this quinidine medication have had anything to do with the occurrences?"

Reply: Yes, it could. Quinidine syncope due to paroxysmal ventricular flutter or fibrillation was seen by Agustin Castellanos's group (University of Miami) in 3 of 111 patients to whom the drug was given for the purpose of preventing the recurrence of a preexistent supraventricular arrhythmia after conversion to sinus rhythm by electrical countershock. The bizarre arrhythmias appeared after only 1.2 Gm. of quinidine sulfate. All of the patients had been adequately digitalized before starting quinidine and none showed clinical or electrocardiographic evidence of digitalis toxicity. One of the earliest detectable effects of quinidine was acceleration of the average ventricular rate due to the appearance of multifocal ventricular activity. It appears that such development should not only contraindicate further use of quinidine in this situation but also the use of electric countershock during the period of quinidine hypersensitivity. None of the patients had any other manifestations of quinidine toxicity, such as skin reactions, gastrointestinal symptoms or cinchonism.

Agustin Castellanos, Jr. Countershock Exposed Quinidine Syncope. Am. J. M. Sc. 250:254, 1965.

"We would like at our hospital to dispense with general anesthesia when converting cardiac arrhythmias by direct-current countershock. Has a feasible method for doing this been devised?"

Reply: At the District of Columbia General Hospital, D. O. Nutter and R. A. Massumi have successfully prepared a number of their patients for the shock with a single intravenous injection of diazepam (Valium). They have premedicated with 200 mg. of quinidine sulfate every 6 hours for three or four doses, and then given 5–20 mg. of diazepam (5 mg./ml.) rapidly intravenously. The countershock is delivered after the onset of sleep, which occurred in 14 of the 15 patients within 1 or 2 minutes. The shock caused transient arousal, muscular contractions of the upper extremities and, in several cases, a brief outcry. The shock was of variable energy, 100–400 watt seconds.

D. O. Nutter and R. A. Massumi. Diazepam in Cardioversion. New England J. Med. 273:650, Sept. 16, 1965.

"In a patient in whom the trial is to be made of conversion of atrial fibrillation to normal sinus rhythm, what should be the preparatory treatment?"

Reply: The program that has evolved during several years' experience at the University of Chicago, as reported by Richard Duchelle, is the following. If a patient has not already been digitalized, this is done, preferably with one of the shorter-acting preparations such as digoxin, until the ventricular response is below 85 at rest and fails to increase above 100 with mild activity. Salt restriction and diuretic therapy are included in the regimen. Then 2 weeks prior to conversion, a course of oral anticoagulant therapy is begun and continued until 1 week following successful conversion. Approximately 1 week before, a maintenance dosage of quinidine sulfate, 0.3 gm. every 6 hours, is started. Perhaps not everyone would use the anticoagulant routinely, but nearly everyone will agree that it is needed in a patient with history of thromboembolism.

Richard A. Duchelle. Indications for Conversion of Atrial Fibrillation to Normal Sinus Rhythm. M. Clin. North America 50:117, 1966.

"I have a patient in his late fifties in whom increasing paroxysms of atrial flutter or fibrillation are requiring increasing rest and incapacitation, and the malady, together with the necessity for frequent injections of high dosage of procainamide (Pronestyl) to terminate the attacks, is beginning to wear everyone out. Do you have any suggestion?"

Reply: I can only tell you what Paul White and George Griffith (Boston and Los Angeles), did in a similar case. They digitalized the patient and slowly increased the dosage to 0.6 Gm. of the leaf daily until constant atrial fibrillation began. At the time of their report the fibrillation was persisting but the clinical improvement, both physical and mental, was described as astonishing. The heart rate was well controlled in the 60's to 70's and this enormous dosage of digitalis was being tolerated without any manifestations of toxicity and with a sense of perfect well-being.

Paul D. White and George C. Griffith. Invalidism Abolished by Transforming Paroxysmal to Permanent Atrial Fibrillation. J.A.M.A. 169:596, Feb. 7, 1959.

"Since there is some degree of inflammatory damage to the conducting mechanism of the heart in Adams-Stokes disease, is anything to be expected of corticosteroid therapy?"

Reply: I really do not know. In the 7 cases reported by Verel and associates (Sheffield, England) there were inconclusive results in 5, but apparently favorable results in 2. That reduction of an inflammatory process was accountable for the salutary effects, when achieved, is rather doubtful because the dosage was very low.

D. Verel, S. J. Mazurkie and F. Rahman. Prednisone in Treatment of Adams-Stokes Attacks. Brit. Heart J. 25: 709, 1963.

"I have recently used isoproterenol (Isuprel) successfully to control recurrent Adams-Stokes seizures in complete atrioventricular heart block; but in another case I failed, probably because of timidity regarding dosage. What dosage plan has proved most effective?"

Reply: There are a number of references to dosage of the following sort: using a solution of 2 mg. of isoproterenol hydrochloride in 500 ml. of 5% dextrose in water, give at the rate of 5 μg./minute to initiate, accelerate and maintain an idioventricular rhythm. With careful monitoring, the rate of infusion may be increased every few minutes in stepwise fashion by 4–8 μg./minute to obtain the desired effect. But be very careful to avoid increasing the idioventricular pacemaker above 50 beats/minute in ventricular asystole, or the appearance of frequent and multifocal premature beats, rapid ventricular rhythms from multiple foci, and cerebral stimulation.

Robert J. Matthews (Los Angeles). Prevention of Ventricular Tachycardia and Adams-Stokes Seizures in Complete Heart Block. Arch. Int. Med. 116:120, 1965.

"What is the best drug to use in treating Adams-Stokes disease?"

Reply: In heart block of this type the most suitable drug, either for treating a syncopal episode or in prophylaxis, is the sympathomimetic amine, isoproterenol (Isuprel). It often performs quite satisfactorily without substantially raising the blood pressure; for example, Schwartz and Schwartz (1959) were able to convert a transient partial or complete block to normal sinus rhythm in all 10 of their patients, although in 5 of them it was not possible to maintain this rhythm for any length of time. Usual practice has been to use the 10 mg. tablets sublingually or to inject 0.2 mg. subcutaneously or intramuscularly.

Thyroid substance, in sufficient dosage to provoke mild hyperthyroidism, has been used successfully when all other drugs have failed to prevent the asystole; so too has molar sodium lactate.

Since it can eliminate the vagal portion of normal heart rate control, one would expect atropine to have considerable usefulness in treating heart block, but this is not the case because vagus tone is greatest under 30 and strikingly decreases after 50 years of age, and most victims of this malady are elderly and have intrinsic heart disease. The instance in which there is a response to the drug is probably one in which some metabolic alteration has rendered the heart transiently exceptionally susceptible to vagal influence. However, the anomalous atrioventricular conduction that characterizes the interesting Wolff-Parkinson-White syndrome may be reverted to normal by atropine.

S. P. Schwartz and L. S. Schwartz. The Adams-Stokes Syndrome During Normal Sinus Rhythm and Transient Heart Block. I. The Effects of Isuprel on Patients with the Adams-Stokes Syndrome During Normal Sinus Rhythm and Transient Heart Block. Am. Heart. J. 57:849, 1959.

"I have heard that dosage of chlorothiazide (Diuril) large enough to lower serum potassium significantly will prevent Adams-Stokes seizures provided the patient does not have permanent complete atrioventricular block between attacks. Is this true?"

Reply: Louis Tobian (University of Minnesota) has been claiming for some years that this is the case, and in another Reply (see bottom p. 44) I have dealt with the matter at some length. Tobian's daily dosage has varied from 500 to 2000 mg., increasing stepwise to achieve a serum potassium level reduction of 1–1.5 mEq./L.

Louis Tobian. Prevention of Stokes-Adams Seizures with Chlorothiazide. Ann. New York Acad. Sc. 111 (art. 3): 855, 1964.

"Has the use of reserpine ever been resorted to in treating a persistent bundle branch block?"

Reply: Yes, in Israel, Joel Pfeiffer reported a case in which the block gradually disappeared while reserpine was administered and returned when the drug was discontinued; the results were reproducible. He gave 0.3 mg. daily for 8 months before toxic symptoms required discontinuance. Each time that administration was resumed thereafter, sometimes in higher than the initial dosage, the toxic symptoms appeared much earlier.

Joel M. Pfeiffer (Malben Hospital Pardess-Katz). Effect of Reserpine on Persistent Bundle-Branch Block. Israel M. J. 20:42, 1961.

"I have a case of sinus tachycardia whose cause I cannot determine, and I have been unable to revert it. Has any measure been devised for control of such a situation?"

Reply: At the University of Oregon, Isidor Brill's group used guanethidine (Ismelin) because of its bradycardic properties. The drug was used successfully in all of their 5 cases in initial dosage of 20 mg. and then 10 mg. daily thereafter.

Isidor C. Brill, John D. Welch, Robert J. Condon and Frank C. Jones. Arch. Int. Med. 115:674, 1965.

"How is it that we can sometimes arrest a paroxysmal atrial tachycardia by the use of phenylephrine (Neo-Synephrine), a sympathomimetic amine? I do not understand this."

Reply: The antiarrhythmic usefulness of this drug derives from the fact that its gross action differs from that of epinephrine in three particulars: (1) myocardial stimulation occurs hardly at all; (2) both systolic and diastolic blood pressures rise without any element of vasodilation entering into the picture; (3) the pulse rate is very much slowed instead of being quickened. It is the striking vasoconstriction that accomplishes the arrest of the tachycardia, for the rapid blood pressure increase, in the aortic arch and carotid sinus simultaneously, activates all the afferent pathways of reflex cardiac slowing. These pathways are the depressor fibers of the vagus (aortic nerve) from the aortic arch and the sinus nerve from the carotid sinus. The efferent pathways causing cardiac slowing are, of course, the vagi. When the drug is injected intravenously, effect is often obtained amazingly rapidly and it may last for 20 minutes or more; it is less likely to be obtained from subcutaneous injection, but if it does occur it may last an hour or more. The preliminary administration of morphine might possibly increase phenylephrine's effectiveness through sensitizing the medullary vagus center.

"One of my associates tells me that he has sometimes resolved a recalcitrant attack of paroxysmal atrial tachycardia through giving 1 or 2 teaspoonfuls of the syrup of ipecac. How would you rationalize such therapy?"

Reply: The action comes about through an increase of cardiac vagal influence simply because central vagal stimulation is an accompaniment of the act of vomiting.

"I have learned through experience not to attempt the arrest of a paroxysmal atrial tachycardia in an elderly individual through carotid sinus pressure or intravenous digitalization, but I have reverted a number of these episodes through use of quinidine or procainamide (Pronestyl) in full dosage. Am I running grave risk by the latter method?"

Reply: No, I do not think that you are; it is the consensus that these two cardiac depressant drugs may be as safely used in the aged as in the younger person, of course with due regard for the side actions, toxicity and contraindications that would apply in any case.

"I have recently seen in consultation 2 cases of atrial tachycardia with block in which digitalis had not been given. But is not digitalis practically always responsible for this arrhythmia?"

Reply: In 1958, the report of Lown and Levine, who found excessive digitalis responsible for this arrhythmia in 73% of 112 episodes, left the facile impression that this is the case, though "practically always" was certainly not implied in their report. More recently, William Morgan and Gerald Breneman (Henry Ford Hospital) reported digitalis intoxication as responsible for only 6 of their 15 cases. As a matter of fact, when digitalis is *not* involved in the causation it may be effectively used to control it.

B. Lown and S. A. Levine. Atrial Arrhythmias, Digitalis and Potassium. New York, Landsberger Medical Books, Inc., 1958. William L. Morgan and Gerald M. Breneman. Atrial Tachycardia with Block Treated with Digitalis. Circulation 25:787, 1962.

"Is it true that digitalis is contraindicated in the Wolff-Parkinson-White syndrome?"

Reply: It has certainly been held that digitalis, by suppressing the A-V node, may actually perpetuate the anomalous conduction in this syndrome; but this viewpoint is no longer generally subscribed to.

Constantine T. Gitsios (Metropolitan Hospital Center, New York). Restoration of Normal Conduction Following Administration of Digitalis in Case of WPW Syndrome. Am. Heart J. 59:283, 1960.

"I have a 20-year-old patient with Wolff-Parkinson-White syndrome whose episodes of paroxysmal tachycardia have not been preventable by digitalis, quinidine, procainamide (Pronestyl), neostigmine (Prostigmin), phenobarbital, diphenylhydantoin (Dilantin), or combinations of these drugs. Reserpine, 0.25 mg. four times daily, was effective for a short time but then failed in even larger doses. What is next?"

Reply: In a quite similar case, W. E. Harris and associates (University of Oregon) gave 10 mg. of guanethidine (Ismelin), with gradually increasing dosage, and 30 mg. of phenobarbital twice daily. At the time of their report the patient had received 50–60 mg. guanethidine daily for 11 months with only rare episodes of tachycardia so long as full dosage of the drug was maintained. In explanation of the effect achieved with guanethidine they suggested that sufficient depressant action on the conduction pathways of the A-V node and the anomalous bundle resulted from predominant vagal influence when sympathetic activity was blocked.

W. E. Harris, Herbert J. Semler and Herbert E. Griswold. Reversed Reciprocating Paroxysmal Tachycardia Controlled by Guanethidine in Case of Wolff-Parkinson-White Syndrome. Am. Heart J. 67:812, 1964.

"I have a patient with ischemic heart disease and a healed myocardial infarct who now has attacks of paroxysmal ventricular tachycardia that I am controlling satisfactorily with procainamide (Pronestyl). How long can I hope to succeed with this?"

Reply: In Jamaica, New York, Albert Douglas has reported such a patient who has been receiving the drug in doses of 9–10.5 Gm. daily for more than 3 years and has tolerated the treatment very well. In Chicago, Paul and Leigh have also used high dosage orally in patients with ventricular tachycardia.

Albert H. Douglas. Procainamide Prophylaxis in Recurrent Ventricular Tachycardia Due to Ischemic Heart Disease. New York J. Med. 65:2476, Oct. l, 1965. Oglesby Paul and Carl G. Leigh. Ventricular Tachycardia: Treatment with Very Large Doses of Procaine Amide. M. Clin. North America 50:271, 1966.

"I have a patient in whom I have stopped intravenous administration of procainamide (Pronestyl) at 1.5 Gm. without reverting the arrhythmia; might I have proceeded to higher dosage with safety?"

Reply: The largest single dosage of Pronestyl that I have seen reported was that of Embree and Levine (Peter Bent Brigham Hospital), in 1959. In a patient with ventricular tachycardia they felt justified in the heroic measure of giving increasing doses of 1, 2 and 3 Gm. on different days without success, and finally going to 4 Gm. The latter dose was given intravenously in 200 ml. of 5% dextrose in water during 36 minutes. During the infusion the pressure fell from 100/80 to 70/60 mm. Hg, and 10 mg. phenylephrine (Neo-Synephrine) was added. When the ventricular rate had dropped from 200 to 140, 1 mg. of atropine was injected intravenously, and several minutes later ventricular tachycardia disappeared; a slow, peculiar nodal rhythm was later replaced by a slow, normal sinus rhythm. The patient was discharged on 0.3 Gm. quinidine twice daily, 0.25 Gm. Pronestyl four times daily and bishydroxycoumarin (Dicumarol).

Larry J. Embree and Samuel A. Levine. Ventricular Tachycardia: Case Requiring Massive Amounts of Procainamide (Pronestyl) for Reversion. Ann. Int. Med. 50:222, 1959.

"I have a patient on routine procainamide (Pronestyl) who is doing very well so far as control of the arrhythmia is concerned, but now she is presenting some evidence of liver function disturbance. Could this be ascribable to the drug?"

Reply: I think that this is unlikely. John King and Robert Blount, Jr. (Rochester, N.Y.) have placed a case on record in which a patient very quickly developed an episode of nausea, vomiting, fever and right upper quadrant pain, together with SGOT elevation each time she ingested procainamide. But this acute reaction, which was probably on a true hypersensitivity basis, seems unrelated to the thing you describe.

John A. King and Robert E. Blount, Jr. An Unexpected Reaction to Procainamide. J.A.M.A. 186:603, Nov. 9, 1963.

"I have a patient with recurrent atrial fibrillation who for the past several months has been on procainamide (Pronestyl) in maintenance dosage of 750 mg. every 6 hours. He has now developed lupus erythematosus. Could it be possible that the drug has induced this?"

Reply: It is certainly possible, though a rare occurrence. Robert Paine, in St. Louis, has collected 12 cases, including 4 of his own, and we have recently had 1 in our own hospital. In the recorded cases the symptoms developed following exposure to the drug in daily oral dosage of 0.5–3.0 Gm. for 3 weeks to 22 months. Perhaps one should bear this drug in mind in any instance in which lupus erythematosus is diagnosed as an apparent complication of another disease, for in addition to the arrhythmias, procainamide has occasionally been used in myotonia dystrophica and congenita, myocardial infarction (prophylactically), angina pectoris, hereditary (Huntington's) chorea, and skeletal pain.

Robert Paine. Procaine Hydrochloride and Lupus Erythematosus. J.A.M.A. 194:23, Oct. 4, 1965.

"I have a patient with chronic atrial fibrillation in whom I cannot use quinidine because she always develops a fever when I try the drug. Is this a common occurrence?"

Reply: No, I should not say common, but it does occur. In fact, several years ago Browning and Heck (Mayo Clinic) emphasized the importance of considering fever as a possible component of a reaction to quinidine because the occurrence might otherwise be taken as evidence of embolism or subacute bacterial endocarditis, which are common in patients with this arrhythmia.

R. J. Browning and F. J. Heck. Fever Secondary to Ingestion of Quinidine. Proc. Staff Meet. Mayo Clin. 35:111, 1960.

"A patient of mine, who has off and on had quinidine for a minor arrhythmia, went into a curare-like state when the drug was administered shortly after recovery from an anesthetic. How explain this?"

Reply: You do not state what anesthetic had been used so I cannot give a precise answer. However, a similar occurrence was reported by Sadove's group (University of Illinois), whose patient became short of breath and developed masked facies and weakness of major and minor muscle groups when given 200 mg. of quinidine sulfate in the recovery room when she had regained motor functions after a 2 hour surgical procedure in which dimethyl tubocurarine (Mecostrin) had been used for muscle relaxation. It was touch and go with this patient for several hours, and the observers felt that she had probably been recurarized by the quinidine since they obtained a similar effect in rabbits in which the same succession of drugs had been employed.

John L. Schmidt, Nicholas A. Vick and Max S. Sadove. Effect of Quinidine on Action of Muscle Relaxants. J.A.M.A. 183:669, Feb. 23, 1963.

"In what type of arrhythmia has quinidine been used with greatest success?"

Reply: In a study of 200 unselected patients, with follow-up, Rolf Rokseth (Bodö, Norway) found the drug achieving the greatest conversion rate in patients with thyrotoxic heart disease and in those with uncomplicated mitral stenosis. The result was poor in individuals with mitral insufficiency, and it was adversely influenced by significant cardiac enlargement, severe congestive failure and fibrillation of several years' standing.

Rolf Rokseth. Clinical Considerations in Quinidine Therapy of Chronic Auricular Fibrillation: Study of 200 Unselected Patients, with Follow-up. Acta med. scandinav. 174:171, 1963.

"My associates tell me that I am too cautious in my use of quinidine, but I think that they are too bold, for this is really a toxic drug. Would you kindly make a statement of acceptable dosage under various circumstances?"

Reply: An ambulant type of therapy, such as would be used in a patient with premature contractions of an apparently otherwise normal heart, is to give 300 mg. of quinidine sulfate orally three times daily. If in 4–5 days when the curve of accumulation will have leveled off the arrhythmia is persisting, the dose must be increased by adding first a fourth daily dose of 300 mg. and thereafter by spreading increments of the same size throughout the four daily doses until effect or toxicity is reached. To maintain the effect it is usually necessary to continue at the dosage at which it was achieved, which may be as high as 4 Gm. daily. Sometimes it is possible to reduce dosage by using intervals of 6 instead of 4 hours and then subtracting 100 or 200 mg. from the dose. In very exceptional cases quite small doses, spaced at 8 hour intervals, will maintain a normal rhythm originally achieved with much higher dosage.

When a more heroic dosage schedule is required in the attempt to convert a serious arrhythmia, some men give a test dose of 100 mg. and wait 12 hours for evidences of hypersensitivity; others wait only an hour, since most allergic reactions can be expected within that time. A great many practitioners, however, consider that the occurrence of serious hypersensitivities is sufficiently rare to justify the use of full dosage initially without preliminary test dosing. The following is an oral dosage schedule often productive of good results: 200 mg. at 4 hour intervals day and night, increasing by 200 mg. per dose every 12 hours until normal rhythm is achieved, toxic symptoms appear or a dose of 800 mg. is reached. Increase in dosage above the latter figure should be made with extreme caution. Some physicians use quinidine more intensively from the first, beginning with 400 mg. at 2–3 hour intervals and increasing to 600 mg. if the effect is not achieved after several doses, in some instances even starting at 600 mg. at 2–3 hour intervals.

"I have sometimes had the experience, during quinidine therapy, of a sudden loss of consciousness in the patient; there is usually cessation of respiration and involuntary skeletal muscular contraction, but recovery is very quick and complete. What is the cause of this?"

Reply: In many instances the episode appears to be triggered by some precipitating factor not yet explained, but sometimes a state of extreme hypoxia, induced by the prolonged cardiac standstill at the moment of conversion, seems to supply a plausible reason for the syncope.

Arthur Selzer and H. Wesley Wray (San Francisco). Quinidine Syncope: Paroxysmal Ventricular Fibrillation Occurring During Treatment of Chronic Atrial Arrhythmias. Circulation 30:17, 1964.

"When is one in most danger in using quinidine?"

Reply: I should say that one probably takes the greatest risk when using high dosage initially in an occlusive coronary episode in a patient who has developed ventricular tachycardia. The heart in this situation may not be able to cope as well with the sudden cut-off of its beat at the source as is one that has been slowed first by lower dosage before the sudden breaking off of the abnormal rhythm.

"Which of the several quinidine preparations now available provides the best maintenance therapy for prevention of recurrence of a reverted arrhythmia, at the lowest dosage and with the least possible side effects?"

Reply: At St. Joseph's Hospital, Hamilton, Ontario, W. M. Goldberg and S. G. Chakrabarti studied the rate of absorption, the blood level obtained and sustained, using both a single and a multiple-dosage schedule of quinidine sulfate, quinidine gluconate, quinidine polygalacturonate (Cardioquin) and dihydroquinidine gluconate. On the assumption that a blood quinidine level of 4–7 mg./L. would have the desired antiarrhythmic effect, it was found that quinidine sulfate and quinidine gluconate best produced this level when 2 tablets, each equivalent to 200 mg. of quinidine sulfate, were given at 8 hour intervals. Serious respiratory arrest occurred in 1 case following quinidine sulfate, which led the observers to believe that quinidine gluconate is the drug to be preferred.

W. M. Goldberg and Siba G. Chakrabarti. The Relationship of Dosage Schedule to the Blood Level of Quinidine Using All Available Quinidine Preparations. Canad. M. A. J. 91:991, Nov. 7, 1964.

"Is it ever admissible to administer digitalis and quinidine simultaneously?"

Reply: Digitalization increases the sensitivity of animals to quinidine, but this fact is possibly not so significant as it seems because cardionormal animals have to be used in such studies, and we must deal with toxic doses of at least one of the drugs in order to obtain measurable effects. The occurrences in the human have not always been explainable upon any simple basis when the two drugs are used together. Quinidine slows atrial conduction, but digitalis may counteract this. Quinidine at times exerts a vagal blocking action which accelerates conduction and would oppose the salutary ventricular slowing induced by the digitalis depression of atrioventricular conduction. Quinidine may also work against digitalis by decreasing the force of muscular contraction. In addition, there is the possibility that digitalis may sufficiently sensitize the heart to quinidine's action to increase the likelihood of occurrence of a quinidine-induced arrhythmia; i.e., that the result of combined therapeutic dosages in man may be like the combination of one therapeutic and one toxic dose in the dog. I doubt if anyone in an authoritative position in cardiovascular work would care at present to declare categorically that neither drug should be used in a patient who is at the time under the full influence of the other, since too much good can sometimes result from just such employments. But certainly the situation is a delicate one and requires the utmost caution in matters of dosage and close supervision and assessment of indications.

"What action is exerted upon the heart by potassium administered as a drug, and what are the evidences of toxic overaction?"

Reply: The potassium ion is intricately involved in the physiologic processes of synaptic transmission and the depolarization of nervous elements, and it is concerned also in the excitation and contraction of voluntary muscle as well as of cardiac muscle, but when potassium chloride is deliberately given as a drug in amounts that transcend those in which it subserves a physiologic function it is a direct depressant of both contractility and conduction in atrial and ventricular myocardial tissue with a less intense effect on nodal tissue. Potassium chloride poisoning of serious degree from oral administration of the drug is practically impossible because excessive dosage is rejected by the stomach. In the presence of renal disease it is theoretically possible to cause potassium poisoning by use of the drug, though actually the kidneys retain the ability to excrete potassium until they are very seriously involved. In the event of intravenous administration of an excessive amount of a potassium salt, the symptoms would comprise paresthesia, muscular weakness, paralysis and excessive myocardial depression with death in cardiac standstill. Molar sodium lactate is antidotal. The artificial kidney will remove potassium.

"I have heard that recalcitrant arrhythmias may sometimes be reverted by reduction of the blood potassium level, but I do not understand this and am therefore chary of trying it. Could you explain?"

Reply: In treating A-V block the objective is to reestablish normal A-V conduction or, failing that, at least to maintain an idioventricular pacemaker at a rate and rhythm that are adequate. But in trying to accomplish this one must be careful not to increase myocardial irritability so much that ventricular tachycardia or fibrillation ensues. This is the danger with the most familiar drugs, the sympathomimetic amines and the parasympatholytic drugs. Several observers have noted that a combination of *hyper*kalemia and acidosis depresses an idioventricular focus and precipitates Adams-Stokes attacks, and it has been observed by Iliescu and Kleinerman in Bucharest, that *reduction* in blood potassium levels, even in the absence of acidosis, is important in prevention of Adams-Stokes attacks. Iliescu and Kleinerman undertook to stabilize the blood potassium level at low physiologic limits through administering thiazide diuretics. In their series there were 13 patients with complete A-V block. Seven displayed frequent Adams-Stokes crises and 4 experienced short fainting episodes due to sudden slowing of the idioventricular focus or to brief intervals of asystole. In 1 patient with complete A-V block the rhythm changed to first degree A-V block with Wenckebach periods after treatment. In all the others with complete A-V block a remarkable stabilization of the rate and rhythm of the idioventricular focus occurred after treatment, accompanied by disappearance of the Adams-Stokes attacks. In 2 patients with partial second degree A-V block, frequent Adams-Stokes crises were abolished through the treatment, and in one of these cases it was necessary to continue the administration of the thiazide diuretic. The authors felt that levels of less than 3.5 mEq./L. and over 5 mEq./L. were the limits within which the blood potassium should be maintained. One must in fact be extremely cautious in adjusting potassium levels because an excessive extracellular titer of the element may induce atrial-ventricular block and decrease myocardial contractile force.

C. C. Iliescu and L. Kleinerman. Effect of Reduction of Blood Potassium Level in Treatment of A-V Block and in Prevention of Adams-Stokes Attacks. Dis. Chest 47:398, 1965.

"In our large municipal hospital we frequently have occasion to resort to some form of temporizing therapy until the primary cause of an arrhythmia can be identified and corrected. Various agents have been used for this purpose, such as the antimalarials, antihistaminics and antispasmotics, and now we are wondering whether definitive trial has ever been made of the antiepileptic drugs that were mentioned some years ago as having antiarrhythmic properties."

Reply: The effect of these agents to which you refer was noted more than 20 years ago, but there have only been sporadic reports of their employment in the intervening years. Recently, however, Robert Conn, in Seattle, tested the acute effects of diphenylhydantoin (Dilantin) in a variety of cardiac arrhythmias in 24 patients, occasionally several different arrhythmias coexisting in the one individual. He analyzed the effects of the drug for each

separate arrhythmia and found it particularly effective in supraventricular and ventricular arrhythmias resulting from digitalis excess. It was also beneficial in controlling paroxysmal atrial and ventricular arrhythmias. There appeared to be no therapeutic effect in patients with atrial flutter and fibrillation. The only evidences of toxicity noted were transient bradycardia and hypotension in one patient and short-term atrial-ventricular block with bradycardia in another. *Dosage:* 250 mg. of diphenylhydantoin sodium in 5 ml. of solvent (usually equivalent to 3.5–5.0 mg./kg.) was given intravenously in 1–3 minutes with continuous electrocardiographic monitoring for approximately 5 minutes, and then at intervals of 5–10 minutes until the effect of the drug could be established. If the arrhythmia recurred the treatment was repeated. After a satisfactory response, maintenance dosage of 200–400 mg. was given intramuscularly or orally daily in divided doses until the problem was solved or other drug therapy was given in place of diphenylhydantoin.

Robert D. Conn. Diphenylhydantoin Sodium in Cardiac Arrhythmias. New England J. Med. 272:277, Feb. 11, 1965. Harold Bernstein, Herbert Gold, Tzu-Wang Lang, Stanley Pappelbaum, Vaclav Bazika and Eliot Corday. Sodium Diphenylhydantoin in the Treatment of Recurrent Cardiac Arrhythmias. J.A.M.A. 191:695, Mar. 1, 1965.

"I have heard that the antihistamines are about as effective as quinidine and procainamide in control of arrhythmias. Is this true?"

Reply: I do not think that one can make the categorical statement regarding the antihistamines, but the antiarrhythmic action of one of them, antazoline (Antistine) has been pretty well demonstrated. Leonard Dreifus and associates (Philadelphia) used the drug effectively in each of 15 patients with atrial premature systoles, 12 of 13 with atrial tachycardia, 6 of 10 with ventricular tachycardia, 64 of 68 with frequent ventricular premature systoles. It failed in 3 patients with atrial flutter, and in 17 of 18 with atrial fibrillation. In paroxysmal atrial tachycardia with block there was failure because the drug enhanced A-V transmission, producing a more rapid ventricular response. Dreifus's dosage: 400–800 mg. daily orally, 10 mg./kg. maximum intravenous dosage. In some refractory cases, George Herrmann's group (University of Texas), when injecting 10 mg./kg. intravenously, did not use a rate of administration higher than 200 mg./hr. They had severe nausea in a few patients and gastrointestinal distress with distention and diarrhea in 2 of them.

Leonard S. Dreifus, Thomas F. McGarry, Yoshio Watanabe, S. Ronald Kline, Morton Waldman and William Likoff. Clinical and Physiologic Effects of Antazoline, A New

Anti-Arrhythmic Agent. Am. Heart J. 65:607, 1963. George R. Herrmann, Charles R. Secrest, Glory J. Vilbig, Robert A. Quint and Anna W. Herrmann. Antiarrhythmic and Antifibrillary Antazoline: Clinical Study. J. Louisiana M. Soc. 116:145, 1964.

"When should one attempt the conversion of an arrhythmia?"

Reply: Orientation in this subject will be appreciably simplified if you will bear in mind that the usefulness of any drug in an arrhythmia, whether of atrial or ventricular site or origin, can be truly judged only on the basis of its relative ability to improve *ventricular* rate, and also that one must sometimes accept improvement in this particular as a sufficiently satisfying achievement under the existing circumstances, even if the arrhythmia has not actually been corrected.

In paroxysmal atrial tachycardia of average moderate degree in young or middle-aged individuals, the attack may be arrested by carotid sinus stimulation through massage or by giving a small dose of quinidine together with a hypnotic drug; on awakening, the patient will often have lost his arrhythmia. Otherwise, cautious intravenous digitalization is tried, and if this fails it is time to resort to full dosage of quinidine and/or procainamide (Pronestyl). However, any of the following may also be helpful: methacholine (Mecholyl), phenylephrine (Neo-Synephrine), neostigmine (Prostigmin), magnesium sulfate, emetics, propylthiouracil, radioactive iodine, chloroquine (Aralen).

If the attack is occurring in an elderly individual, greater caution is enjoined; carotid sinus massage is generally considered potentially dangerous in such patients, and precipitous digitalization is to be avoided if there is suspicion of recent myocardial infarction. Quinidine and procainamide may be used in full dosage, however. These drugs often arrest the arrhythmia quite abruptly, though there may be a preliminary period of gradual slowing of the rate.

The first drug to be thought of and used in atrial fibrillation is digitalis to slow the ventricular rate; sometimes when this happens conversion to a regular sinus rhythm will follow. But regardless of whether conversion has occurred, the emergency has passed once the ventricles are sufficiently slowed – provided, that is, that the fibrillating atria are not throwing off emboli. This latter situation justifies use of quinidine or procainamide in "a vigorous attempt at conversion," in the words of Prinzmetal and Kennamer. Chloroquine sometimes succeeds when both these drugs have failed.

Whether to attempt conversion after successful digitalization when there have been no embolic episodes has been a controversial question all the while that I have been in medicine. The present consensus, but by no means the unanimous opinion, is that if there is much atrial dilation and some degree of failure the situation should not be disturbed; furthermore, it is generally believed that if there is bundle branch block the drugs should not be used.

Sokolow has authoritatively listed the following as individuals in whom he attempts conversion of an arrhythmia: those whose fibrillation has been of less than 6 months' duration; those continuing to fibrillate after adequate treatment for thyrotoxicosis; those who had a technically successful mitral valvulotomy and who still fibrillate, or who previously had sinus rhythm and then fibrillate postoperatively; those whose ventricular rate is uncontrolled while they are fibrillating, despite full doses of digitalis; those who have cardiac failure that is not improved despite full treatment of the usual variety.

In the case of atrial flutter, which is practically always superimposed upon organic heart disease, treatment should be directed primarily toward protection of the ventricular myocardium by slowing the rate through digitalization. The advisability of attempting regularization through use of quinidine or procainamide may then be considered. I believe it is generally thought advisable not to attempt conversion if there is congestive failure and considerable cardiac enlargement.

In premature contractions (extrasystoles) both quinidine and procainamide are effective, and usually only relatively low dosage is needed. Most experience has been had with quinidine; usually only 2 to 5 days are required to effect termination of the irregularity, though the patient may be kept on low maintenance dosage practically indefinitely in selected cases.

In the emergency of ventricular tachycardia there should be no hesitancy in using quinidine and/or procainamide (Pronestyl) parenterally in sufficient dosage to accomplish reversion quickly. The drug or drugs should then be stopped but resumed on a prophylactic basis if reappearance of extrasystoles hints at probable recurrence of the episode. When these two drugs have failed and the third myocardial depressant, potassium chloride, has also not been helpful, magnesium sulfate may be tried and then atropine as a last resort.

In ventricular fibrillation as encountered in the operating theater the use of procainamide or quinidine is indicated while cardiac massage is being performed, but nowadays the electric defibrillator is saving more hearts than the drugs ever did. If a paroxysm of ventricular fibrillation occurs in a patient with heart block, the myocardial depressant drugs are contraindicated because of their depressing action on the idioventricular pacemaker.

In sinus and nodal tachycardia, neostigmine (Prostigmin) may occasionally effect a conversion to normal rhythm.

M. Prinzmetal and R. Kennamer. Emergency Treatment of Cardiac Arrhythmias. J.A.M.A. 54:1049, 1954. M. Sokolow. Panel Discussion of Arrhythmias. Circulation 20:286, 1959.

"In what sort of dosage may quinidine be administered to a child?"

Reply: There are few indications for the use of quinidine in cardiac disorders of childhood. Atrial fibrillation is rare, but possibly paroxysmal atrial tachycardia occurs more often in infancy than is suspected. In one such reported case in a 4-month old infant, oral dosage of quinidine was begun at 20 mg., increased in 2 hours to 40, then 60, then 80, then 100 and finally to 120 mg. before the attack subsided. Subsequent attacks were stopped with amounts of 100, 140 and 180 mg. at a single dose. Newton and Crawford say that a child may be given 5 mg./kg. orally every 2 hours and that the capillary blood level 1 hour after the second and third doses should represent about half the maximum (average about 10 mg./L.) to be attained. Thick soda fountain chocolate syrup disguises quinidine's bitter taste fairly well.

G. Newton and E. J. Crawford. A Study of Quinidine Dosage in Infants and Children. J. Pediat. 47:700, 1955.

"After cardiac massage and adequate ventilation have terminated an episode of cardiac arrest, but the re-established heartbeat is very feeble, are there any drugs that may improve the situation?"

Reply: I take it you mean drugs used as an emergency measure. Yes, you can give an intracardiac injection of 1 : 10,000 solution of epinephrine (Adrenalin) in dosage of 2–5 ml. (remember that the commercial preparation is a 1 : 1000 concentration, thus requiring dilution with 9 parts of physiologic saline). Isoproterenol (Isuprel) could also be used in the same dosage of a 1 : 50,000 solution. Then there are the calcium salts: 2–5 ml. of 10% calcium gluconate or chloride or lactate. Intracardiac injections are best made near the left edge of the sternum in the fourth intercostal space, which should allow the needle to enter the left ventricle.

ASTHMA

"I have a number of asthmatics with whom I am certainly not accomplishing very much, and yet I hesitate to begin corticosteroid therapy in them. What are the criteria for initiating this therapy, and do the benefits outweigh the risks?"

Reply: One simply cannot answer this question categorically. Many men certainly feel, however, that no asthmatic should be embarked upon what is expected to be a long-term corticosteroid journey without realization on the physician's part that it might be difficult to terminate the thing. Even with strict vigilance in the matter of dosage, the accomplishment of satisfactory therapeutic effect without a cushingoid state is difficult to achieve, though switching from one compound to another is sometimes quite helpful. Undeniably the relief afforded is often very great, but then the depression that follows necessary withdrawal of the drug is often of considerable proportion also. Hold off as long as possible in any case, and don't begin the use of these drugs unless the case is severe and resistant to all other therapy.

"A veritable wave of enthusiasm has swept through our hospital for the use in asthmatics of a relatively new corticosteroid that is said to be much more potent, milligram for milligram, than those we have been customarily using. Is anything gained by switching to a compound merely because it is alleged to be more potent than other compounds?"

Reply: I do not know what the gain could be unless your associates are accomplishing what they want for their patients with fewer side effects than accompanied the use of the earlier preparations. Certainly it means nothing to the patient in these days of precompounded medication, that he is ingesting a different number of milligrams in one tablet than in another. However, if the new preparation, whose greater potency is making the detail man ecstatic, is much more costly than the older one, this is going eventually to interest the patient very much.

"It has been my experience that once I put an asthmatic patient on corticosteroids it is difficult ever to get him off again, so that the subsequent history is one of a constant wrestle with dosage in the attempt to avoid cushingoid symptoms. Is there any solution to this; what has been experienced?"

Reply: I think that there just is no solution other than the attempt to avoid the initiation of corticosteroid therapy through meticulous use of the other available drugs–antispasmodics, sympathomimetic amines, theophylline, tranquilizers, etc. A helpful thing to remember is that in acute, self-limited, recalcitrant attacks, one or two parenteral doses of a steroid may be all that is needed to bring about a remission; this was nicely documented by Friedlaender and Friedlaender, in 1961.

As for weaning the patient away from the drugs, this is no simple matter surely. At the University College Hospital, London, J. P. Knowles investigated the long-term steroid requirements of 135 patients, with a follow-up of 8 years or less (average 27.7 months). When last seen, 102 of these patients (76%) were still taking the drugs, although in 42 of them (31.9%) intermittent therapy was sufficing. His conclusion was that the only patients with asthma likely to remain off steroid therapy for any predictable period are those who do not benefit from treatment.

J. P. Knowles. Difficulties in Weaning in Steroid Treatment of Asthma. Brit. M. J. 2:1396, Nov. 25, 1961. Sidney Friedlaender and Alex S. Friedlaender (Detroit). Parenteral Steroids in Management of Acute Allergic States. Am. Pract. Digest Treat. 12:175, 1961.

"I am seriously thinking of changing some of my chronic patients who have severe respiratory handicaps to aerosol instead of oral corticosteroid therapy. They are principally asthmatics, but a few of them have complicating bronchiectasis and a larger number complicating pulmonary emphysema. Since the therapeutic effect of inhalational corticosteroids is considered to result principally from topical deposition on the tracheobronchial mucosa, may I really expect to be able to take most of these patients off of the orally administered drugs? In other words, is there much to be gained by the contemplated change?"

Reply: In the 54 patients of Bickerman and Itkin (Columbia University), it was possible to discontinue oral prednisone in 21 and to lower the average maintenance dose in the others from 14.4 mg. to 5.6 mg. daily. And the patients with associated disease states showed no evidences of exacerbation or reactivation. Furthermore, signs of hypercortisonism regressed in 12 individuals who were able to replace oral prednisone with inhalational steroids. A modicum of systemic effect is to be expected, however, even though the major action is the result of topical deposition of the material on the tracheobronchial mucosa; some of the material is absorbed from the gastrointestinal tract when saliva and sputum are swallowed, and doubtless some is directly absorbed through the lungs. A note should be taken, however, of the experience of Crepea, in a school for disabled, intractably asthmatic children. He found that when the child's ability to inhale adequately during viral-respiratory epidemics is impaired, the efficiency of the inhalational method decreases. He also felt that the possibility of chronic irritation should be extensively investigated although there appeared little evidence of acute bronchial irritation during his study.

Hylan A. Bickerman and Sylvia E. Itkin. Aerosol Steroid Therapy and Chronic Bronchial Asthma. J.A.M.A. 184: 533, May 18, 1963. Seymour B. Crepea. Inhalation Corticosteroid (Dexamethasone) Management of Chronically Asthmatic Children. J. Allergy 34:119, 1963.

"Could you supply a brief statement of the nature of action of the respective mucolytic agents that are available nowadays?"

Reply: One of the earlier ones to make a place for itself was Alevaire, an aqueous mixture of the detergent, Superinone, with sodium bicarbonate to promote cleavage of large molecules, and glycerin to stabilize the size of droplets and prevent their evaporation while allegedly assuring their actual carriage into the bronchial passages. Tergemist and Tween 80 are detergents of more or less this nature. Varidase, an enzymatic agent, allegedly lyses fibrin through the action of its contained streptokinase while liquifying the DNA of purulent secretions through its streptodornase; it appears that mucus as such is not directly acted on. The action of Dornavac, pancreatic dornase, is much like that of streptodornase; i.e., it reduces the tenacity of pulmonary secretions through depolymerizing action on DNA; however, the process appears not to be carried quite so far. Acetylcysteine (Mucomyst) is alleged to liquify mucus and DNA without having effect on fibrin or blood clots; it appears that the sulfhydril group in this compound opens disulfide bonds that are present in mucus, allegedly without disrupting peptide linkages in proteins and consequently not eroding living tissues.

Additional enzymatic agents are trypsin (Tryptar) and chymotrypsin (Chymar), which liquify clots and pus and digest fibrin deposits and necrotic tissues but do not affect living tissue because there are both specific and nonspecific trypsin inhibitors in serum.

It is said, with regard to expulsion of the debris by the two types of agents, that the detergents emulsify the exudate but do not thin it out and that vigorous coughing is therefore still required, whereas the enzymatic agents facilitate coughing through their thinning action. But it does not always work out this way.

"In a patient with severe chronic bronchopulmonary disease with respiratory distress from bronchospasm or the retention of tenacious secretions, would it be rational to give heparin when maximal conventional therapy has failed?"

Reply: There does appear to be an anti-inflammatory and antiallergic aspect to heparin's action at times, which might be helpful in eliminating bronchospasm and obstructive secretions. Boyle's group (University of Southern California) used the drug for this purpose, giving 20,000 units intravenously at once and following this by 10,000 units at 12 hour intervals for three more doses. They obtained complete, or almost complete subjective relief in 58% of their cases, in comparison with only 23% response in those who had been given placebo.

Joseph P. Boyle, Reginald H. Smart and John K. Shirey (University of Southern California). Heparin in Treatment of Chronic Obstructive Bronchopulmonary Disease. Am. J. Cardiol. 14:25, 1964.

"Can the linear growth rate of asthmatic children under treatment with corticosteroids actually be retarded by this therapy?"

Reply: Yes. At Johns Hopkins, Van Metre and Pinkerton found that the degree of retardation was roughly proportional to dosage and that when therapy was stopped the rate of growth accelerated. However, growth was retarded in no instance in which the average dose for 6 months or longer exceeded 5 mg./sq.m. of body surface daily.

Thomas E. Van Metre, Jr., and Herman L. Pinkerton, Jr. Growth Suppression in Asthmatic Children Receiving Prolonged Therapy with Prednisone (Delta-Cortef) and Methylprednisolone (Medrol). J. Allergy 30:103, 1959.

"In some of my asthmatics the only thing that will keep them reasonably active is corticosteroid therapy. I am aware of the usual dangers in connection with such therapy, but in doubt about the possibility of inducing cataracts. What is the risk?"

Reply: Clear cut answer cannot be made presently. Leibold and Itkin (National Jewish Hospital, Denver) studied their material and felt that treatment with oral steroids is *not* likely to cause cataracts in asthmatic patients; whereas Conrad Giles and associates (University of Michigan) felt that their observations confirmed the impression that posterior subcapsular cataracts may be associated with long-term systemic corticosteroid therapy. Obviously, more studies need to be made.

Conrad L. Giles, Gordon L. Mason, Ivan F. Duff and James A. McLean. Association of Cataract Formation and Systemic Corticosteroid Therapy. J.A.M.A. 182:719, Nov. 17, 1962.

"I have a young asthmatic patient who has severe intermittent attacks that are no longer benefited by isoproterenol (Isuprel) inhalations or ephedrine preparations. May I safely put him on corticosteroids?"

Reply: Yes, but do so as Donald Unger and associates did in Chicago. To 15 patients of this sort they gave 41 short courses of betamethasone (Celestone); from 3 to 6 tablets (0.6 mg./tablet) were given the first day and the dosage was then decreased by 1 tablet/ day until the drug was completely eliminated. In these children, and indeed in most of their adults, they also gave full therapeutic dosage of tetracycline to hedge against the possible worsening of infections by the corticosteroids. All of the patients were much improved in 2–4 hours after initiation of therapy and remained practically symptom-free even when the dosage was decreased. They stated that rebound asthma almost never occurred and that no side effects were observed.

Donald L. Unger, Leon Unger and Gerald Cohen. Rapid Therapy with Betamethasone (Celestone) in Severe Intermittent Asthma. Illinois M. J. 126:349, 1964.

"I have had good success with the use of aerosolized corticosteroids in asthma but invariably the patients finally develop some elements of the Cushing syndrome. Is this because of something I do not know in the matter of dosage regulation or is the thing inevitable?"

Reply: I am afraid that all the findings militate against the view that an exclusively local action can be obtained with aerosolized corticosteroids, and hence cushingoid evidence of systemic action is to be expected. Witness the experience of Harold Novey and Gildon Beall, at the University of California, Los Angeles, whose patients were told to take four inhalations every 8 hours for a dose of 1 mg. of dexamethasone (Decadron) daily. Most patients could be maintained free from asthma with this dosage, but signs of Cushing's syndrome persisted in all of them save one.

Harold S. Novey and Gildon Beall. Aerosolized Steroids and Induced Cushing's Syndrome. Arch. Int. Med. 115:602, 1965.

"I have recently used dexamethasone (Decadron, Deronil) aerosols in chronic 'intractable' asthmatic children with good effect. May I assume that the untoward effects of steroid therapy are less likely to occur with the aerosol than with the oral route of administration?"

Reply: At the University of California, Los Angeles, Sheldon Siegel and associates found this not to be the case. It was their feeling that only patients who had failed to respond to orthodox allergic management should be selected for this type of aerosol therapy, and that when discontinuing it, the dose should be carefully tapered. Furthermore, they advocated supplementing this form of therapy with oral steroids in the event of any stressful illness or injury.

Sheldon C. Siegel, Ernest M. Heimlich, Warren Richards and Vincent C. Kelley. Adrenal Function in Allergy: IV. Effect of Dexamethasone (Decadron, Deronil) Aerosols in Asthmatic Children. Pediatrics 33:245, 1964.

"Does superimposed infection of the upper respiratory tract occur as a hazard in connection with the use of dexamethasone (Decadron, Deronil) aerosol?"

Reply: It may. In the 25 patients of Dennis and Itkin (National Jewish Hospital, Denver) there were five clinical infections of the oropharynx with *Candida albicans*.

Macey Dennis and Irving H. Itkin. Effectiveness and Complications of Aerosol Dexamethasone Phosphate (Decadron, Deronil) in Severe Asthma. J. Allergy 35:70, 1964.

"Should corticosteroid aerosols be used in treating status asthmaticus, and is it necessary to use any unusual vigilance when the patient is a child?"

Reply: In the opinion of Sheldon Siegel and associates (University of California, Los Angeles) the aerosols should not be used in status asthmaticus. As for the use of corticosteroids in children, one should certainly remember that the ordinary virus diseases may be converted into serious affairs by these drugs.

Sheldon C. Siegel, Ernest M. Heimlich, Warren Richards and Vincent C. Kelley. Adrenal Function in Allergy: IV. Effect of Dexamethasone (Decadron, Deronil) Aerosols in Asthmatic Children. Pediatrics 33:245, 1964.

"I have been tempted to resort to dexamethasone (Decadron, Deronil) aerosol therapy in some of my more resistant cases of bronchial asthma. Has this therapy been generally effective?"

Reply: I should say that its role should so far be considered a limited one. Gordon Snider's group, in Chicago, evaluated the bronchodilator effect in 26 patients, none of whom had received steroid therapy in the preceding 3 months. One had allergic bronchial asthma, 4 infectious and 21 mixed asthma. The results certainly were not dramatic, although most of the patients who responded satisfactorily had the more severe degrees of airway obstruction.

Gordon L. Snider, Michael I. Frank, A. L. Aaronson, David B. Radner, Morris A. Kaplan and Milton M. Mosko. Effect of Dexamethasone (Decadron, Deronil) Aerosol on Airway Obstruction in Bronchial Asthma: Study Using Forced Expiratory Volume for One Second. Dis. Chest 44:408, 1963.

"What is the risk to bone in asthmatics with continual dyspnea for whom it is often essential to employ corticosteroid therapy?"

Reply: J. Charpin and associates (Marseilles, France) observed spontaneous fractures of the spine in 5 of their 256 patients during a 2 year period. Among 33 patients (28 women), all but 1 over 40 years of age, who had received corticosteroids for long periods, there were 15 with definite signs of osseous rarefaction when closely studied. Daily doses of cortisone had varied, but the average was 10.3 mg. (expressed as dosage of delta-hydrocortisone), and none had received this dosage for less than 3 years; 23 of the 33 for 3–6 years and 7 for over 6 years. These observers felt that in therapy of this sort one should give calcium, vitamin D_2 and 30 mg. of norethandrolone (Nilevar) daily for 10 days in each month. This supplemental therapy is rational, because osteoporosis is a reflection of protein depletion that weakens the connective tissue stroma on which calcium and phosphorus are deposited.

J. Charpin, H. Payan, R. Luccioni, R. Lieutaud, Ph. Ohresser and J. Nicolino. Attempt at Evaluation of Risk to Bone in Asthmatics Subjected to Prolonged Treatment with Cortisone. Semaine hop. Paris 39:2129, Oct. 14, 1963.

"Is there a greater frequency of thromboembolic episodes in patients on corticosteroid therapy while in status asthmaticus than has been brought to general attention? I have consulted in an episode recently that provoked the question."

Reply: I think it may be so. Milton Hartman (Presbyterian Medical Center, San Francisco) has stated that patients with status asthmaticus tend to have low clotting times or protamine titration values, or both. Corticosteroids or ACTH may lower these values to pathologic levels, an action which he attributes to direct ACTH-heparin antagonism and reduction of mast cell activity by corticosteroids. He found it of advantage to give heparin to patients with status asthmaticus who are receiving ACTH or corticosteroids. In such cases he added heparin on the fifth day of the steroid therapy, most patients receiving 100 mg. every 8 hours or 150 mg. every 12 hours initially, the dosage and frequency being reduced as the steroid requirements decreased.

Milton M. Hartman. Thromboembolic Phenomena in Severe Asthma: Use of Heparin for Prevention and Treatment in Patients Receiving ACTH or Glucosteroids. California Med. 98:27, 1963.

"Theophylline is frequently very efficacious in relieving the acute asthmatic attack, but often it unaccountably fails. Has an exact study ever been made of the theophylline serum levels required to produce clinical benefit?"

Reply: The correlation of pulmonary function studies in asthmatics and theophylline serum levels was carefully studied by Richard Jackson and associates (Houston), whose findings indicated that a theophylline concentration of about 1000 μg./100 ml. of serum is required to effect relief in the acute episode. Their drug was given orally, so the assumption is probably admissible that the rate and extent of absorption from the intestinal tract is the determinant of efficacy in the individual case.

Richard H. Jackson, John I. McHenry, Ferrin B. Moreland, Warren J. Raymer and Richard L. Etter. Clinical Evaluation of Elixophyllin with Correlation of Pulmonary Function Studies and Theophylline Serum Levels in Acute and Chronic Asthmatic Patients. Dis. Chest 45:75, 1964.

"In reviewing the drugs dispensed by our hospital pharmacy during the past year I have found that a quite tremendous amount of theophylline ethylenediamine (Aminophylline) is being prescribed by the staff. Since we do not have a disproportionate amount of asthma under treatment, a certain amount of the drug must be in use for other purposes. Are there really many legitimate uses for theophylline; in other words, what are the actions of this drug that would warrant its large-scale employment?"

Reply: Theophylline causes generalized vasodilation by direct relaxing action on vessel walls, including the coronary arteries; slows the heart through stimulation of the vagal nuclei in the medulla; opposes through central vasomotor stimulation the blood pressure–lowering effect which would result from vascular dilatation; and directly stimulates the myocardium. The result of these several opposing actions is usually an increase in cardiac output, which probably improves coronary circulation because the coronary vessels are not affected by the central vasomotor stimulation. Thus we can rationalize several frequent clinical employments of the drug: in coronary disease to effect dilatation of the coronary vessels while simultaneously improving cardiac output (both of which occurrences are doubted by some observers); in the pulmonary crisis of left ventricular failure; in heart failures of acute glomerulonephritis and of terminal uremia; and to oppose the sudden coronary insufficiency that is one of the features in the complete circulatory dissolution characterizing pulmonary embolism. These things, however, do not comprise the full list of the clinical uses of theophylline for its beneficent circulatory actions, for Moyer and associates, confirming the general clinical impression that severe hypertensive headaches can often be relieved by the use of theophylline, found an average drop in cerebrospinal fluid pressure from 210 to 132 mm. with use of the drug and an average fall in cerebral blood flow from 53 to 36 ml./100 gm. brain/minute. This fall in cerebral blood flow results from another specialized cardiovascular action of the drug, namely a direct stimulating action on cerebral arteriolar musculature, according to the findings of Wechsler's group. This work of Wechsler has forced a search for a new explanation of another of theophylline's observed effects: the arresting of Cheyne-Stokes respiration in cardiac failure. Moyer, in confirming Wechsler's findings, concluded that respiratory improvement in these cases is the result of a stimulating action on the respiratory center, being either a direct action there or an indirect one secondary to the depressed cerebral circulation and the resultant rise in tissue carbon dioxide.

Theophylline is useful in another respiratory malady, too, i.e., that which you mention, bronchial asthma, particularly in the critical condition known as status asthmaticus. The antihistaminic nature of this action has been demonstrated experimentally in both rabbits and man. The interesting speculation has also been offered in connection with this use of the drug, which is sometimes a lifesaving measure, that perhaps in bronchial asthma there is a reversible pulmonary arteriolar spasm and that aminophylline's effect may be partially explained on the basis of its relaxation of this spasm. However, there is also another pharmacologic rationalization of the action, since theophylline can be shown under experimental conditions in the laboratory to be a relaxant of smooth muscle in general. This would include the smooth muscles of the bronchioles, which are spasmodically contracted in the asthmatic attack.

The extent of the relaxant action in the gastrointestinal tract usually is not sufficient to be of clinical importance except that parenteral use of the drug during an attack of gallstone colic may relax the sphincter of Oddi and bring relief.

Theophylline has a certain diuretic efficacy but is not much used alone for the purpose at present because dosage productive of results in congestive failure causes a prohibitive amount of gastrointestinal disturbance and nervousness, and the effects are inferior to those obtainable with less disturbing drugs. There is experimental evidence that theophylline depresses tubular reabsorption, thus accounting for the diuretic action under usual circumstances. But there is a situation in which more potent diuretics fail to produce urine because of a very low glomerular filtration rate, and it may be that under these circumstances the circulatory actions of theophylline are of supplementary value. At any rate, the drug's greatest practical diuretic usefulness is to supplement the action of other diuretics rather than as a diuretic agent per se.

One last clinical use of theophylline needs to be mentioned, though we have no adequate pharmacologic rationalization of it: the drug is often strikingly effective in allaying pruritus and in bringing relief to patients suffering from sensitization dermatoses.

J. H. Moyer, S. I. Miller, A. B. Tashnek, and R. Bowman. Effect of Theophylline with Ethylene Diamine (Aminophylline) on Cerebral Hemodynamics in Presence of Cardiac Failure with and Without Cheyne-Stokes Respiration. J. Clin. Invest. 31:267, 1952. J. H. Moyer, A. B. Tashnek, S. I. Miller, H. Snyder and R. O. Bowman. The Effect of Theophylline with Ethylene Diamine (Aminophylline) and Caffeine on Cerebral Hemodynamics and Cerebrospinal Fluid Pressure in Patients with Hypertension Headaches. Am. J. M. Sc. 224:377, 1952. R. L. Wechsler, L. M. Kleiss and S. S. Kety. The Effects of Intravenously Administered Aminophylline on Cerebral Circulation and Metabolism in Man. J. Clin. Invest. 29: 28, 1950.

"I am currently getting better results in some of my asthmatics with the hydroalcoholic solution of theophylline, Elixophyllin, than with aminophylline. Is this due to the more effective absorption of the active agent from the elixir?"

Reply: Could be. Some years ago, A. Oscharoff, when studying the efficacy of Elixophyllin in comparison with aminophylline in relieving severe angina pectoris, obtained suggestive evidence of the more rapid absorption of the alcoholic solution, but he also thought it possible that the tranquilizing effect of the alcohol it contained may have been of some importance. I presume you are prescribing for an adult a tablespoonful before meals and possibly again on retiring. Four or 5 tablespoonfuls of the preparation will contain an amount of alcohol roughly equivalent to 1 oz. of whiskey. I do not know that this would actually have a therapeutic effect but do recall that an old remedy, that often worked well in asthma, was aspirin and whiskey; this, however, was before the allergists began going into a state of shock at the mere mention of aspirin and frightened us all into giving it up in the aspirin-alcohol combination.

Alexander Oscharoff (Long Island City, N.Y.) Therapeutic Effectiveness of Elixophyllin as Compared with Aminophylline in Severe Angina Pectoris. New York J. Med. 57:2975, Sept. 15, 1957.

"For the second time in our group we have had a frightening reaction to aminophylline given to an asthmatic child in a rectal suppository. Both times we had used the 'pediatric' suppository. Have others had this experience?"

Reply: Yes, this has occurred a number of times and been documented and recorded. Some years ago, Veum and Schwartz pointed out that aminophylline dosage for a child under age 3 should not exceed one-fifth the adult dose, i.e., 0.100 Gm. instead of the 0.250 Gm. available in the "children's" suppository. It does not seem to be generally known in the profession that there is a truly "pediatric" suppository available that contains only 0.125 Gm.

Even for older children one should increase this dosage only very cautiously.

Roy Pollack (Englewood, N. J.). Aminophylline Poisoning in Childhood. J. M. Soc. New Jersey 56:550, 1959. James Veum and Abraham B. Schwartz (Milwaukee Children's Hospital). Toxic Effects of Half-Strength Aminophylline Suppositories in Asthmatic Children. J. Pediat. 49:703, 1956.

"Is there available a satisfactory liquid preparation of theophylline for use in asthmatic youngsters?"

Reply: Yes, there is the preparation oxtriphylline-glyceryl guaiacolate elixir (Brondecon), each 5 ml. of which contains 100 mg. of oxtriphylline, which is choline theophyllinate, and 50 mg. of glyceryl guaiacolate in 20% alcohol. In Dallas, Frederick Grover found this preparation an effective, safe, well tolerated one suitable for use in the management of mild and moderate allergic bronchial disorders in infants and children.

Frederick W. Grover. Oxtriphylline-Glyceryl Guaiacolate Elixir (Brondecon) in Pediatric Asthma. Ann. Allergy 23: 127, 1965.

"In those of my asthmatic patients who remain sufficiently sensitive to the therapeutic effect of epinephrine but cannot for one reason or another take it in aerosol form, I still use it subcutaneously of course. However, it is often necessary to give such large dosage in relief of an acute attack that the patient experiences considerable unpleasantness from the drug. Can this be remedied in any way?"

Reply: It has often been observed that small subcutaneous doses repeated at brief intervals have a cumulative therapeutic effect without a cumulative toxic effect. Try injecting 0.2 or 0.3 mg. at 20 minute intervals.

Milton M. Moxko, M. C. Arkin, B. H. Miller and G. L. Snider (Michael Reese Hosp.). Studies on Effects of Sympathicoamines in Asthma: Variability of Effect from Differing Routes of Administration. Dis. Chest 38:264, 1960.

"I have a number of asthmatic patients under treatment with several of the epinephrine-like analogues, but their responses are not predictable. One patient will do well on ephedrine and another not at all, and neither may respond to Orthoxine, although they both do well on Alupent. Is this general experience?"

Reply: Yes, I think one may say so. Kennedy and Jackson (City General Hospital, Stoke-on-Trent, England) initiated oral sympathomimetic amine therapy in 12 patients who had generally had a consistently good response to aerosol epinephrine, and found that 5 responded best to 20 mg. metaproterenol (Alupent), 4 to 10 mg. metaproterenol, 1 to 30 mg. ephedrine, 1 to 100 mg. methoxyphenamine (Orthoxine) and 1 to 10 mg. isoprenaline (Isuprel, etc). Isuprel gave the quickest but most transient action, ephedrine and Orthoxine the slowest and most prolonged. It would seem that the only thing to do is switch about among these compounds to find the one most suitable for the individual patient.

M. C. S. Kennedy and S. L. O. Jackson. Oral Sympathomimetic Amines in Treatment of Asthma. Brit. M. J. 2:1506, Dec. 14, 1963.

"I have been using the tablet form of metaproterenol (Alupent) upon the whole quite favorably, but I now hear some mention of the aerosol preparation; has it been giving satisfaction?"

Reply: I have seen several favorable reports. The dose of this preparation varies from 1 to 4 puffs, each containing 0.75 mg. Patients who obtain good response with it seem to be enthusiastic about it because they claim quick relief and the expelling of thick mucus; in some instances it seems necessary to use the inhaler only every few days rather than daily. But, as with most asthma remedies, the older, chronically ill patients obtain less prompt and briefer relief than the individuals whose cases are of shorter duration.

Frederick Kessler. Clinical Trial of Metaproterenol (Alupent) Aerosol in Bronchial Asthma. Ann. Allergy 22:588, 1964. William C. Grater. Treatment of Acute Asthma by Aerosolized Metaproterenol (Alupent) Measured by Pulmonary Ventilatory Studies. Ann. Allergy 23:23, 1965.

"I sometimes think that if I used initially higher dosage of epinephrine in my status asthmaticus patients I would get better results; how high dare I go?"

Reply: I do not know how high *you* would dare to go, but I would have some qualms myself about using the dosage that Bryan Broom (Middlesex Hospital, Medical School, London) has advocated. In 24 patients he gave 1 : 1000 epinephrine, 2–5 ml. in 5–15 minutes, rapidity of response serving as a guide to total dosage. Three of these patients required a second injection, and 2 had to be hospitalized after 10 and 8 ml., respectively, failed to produce improvement. He had side effects, "often unpleasant" (I use the British terminology), in all but 6 individuals: tachycardia in 18, vomiting in 16, pallor with headache and sweating in 10, extrasystoles in 5, and tremors and anxiety in 2. He very carefully advocates that when one gives intramuscular injections of this size during a period of as long as 5–15 minutes, one must make sure at 1 minute intervals that the syringe is not in a vein. A few instances of an excessively high rise in blood pressure and even hemiplegia were reported from Copenhagen a great many years ago in association with somewhat higher than

ordinary dosage of epinephrine subcutaneously, but I have seen nothing of this sort in the literature since.

Bryan Broom. Adrenaline and Status Asthmaticus. Lancet 2:1174, Nov. 25, 1961. L. S. Fridericia. Ugesk. laeger 49: 1915, Dec. 9, 1915, (abstracted in J.A.M.A. 66:466, 1915).

"Occasionally one or another of my colleagues will say 'I am tempted to go back to the iodides again in some of my asthmatics.' Is there really any justification for this? What is the position of iodide therapy in asthma?"

Reply: It seems to me very doubtful that the iodides have any real efficacy in the treatment of asthma. At the Mount Sinai Hospital in New York, Sheppard Siegal, who has devoted many years to the study of this disease, provoked considerable instructive comment among other authorities on the subject when he reported his results in 200 cases. His dosage was potassium iodide in 0.3 Gm. enteric-coated tablets, 2 tablets four times daily, and he admitted that the suppressive effect could probably not be anticipated in more than 5–10% of the cases. The outstanding weakness of the claim, in my view, is that as many as 5–12% of individuals are often recorded as responding to the oral administration of placebos. However, in some of Siegal's cases the iodide dose level appeared to be critical, and a noniodide placebo tablet was ineffective. A very long shot therefore, if the nag is to be entered at all.

Sheppard Siegal. Asthma-Suppressive Action of Potassium Iodide. J. Allergy 35:252, 1964.

"I have an asthmatic patient who, on her own responsibility, has been taking a proprietary preparation containing inorganic iodide for many years. She has a goiter and is hypothyroid. If I discontinue this medication, is prescription of thyroid hormone indicated?"

Reply: Among the 9 patients of T. B. Begg and R. Hall, in England, in whom iodide medication was discontinued and thyroid hormone was not given, or given for only a short time, there was complete resolution of the goiter in 3–29 months and of hypothyroidism, where it had existed, in 5 of the patients; in 1 patient the goiter enlarged a little and thyrotoxic signs appeared. In 6 other patients, to whom thyroid hormone was given after the omission of iodide, the existing hypothyroidism was corrected, and the goiter decreased in 3, remaining unchanged in the other 3.

T. B. Begg and R. Hall. Iodide Goiter and Hypothyroidism. Quart. J. Med. 32:351, 1963.

"I have a patient who has been taking moderate doses of potassium iodide for a prolonged period

in the treatment of her asthma and has now been detected in the early stage of myxedema. Could the iodides be incriminated?"

Reply: Certainly in most euthyroid individuals the taking of iodides in moderate dosage does not provoke thyroid derangement, but in an occasional patient it will do so. At the University of Chicago, Benjamin Burrows and associates reported four instances of goiter and myxedema which they attributed to iodide administration.

Benjamin Burrows, Albert H. Niden and William R. Barclay. Goiter and Myxedema Due to Iodide Administration. Ann. Int. Med. 52:858, 1960.

"When epinephrine, aminophylline and corticosteroids have failed in status asthmaticus, is it rational to try alkaline therapy?"

Reply: A number of years ago, J. S. Blumenthal and associates suggested that there may be a depression of epinephrine response by acidosis in these cases and proposed the use of sodium lactate in treatment; more recently they have confirmed their original therapeutic success with this agent. It appears necessary to give the drug fairly rapidly in concentrated solution and early, before the thick tenacious secretions become increasingly more important than muscle spasm. *Dosage:* one molar sodium lactate, 120–300 ml. given during about 30 minutes. The response to this treatment was sometimes dramatic. Another approach has been that of John Mithoefer's group at the Mary Imogene Bassett Hospital, Cooperstown, who successfully reversed the declivitous course in 6 patients by correcting respiratory acidosis with sodium bicarbonate intravenously. When they found in these patients that significant respiratory acidosis was demonstrated by measurements of arterial blood pH and carbon dioxide tension, they gave 100 ml. of 0.9M solution of sodium bicarbonate during a 5 minute period; subsequently, this or half-dosage is given at 5 or 10 minute intervals, each preceded by proper measurements until the pH has returned to near normal value or satisfactory clinical improvement has occurred. However, the investigators feel that these measures can be employed safely without the pH and carbon dioxide tension measurements, through spacing subsequent doses after the initial one preferably at intervals of 15 to 30 minutes. The therapy has not been employed by them in children.

John C. Mithoefer, Richard H. Runser and Monroe S. Karetzky. The Use of Sodium Bicarbonate in the Treatment of Acute Bronchial Asthma. New England J. Med. 272:1200, June 10, 1965. J. S. Blumenthal, M. N. Blumenthal, E. B. Brown, G. S. Campbell and A. Prasad. Effect of Changes in Arterial pH on Action of Adrenalin in Acute Adrenalin-Fast Asthmatics. Dis. Chest 39:516, 1961.

"One of my associates has just returned from a meeting at which he heard it said that the use of an antiserotonin agent could be helpful in the treatment of asthma. What is the rationale of this?"

Reply: In this confusing field of allergy it is now increasingly the belief that the reaction comprises not merely the release of histamine alone but also of all the following substances: acetylcholine, heparin, plasma kinins, slow-reacting substances, permeability factors, leukotaxine and serotonin. Trial of an anti-serotonin agent would therefore be rational. In fact, at Johns Hopkins Hospital, Arnold Lavenstein and associates studied such an agent, cyproheptadine (Periactin), in asthmatic children, comparing its efficacy with an antihistaminic compound. They found it to be no more effective than the latter, but did observe that there was both an increase in appetite and a gain in weight by the children given the cyproheptadine.

Arnold F. Lavenstein, Eleanora P. Dacaney, Louis Lasagna and Thomas E. Van Metre. Effect of Cyproheptadine (Periactin) on Asthmatic Children: Study of Appetite, Weight Gain and Linear Growth. J.A.M.A. 180:912, June 16, 1962.

"Recently I have been using in my asthmatics a compounded tablet (elixir for the youngsters) containing ephedrine, theophylline, thenyldiamine, glyceryl guaiacolate and phenobarbital. The results have been quite good, and I have been wondering what is the real objection to using a preparation of this sort rather than trying one drug after another to see which one best suits the individual case?"

Reply: This is a very rational preparation, for you have in it not only the somewhat specific agents ephedrine, theophylline and thenyldiamine (an antihistaminic) but also an expectorant in glyceryl guaiacolate and a sedative barbiturate. An objection to its use, however, from the standpoint of the purist, is precisely that which may be brought against any shotgun preparation, namely, that the possibility of adjustment in dosage of any one of the ingredients is lost. There will of course be some patients who will not respond well at all to this preparation because the ingredient to which they are most responsive is present in dosage which is too low for their needs. How are you going to know which ingredient this is? And then, too, when eventually they all begin to fail to obtain the relief that they did in the beginning, you cannot simply double or triple the dosage of all these ingredients by ordering the taking of multiple units without risking overaction of some of them in sensitive patients. I am not wishing to doubt that you are getting good results presently, but I do wonder whether in the long run it is not going to be of greater value to know that this or that patient gets his greatest relief from this or that individual drug, or from this or that combination of several drugs deliberately reached through trial and error, than merely to effect relief in him in the beginning with dabs of all the drugs. One of the ingredients in this preparation is phenobarbital, you have said. Since this is definitely a drug of habituation, I should think you would want to take your patient off of it much sooner than you might want to withdraw some of the other ingredients of the mixture—but admittedly this is just because of my crotchety belief that altogether too many people are being barbiturate-dosed nowadays.

"In our area there is a good deal of self-medication of asthmatics with a proprietary preparation containing belladonna alkaloids. What is really the efficacy of the belladonna compounds in asthma?"

Reply: Actually, there has not been much critical assessment of the matter, though it appears that stramonium smoking was introduced into England from India as long ago as 1802. When I was a student, not quite that long ago, it was customary among asthma patients to burn nightly in their bedrooms an "asthma powder," which contained stramonium and belladonna or hyoscyamus leaves. In Germany, in 1959, Herxheimer studied the effect of atropine smoke on lung function in asthmatic and emphysematous patients. In almost all of them, vital capacity increased after smoking the cigarettes, but there was considerable variation in the amount of this increase, and there was no increase in those in whom the control vital capacity was normal. In 52 of the 62 experiments, the increase was 10% or more, often noted immediately after smoking and maintained for as long as 3 hours in one patient and for at least 1 or 1½ hours in almost all. At the Brompton Hospital, London, Chamberlain's group, in 1962, found that the addition of atropine methonitrate (Harvatrate, etc.) to isoprenaline (Aludrine, etc.) in inhalation therapy in asthmatics considerably increased and prolonged the effect.

H. Herxheimer (Free University of Berlin). Atropine Cigarettes in Asthma and Emphysema. Brit. M. J. 2:167, Aug. 15, 1959. D. A. Chamberlain, D. C. F. Muir and K. P. Kennedy. Atropine Methonitrate (Harvatrate, etc.) and Isoprenaline (Aludrine, Isuprel) in Bronchial Asthma. Lancet 2:1019, Nov. 17, 1962.

"I have recently had as a new patient a moderately severe asthmatic who was hallucinating slightly when first seen. He confessed to taking an over-the-counter preparation, very popular in our area, that contains, I believe, about 50% stramonium and 4% or more of a belladonna preparation. Could this nostrum have accounted for the hallucination?"

Reply: Indeed, yes. Stramonium has long been known as a hallucinating, confusing and stupidifying poison with a considerable criminal record. Edward Dean (San Francisco General Hospital) has reported three young men who deliberately self-induced intoxication with a proprietary preparation similar to the one you describe. Diagnosis in his cases was aided by the evidence of atropinism: dilatation of the pupil when a drop of the patient's urine is placed in a cat's eye.

Edward S. Dean. Self-Induced Stramonium Intoxication. J.A.M.A. 185:882, Sept. 14, 1963.

"What are the principal monoamine oxidase inhibitor agents; and if their use is to be shunned in asthmatics because of possible worsening of the symptoms, is there any central nervous system stimulant that may be used with greater safety?"

Reply: The principal monoamine oxidase inhibitors currently available are pargyline (Eutonyl), isocarboxazid (Marplan), nialamide (Niamid), phenelzine (Nardil) and tranylcypromine (Parnate). Arthur Goldfarb and Felix Venutolo (Holy Name Hospital, Teaneck, N. J.) reported that after 6 weeks of therapy in a group of 100 patients with various major allergies of long duration, 44 had improved on imipramine (Tofranil) but not on placebo or atropine. There was no mention of the asthma having been worsened in any of these patients. Since depression is not an infrequent ingredient in the total congeries of symptoms comprising asthma, the use of this drug in attempting to overcome it is at least rational.

Arthur A. Goldfarb and Felix Venutolo. Use of an Antidepressant Drug in Chronically Allergic Individuals: Double-Blind Study. Ann. Allergy 21:667, 1963.

"I have had occasion to use nialamide (Niamid), which is a monoamine oxidase inhibitor, for central nervous system stimulation in a patient who is rather severely asthmatic. It has seemed to me that her asthma is worsened; is this effect characteristic of this group of drugs?"

Reply: Perhaps one should not say characteristic, but Enrique Mathov (Buenos Aires) certainly had the same experience. In a controlled study, about one third of the treated and none of the untreated patients became worse. The aggravation of the asthmatic symptoms might be due to accumulation of histamine in the tissues under influence of the drugs, or to accumulation of catechols.

Enrique Mathov. Risks of Monoamine Oxidase Inhibitors in Treatment of Bronchial Asthma. J. Allergy 34:483, 1963.

"When all the usual methods have failed in a severe case of status asthmaticus and the patient is moribund, is there anything 'new' to which one may turn in desperation?"

Reply: Lewis Beam and associates have reported from the Children's Hospital of Pittsburgh that they saved 3 children in apparently irreversible status asthmaticus through resort to paralysis and controlled respiration. The drug used to accomplish muscle paralysis and facilitate endotracheal intubation and controlled respiration was gallamine triethiodide (Flaxedil), being preferred to other drugs of this nature because it does not cause bronchospasm and possesses no histamine-like action. The advantages claimed for this method of therapy in comparison with inhalation anesthesia and controlled respiration in the agitated, struggling child is that the control of respiration is immediate, there is lack of increased mucous secretion caused by anesthetics, and recovery is relatively rapid upon discontinuing the drug. However, one must be cautious in the use of gallamine if there is impaired renal function since this may prolong the curarization; and possibly iodide sensitivity should also be considered. Another thing that might lead to prolonged muscular paralysis would be the concomitant employment of neomycin, streptomycin or kanamycin. The drug also has a vagus-inhibiting action, which may result in tachycardia. The effective antidote for gallamine is edrophonium chloride (Tensilon).

Lewis R. Beam, Joseph H. Marcy and Herbert C. Mansmann, Jr. Medically Irreversible Status Asthmaticus in Children. J.A.M.A. 194:968, Nov. 29, 1965.

"I have heard that ipecac is useful in the treatment of asthma but cannot understand how this could be true. Is this merely an old wives' tale?"

Reply: No, it is not. In the asthmatic attack, when the bronchi are blocked with accumulations of mucus, forceful vomiting will release the plugs and often afford truly dramatic relief. It is possible that the retching and vomiting induce a peristaltoid action in the trachea and release the obstructing plugs in what has been called "tracheal vomiting." Usual dosage of syrup of ipecac for infants and young children is ½–1 teaspoonful (2.5–5.0 ml.) followed by tepid water; 2–4 teaspoonfuls (10–20 ml.) may be given, and repetition of dosage may be made at intervals of a few minutes in older children and adults until effect is obtained.

"Is it acceptable to use morphine in the patient with a severe asthmatic attack?"

Reply: Individuals with severe asthma are often gasping for breath; their respirations are labored but are not always rapid. The temptation to use morphine is great and often yielded to. The patient is quieted by the drug and his apprehension is relieved, but the asthma itself is usually not helped, and the wheezing continues. Most allergists consider morphine dangerous for two reasons: (1) its depression of the respiratory center in an individual already handicapped in breathing; (2) the decrease it effects in the cough reflex, which opposes rather than aids getting rid of bronchial secretions. I think that morphine has probably accounted for a good many asthmatic deaths.

"Is meperidine (Demerol) safer than morphine to use in an acute asthmatic attack?"

Reply: It has not been established to be.

"It is alleged that exercise increases the efficacy of bronchodilator drugs in the asthmatic child. Is this true?"

Reply: R. S. Jones and associates (University of Liverpool) studied this matter and concluded that prolonged continuous exercise is unsuitable for the asthmatic child, even at levels not causing undue breathlessness. They felt, however, that games in which the exercise occurs in short bouts may have therapeutic value. For the most part, baseball provides that sort of exercise, but I would warn against permitting a young asthmatic to participate in Little League activities. The people who are fostering this movement have built an amount of stress and tension into the thing which is altogether taboo for the asthmatic — and as a matter of fact it seems to me altogether ridiculous to introduce so much serious competition into the "fun" of kids.

R. S. Jones, M. J. Wharton and M. H. Buston. Place of Physical Exercise and Bronchodilator Drugs in Assessment of the Asthmatic Child. Arch. Dis. Childhood 38: 539, 1963.

"I am sometimes tempted to prescribe tranquilizing drugs for the parents of my young allergic patients as well as for the children themselves during periods of the sort of stress that seems provocative of attacks. What would you think of this?"

Reply: And so why not the school teacher and the child's fellow pupils and the neighbors too? I know that a group deep in the heart of Texas, McGovern and associates, say that they did find it frequently advantageous to tranquilize the parents also, but I am just an old-fashioned fellow and the thought of such a thing gives me goose pimples.

John P. McGovern, Kemal Ozkaragoz, Gilbert Barkin, Theodore Haywood, Thomas McElhenney and Albert F.

Hensel, Jr. (Houston). Studies of Chlordiazepoxide (Librium) in Various Allergic Diseases. Ann. Allergy 18: 1193, 1960.

"In a certain type of patient I customarily give influenza vaccine seasonally, but if the patient is an asthmatic he often becomes less responsive to the antiasthmatic drugs for a brief period. Why is this?"

Reply: I do not know. At the University of Wisconsin, John Ouellette and Charles Reed studied the matter and could only produce a speculative answer. The chief respiratory infections will often provoke attacks in asthmatic patients too, as I am sure you know.

John J. Ouellette and Charles E. Reed. Increased Response of Asthmatic Subjects to Methacholine after Influenza Vaccine. J. Allergy 36:558, 1965.

"In a patient with intractable chronic bronchial asthma, i.e., one in whom relief can no longer be obtained through the use of drugs, would you recommend glomectomy, which is removal of the right carotid body and excision of the wall of the carotid bulb and the carotid sinus?"

Reply: As with any radical surgical procedure, the measure has its enthusiastic advocates, but I should like to bring to your attention the editorial remarks regarding the matter made by Francis Rackemann, whose vast experience in asthma is everywhere recognized. He points out that before one can fully appraise any sort of treatment in asthma it should be recognized that results can be expected to differ among the variety of forms of the disease, and that the surgical enthusiasts have said very little on this point. Furthermore, he questions the specificity of the carotid operation since many other types of surgical procedure, as well as accidents, fractures, wounds, pregnancy and parturition, have also been observed to initiate a period of relief in asthma.

F. M. Rackemann. The Carotid Sinus and the Carotid Body. J.A.M.A. 191:593, 1965.

"I have heard that, of all outlandish things, they are treating asthma with vermifuges down in Mexico. Is this true?"

Reply: It is certainly not true that "they" are doing so, but Mario Mallén, who is Chief of the Allergy Service at the General Hospital in Mexico City, has reported the effective use of diethylcarbamazine citrate (Hetrazan) in a small group of cases after observing the excellent antiasthmatic effect of the drug in a patient in whom it was being used in the treatment of tropical eosinophilia. Daily dosage of the drug was 10 mg./kg., with half this dosage sometimes sufficing later.

Mario S. Mallén. Treatment of Intractable Asthma with Diethylcarbamazine Citrate. Ann. Allergy 23:534, 1965.

"What is probably the ultimate that can be achieved in the treatment of childhood asthma under ideal circumstances?"

Reply: C. J. Falliers, who is Medical Director of the Children's Asthma Research Institute in Denver, reported that during a 6 year period, 38% of the 515 children admitted to that institution showed remarkable recovery, either remaining entirely free of asthma or experiencing only mild, brief episodes of wheezing on an average of less than once a month. Another 40% showed varying degrees of improvement, but each still required intermittent therapy with inhaled, oral or injected bronchodilators and, in almost half of the cases, occasional brief courses of corticosteroids. The remaining 22% received antiasthmatic therapy, including small maintenance doses of corticosteroids, practically without interruption throughout their stay in the hospital; efforts to discontinue the corticosteroids in this group, or reduce the dosage below a critical level for each patient, invariably caused exacerbations of the disease. The average time of residence for the children in the survey period was 19 months, with a range of 12–24 months.

Constantine J. Falliers. Corticosteroids and Anabolic Hormones for Childhood Asthma. Clin. Pediat. 4:441, 1965.

"While not subscribing to the belief that asthma is a psychoneurosis, I have seen patients who were very much helped by the use of tranquilizing agents and in 1 case even an antidepressive drug. Have agents of the latter type been given thorough study in this malady?"

Reply: No, I do not think so, although in Japan, Sugihara and associates reported quite favorably on the use of amitriptyline (Elavil) in 60 patients, 8 of whom had an "excellent" and 29 a "good" therapeutic effect. It was notable, however, that in this series 38% of the patients experienced an hypnotic effect from the drug and that the best results were achieved when this drowsiness was experienced.

H. Sugihara, K. Ishihara and H. Moguchi. Clinical Experience with Amitriptyline in the Treatment of Bronchial Asthma. Ann. Allergy 23:422, 1965.

ATELECTASIS

"What is to be done in a case of postoperative atelectasis that is resistant to all standard measures: the use of aerosols, bronchodilator drugs, mucolytic agents and intermittent positive pressure breathing?"

Reply: In California, Jacob Robbins and associates have reported 4 consecutive cases of this sort that cleared dramatically following rapid intravenous injection of aminophylline. The drug is injected in 125–150 mg. dosage through a 22 gauge needle as rapidly as possible, relief of bronchospasm being heralded by the occurrence of paresthesia of the face and/or fleeting nitritoid reaction in the lapsed interval of the circulation time. Immediately or shortly thereafter it is said that the patient, either spontaneously or on suggestion, coughs up a quantity of obstructing mucus. It has always seemed advisable to most observers to shun the rapid intravenous administration of aminophylline because of fear of the nitritoid reaction, but Robbins' group say that they have not found such reaction, in their more than 5000 injections, to be more than evanescent and not alarming when the patient is warned of its imminence.

Jacob John Robbins, Stanley H. Schonberger, Sidney C. Jackson and Desi Handra. Successful Treatment of Post-operative Atelectasis by Intravenous Injection of Amino-phylline. J. Thoracic & Cardio. Surg. 49:874, 1965.

"Patients with chronic bronchopulmonary disease, pulmonary fibrosis, emphysema, heavy smokers, and obese short-necked individuals are prone to develop serious pulmonary complications, primarily atelectasis, after pulmonary surgery. Ordinary expectorants as used in combating cough do not suffice for relief of these symptoms. Is pancreatic dornase (Dornavac) being used effectively?"

Reply: At Cornell University, Eugene Cliffton and associates reported the treatment of 406 patients with this agent, with rapid clearing of atelectasis or other pulmonary complications in 90% of them. Of 92 patients with serious postoperative atelectasis after thoracic procedures, 83 were completely relieved within 48 hours. In the 72 patients with lobar or segmental atelectasis, pneumonitis or both, after head and neck, breast, abdominal or pelvic operations, relief was obtained in a few hours to 2 days in over 90%. There was also relief of over 90% of the 119 patients with severe tracheitis sicca with relief usually noted in 30 minutes and return to normal within 24 hours. Finally, excellent results were obtained in 52 of 59 patients with a wide variety of chronic bronchopulmonary diseases. The drug is administered as an irrigating solution or as an aerosol, but ordinary hand nebulizers will not deliver sufficient amounts. The mouth and oral pharynx should be rinsed after each treatment in order to prevent pharyngeal irritation; there

have been a few hypersensitivity reactions due to the beef protein in the preparation. I am unaware of a satisfactory comparative study of this agent with other competing preparations, but I would draw your attention to two of these, acetylcysteine (Mucomyst) and Alevair.

Eugene E. Cliffton, Caro E. Grossi and Ernest R. Esakof. Management of Pulmonary Complications of Surgical Operations (Primarily Atelectasis) with Pancreatic Dornase Inhalations. Surgery 50:176, 1961.

"It is the general impression, which I believe to be warranted, that postoperative atelectasis is high in individuals who have been heavily morphinized, but our residents have been studying the rate and volume of respiration in a small group of patients and have not found these parameters greatly affected by the drug. How then explain the atelectasis?"

Reply: In studying this matter at the Massachusetts General Hospital, L. D. Egbert and H. H. Bendixen found that the principal difference between the morphinized and the non-morphinized postoperative patient is that the former sighs much less often than does the latter. It appears that periodic deep breaths is a component of normal respiratory function.

L. D. Egbert and H. H. Bendixen. Effect of Morphine on Breathing Pattern: Possible Factor in Atelectasis. J.A.M.A. 188:485, May 11, 1964.

ATHEROSCLEROSIS

"How is any individual practitioner ever to know whether he is achieving anything with anticholesteremic agents in atherosclerotic patients? Of course he may bring down the cholesterol level, but does that mean that he is really affecting the atheromatous lesion? And it is said that the early lesion responds better than the later one; but how is he to sort out his patients on that basis?"

Reply: It seems to me that you simply have to take the whole thing on faith as it applies to your individual practice, or not at all. Even in the attempts to submit the matter to careful clinical investigation the statistical limitations have been very great. For example, in order to obtain 63 patients with pedigreed hypercholesterolemia satisfactory for his purpose, Burton Cohen (Seton Hall College of Medicine) had to screen 641 adults. The average pretreatment cholesterol level in this group was 338.4 mg./100 ml. In the final tally, 28 patients had finished 108 weeks of medication with an average decrement of 30.3% and 14 treated for 156 weeks had an average drop of 34.4%. But 9 of the 28 patients had higher levels at 108 weeks than at 52 weeks, the average increment being 15.5% (Cohen's dosage: sodium dextrothyroxine, one 2 mg. tablet on arising, increased by 2 mg. at a time in the first 20 weeks; total period of administration 28–156 weeks). It seems to me, furthermore, that an additional fact to be weighed in the balance is that, even though it may be easily shown that estrogens, nicotinic acid, dextrothyroxine, the sitosterols and cholestyramine, administered to men will considerably reduce their blood cholesterol levels, it has not been possible to present statistically satisfactory evidence that the infarction morbidity or mortality has been favorably reduced by this.

Burton M. Cohen. Sodium Dextrothyroxine Therapy for Hypercholesteremia: Three Years of Administration to Cardiovascular Subjects. Geriatrics 19:585, 1964.

"As far as I am concerned, the question is still wide open whether reduction in the levels of triglycerides or cholesterol truly confers protection against coronary sclerosis; but now I make bold to ask whether we really know if it is the elevated level of triglyceride or of cholesterol that best correlates with ischemic heart disease?"

Reply: *I* do not know, at any rate.

Maurice M. Best and Charles H. Duncan (Univ. of Louisville). Effects of Cholesterol-Lowering Drugs on Serum Triglycerides. Proc. Soc. Exper. Biol. & Med. 115:718, 1964.

"What is the position of cholestyramine resin (Cumid) in the treatment of hypercholesteremia?"

Reply: This drug, a bile acid–sequestering agent, promotes fecal excretion of bile acids and thus induces an increase in the rate of cholesterol conversion to bile acids in the liver, which in turn results in a diminution of plasma cholesterol levels. During treatment with 13.3 Gm. of the drug daily in four equally divided doses after each meal and at bedtime, Hashim and Van Itallie (St. Luke's Hospital, New York) were able to lower serum total cholesterol levels in 8 of 9 patients to the extent of 20–50%, the decreases being sustained for the duration of treatment. In 2 patients treatment was discontinued and started again to establish the reproducibility of the cholesterol-lowering effect. The drug occasionally produced gastrointestinal discomfort, ranging from slight distention to manifest peptic distress, but these symptoms tended to disappear after the first few weeks of therapy. The patients often preferred to mix the powder with a variety of foods such as fruit juices and applesauce, and some took it in capsule form. Some patients complained of constipation. Serum calcium, chloride, carbon dioxide values and serum alkaline phosphatase, prothrombin activity and serum proteins all remained at normal levels while the drug was being taken, and x-ray films of the liver of all 9 patients did not disclose evidence of enlargement or abnormal calcification. I think it should be added that in England, D. V. Datta and Sheila Sherlock felt it advisable to inject the fat-soluble vitamins A, D and K intramuscularly at 2 week intervals while using the resin because there have been a few instances of hypoprothrombinemia.

In familial cases, some investigators have found the drug effective, but often at the price of severe gastrointestinal side effects. The dosage has to be quite high; Horan's group (University of Tennessee) gave 15 Gm. daily to obtain much effect.

Sami A. Hashim and Theodore B. Van Itallie. Cholestyramine Resin Therapy for Hypercholesteremia. J.A.M.A. 192:289, Apr. 26, 1965. D. V. Datta and Sheila Sherlock. Treatment of Pruritus of Obstructive Jaundice with Cholestyramine. Brit. M. J. 1:216, Jan. 26, 1963. J. M. Horan, N. R. DiLuzio and J. N. Etteldorf. Use of Anion Exchange Resin in Treatment of Two Siblings with Familial Hypercholesteremia. J. Pediat. 64:201, 1964.

"Is there any basis for the rumor that alcohol is harmful in an individual with elevated serum cholesterol?"

Reply: At the University of Minnesota, several years ago, Grande and Amatuzio found that alcohol produced a significant increase of serum cholesterol concentration in dogs, particularly when they were given a high-fat diet. They then experimented with normal male prison inmates, who were taking a normal diet containing 38% fat calories. Fifty-nine individuals who received 3 oz. of 100 proof whiskey daily did not increase their serum cholesterol, but when the alcoholic supplement was raised to 9 oz. there was a small increase in serum cholesterol. These observers felt that the increase of 18 mg./100 ml. was statistically significant, but I think one may wonder whether our cholesterol determination methods are sufficiently refined to justify such a conclusion. At any rate, it certainly does not appear that the ingestion of alcohol *lowers* serum cholesterol.

Francisco Grande and Donald S. Amatuzio. Influence of Ethanol on Serum Cholesterol Concentration. Minnesota Med. 43:731, 1960.

"If one gives the rather new drug paromomycin (Humatin) orally for a number of weeks an abnormally high serum cholesterol can be brought down significantly in most patients, and the same thing can be accomplished with neomycin and kanamycin (Kantrex). How is this effect produced and does it have any significance regarding the etiology of atherosclerosis?"

Reply: The cholesterol-lowering effect is probably the result of an action on the intestinal flora; whether this also means reduction in atherosclerosis is *sub judice*. Thinking on this subject, Samuel's group (Long Island Jewish Hospital, New Hyde Park, N. Y.) has ingeniously suggested that the geographic differences in serum cholesterol levels of different populations may reflect environment-induced differences of normal intestinal bacteria.

Paul Samuel, Olya B. Shalchi and Charles M. Holtzman. Reduction of Serum Cholesterol Concentrations by Paromomycin (Humatin) in patients with Arteriosclerosis. Proc. Soc. Exper. Biol. & Med. 115:718, 1964.

"Granting that nicotinic acid reduces blood cholesterol levels pretty consistently, and usually does so without much accompanying deleterious side action, does it follow that the patient's life expectancy is increased as a result?"

Reply: I will counter with a question: Is it really established that "abnormal" cholesterol levels are accountable for untimely demise? As a matter of fact, in the institutionalized patients of Murray Mahl and Kurt Lange (New York Medical College) there was very poor correlation between cholesterol levels and evidence of peripheral or coronary arteriosclerosis, though admittedly in ambulatory groups with these diagnoses there was an elevation of cholesterol in 83% of cases. The necropsy analysis of the matter made by Wilens and Plair (New York University) disclosed that in the aortas of two of every three men examined, the sclerotic process is roughly commensurate with age, including persons with both abnormally high and low blood cholesterol values and obese as well as cachectic ones, hypertensives and prolonged diabetics. However, it appeared also to be evident in this study that the blood cholesterol levels and state of nutrition can be minor factors in retarding or accelerating the rate of development of the process at least in certain individuals.

Murray Mahl and Kurt Lange. Long-Term Study of Effect of Nicotinic Acid Medication on Hypercholesteremia. Am. J. M. Sc. 246:673, 1963. Sigmund L. Wilens and Cassius M. Plair. Blood Cholesterol, Nutrition and Atherosclerosis. Arch. Int. Med. 116:373, 1965.

"I have transferred one of my atherosclerotic patients, an individual with peripheral arterial insufficiency and a high serum cholesterol, to sitosterol (Cytellin) with excellent results so far as lowering of the hypercholesteremia is concerned. I am considering a trial in a few other patients; why is the agent not more generally used?"

Reply: The drug is somewhat more expensive than some of the others, perhaps not as effective in lowering cholesterol in all instances, and some people undeniably grow tired of taking a tablespoonful of the suspension before each meal. Some individuals object to the taste also, but certainly the few complaints of anorexia and slight diarrhea that are made should not militate against use of the drug.

Charles H. Duncan and Maurice M. Best (Univ. of Louisville). Long-Term Use of Sitosterol (Cytellin) as a Hypocholesteremic Agent. J. Kentucky M. A. 61:45, 1963.

"I am trying, in such time as I have, to keep abreast of the tremendously interesting ideas that are developing with regard to the pathogenesis of atherosclerosis, but from a practical standpoint I want very badly to know whether there is any way of predicting in the individual patient which, if any, of his various arterial systems is going to become involved with the process. I do not feel that any of the drugs or other measures designed to reduce hypercholesteremia has been convincingly shown to influence atherosclerosis, but I shall resort to their use if I can learn that my patient really is threatened. Have criteria developed upon which to base a prediction?"

Reply: No.

ATHLETIC PERFORMANCE

"What is truly the position of the amphetamines, such drugs as Benzedrine and Dexedrine, with relation to athletic performance?"

Reply: In studies in man it has been easy to show the promotion of wakefulness by the drugs and evidences of increased alertness and attentiveness as well as quantitatively better work performance. But it has been apparent that this stimulation, which may amount to euphoria, reflects more an increased incentive to work than an increase in work efficiency. However, Smith and Beecher were able to show in carefully executed studies that the performance of highly trained athletes is significantly improved, and they thought it likely that this was due to the psychic stimulation, improved coordination and form, increased strength and endurance, and increased mental and physical activation. Whether the drugs produced judgment distortion was open to question. These findings regarding improvement in athletic performance under the influence of amphetamines certainly should not be construed as sanctioning their use for that purpose, since such use may not only lead to overexertion with consequences that may be very unfortunate but would also imply a flouting of the traditions of true sportsmanship which brand such practices as ethically undesirable and dishonorable.

G. M. Smith and H. K. Beecher. Amphetamine Sulfate and Athletic Performance. I. Objective Effects. J.A.M.A. 170: 542, 1959.

"Is there reliable evidence that use of an anabolic steroid improves athletic performance?"

Reply: At the University of California, Fowler's group studied this matter in both trained and untrained college students and found no justification for use of such drugs to improve the efficiency of physical performance.

William M. Fowler, Jr., Gerald W. Gardner and Glen H. Egstrom. Effect of an Anabolic Steroid on Physical Performance of Young Men. J. Appl. Physiol. 20:1038, 1965.

ATOPIC DERMATITIS

"In atopic dermatitis might one be justified in trying adrenergic-blocking drugs because of the abnormal and excessive vasoconstrictor responses of the cutaneous vessels that have sometimes been demonstrated in these patients?"

Reply: In India, B. S. Verma and associates felt that the following things suggest a possible defect in adrenergic mechanisms in atopic dermatitis: (1) a low blood pressure during exacerbation of the disease, (2) a "flat" glucose tolerance curve, (3) delayed accommodation to variations in environmental temperature, (4) disturbances in sweating and (5) epinephrine-resistant eosinophilia during stress. They therefore used guanethidine (Ismelin) for antagonism of the excessive acetylcholine present in the skin of these patients, and phenoxybenzamine (Dibenzyline) to annul the excessive vasoconstrictor action of the cutaneous vessels. The results were gratifying, but the series of cases was very small and much more work will be needed to establish the usefulness of such therapy.

B. S. Verma, O. D. Gulati, S. D. Gokhale and K. C. Shah. Guanethidine (Ismelin) and Phenoxybenzamine (Dibenzyline) in Atopic Dermatitis: Clinical Trial. Arch. Dermat. 90:414, 1964.

AVITAMINOSES

"In our part of the country there is a great deal of vitamin A prescribing, and most of it does not seem justified to me. Would you kindly supply a statement regarding the uses of vitamin A?"

Reply: Vitamin A is essential to the growth and development of children and is therefore given to them as a dietary supplement in economically favored countries. True vitamin A deficiency is characterized principally by night blindness (nyctalopia), changes in the skin and certain corneal symptoms to which are applied the term "keratomalacia." Sometimes in xerophthalmia, a designation for vitamin A deficiency that perhaps overstresses the eye symptoms, vaginitis is also present as well as keratinization of the bronchial epithelium. The latter causes atelectasis and bronchiectasis and complicates pneumonia.

Vitamin A deficiency is easily cured by placing the patient on a diet containing sufficient vitamin A or its precursor, carotene, or by giving vitamin A or carotene as drugs. The eye symptoms usually abate in a few days and are soon completely gone, but some of the other manifestations require several months to disappear. Vitamin A administration will not improve night vision in individuals who are not suffering from deficiency of the vitamin, nor has it been established that vitamin A will prevent upper respiratory tract infections or, indeed, any other infections. Its alleged value in preventing the formation of renal calculi or in the treatment of anemia, thyrotoxicosis, neuropathies, burns or ulcers has not been proved.

This agent is being widely employed nowadays in the therapy of a diverse group of maladies in which there is believed to be abnormal keratinization as a reflection of disturbed vitamin A metabolism. The principal diseases, as listed by dermatologists currently enthusiastic about this therapy, are ichthyosis, pityriasis rubra pilaris, keratosis follicularis (Darier's disease), pachyonychia congenita, keratoderma palmaris et plantaris, phrynoderma, xerosis, lichen spinulosus, porokeratosis, keratosis pilaris, lichen lividus, ichthyosis follicularis, senile keratoses, chronic actinic dermatitis, acne vulgaris, keratoderma climactericum, abnormal callous formation, buccal leukoplakia and kraurosis vulvae. It is not difficult to be somewhat less convinced of the efficacy of this therapy than are some of those who are practicing it. Oftentimes 18–24 months are required to bring results, and some of the patients have not had low plasma–vitamin A titers to begin with. It may be that faulty utilization is the basic trouble, or that the vitamin in these cases is not endowed with full biologic properties, or that the tissues are somehow handicapped in their utilization of it, but none of these things is established. There have been reports from the Continent of effective use in the distressing nasal maladies, ozena and rhinopharyngitis chronica sicca.

"What symptoms are caused by the excessive ingestion of vitamin A?"

Reply: The minimum daily requirement of vitamin A is not known with certainty but appears to be 1500 U.S.P. units for infants, 3000 for children and 4000 for adults. It is customary to provide about twice the usual adult requirement to women during pregnancy and lactation, but I do not know that this is necessary. Therapeutic dosages should probably be at least three times as high as the minimal daily requirements. Dosage of the order of 100,000–300,000 units daily is often used in the empiric employments of vitamin A for maladies other than avitaminosis A, but I doubt that dosage above 25,000 units is rational in many instances.

When vitamin A is ingested in highly excessive quantities during long periods, a state of hypervitaminosis A may develop with such symptoms as irritability, miosis, anorexia, loss of hair, dry skin, pruritus, tender extremities, hepatomegaly and splenomegaly, roentgenographic evidence of elevation of the periosteum of the long bones, high serum vitamin A, increased serum lipids, hypoplastic anemia, leukopenia, clubbing of the fingers and advanced skeletal development. Uniquely, Marie and Sée reported a bulging fontanel in association with this syndrome. The symptoms regress slowly during several months after administration of the vitamin is stopped. Most of these cases have resulted from administration by overanxious mothers of enormous doses of vitamin A preparations to infants or young children, dosage of the order of 200,000 units or more daily. However, the case of Elliott and Dryer was that of a 21-year-old woman who took 160,000–180,000 units daily for 7 months (without curing her acne!).

Overdosage with carotene causes carotenemia and accumulation of the yellow material in the skin, the latter being in itself not harmful. The patient of Reich and associates was a middle-aged woman who drank 2 quarts of tomato juice daily for several years. It is of interest that the severe illness caused by eating polar bear liver — learned the hard way by arctic explorers — is due to the extremely high vitamin A content of this tissue.

J. Marie and G. Sée. Acute Hypervitaminosis A of the Infant: Its Clinical Manifestation with Benign Acute Hydrocephalus and Pronounced Bulge of Fontanel; Clinical and Biologic Study. Am. J. Dis. Child. 87:731, 1954. R. A. Elliott, Jr. and R. L. Dryer. Hypervitaminosis A; Report of a Case in an Adult. J.A.M.A. 161:1157, 1956. P. Reich, H. Shwachman and J. M. Craig. Lycopenemia. A Variant of Carotenemia. New England J. Med. 262:263, 1960.

"When is it advisable to use the total vitamin B complex rather than the individual constituents?"

Reply: Eleven of the 12 known nutritive factors of the B complex have been obtained in crystalline form: thiamine, riboflavin, nicotinic acid, pyridoxine, pantothenic acid, choline, biotin, inositol, para-aminobenzoic acid, pteroylglutamic acid (folic acid) and cyanocobalamine (vitamin B_{12}). However, naturally occurring deficiency syndromes associated with lack of only six of these ingredients are known,

namely thiamine, riboflavin, nicotinic acid, pyridoxine, pteroylglutamic acid and cyanocobalamine. In the macrocytic anemias expressive of folic acid and vitamin B_{12} lack, it is customary to use these two agents themselves and not to give them in the form of the B complex. But in thiamine, riboflavin or nicotinic acid deficiencies it is probably good practice to use the complex, supplemented with the predominantly deficient vitamin, because these deficiencies rarely occur singly. Pyridoxine deficiency has been reported as an isolated entity.

"What untoward reactions have been associated with administration of vitamin B complex or its constituents?"

Reply: An instance of circulatory collapse following intravenous administration of a vitamin B complex preparation was reported by Chitwood and Moore, the only such occurrence that has come to my attention. But several reports have appeared of an anaphylactic type of reaction in patients apparently sensitized by repeated injections of thiamine. Skin tests are fairly reliable in detecting thiamine sensitivity, the scratch being superior to the intradermal test. Symptoms resembling those of hyperthyroidism have also been reported, and it has often been observed that thiamine administration is followed by an unexplained transitory increase of riboflavin excretion in the urine.

Nicotinamide does not cause any deleterious effects, but nicotinic acid, in addition to the flushing which manifests its selective vasodilator action, sometimes causes urticaria, nausea and vomiting, occasionally circulatory collapse or a severe anaphylactic reaction, the two latter occurrences being associated with intravenous administration. Barker reported slight and reversible alterations in liver function tests in a few individuals receiving the high dosage that is used in treating hypercholesterolemia; many persons have had a slight elevation in blood sugar and a positive glucose tolerance test, both also reversible.

No instances of riboflavin or pyridoxine toxicity have been reported to my knowledge.

W. R. Chitwood and C. D. Moore. Anaphylactic Shock Following Intravenous Administration of Vitamin B Complex. J.A.M.A. 148:461, 1952. N. W. Barker. The Effect of Niacin on the Blood Cholesterol. Illinois M. J. 116:138, 1959.

"Are there legitimate uses of vitamin C (ascorbic acid) other than in the therapy of scurvy?"

Reply: Defective formation of intercellular ground substance in the capillaries is presumed to underlie the bleeding in scurvy, and since vitamin C quickly terminates such bleeding it is assumed to promote collagen and reticulum formation. Regeneration of connective tissue can actually be demonstrated within 40 hours. It is probably this same action that makes vitamin C useful to hasten wound healing. Deposition of lime salts in osteoid tissues appears to be increased also, and the hematopoietic activity of folic acid is promoted by the vitamin in scorbutic patients as in normal individuals.

On the experimental level ascorbic acid effects complement and antibody production and possibly thus increases resistance to infection, especially with viruses. In fact, a virucidal effect can be demonstrated in vitro. Ascorbic acid stores may be severely depleted during the course of infectious diseases; capillary resistance decreases and susceptibility to the action of certain toxins appears to increase. These things seem to justify the use of ascorbic acid as a drug in severe infections and in individuals otherwise seriously ill. There is some evidence that animals with low vitamin C level are more susceptible to shock than normal animals, and since the vitamin C level is said to diminish in the human after the performance of major surgical procedures, the suggestion has been made that the preoperative intravenous administration of vitamin C might be of value in preventing shock. In fact, Crandon and associates found an average fall of 17% in plasma ascorbic acid in 105 patients during operation.

J. H. Crandon, B. Landau, S. Mikal, J. Balmanno, M. Jefferson and N. Mahoney. Ascorbic Acid Economy in Surgical Patients as Indicated by Blood Ascorbic Acid Levels. New England J. Med. 258:105, 1958.

"Have untoward symptoms ever been associated with the administration of vitamin C (ascorbic acid)?"

Reply: Not to my knowledge. I believe that as much as 10 Gm. has been given in a single dose without causing trouble.

"Other than in certain of the tetanies, what uses of vitamin D have been found profitable?"

Reply: We have no effective therapy in renal rickets unless the condition can be corrected by surgical measures. But ordinary rickets and osteomalacia are caused by deficiency in vitamin D (with associated calcium-phosphorus imbalance), in some other factor not yet determined, and, in the case of rickets, by insufficient exposure to sunlight during the winter months. Both maladies are successfully prevented and treated by the use of vitamin D preparations. The administration of such preparations to nursing mothers much lessens the incidence of rickets in breast-fed infants, although Pincus's group noted paradoxically that vitamin D worsens the tendency to hypocalcemia when given to infants during the first week of life. Administration of phosphorus is not indicated, because we are dealing with failure of the calcifying mechanism rather than faulty absorption of bone salts.

The use of calciferol faithfully for a number of months appears to cure the tuberculous lesion, lupus vulgaris, in a considerable proportion of instances. For best results treatment should be prolonged for several months after complete clinical recovery. Skin lesions closely resembling those of lupus vulgaris are found in Boeck's sarcoidosis, a diffuse reticuloendotheliosis with formation of folliculoid tissue affecting particularly lymphoid and hematopoietic structures. Calciferol has been used effectively in a few of these cases also. Unfortunately, there is usually considerable residual scarring after the lupus lesions are arrested. A bacteriostatic action of calciferol on the bacillus of tuberculosis cannot be demonstrated in vitro, and as an active tuberculous process seems often to be demonstrable by laboratory methods in patients apparently clinically cured by calciferol, perhaps we should not too enthusiastically speak of "cures" in these cases. Some men now prefer to use both calciferol and streptomycin, and it would appear that the full antituberculosis treatment, employing isoniazid and p-aminosalicylic acid, is entirely superseding calciferol therapy. The thing that initiated trial of calciferol was the observation that measures used off and on throughout the years, such as specialized diets, cod liver oil and ultraviolet irradiation, all supply large amounts of vitamin D.

It has frequently been both affirmed and denied that the vitamin D carrier, cod liver oil, sprayed from an ordinary atomizer, is analgesic in instances of laryngeal pain in the tuberculous patient who is not responding to the systemic administration of chemotherapeutic agents.

Whether the local application of cod liver oil is helpful in promoting wound healing in man is not clearly decided, but animal experimentation is rather suggestively in favor of it. The oil, in the form of a 70% ointment, is often applied freely to burns of the face, head, neck, genitalia and anal regions, where compression bandages are not applied and the dressings are therefore changed frequently; however, Grayzell and Schapiro reported good results in severe burn cases when the cod liver oil pressure dressings had remained in place for a week.

J. B. Pincus, I. F. Gittleman and A. E. Sobel. Influence of

Vitamin D on Serum Calcium and Inorganic Phosphate in the Neonatal Period. Ann. New York Acad. Sc. 64:424, 1956. H. G. Grayzell and S. Schapiro. Wound Healing with Cod Liver Oil Ointment. West. J. Surg. 64:558, 1956.

"There does not appear to be clear understanding in our group of the respective positions of calcium, vitamin D, parathyroid and dihydrotachysterol in the therapy of tetany of various types. Would you kindly set out the problem clearly?"

Reply: Tetany, characterized by carpopedal spasm and laryngospasm, sometimes by edema of the dorsal surfaces of the hands and feet and in severe cases by generalized convulsions and unconsciousness, is most frequently seen in association with rickets in young children, probably as the result of decreased absorption of calcium in the absence of sufficient vitamin D. The tetany of sprue is likely of the same nature. Frank tetany during pregnancy and lactation is rare, but tetanoid manifestations, such as irritability, painful leg cramps, insomnia, transient paresthesias and edemas occur commonly. This type may be due to loss of calcium, first to the fetus and then in the milk, but it is also possible that in these cases a latent tendency to parathyroid deficiency is merely uncovered. True postoperative tetany, rarely seen nowadays, does not necessarily mean that the surgical technique has been poor since the parathyroid glands are often eccentrically located and easily damaged. Tetany associated with alkalosis occurs when there has been persistent vomiting, hysterical hyperpnea or excessive administration of alkali. A type of idiopathic tetany is recognized in adults, but most of these cases are probably due to vitamin D deficiency and hence are of the infantile type. Transient tetany may also unquestionably appear at the height of serious toxic attacks such as acute poisoning or a febrile state. The rare tetany of the newborn is due to temporary hypofunction of the parathyroid glands, or in some instances to prelactational feeding of alkaline mixtures. Tetany occurs commonly in osteomalacia.

Most of these tetanies are characterized by a decrease in blood calcium during the period of active symptoms and a rise in blood calcium as improvement takes place. The exceptions are the gastric (excessive vomiting), excessive alkali and hyperpneic forms, in all of which there is a state of alkalosis but normal blood calcium. The important matter in tetany seems to be not how much calcium there is in the blood but how much of it is ionized. A shift to the alkaline side is thought to decrease ionization. There are undoubtedly other factors of etiologic importance in tetany, however, because calcium deficiency and the full symptomatology of the malady are not necessarily parallel phenomena. A low plasma magnesium content has been reported in the etiologic role in tetany also. Probably full understanding will come only when we can properly interpret relationships between calcium, magnesium, phosphorus, carbohydrate and protein metabolisms.

Of course, in the alkalotic cases the principal indication is to overcome the alkalosis, usually easily accomplished if overdosage of alkalies has been at fault. If the trouble has been excessive vomiting, physiologic saline solution should be given intravenously to compensate for the chloride loss. In fact, chlorides are lost from the system in any type of alkalosis even though there is no vomiting. Ammonium chloride, to increase the ionization of calcium, may be given by mouth in 1 Gm. dosage or intravenously in amounts of 300–500 ml. of 0.82% solution, the latter first being tested to see whether it causes hemolysis. In the hyperpneic cases it may be difficult to control the causative hysterical breathing, but inhalation of 5% carbon dioxide and 95% oxygen will often do it, or the patient may be asked to breathe into a paper bag to increase the carbon dioxide content of the inhaled air.

Parathyroid was formerly much used in treating postoperative tetany but has been superseded almost completely by dihydrotachysterol unless very quick action is required. The reasons for this are its excessive potency, the considerable individual variations in response to it and the fact that after a few weeks of therapy the effectiveness of the drug often diminishes strikingly. Instances of the latter sort may not reflect so much the development of true resistance as the introduction of factors conducive to increase in phosphorus intake. In infantile tetany the use of parathyroid has been extremely variable and perhaps, on the whole, unsatisfactory. It has been used in small dosage with more satisfaction in the maternal cases but not in sprue. In the gastric, hyperpneic and excessive-alkali forms of tetany, in which serum calcium is normal, parathyroid has not been effectively used. It is definitely contraindicated to combat the tetanoid symptoms of uremia because there is evidence that the activity of the parathyroid glands is increased in chronic nephritis.

The advantages of dihydrotachysterol over parathyroid are that it may be given by mouth and that patients do not become refractory to it. It is used as a substitute for parathyroid extract in all situations in which that drug is effective and, being slower in action, the likelihood of a dangerous degree of hypercalcemia is less. Full effects are usually not achieved under 7–10 days when the drug is administered by mouth daily; it is not given by injection. Administration of both calcium and vitamin D along with the dihydrotachysterol is advisable; perhaps in some cases ammonium chloride should be given also.

Most patients with tetany with a low blood calcium, which excludes the alkalotic cases, can be handled through use of calcium salts without resorting to such potent agents as dihydrotachysterol or parathyroid extract.

Bed rest causes decalcification, with the threat of urolithiasis as a result of the large amounts of calcium being excreted. The indication is to administer fluids and not calcium and to terminate bed rest as soon as possible.

Some loss of calcium from the bones occurs at times in menopausal women, but this loss is apparently due to some elusive endocrine dysfunction and is not made good by administration of calcium. Demineralization of the bones occurs to some extent in severe hyperthyroidism, but remedial measures must be directed primarily toward cure of the hyperthyroidism rather than of the demineralization. Administration of calcium salts may be helpful, however. The osteoporosis of old age is due to lessened activity of the osteoblasts, which lay down new bone, in comparison with that of the osteoclasts, which destroy bone. Calcium is therefore not the remedy for this malady.

The administration of calcium, vitamin D and dihydrotachysterol is advisable in attempting to raise the serum calcium level in sprue, but since this complex malady apparently reflects a functional interference with absorption of many things and thereby the establishment of a vicious circle of symptoms, it is not to be expected that the mere supplying of these agents will in itself effect a cure of the disease.

"I am aware that dihydrotachysterol, sometimes used in the treatment of tetany, is a dangerous drug because it can easily cause hypercalcemia. But what of calcium itself; may it not cause some trouble also?"

Reply: Intravenous administration of a calcium salt will cause nausea and vomiting, and a too rapid rise in serum calcium titer may plunge the heart into ventricular fibrillation. Even slow administration is likely to make the patient feel that he is on fire and to cause his blood pressure to fall moderately, both effects being the result of vasodilatation from calcium's local action on the vessels, which is probably effected through alterations in the permeability of cell membranes.

Calcium salts tend to precipitate locally when injected intramuscularly in infants. Cases have indeed been reported in which calcium salts were not only precipitated at the sites of injection but also at remote points in the body. Accidental injection outside the vein induces an unpleasant reaction and occasionally slough. Calcium and digitalis should probably not be used together because calcium allegedly synergizes digitalis and may possibly increase its toxicity.

"What are the evidences of vitamin D intoxication and how might it be combated?"

Reply: Practically all the instances of severe vitamin D toxicity have occurred when high dosage was being employed during long periods in the treatment of either rheumatoid arthritis or lupus vulgaris. I have seen no reports of toxicity in association with the use of high dosage in the rare cases of "refractory" rickets, even though as much as 1,000,000 units daily may be used for cure in such instances and half as much for maintenance.

There is usually an excessively high blood calcium and sometimes a low blood phosphorus titer, the latter possibly reflecting secondary hyperparathyroidism. Sometimes the hypercalcemia persists for weeks after vitamin D administration has been stopped, and during the period of its presence the walls of blood vessels and adjacent tissues become involved in a process of fibrinous degeneration, necrosis and calcification. The special vulnerability of the kidneys to this sort of reaction, as demonstrated both in the laboratory and clinically, is conceivably a reflection of the necessity to excrete urine with a very high calcium content. Widespread metastatic calcification has been found in some cases coming to necropsy. Treatment of vitamin D intoxication had been largely symptomatic prior to the recognition of an apparent antagonism of vitamin D and the adrenal glucocorticoids. Nowadays very quick recoveries are accomplished with the use of corticosteroids; for example, in the 2 patients of Verner and associates, who presented clinical syndromes of mental confusion, dehydration, polyuria and hypokalemic alkalosis, there was sharp improvement in mental status in 48 hours and return of serum calcium to normal in 8 and 13 days, respectively.

J. V. Verner, F. L. Engel and H. T. McPherson. Vitamin D Intoxication: Report of Two Cases Treated with Cortisone. Ann. Int. Med. 48:765, 1958.

BACTERIAL ENDOCARDITIS

"There is surprisingly little information available on the problem of therapy in subacute bacterial endocarditis due to a gram-positive coccus in a hypersensitized patient. But I happen to have such a patient at the moment. What do I do?"

Reply: Thomas Theobald and William Grace (St. Vincent's Hospital, New York) found the combined use of an antihistaminic and a corticosteroid, while continuing administration of penicillin in the necessarily high dosage, entirely satisfactory in handling the situation in their patient. Parabromdylamine maleate (Dimetane) was given three times daily in 12 mg. dosage with 100 mg. prednisone (Meticorten, etc.) daily in divided doses. Intravenous penicillin was given in dosage of 120,000,000 units daily in continuous infusion for 40 consecutive days, and another 450 mg. parabromdylamine was given daily with the penicillin. In Columbus, Ohio, Michael Apicella's group used cephalothin (Keflin) effectively in 1 of their patients, infusing 2 grams during 20 minutes every 6 hours for 22 days and thereafter 1 gram every 6 hours for 6 days.

Thomas John Theobald and William J. Grace. Subacute Bacterial Endocarditis in Patients Allergic to Penicillin: Possible Immunologic Mechanisms. New York J. Med. 63:3570, Dec. 15, 1963. A. Jarrell Raper and V. Eric Kemp. Use of Steroids in Penicillin-Sensitive Patients with Bacterial Endocarditis. New England J. Med. 273: 297, Aug. 5, 1965. Michael A. Apicella, Robert L. Perkins and Samuel Saslaw. Treatment of Bacterial Endocarditis with Cephalosporin Derivatives in Penicillin-Allergic Patients. New England J. Med. 274:1002, May 5, 1966.

"How should I treat my case of Streptococcus faecalis endocarditis?"

Reply: Penicillin alone will rarely kill this enterococcal organism, and it is also usually resistant to streptomycin. However, the combined use of these two antibiotics has often been effective. Eight of the 9 patients of Ernest Jawetz and Minetta Sonne were bacteriologically cured by the combination. Dosage was 20 million to 60 million units of penicillin G and 1–2 grams of streptomycin daily, parenterally.

Ernest Jawetz and Minetta Sonne. Penicillin-Streptomycin Treatment of Enterococcal Endocarditis. New England J. Med. 274:710, Mar. 31, 1966.

BACTEROIDES INFECTION

"Our laboratory has just returned the diagnosis of bacteroides septicemia in a patient of mine who is very ill. The organism appears to be sensitive to both tetracycline and chloramphenicol. In addition to using these agents, is there any other drug that you might suggest?"

Reply: In the series of Tynes and Frommeyer, at the University of Alabama, the 9 patients who received sulfonamides in addition to antibiotics all recovered, whereas the overall mortality was 20% in the 25 patients. In in vitro studies more recently, Keusch and O'Connell, in Buffalo, have found cephalothin

(Keflin) and, to a lesser extent, ampicillin (Polycillin) effective; penicillin G also in very large quantities.

Bayard S. Tynes and Walter B. Frommeyer, Jr. Bacteroides Septicemia: Cultural, Clinical and Therapeutic Features in Series of 25 Patients. Ann. Int. Med. 56:12, 1962. Gerald T. Keusch and Cornelius J. O'Connell. The Susceptibility of Bacteroides to the Penicillins and Cephalothin. Am. J. M. Sc. 251:428, 1966.

BALANTIDIASIS

"We have understandable satisfaction. The pathologist in our northern small town hospital has just made the diagnosis of balantidiasis in a young patient who has flown in from the West Indies with dysentery. What is the latest drug magic in this tropical disease?"

Reply: At the Hospital for Tropical Diseases, in London, Bell has treated a boy of 5 years very satisfactorily with 250 mg. of ampicillin (Penbritin) every 6 hours for 10 days.

S. Bell. Trial of Ampicillin (Penbritin) in Balantidial Dysentery. J. Trop. Med. & Hyg. 66:309, 1963.

BEHÇET'S SYNDROME

"I have a case of the rare malady comprising recurrent oral and genital ulcerations and hypopyon iritis, known as Behçet's syndrome. What is the most promising therapy?"

Reply: This disease runs such a variable course that it is dangerous to assert the ameliorative value of any agent. However, Norman Sigel and Roger Larson, in Fresno, California, have reported a very interesting case in a 23-year-old Negro female in which there were serious neurologic involvements that appeared to be reversed and suppressed by the use of corticosteroids.

Norman Sigel and Roger Larson. Behçet's Syndrome. Arch. Int. Med. 115:203, 1965.

BELL'S PALSY

"Is there any rationale for using the corticosteroids or corticotropin in treatment of Bell's palsy?"

Reply: Well, if it is assumed that there is some swelling of the facial nerve in the facial canal, which I believe has been sometimes demonstrated, then it is rational to invoke the antiphlogistic action of the corticosteroids. But clinical evidence of their efficacy is not very impressive. The recent claim of fine results from using corticotropin (ACTH), made by Taverner and associates, in England, is interesting but needs independent confirmation.

D. Taverner, M. E. Fearnley, F. Kemble, D. W. Miles and O. A. Peiris. Prevention of Denervation in Bell's Palsy. Brit. M. J. 1:391, Feb. 12, 1966.

BENIGN RECURRENT INTRAHEPATIC CHOLESTASIS

"A patient has just entered my practice with the very rare malady, benign recurrent intrahepatic cholestasis. Has effective therapy been developed?"

Reply: In Cincinnati, Earl Spiegel's group has reported the case of a 14-year-old girl with this malady in whom cholestyramine in daily dosage of 16 Gm. divided into four portions effected considerable clinical improvement. There was a decrease in the abnormally increased serum bile acid concentration and the pruritus was relieved, these changes being accompanied by a decrease in the serum alkaline phosphatase and total bilirubin; bromsulfalein retention was no longer abnormal, and there was no histologic evidence of cholestasis.

Earl L. Spiegel, William Schubert, Eugene Perrin and Leon Schiff. Benign Recurrent Intrahepatic Cholestasis, with Response to Cholestyramine. Am. J. Med. 39:682, 1965.

BILIARY DYSKINESIA

"Why is it that we can accomplish so little with drugs in biliary dyskinesia?"

Reply: In this distressing entity, in which after removal of the gallbladder the patient suffers considerable pain from a spastically contracted sphincter of Oddi and the damming back of bile into biliary ducts that have not sufficiently dilated, there is the pure and simple pharmacologic indication to provide drugs to effect continuous relaxation of the sphincter. We do not meet the situation with conspicuous success, probably because the sphincter of Oddi is under both sympathetic and parasympathetic influences as well as that of the hormone, cholecystokinin. Epinephrine will completely relax it under experimental conditions, but this fact is of no clinical importance because the duration of the effect is very brief and there is a considerable accompanying blood pressure rise. Papaverine relaxes the sphincter also, in this case through action directly exerted on the musculature, but this action too is very fleeting and accompanied by some depression of blood pressure and increase in respiratory volume under experimental circumstances. Atropine relaxes the sphincter beautifully and for a prolonged period in the anesthetized dog, when it is under

the stimulating influence at the moment of a continuous intravenous drip of neostigmine (Prostigmin), but the dosage is out of all proportion to what could be considered therapeutic. In man this is the case also; atropine is effective but the side effects of the dosage required are prohibitive.

"In the (fortunately!) rather rare case of biliary dyskinesia in our practice we have not had success with conventional analgesic measures; is there any 'unorthodox' therapy that has been used successfully?"

Reply: I have not seen any further reports of the following, but a few years ago George Parson (Southern Clinic, Texarkana, Texas) observed several patients in whom this pain was relieved almost immediately and without emesis by 1/40 gr. apomorphine hydrochloride given subcutaneously.

George W. Parson. Specific for Relief of Pain in Biliary Dyskinesia. Ann. Int. Med. 52:444, 1960.

"It seems to me that papaverine with its directly exerted relaxing effect on smooth musculature should be an excellent drug for relief of the symptoms of biliary dyskinesia, in which drugs are needed to effect continuous relaxation of the sphincter of Oddi, but I have not been able to use it with satisfaction. Why does it fail, and could this failure be remedied?"

Reply: It is unreasonable to expect very much effect from this drug when given orally because it is very quickly bound inactively to plasma proteins and thus rendered therapeutically ineffective. However, if one were to administer it in a rectal suppository so that it was being continuously absorbed into the blood stream it might be expected that there would always be some arriving there and able to exert therapeutic action before being pocketed away in the protein binding. I would suggest trial of a rectal suppository containing 200 mg. at 3 hour intervals throughout the day and one of 600 mg. the last thing at night. This therapy might just possibly turn the trick; it is sometimes effective in an individual with a recent coronary infarction.

BRONCHIECTASIS

"In many of my patients with moderate degrees of bronchiectasis I am able to afford considerable relief through use of Tedral, which contains ephedrine, theophylline and phenobarbital, the two latter ingredients apparently counteracting the 'nervousness' and tachycardia and sweating that ephedrine often causes when used in effective dosage alone. But in a patient who is also hyper-

tensive I am fearful of using any type of sympathomimetic drug such as ephedrine, or even isoproterenol (Isuprel) administered from a nebulizer. What would you recommend in such a case?"

Reply: Simply to stay away from the sympathomimetic amines, as you are doing, foregoing attempt to reduce mucosal congestion, and attempting to lessen the muscle spasm through use of aminophylline, well administered as rectal suppository (125, 250, 500 mg. sizes) or orally as Elixophyllin in dosage of 5 teaspoonfuls or more several times daily (bear in mind that the patient is getting a good deal of alcohol in this preparation). Choledyl, which is choline theophyllinate, is also sometimes effectively used in dosage of 100–200 mg.

"What is the preferred antibiotic in the treatment of bronchiectasis?"

Reply: This is simply a matter of determining the sensitivity of the organisms cultured and being guided thereby in choice of the drug.

"What are the principal mucolytic agents that might be helpful in bronchiectasis?"

Reply: Alevaire, Tergemist, Tween 80, Mucomyst, Varidase, Dornavac, Tryptar, Chymar. The nature of action of these various agents is discussed in a Reply in the section on asthma in this volume.

BRONCHITIS—EMPHYSEMA

"Now that we are beginning to recognize here in the United States a higher morbidity from chronic bronchitis than in former times, we must of course face up to the therapy. What has been the experience with antibiotic regimes?"

Reply: The earlier reports came from Britain of course, where the disease has long been recognized as one of both high incidence and contributory mortality. In 1958, Buchanan and associates reported favorably on the use of tetracycline at least from the standpoint of subjective improvement. Then in 1961, the Bronchitis Subcommittee of the British Tuberculosis Association published a second favorable report on the daily administration of either tetracycline or potassium penicillin V. More recently, Fear and Edwards found a statistically significant result in favor of antibiotic-treated groups. There have also been favorable reports in the United States. I cite that of Norman's group (Johns Hopkins University), and Dowling's group (University of Chicago); tetracycline had been used in both

of these studies. However, not all of the studies have resulted in favor of antibiotic therapy. For example, Pridie and associates, in London, performed a double-blind study of oxytetracycline, a penicillin-sulfonamide combination and a placebo, and were unable to recommend any of these drug regimens for the control of winter bronchitis. It appears, therefore, that more study must be done, even though there is presently a preponderance of favorable observations; I say advisedly that more investigation needs to be undertaken because it is quite a responsibility to embark a patient upon an onerous course of therapy with expensive drugs unless one is sure of one's ground.

E. C. Fear and Gordon Edwards. Antibiotic Regimens in Chronic Bronchitis. Brit. J. Dis. Chest 56:153, 1962. John Buchanan, W. Watson Buchanan, A. G. Melrose, J. B. McGinness and A. U. Price. Long-Term Prophylactic Administration of Tetracycline to Chronic Bronchitics. Lancet 2:719, 1958. British Tuberculosis Association, Bronchitis Subcommittee, R. S. Francis, J. R. May and C. C. Spicer. Chemotherapy of Bronchitis: Influence of Penicillin and Tetracycline Administered Daily or Intermittently for Exacerbations. Brit. M. J. 2:979, Oct. 14, 1961. Phillip S. Norman, Edward W. Hook, Robert G. Petersdorf, Leighton E. Cluff, Malcolm P. Godfrey and Allan H. Levy. Long-Term Tetracycline Treatment of Chronic Bronchitis. J.A.M.A. 179:833, March 17, 1962. Harry F. Dowling, Mark H. Lepper and George Gee Jackson. Suppressive Therapy of Chronic Bronchial Infections. Clin. Pharmacol. & Therap. 3:564, 1962. Ronald B. Pridie, Naomi Datta, D. G. Massey, Graham W. Poole, J. Schneeweiss and Peter Stradling. Trial of Continuous Winter Chemotherapy in Chronic Bronchitis. Lancet 2: 723, Oct. 1, 1960.

"My own experience has not convinced me that the use of antibiotics in the treatment of exacerbations of chronic bronchitis is really profitable, but I have not tried the newer penicillins. Has anyone assessed their position in this area?"

Reply: In Belfast, P. C. Elmes and associates carefully studied the matter, using ampicillin (Polycillin). Twenty-eight pairs of patients were included in a sequential trial in which all patients were treated intensively with bronchodilator drugs and physiotherapy. One member of each pair received bacteriologically effective doses of ampicillin for 7 days, while the other member of the pair received a placebo. Sequential analysis of the results yielded no conclusive evidence that ampicillin was beneficial.

P. C. Elmes, T. K. C. King, J. H. M. Langlands, J. A. Mackay, W. F. M. Wallace, O. L. Wade and T. S. Wilson. Value of Ampicillin in the Hospital Treatment of Exacerbations of Chronic Bronchitis. Brit. M. J. 2:904, Oct. 16, 1965.

"The teaching has long been that one should not attempt to relieve the intense dyspnea in patients with chronic bronchitis and/or emphysema with opiates. Is this attitude justified?"

Reply: Yes, I believe that it is, for not only is the view derived from clinical impressions but it is also fully supported by the recent observations of Murray and Grant in Edinburgh. The scientifically controlled study of these investigators caused them to conclude that opiates should not be given to patients with chronic ventilatory failure, even for the relief of severe dyspnea.

W. D. Murray and I. W. B. Grant. Effect of Opiates in Chronic Bronchitis. Thorax 21:57, 1966.

"Sometimes when a painful episode is superimposed in a patient with limited pulmonary reserve, such as in a case of emphysema, one would wish to give a potent narcotic but is reluctant to do so because of the respiratory depressant action of such drugs. Might one of the new narcotic-antagonist agents be rationally used in such a situation?"

Reply: Employment of such a drug would of course be theoretically acceptable, but actually some years ago Reidt and associates (Albany, New York) found that this sort of narcotic antagonism could not be relied upon to prevent respiratory depression under such circumstances. The combination of drugs they used was Meperidine (Demerol) and Levallorphan (Lorfan), but doubtless the antagonism would fail also if morphine were employed.

William U. Reidt, James H. Cullen and Lawrence H. E. Smith. Effects of Meperidine Alone and in Combination with Levallophan in Patients with Pulmonary Emphysema. Am. Rev. Resp. Dis. 83:481, 1961.

"Have the sulfonamides or the antibiotics proved the more effective in reducing the acute exacerbations of bronchitis?"

Reply: The Research Committee of the British Tuberculosis Association compared a number of antibiotics with sulfamethoxypyridazine (Kynex) and found the sulfonamide the least effective of the lot. In fact they felt there is no justification for its use. Tetracycline was found to be the only antibiotic of those tested that was capable of suppressing both pneumococci and *Hemophilus influenzae*, which was felt to be the most desirable accomplishment under the circumstances. 1 Gm. tetracycline was used by them daily.

R. S. Francis, J. R. May and C. C. Spicer (London). Brit. M. J. 1:728, Mar. 21, 1964.

"I am aware of only two main types of obstructive airway disease: asthma and the bronchitis-emphysema complex. And I sometimes have considerable difficulty in distinguishing between them. Is there any drug that is helpful in making this differential diagnosis?"

Reply: Put the patient for a short period on corticosteroids; the asthmatic will nearly always improve at least temporarily, the emphysematous patient rarely, at least objectively though there may be some subjective improvement.

W. K. C. Morgan and E. Rusche (University of Maryland). Controlled Trial of Effect of Steroids in Obstructive Airway Disease. Ann. Int. Med. 61:248, 1964.

"I have been using intermittent tetracycline administration as a prophylactic measure in some of my emphysema patients, but without appreciable effect. Has the usefulness of prophylactic antibiotics been carefully studied?"

Reply: At Bellevue Hospital, Anne Davis and associates assigned patients randomly to one of two groups, one receiving 0.5 Gm. tetracycline four times daily for 48 hours each week and the other a similar number of placebo capsules. All patients were followed for 11–14 months of treatment. They found the regimen of intermittent tetracycline prophylaxis of questionable value because (a) the infection rate was so high that the reduction effected by the drug was of minimal importance; (b) there was subjective improvement only slightly more often in the treated than in the untreated group; (c) no significant change in either group was observed in an objective evaluation of pulmonary function. The more recent report of these same investigators on daily 1 Gm. dosage of chloramphenicol (Chloromycetin) did not reveal this drug to be indicated for the majority of patients. Your answer is, then, that the beneficial effects of prophylactic antibiotic administration in chronic emphysema are certainly dubious.

Anne L. Davis, Evelyn J. Grobow, Ralph Tompsett and John H. McClement. Bacterial Infection and Some Effects of Chemoprophylaxis in Chronic Pulmonary Emphysema: I. Chemoprophylaxis with Intermittent Tetracycline. Am. J. Med. 31:365, 1961. Anne L. Davis, Evelyn J. Grobow, Theresa Kaminski, Ralph Tompsett and John H. McClement. Bacterial Infection and Some Effects of Chemoprophylaxis in Chronic Pulmonary Emphysema. Am. Rev. Resp. Dis. 92:900, 1965.

"I have used the respiratory stimulant agent, ethamivan (Emivan) with fair success in a case of severe pulmonary emphysema, but I was obliged to stop use of the drug because the patient developed a generalized pruritus. Has this reaction occurred often in the experience of others, and what is the overall toxicity of this agent?"

Reply: In connection with ethamivan administration there has been a fairly high incidence of restlessness, muscular twitching, sneezing and general pruritus, but these things have usually been controlled by slowing the infusion.

"I am being urged by one of my residents to try dichlorphenamide (Daranide) in a case of severe respiratory acidosis associated with chronic obstructive pulmonary emphysema, but I am hesitating because it is always touch-and-go with such patients. What is the drug's record in this situation?"

Reply: The record provides little to commend the carbonic anhydrase inhibitors, of which this drug is one, in your situation.

"What is the efficacy of the corticosteroids in treatment of the bronchitis-emphysema complex?"

Reply: The reports certainly vary considerably: some observers feel that these drugs are never effective in obstructive airway disease, others that some benefit is always to be obtained from them, and the third, perhaps the largest group, believes that they help only occasionally. In a carefully controlled study, Morgan and Rusche, at the University of Maryland, failed to obtain evidence that a small group of emphysematous patients obtained improvement of airway obstruction while receiving 3.6 mg. of betamethasone (Celestone) daily for 3 days and then 1.8 mg. daily during the remainder of a 4 week period, the conclusion being based upon alterations in the mean forced expiratory volumes and maximal midexpiratory flow rates obtained. However, J. J. Robbins, of Hayward, California, in commenting to me regarding this study of Morgan and Rusche, has expressed the belief that the findings might have been different had adequate toilette of the bronchial tree been accomplished through rapid intravenous administration of aminophylline, as practiced by him and his associates and discussed elsewhere in these Replies. He feels that, while corticosteroids have little value in producing bronchodilatation, they are effective in preventing recurrence of spasm and inflammatory reaction.

W. K. C. Morgan and E. Rusche. Controlled Trial of Effect of Steroids in Obstructive Airway Disease. Ann. Int. Med. 61:248, 1964. J. J. Robbins. Personal Communication to the author, Mar. 15, 1966.

"In the treatment of pulmonary emphysema the corticosteroids have been rather widely recommended and much used. I understand that this is on the basis of alleged subjective benefit that is not reflected in objective changes as determined by pulmonary function studies. What is the present state of affairs?"

Reply: The answer can certainly not be clear cut. Among the recent authoritative reports based upon careful study, that of Frederick Beerel and associates (Lemuel Shattuck Hospital, Boston) provided some evidence that objective improvement may sometimes occur, but these investigators were unable to substantiate the alleged subjective improvement. They divided their 10 patients randomly into two groups. The first group received 60 mg. prednisone on the first day, 45 mg. on the second day and 30 mg. daily thereafter for the remainder of 2 weeks; then during the next 2 weeks they received identical capsules containing 0.01 mg. prednisone as a placebo. Patients in the other group received the placebo first and then the active drug during the second 2 weeks. When the results in the 10 patients were analyzed together it was found that prednisone did not produce a statistically significant increase in timed vital capacity, but 2 of the 10 patients behaved as if they belonged to a different population since they showed sizeable and significant increases in vital capacity under the drug. This would indicate that at least a trial might be in order in patients with emphysema in the hope that now and then the individual would prove to be one of these "wild" cases – a long chance, to be sure. So far as subjective benefit is concerned, Cullen and Reidt were also unable to observe it. See also the immediately preceding Reply.

Frederick Beerel, Hershel Jick and John M. Tyler. Controlled Study of Effect of Prednisone on Air-Flow Obstruction in Severe Pulmonary Emphysema. New England J. Med. 268:226, Jan. 31, 1963. J. H. Cullen and W. U. Reidt. Study of Respiratory Effects of Prednisone in Diffuse Airway Obstruction. Am. Rev. Resp. Dis. 82:508, 1960.

"Granting that the therapy of emphysema is controversial, each of us has a drug or two with which he usually obtains some success. Would you care to list the drugs that most men find helpful?"

Reply: Edward Gaensler and William Graham, at Boston University, say that the following drugs have proved their worth and are no longer controversial: specific antibiotics for infectious exacerbations, digitalis and other measures to combat right heart failure, sympathomimetics (epinephrine type of drugs), xanthine derivatives (theophylline compounds) and oxygen therapy, though the latter provides problems of its own. Other measures whose value it is not easy to support with objective data are the use of expectorants, cessation from smoking, removal from an irritating environment and transfer to a warmer or dryer climate, limitation of physical activity.

Edward A. Gaensler and William G. B. Graham. Treatment of Emphysema: Fact or Fancy? *In* F. J. Ingelfinger, A. S. Relman and M. Finland, eds., Controversy in Internal Medicine. Phila., W. B. Saunders Co., 1966, p. 399.

"Is there any reason for not using morphine in an individual with chronic lung disease?"

Reply: There is some reason to believe that any chronic lung condition in association with cardiac decompensation should be considered a contraindication to the use of morphine. In chronic cor pulmonale, for example, very severe respiratory depression has followed therapeutic morphine dosage. A patient with kyphoscoliosis, with a respiratory embarrassment of any sort, is often very sensitive to the drug; such patients frequently have heart failure, but even without it their vital capacity is low.

"In our hospital we have the definite impression that the traditional use of aminophylline is rewarding in the treatment of cor pulmonale. Have the hemodynamic effects of this drug ever been fully explored?"

Reply: Yes, the matter was studied in the cardiopulmonary laboratory at Queen's University in Canada by John Parker and associates, the subjects being 9 patients with chronic bronchitis or obstructive pulmonary emphysema with complicating cor pulmonale. The evidence obtained was certainly suggestive that the decrease in pulmonary artery pressure observed was due to pulmonary arteriolar dilatation. The dosage used in the study was greater than that usually employed clinically, but the changes induced were nevertheless evident after the administration of only therapeutic dosage.

John O. Parker, Kumar Kelkar and Roxboy O. West. Hemodynamic Effects of Aminophylline in Cor Pulmonale. Circulation 33:17, 1966.

"After discharging patients from the hospital, where they have been receiving isoproterenol (Aludrine, Isuprel), 1%, delivered by a nebulizer driven by an oxygen cylinder at 6 L./minute for 3 minutes, I customarily place them on Medihaler of the same compound. My impression is that they do just as well or better on the latter than on the former therapy; has anyone made an exact study of the matter?"

Reply: Feinmann and Newell (Newcastle-upon-Tyne) did make a careful forced expiratory volume and vital capacity study and found greater improvement in both of these parameters with Medihaler than with the standard spray. They felt that the superiority of the Medihaler probably lies in the preparation of the drug, i.e., that most of the particles are within optimal size range for inhalation therapy.

L. Feinmann and D. J. Newell. Isoprenaline in Treatment of Chronic Bronchitis. Controlled Trial of Different Methods of Administration. Brit. J. Dis. Chest 57:140, 1963.

"What would you do in a case in which the clinical features are those of chronic bronchial

asthma with chronic bronchitis, but in which there is no response to bronchodilators or corticosteroids?"

Reply: If you had added that there are also signs of possible cardiovascular etiology but with negative physical and radiological signs of left ventricular failure, you would have described a type of case that is sometimes seen and that responds to digitalis and diuretics even though the classical picture of acute pulmonary edema is not present.

"Is there any drug that will abolish Cheyne-Stokes respiration and restore a normal breathing pattern?"

Reply: Yes, it has been known for a long time that aminophylline will do this. In studying the matter at Duke University, Dowell's group found that the drug rapidly abolishes periodic breathing, increases ventilation, lowers the arterial carbon dioxide tension and increases arterial blood pH significantly. These workers suggested that aminophylline abolishes Cheyne-Stokes respiration through lowering the threshold of carbon dioxide tension so that the respiratory response occurs more promptly when the blood carbon dioxide tension rises.

A. R. Dowell, A. Heyman, H. O. Seiker and K. Tripathy. Effect of Aminophylline on Respiratory-Center Sensitivity in Cheyne-Stokes Respiration and in Pulmonary Emphysema. New England J. Med. 273:1447, Dec. 30, 1965.

BRUCELLOSIS

"Two cases of acute brucellosis caused by Brucella melitensis *have just come into my practice and have been quickly controlled with a combination of antibiotics, which is usual experience in this area. Is there a recent authoritative report of the ideal treatment for prevention of relapse?"*

Reply: At a U.S. Naval Medical Research Unit in Cairo, Farid and associates compared several different regimens in treating their 86 patients with acute and 8 with subacute brucellosis. As in your own experience, and that of numerous other reporting groups, there was excellent immediate clinical response, but relapse rate ranged from 10 to 14%. I do not know anything more "authoritative" than the 1960 review of Spink, who recommended as the treatment of choice 500 mg. of a tetracycline drug orally every 6 hours for at least 3 weeks, repeating the course within 6–8 weeks if relapse occurs. In the more severe cases, he recommends as additional therapy the intramuscular administration of 1–2 Gm. streptomycin daily for 2 weeks.

Z. Farid, A. Miale, Jr., M. S. Omar and P. F. D. Van Peenen. Antibiotic Treatment of Acute Brucellosis Caused by Brucella Melitensis. J. Trop. Med. & Hyg. 64:157, 1961.

BURNS

"I have recently had a patient who, during the period of sustained stress following an extensive burn requiring multiple debridement and grafting, developed the syndrome of dehydration, coma and severe hyperglycemia without ketosis. Insulin, and later tolbutamide, adequately handled the situation, and the latter was subsequently withdrawn before the patient's discharge. Now I have lost track of him and am concerned to know whether it is likely that he may slide unawares into a low grade diabetes?"

Reply: Doubtless your patient, like all of the 6 cases that have been reported to my knowledge, was receiving a diet very high in calories and carbohydrates when the episode occurred. In discussing their case, Steven Rosenberg's group at the Peter Bent Brigham Hospital, Boston, felt that the prolonged high carbohydrate intake led to beta cell exhaustion and an inability to metabolize excess glucose until this stimulus was removed. Actually, it does not appear that the burn state itself is a necessary component of this syndrome since a similar syndrome may ensue in any patient chronically given a high carbohydrate diet. However, it is not definitely known whether the prediabetic state is a necessary element in the pathogenesis of this malady, and therefore one cannot categorically supply a negative answer to your question.

Steven Rosenberg, Donald K. Brief, John M. Kinney, Manuel G. Herrera, Richard E. Wilson and Francis D. Moore. The Syndrome of Dehydration, Coma and Severe Hyperglycemia without Ketosis in Patients Convalescing from Burns. New England J. Med. 272:931, May 6, 1965.

"The high hopes for the control of burn sepsis engendered with the development of such synthetic penicillin analogues as oxacillin (Prostaphlin, Resistopen) and methicillin (Staphcillin, Dimocillin-RT) have not been fulfilled and we still have patients dying from gram-negative infections, of which that with *Pseudomonas aeruginosa* is the most prevalent and lethal pathogen. Is there any hopeful new development in this field?"

Reply: H. Harlan Stone's group, at Emory University, have reported the treatment of *Pseudomonas* sepsis in 13 burn patients, with control of the infection in 12 and eventual survival in 10. Treatment consisted in intramuscular administration of gentamicin (Garamycin), 3 mg./kg./day (4 mg. in near-terminal patients), blood transfusions, early energetic debridement, application of fine mesh gauze impregnated with gentamicin ointment beneath bulky pressure dressings, wound coverage with autografts and/or homografts as soon as possible, and continuation of the gentamicin gauze until almost total wound closure was accomplished; systemic administration of the drug was interrupted after 14–16 days and followed by a 2 week respite before reinstitution.

H. Harlan Stone, J. D. Martin, Jr., William E. Huger, Laura Kolb. Gentamicin Sulfate in the Treatment of Pseudomonas Sepsis in Burns. Surg. Gynec. & Obst. 120:351, 1965. H. Hailan Stone. Review of Pseudomonas Sepsis in Thermal Burns: Verdoglobin Determination and Gentamicin Therapy. Ann. Surg. 163:297, 1966.

"I am aware that antibiotic prophylaxis generally has been widely condemned in surgery as likely to increase the population of resistant staphylococci and other organisms in the environment, and that this interdiction has usually been made to apply also to the local use of these agents in the treatment of burns. But has this latter aspect of the matter been looked into in recent years?"

Reply: Yes, it has. In Birmingham, England, E. J. L. Lowbury and associates treated a group of 31 patients with fresh burns of up to 30% of the body surface with "tulle gras" that was prepared by impregnating gauze strips with paraffin moll. flav. B. P. (yellow soft paraffin) containing 5 mg./Gm. of neomycin sulfate and 5 mg./Gm. of chlorhexidine diacetate. Another group of 29 patients was treated with penicillin cream (1000 units/Gm.) in a lanette wax base, as controls. For burns of 15% or more (10% or more in children) the first dressings were applied after completion of treatment for the shock period, about 48 hours; for less extensive burns, on the day of admission. Split-skin grafts were supported on tulle gras or on neomycin-chlorhexidine tulle gras in the treatment group, and on tulle gras containing no antibacterial agent in the control group. No growth was obtained in 25% of 255 cultures from burns in the treatment group but in only 5% in 287 cultures from the control group, *Staphylococcus aureus, Pseudomonas aeruginosa,* proteus and coliform bacilli being significantly more common in the control group. But once the exudate had dried, there was a longer period between dressings in the treatment group and the dressings tended to stick to the eschar; slough separation was also considerably prolonged in some patients. There were 19 successful (80% or more graft "take") operations among 35 in the treatment group and 29 among 37 in the control group. It appeared that the treatment method was acceptable as a backing for split-skin grafts and as dressing for burns of partial skin thickness. Mean healing time in the treatment group was 66 days and in the control group 76 days.

Temperatures and respiratory rates were consistently lower in the treatment than in the control group. In patients suitable for treatment by the exposure method, a spray was used containing a suspension of polymyxin, neomycin and bacitracin in dichlorofluroethane, with penicillin-lactose powder (10,000 units/Gm.) or with no antibacterial application. Cultures from the sprayed burns remained sterile in 22% of instances as against 2% from those treated with no antibiotic; the penicillin powder did not improve this picture very much. The temperature remained significantly lower in the sprayed group also, and split-skin grafts were successful as follows: sprayed group, 5 of 6; penicillin powder group, 3 of 7; controls, 3 of 3. In earlier studies, Cason and Lowbury showed that the most obviously important pathogens in burns do not appear to produce resistant variants in the agents that they apply locally.

J. S. Cason and E. J. L. Lowbury. Lancet 2:501, 1960. E. J. L. Lowbury, R. W. S. Miller, J. S. Cason and D. MacG. Jackson. Local Prophylactic Chemotherapy for Burns: Treated with Tulle Gras and by the Exposure Method. Lancet 2:958, Nov. 10, 1962.

BURSITIS

"In a patient with subacromial bursitis, who has gotten only temporary relief from topical corticosteroid injections, would it be advisable to resort to the x-ray therapy that is strongly advocated by one of our local people?"

Reply: I do not think so. Nathan Abrams has said that, at the University of Cincinnati, roentgen-ray therapy with a lead filter inserted to block the rays has been found fully as beneficial as conventional roentgen-ray therapy.

Nathan R. Abrams. Subacromial Bursitis. *In* H. F. Conn, ed., Current Therapy, 1966. Phila., W. B. Saunders Co., 1966, p. 654.

CARDIOSPASM

"I have a patient with cardiospasm in whom I am unable to effect relief through use of either glycopyrrolate (Robinul) or isopropamide (Darbid), though one would expect these drugs to be effective. Why is this?"

Reply: I think it likely that you could run through a whole series of these anticholinergic agents, such as the ones you mention and other newer and the older ones, and atropine itself without obtaining the effect you desire because these drugs are not able to relax the esophagogastric sphincter. I should think that you would get some relaxation of painful esophageal spasms, however. The nitrites will relax

that sphincter and might therefore give you better effect. Of course the relief provided by amyl nitrite inhalation will only be fleeting, but why not have your patient try nitroglycerin under the tongue?

CAROTID SINUS SYNDROME

"Would you kindly discuss the carotid sinus syndrome from the standpoint of its drug therapy?"

Reply: The carotid sinus is situated in the neck at the beginning of the internal carotid artery just above the bifurcation of the common carotid artery. A rise of blood pressure in the sinus stimulates the delicate sympathetic carotid sinus nerve, which proceeds afferently from the sinus to the glossopharyngeal nerve, and causes a striking decrease in heart rate and fall in blood pressure. Decrease in rate is the vagal reflex response to the stimulus. The blood pressure fall is due both to the rate decrease and to stimulation of the parasympathetic vasodilator influence and inhibition of the sympathetic vasoconstrictor centers in the medulla. Reduction of pressure in the sinus causes just the opposite effects: acceleration in rate and rise in pressure. This sort of thing is occurring all the time in the reflex regulation of blood pressure and heart rate. In the carotid sinus syndrome there is overactivity of the sinus, with a resultant fall in cerebral blood pressure that causes attacks of dizziness, syncope and even convulsions and sometimes extrasystoles and atrioventricular conduction disturbances as well. The challenge of the malady is met pharmacologically with only partial satisfaction because not only are the patients usually in advanced years with complicating hypertension or considerable arteriosclerosis, but also because only incomplete or transient action can be obtained from drugs in a situation in which prolonged action is required. For example, atropine subcutaneously in somewhat greater than usual dosage will eliminate the parasympathetic portion of the action temporarily, but it will not affect the sympathetic portion. Conversely, adrenergic (sympathomimetic) drugs such as ephedrine, which has a longer lasting action than epinephrine itself, will partially overcome the sympathetic portion of the action, but usually higher than feasible dosage is required. Tetraethylammonium chloride, which paralyzes the ganglia in both the parasympathetic and the sympathetic systems, will prevent both efferent portions of the reflex response, but the effect is of only relatively short duration, and the drug causes more widespread autonomic effects than are desirable in such a situation. Anesthetization of the sinus with procaine will temporarily impede the reflex, but surgical denervation of the sinuses or intracranial section of the glossopharyngeal nerves is really the best remedial measure in cases of real severity.

CAT-SCRATCH DISEASE

"Has specific therapy been devised for cat-scratch disease?"

Reply: No it has not, though it appears that the corticosteroids are being used rather effectively in some instances. The etiology of this entity remains elusive, for the evidence against an acid-fast bacillus has not been convincing. The disease sometimes assumes quite bizarre forms, and it is a difficult though fascinating entity to study because the cases are few and widely scattered.

William F. Eckhardt, Jr. and Abraham I. Levine. Corticosteroid Therapy of Cat-Scratch Disease: Results of Treatment in Three Cases with Rapid Resolution of Painful Lymphadenopathy; Tietze's Syndrome and Bilateral Cervical Adenitis as New Complications. Arch. Int. Med. 109:463, 1962.

CAUSALGIA

"Is there any sort of systemic drug therapy that will relieve the suffering of a patient with causalgia? I mean the true causalgia and not the hand-shoulder syndrome that is sometimes incorrectly referred to under this title."

Reply: No. Unless he can be relieved by procaine injections of the sympathetic ganglia, the only hope for this patient lies in surgery.

CEREBROVASCULAR DISORDERS

"With what drugs may one hope to relieve the episodes of vertigo, tinnitus, the 'little stroke' and things of that sort that are due to spasm of arteriosclerotic cerebral vessels?"

Reply: In the first place, I do not know that episodes of the sort you mention are really due to cerebrovascular spasm; this has not been proved, you know. And as for selectively dilating such vessels there is not much substantiated evidence either. The trouble with all vasodilators is that they dilate all vessels and hence produce a generalized lowering of blood pressure. However, claims have been made, though upon the basis of unconvincing studies, for effective action in the situations you have in mind by cyclandelate (Cyclospasmol), isoxsuprine (Vasodilan) and nylidrin (Arlidin). Cyclospasmol is usually used in dosage of 200 mg. (3 gr.) four times daily, with maintenance dosage of 100 mg. four times daily. Vasodilan dosage is 10–20 mg. three or four times daily. Arlidin is given orally in dosage of 1–2 of the 6 mg. tablets three or four times daily. The preparation known as C.V.P., which is a mixture of bioflavonoid compounds and ascorbic acid, has also been claimed to be useful in these cerebrovascular disorders, but none of the evidence favorable to the use of this preparation is based upon soundly controlled studies. I do not believe that C.V.P. has value. Actually, this preparation is promoted to counteract capillary oozing rather than to oppose arteriolar spasm, but such claims would bring it into the realm of treatment of the "little stroke" and I therefore mention it in this context. Breathing of 5% carbon dioxide for a brief period will sometimes increase cerebral blood flow, and in Boston, Donald Ehrenreich and associates found that the intravenous administration of 1 Gm. of acetazolamide (Diamox) during a 10 minute period usually increased cerebral blood flow more strikingly than did 5 minutes of 5% carbon dioxide inhalation and that the change persisted for at least an hour after administration of the drug.

Donald L. Ehrenreich, Rosalie A. Burns, Ralph W. Alman and Joseph F. Fazekas. Influence of Acetazolamide on Cerebral Blood Flow. Arch Neurol. 5:227, 1961.

"I have heard dimenhydrinate (Dramamine) praised for its usefulness in treating dizziness, nausea and vomiting in geriatric patients, but have had very little success with it myself. What could be at fault?"

Reply: I really think that it is not you but the drug that is to blame. In treating symptoms due to vascular dysfunction in the geriatric patient, one may expect the best result with preparations containing an antiemetic and a vasodilator. Dramamine does not have both of these characteristics to a notable degree. In a study of patients with these symptoms, whose age averaged 72 years, Francis Stern (Philadelphia) found both Tigacol and Antivert quite effective agents and Dramamine much less useful. Both Tigacol and Antivert contain a vasodilator and Dramamine does not.

Francis H. Stern. Comparison of Three Agents (Tigacol, Dramamine and Antivert) for Control of Dizziness in Geriatric Patients. J. Am. Geriatrics Soc. 11:884, 1963.

"Is anticoagulant therapy justified in occlusive cerebrovascular disease?"

Reply: R. N. Baker and a number of associates, at the Massachusetts General Hospital, studied this matter quite thoroughly in a group of 443 patients, practically equally divided randomly between anticoagulant-treated and nonanticoagulant control groups. The conclusions they reached were quite clear cut: from the standpoint of mortality, long-term anticoagulant therapy is not beneficial in thrombotic cerebrovascular disease and may be harmful through increasing the incidence of hemorrhagic complications; in transient ischemic attacks, short-term anticoagulant therapy may reduce the incidence of attacks; and in thrombosis-in-evolution it may reduce morbidity from neurologic illness though not reducing mortality. Unfortunately, there is one outstanding fact that severely limits the usefulness of this information, namely, that classification of the individual case is not always easy to make.

R. N. Baker, J. A. Broward, H. C. Fang, C. M. Fisher, S. N. Groch, A. Heyman, H. R. Karp, E. McDevitt, P. Scheinberg, W. Schwartz and J. F. Toole. Anticoagulant Therapy in Cerebral Infarction: Report on Cooperative Study. Neurology 12:823, 1962.

"Is hypertonic mannitol solution useful whenever lowering of cerebrospinal fluid pressure and decrease of brain mass are required?"

Reply: Burton Wise and Norman Chater (University of California) decided that this is so, as the result of a considerable study of the matter, but they had certain reservations, namely, that its use would probably be unwise in patients with active intracranial bleeding, except during craniotomy, and that it should be used cautiously in patients with cardiac disease or cardiac failure. Barry and Malloy (Washington, D.C.) reported successful use of the agent in acute functional renal failure but poor results when there was total organic renal failure. They felt, however, that since the result cannot be unfailingly predicted, an innocuous 12.5 Gm. dose may be tried in any acutely oliguric patient. Dosage of Wise and Chater: 2.5–3 Gm./kg. of 20% solution in distilled water, going as high as 4.25 Gm./kg. in some instances. Usually, 1–1½ hours is required to complete the infusion.

Burton L. Wise and Norman Chater. Value of Hypertonic Mannitol Solution in Decreasing Brain Mass and Lowering Cerebrospinal Fluid Pressure. J. Neurosurg. 19:1038, 1962. Kevin G. Barry and John P. Malloy. Oliguric Renal Failure: Evaluation and Therapy by Intravenous Infusion of Mannitol. J.A.M.A. 179:510, Jan. 17, 1962.

"Should arteriography be performed unless the decision to operate has already been made?"

Reply: A very important question to which the answer has not yet been supplied, so far as I am aware.

"Is the patient with completed stroke a candidate for either anticoagulant or surgical therapy?"

Reply: According to Siekert and associates (Mayo Clinic) he is not unless new ischemic phenomena occur. In their experience, however, those with evolving stroke respond well to anticoagulant therapy. In patients with actively advancing stroke in the carotid system, the proportion of those with hemiplegia or those who did not survive was reduced in their series from 35 to 6%, and in those with actively advancing stroke in the vertebrobasilar system, the mortality was reduced from 58 to 8%. They found that surgical therapy did not appear to improve statistical results in patients with evolving stroke. But they found both surgical therapy and anticoagulant therapy useful in prevention of cerebral infarction in patients with intermittent insufficiency: a follow-up of 3–8 years after patients with transient ischemic attacks were put on long-term anticoagulant therapy revealed 74.9% of the treated and 51.9% of the untreated patients to be normal. Nonfatal infarction occurred in 2.3% of the treated and in 20.6% of the untreated patients, and fatal cerebral infarction in 1.7% of the treated and 11.2% of the untreated. The incidence of fatal cerebral hemorrhage was higher in treated (7.4%) than in untreated (4.4%), but this increase was minimal compared with the incidence of fatal thrombotic infarcts. As for surgical treatment in a highly selected group of patients, with transient ischemic attacks and a well-defined occlusive lesion in an extracranial artery, the advantage was definitely with the surgically treated individuals, but it appeared that there was about a 10% mortality associated with the surgery itself. I think we would all like to see a statistically significant study of operation immediately as the stroke is occurring.

Robert G. Siekert, Jack P. Whisnant and Clark H. Millikan. Surgical and Anticoagulant Therapy of Occlusive Cerebrovascular Disease. Ann. Int. Med. 58:637, 1963.

"In cerebrovascular thromboembolism with cerebral infarction (catastrophic stroke, progressive stroke, or stroke in evolution), might it not be advisable to direct therapy toward increasing the cerebral collateral circulation during the first few days? Has anyone approached the subject in this manner?"

Reply: Yes, at Harper Hospital, Detroit, John Meyer and associates presented data showing that intravenously administered papaverine increases cerebral blood flow and oxygenation both in subjects with and without occlusive cerebrovascular disease. The drug was used in an infusion of 500 mg. in 1000 ml. of 5% dextrose in 0.2 N sodium chloride during an 8 hour period; such periods were alternated with 8 hour periods without therapy during 10 days. Thirty-four patients received the drug and 36 acted as controls. It was said that the treated group experienced greater neurological recovery than did the untreated group. All the patients had suffered a stroke within 72 hours of acceptance into the study, and to minimize the risk of treating patients with intracerebral hemorrhage, only patients with systolic blood pressure below 100 mm. Hg and with clear cerebrospinal fluid were considered to be suitable candidates.

John S. Meyer, Fumio Goth, John Gilroy and Nasaharu Nara. Improvement in Brain Oxygenation and Clinical Improvement in Patients with Strokes Treated with Papaverine Hydrochloride. J.A.M.A. 194:957, Nov. 29, 1965.

"In progressive cerebral thrombosis, the state that we are now calling 'stroke in evolution,' is thrombolytic therapy feasible?"

Reply: John Meyer's group (Wayne State University) studied 40 patients who fitted into this category. Thrombolysin, 200,000 units, or placebo was given by intravenous infusion in 1000 ml. of 5% dextrose in water, cooled to about 4° C., over a 4 hour period daily for 3 days. The thrombolytic treatment did not seem to be helpful except possibly in patients over age 65.

John S. Meyer, John Gilroy, Marion I. Barnhart and J. Frederick Johnson. Therapeutic Thrombolysis in Cerebral Thromboembolism: Double-Blind Evaluation of Intravenous Plasmin Therapy in Carotid and Middle Cerebral Arterial Occlusion. Neurology 13:927, 1963.

"Does streptokinase therapy have a place in the treatment of progressive stroke?"

Reply: John Meyer and associates (Detroit) found its use contraindicated.

John S. Meyer, John Gilroy, Marion I. Barnhart and J. Frederick Johnson. Anticoagulants Plus Streptokinase Therapy in Progressive Stroke. J.A.M.A. 189:373, Aug. 3, 1964.

"One hears of or reads, as in the article of John Meyer and associates (Detroit), that the use of anticoagulants is a part of the 'best possible medical treatment' of progressive stroke. Is this really the case?"

Reply: I know that there is some vogue for the use of anticoagulants in this situation nowadays, but I wonder if we should overlook C. M. Fisher's report, in 1961, on a national cooperative study of the matter in cerebral thrombosis and cerebral embolism? His conclusion was that long-term anticoagulant therapy does not apparently reduce mortality in occlusive cerebrovascular disease and that,

in fact, it is associated with an increase in the risk of death through hemorrhagic complications.

C. Miller Fisher (Massachusetts General Hospital) Anticoagulant Therapy in Cerebral Thrombosis and Cerebral Embolism: National Cooperative Study, Interim Report. Neurology 11 (Part 2):119, 1961. John S. Meyer, John Gilroy, Marion I. Barnhart and J. Frederick Johnson. Anticoagulants Plus Streptokinase Therapy in Progressive Stroke. J.A.M.A. 189:373, Aug. 3, 1964.

CHOLANGITIS

"In cholangitis due to incomplete obstruction of the common hepatic or common bile duct the treatment is surgical, because short courses of chemotherapy often fail and have often been observed to fail in patients who refuse surgery or are unsuitable for operation. But has the last word necessarily been said here? Might it not be advisable to try some of these patients on long-term therapy?"

Reply: Precisely this has been done by P. C. Reynell, in England, in 3 patients who had had Charcot's intermittent fever for 12–30 months, and in 2 of whom short courses of chemotherapy had been totally ineffective. All were apparently cured by at least 4 weeks' treatment with antibiotics and had no further illness after 48, 42 and 18 months, respectively. One patient was cured by streptomycin with penicillin when tetracycline had failed.

P. C. Reynell. Antibiotics in Recurrent Cholangitis. Brit. M. J. 1:1288, May 15, 1965.

CHOLECYSTITIS

"Should one use chemotherapeutic or antibiotic agents in the treatment of cholecystitis?"

Reply: I think there is considerable reason to be doubtful of the rationale of such therapy because many observers feel that cholecystitis is not primarily an infectious process but a chemical inflammation. Some years ago, Jerry Zaslow found the use of antibiotics not helpful in mild cases of acute obstructive cholecystitis and that they did not appear to affect the local process in gravely ill patients, though in the latter the systemic manifestations were often relieved. A few years later, E. Christoffersson and associates reported that one of the two sulfonamides they tried was superior to placebo, which is certainly not striking testimony in favor of chemotherapy.

W. van der Linden. Sulfonamide in Treatment of Acute Cholecystitis: Sequential Clinical Trial. Acta chir. scandinav. 127:652, 1964. Jerry Zaslow. Antibiotics in Diseases of the Biliary Tract. J.A.M.A. 152:1683, 1953. E. Christoffersson, Y. Edlund, R. Gamklou and L. A. Nilsson. The Effect of Dosulfin in Acute Cholecystitis. Acta chir. scandinav. 123:44, 1962.

CHOLERA

"We had as well learn what to do about cholera as any of the other 'exotic' diseases, the world having become the small round ball that it is. What is the specific antibiotic?"

Reply: There is none, though in India they seem to be getting good results, so far as diminishing diarrhea is concerned, through use of 500 mg. of tetracycline orally every 6 hours. But of course the important thing in this disease is fluid replacement.

CHOLERETICS

"What is the position of the choleretic drugs in the treatment of chronic liver and gallbladder disease?"

Reply: Choleretics are drugs that increase the liver's production of bile. The bile salts themselves, i.e., ox bile extract, in addition to this choleretic action promote absorption of fatty foods and of the fat-soluble vitamins A, D, E and K. Allegedly they are occasionally mildly laxative also. There is no reason to believe, however, that any of these actions makes them useful in treating chronic gallbladder disease (cholecystitis and cholelithiasis), because the patient with this malady is not functioning faultily in any of these respects. The exception might be in the case of the promotion of bile production, not for its own sake but merely as a means of increasing the current of fluid away from the liver and toward the gallbladder and intestine as a cleansing and protective measure against ascending infection. Of course, if there is sufficient associated hepatitis to diminish bile salt synthesis but not to prevent bile pigment excretion, i.e., in instances of bile salt deficiency in the presence of pigmented feces, the additional activities of the bile salts would be profitably invoked by giving these extracts. But this must be a very infrequent occurrence.

It therefore appears that the best bile salt to use in chronic gallbladder disease would be the one that produced the most copious flow of secretion from the liver irrespective of the constituents of the fluid. In short, *hydro*choleresis would be advantageous, if achievable. And it is, for dehydrocholic acid (Decholin, etc.) though having a very doubtful effect on production of bile salts, does considerably increase the volume output of a bile of relatively high water content and low viscosity. This drug is therefore a good "flusher," and is effectively used in treating both the chronic unoperated patient and the patient who has a T-tube drainage of an infected common bile duct. It is sometimes also employed to float a small obstructing stone out of the common bile duct, usually being used in such instances together with a cholagogue such as magnesium sulphate.

Of course when a biliary fistula is draining bile away from the intestinal lumen, the bile salts themselves should be used (Bilein, etc.), whether dehydrocholic acid is being given or not, because they are much better promoters of digestion and absorption than the partially synthetic compound. The desirability of administration of bile salts might also arise in some cases of obstructive jaundice, when it will be necessary to weigh the advantage of promoting fat-soluble vitamin absorption against the possibility of increasing the amount of bile in circulation. Their usefulness in cirrhosis is very doubtful.

Both the bile salts and dehydrocholic acid are given in dosage of 1 or 2 of the commercially available tablets two or three times daily.

CIRRHOSIS

"How may one best combine the diuretic agents in combating ascites in cirrhosis?"

Reply: Steigmann's group (Cook County Hospital) have described their use of combinations of diuretic agents in 40 patients with "intractable" ascites, all patients being on a 2000 calorie diet with no more than 200 mg. sodium and receiving daily a 3 Gm. potassium chloride supplement. The first therapy was with 300 mg. hydrochlorothiazide (Hydro-Diuril, etc.) or 30 mg. bendroflumethiazide (Naturetin) daily—5 patients responded satisfactorily. If no response was noted in 3–5 days, 400 mg. spironolactone (Aldactone) was added to the regimen—21 responded satisfactorily. If there was insufficient response to this last therapy within 1 week, 30 mg. prednisone (Meticorten, etc.) daily or a daily intramuscular injection of 250 mg. hydroxyprogesterone caproate (Delalutin, Prodox) was given—6 patients responded to each of these latter combinations. In 2 patients it was necessary to use a combination of bendroflumethiazide, spironolactone, prednisone and hydroxyprogesterone in order to obtain relief.

Frederick Steigmann, Alfredo Sison and Alvin Dubin. "Intractable" Ascites in Cirrhosis: Management by a Multiple Diuretic Approach. Am. J. M. Sc. 245:521, 1963.

"When treating hepatic coma with antibiotics it is usually a practice in our area to eliminate protein completely from the diet and to wash out nitrogenous materials from the colon by enemas and flushing with cathartic salts given orally.

Might one not do just as well to omit all this protein elimination and rely principally on the use of antibiotics orally to wipe out the microorganisms in the gut whose bacterial enzymatic action on nitrogenous compounds there provides most of the undesired ammonia?"

Reply: Actually, Faloon and Fisher (State University of New York, Syracuse) satisfied themselves, at least, that such a program is perfectly feasible. They followed 22 patients with alcoholic cirrhosis through 25 episodes of coma or impending coma with a treatment that consisted only of oral neomycin while oral protein was continued. Protein to the extent of 20–40 Gm. was given orally or by gastric tube in divided feedings, and neomycin, 12 Gm. daily in a schedule of 3 Gm. every 6 hours orally or by tube. Other measures were the intravenous administration of dextrose, usually containing vitamins and potassium chloride; insertion of a Sengstaken tube when indicated; and the administration of penicillin and streptomycin to prevent pneumonia. Emptying of the intestinal tract by enemas and cathartics was not resorted to routinely. Eleven of the 22 patients died, but 9 of these had improved before death; indeed improvement was noted in 23 of the 25 episodes of hepatic coma. There was a decrease in blood ammonia during therapy in 16 of the 18 patients in whom it was determined. There was no significant difference in survival rate between patients receiving more than 25 Gm. of protein and those receiving less than 25 Gm.

W. W. Faloon and Curtis J. Fisher. Clinical Experience with Use of Neomycin in Hepatic Coma. Arch. Int. Med. 103: 43, 1959.

"Some of my friends are using an androgen together with corticosteroids in treating cirrhosis; has the usefulness of such a combination been established?"

Reply: It seems to me that the evidence favoring the use of such a *combination* is only suggestive, though the two drugs used alone appear to have established merit. A suitable series to cite is that of Ronald Wells (General Hospital, Singapore); of his 80 cirrhotic patients, 27 were treated with prednisolone, 26 with testosterone, and 27 served as controls. All patients were given an adequate diet, supplemented by intragastric drip when necessary, and vitamin supplements; and those with severe edema or ascites also received a thiazide and potassium chloride daily. The prednisolone-treated patients received an initial 4 week course of 20 mg. daily, and then after the sixth week 1 week of prednisolone dosing was given only every 4 weeks. These patients also received 40 units of long-acting corticotropin every 2 weeks. The testosterone patients were injected with 100 mg. testosterone propionate on alternate days for the first 4 weeks and then 300 mg. every 2 weeks thereafter. The observation periods ranged between 14 and 86 weeks, and during the study there was a mortality of 26% in the prednisolone group, 31% in the testosterone group and 55% in the control group. Fourteen prednisolone patients, 13 testosterone patients and only 4 control patients could be certified as fit for work.

Ronald Wells. Prednisolone and Testosterone Propionate in Cirrhosis of Liver: Controlled Trial. Lancet 2:1416, Dec. 31, 1960.

"To what drugs other than ammonium chloride, the thiazide diuretics and carbonic anhydrase inhibitors is a patient with advanced cirrhosis of the liver likely to be particularly sensitive?"

Reply: To those drugs you have listed I should certainly add the opium alkaloids and derivatives of the same, the oral anticoagulants, ergotamine (Gynergen), barbiturates, paraldehyde and the phenothiazine derivatives of the type of chlorpromazine (Thorazine), mepazine (Pacatal), prochlorperazine (Compazine), etc.

"Being dissatisfied with my results in the treatment of bleeding esophageal varices in cirrhosis, I am tempted to return to the use of posterior pituitary extract that had some vogue a few years ago. What was the rationale of this treatment and what results were obtained?"

Reply: The reason for our using Pituitrin is to attempt to control bleeding from the varices by reducing portal venous pressure. Harold Conn and Donald Dalessio (VA Hospital, West Haven, Connecticut) administered intravenously 20 units of surgical Pituitrin in 100–200 ml. of 5% dextrose in water over 15–30 minutes to 16 cirrhotic patients who had 25 episodes of hemorrhage from esophageal varices. Bleeding ceased and did not recur for at least 24 hours in 10 of the 25 episodes; in 4 others there was success when the therapy was used in conjunction with the Sengstaken-Blakemore tube. Late in this experience it was felt that best results were achieved when the drug was given more frequently, more rapidly and more regularly. S. I. Schwartz and associates repeated injections at 4 hour intervals if bleeding continued or recurred.

Harold O. Conn and Donald J. Dalessio. Multiple Infusions of Posterior Pituitary Extract in Treatment of Bleeding Esophageal Varices. Ann. Int. Med. 57:804, 1962. Seymour I. Schwartz, Harold W. Bales, George L. Emerson and Earle B. Mahoney (University of Rochester). Use of Intravenous Pituitrin in Treatment of Bleeding Esophageal Varices. Surgery 45:72, 1959.

"What is the position of sodium glutamate (Glutavene) in combating hepatic coma?"

Reply: This drug has been shown to lower blood ammonia in the experimental animal, but since it has also been found to increase plasma bicarbonate, this fact alone may account for its beneficial effect in the treatment of hepatic coma, since an elevation in plasma bicarbonate increases urea production and thus lowers the blood ammonia level. However, be the mechanism what it may, the use of sodium glutamate is occasionally provocative of dramatic release of the patient from coma. High dosage is necessary. Vanamee and Poppell give 120 Gm. in 3 liters of 10% glucose during 24–36 hours; this causes metabolic alkalosis and hypokalemia, and so 40 m Eq. of potassium chloride is added to each liter of solution.

P. Vanamee and J. W. Poppell. Hepatic Coma. M. Clin. North America 44:765, 1960.

"In a patient with cirrhosis in whom I want to induce more diuresis than I can get with hydrochlorothiazide (Hydro-Diuril, Esidrex) without significantly increasing potassium loss, is there anything that I can turn to?"

Reply: In a small series of patients at Western Reserve University, David Ginsberg and associates made effective use of triamterene (Dyrenium) to supplement the thiazide diuretic. Dosage was 100 mg. twice daily for 3 days, which produced a consistent, significant diuresis and natriuresis accompanied by decreases in potassium and net hydrogen ion excretion. You should be advised, however, that there is not as yet as much information available regarding triamterene's possible serious effects on the kidneys, liver and bone marrow as would be desirable.

David J. Ginsberg, Atif Saad and George J. Gabuzda. Metabolic Studies with the Diuretic Triamterene (Dyrenium) in Patients with Cirrhosis and Ascites. New England J. Med. 271:1229, Dec. 10, 1964.

"I am aware that a patient with cirrhosis of the liver may become comatose when given ammonium chloride; are there other drugs that might have this effect?"

Reply: Yes, the thiazide diuretics (such as chlorothiazide [Diuril], bendroflumethiazide [Naturetin], cyclothiazide [Anhydron], hydrochlorothiazide [Esidrix, Hydro-Diuril, Oretic], hydroflumethiazide [Saluron], polythiazide [Renese], trichlormethiazide [Naqua], benzthiazide [Exna], methyclothiazide [Enduron]) and the carbonic anhydrase inhibitors (such drugs as acetazolamide [Diamox], dichlorphenamide [Daranide], ethoxzolamide [Car-drase], methazolamide [Neptazane]) may do it; so also may the barbiturates, the opiates and derivatives, paraldehyde and the phenothiazide-derivative major tranquilizers of the chlorpromazine (Thorazine, etc.) type.

"Use of the aldosterone antagonist, spironolactone (Aldactone) is being rather heavily promoted in our area for reduction of ascites in cirrhosis. Is this soundly based?"

Reply: Yes, I believe so. The importance of aldosterone in the retention of fluid complicating cirrhosis is indicated by the low sodium content of urine, saliva, sweat and feces in patients with ascites. Additional evidence, cited by Clowdus and associates (Mayo Clinic) is the fact that bilateral adrenalectomy effects re-establishment of sensitivity to diuretics or by suppression of adrenocortical function and aldosterone secretion by administration of amphenone. Henley's group, in 1960, pointed out that there is a factor operating in cirrhosis to stimulate persistent increase in aldosterone production. In fact, total blood volume decrease might in itself account for the aldosterone increase in production through homeostatic mechanisms, though such a blood volume decrease is not a distinguishing characteristic of cirrhosis, but we cannot be certain that a local volume alteration in an area responsible for the promotion of aldosterone secretion might not be occurring when there is a pooling of blood in the splanchnic area. At any rate, there is an increase in the urinary excretion of aldosterone in cirrhotic patients with ascites, as shown by Wolff's group in Germany in 1956, and an effort to combat what seems to be patently an excessive aldosterone activity in the body appears rational.

Bernard F. Clowdus, John A. Higgins, John W. Rosevear and William H. J. Summerskill. Treatment of "Refractory" Ascites with New Aldosterone Antagonist in Patients with Cirrhosis. Proc. Staff Meet. Mayo Clin. 35:97, Mar. 2, 1960. H. P. Wolff, Kh. R. Koczorek, W. Jesch u. E. Buchborn. Untersuchungen U. d. Aldersteroneausscheidung bei Leberkranken. Klin. Wchnschr. 34:366, 1956. K. S. Henley, D. H. Streeten and H. M. Pollard. Gastroenterology 38:681, 1960. Chas. H. Lockwood. Spironolactone Therapy for Ascites Due to Cirrhosis of Liver. Canad. M. A. J. 85:631, Sept. 9, 1961.

"I have tried progesterone as aldosterone antagonist in a few cases of hepatic cirrhosis with good early results but the patients all escaped very quickly from the drug's influence; has this been the experience of others?"

Reply: Yes, it has. Progesterone seems to be useful only in combination with a diuretic drug and even when thus combined its effect is quite fleeting. It seems usually to require only 5–10 days for the biologic competitive action of progesterone to be blocked by an increase in aldosterone production. As most effective use of a combination of progesterone with a diuretic, Hempel-Jørgenson and Eilersen (Hillerød, Denmark) suggested the use of a diuretic once or twice weekly with a dose of progesterone on the same day; some such scheme as 50–100 mg. progesterone intramuscularly in the morning and on the same day 50 mg. of hydroflumethiazide (Saluron) morning and noon, or 1 or 2 ml. of mercaptomerin (Thiomerin) in the morning.

Povl Hempel-Jørgensen and Preben Eilersen. Antagonism of Aldosterone by Progesterone: Effect of Progesterone in Two Cases of Hepatic Cirrhosis. Acta med. scandinav. 168:55, 1960.

"I have heard of the administration of arginine in chronic liver disease. What is its rationale and effectiveness?"

Reply: The elevation of blood ammonia levels is believed to remove substances from the brain that are essential to its metabolism; so effort is made to diminish ammonia formation in the intestinal tract by restricting protein intake, controlling gastrointestinal bleeding, and giving antibiotics orally. Arginine and glutamic acid, in the form of arginine glutamate, is given parenterally in the attempt to bind blood ammonia. Actually, however, the efficacy of this latter measure is still undetermined. At the University of Adelaide, Davey gave the drug to 2 patients with chronic cerebral dysfunction associated with severe liver disease. In 1 of these there was no effect either mental or physical; the other improved mentally for about a week. Arginine glutamate (Modumate) was used as a 25% solution in water, and each 100 ml. dose was brought up to 500 ml. with 5% glucose. Intravenous infusion dosage was 50 Gm. initially and three doses of 25 Gm. each at 8 hour intervals; both patients became nauseated when the infusion rate exceeded 25 Gm./hour and 1 complained of facial stiffness and paresthesias at the beginning of each infusion.

M. G. Davey. Effect of Arginine Glutamate (Modumate) on Elevated Blood Ammonia Levels in Chronic Liver Disease. Australasian Ann. Med. 13:72, 1964.

"Is it admissible to use morphine in a patient with liver disease?"

Reply: Use of morphine is to be avoided in disturbances of the liver, such as infectious hepatitis and cirrhosis, because when liver function is disrupted the rate of morphine conjugation is drastically reduced. Disregarding this admonition has sometimes been fatal.

"A number of men in our area are trying the sort of intermittent corticosteroid therapy that is nowadays being promoted from some research centers. Would you advocate this type of therapy in an individual with serious liver disease?"

Reply: I take it that you have had some sort of experience that provoked this question? I should be inclined myself to let a little more time pass before using this treatment method in an individual with known hepatic pathology. In Germany, H. Lindner has observed a number of recurrences or exacerbations of liver disease upon the withdrawal of corticosteroid therapy, and he points out that these occurrences are seldom noted because shortly after stopping the therapy the patient is released in good general condition and with objective improvement in laboratory findings. He cites, for example, the case of a woman who had a recurrence of acute hepatitis a few weeks after leaving the hospital and her physician interpreted the condition as recurring epidemic hepatitis and continued the corticosteroid that she had been taking; then against his advice she stopped the drug suddenly and shortly afterward, in a final fatal attack, the transaminase activity was reduced more than it had ever been before and bilirubin was increased. Necropsy showed a scarred liver with acute hepatitis. This is of course proof of nothing, but the evidence appears to me to be sufficiently suggestive to engender caution.

H. Lindner. Dangers in Withdrawal of Glucocorticoid Therapy of Acute and Chronic Liver Diseases. Deutsche med. Wchnschr. 89:1622, Aug. 28, 1964.

"When you have a patient with cirrhosis under treatment with corticosteroids, is there any point in making repeated determinations of serum transaminase activity?"

Reply: Yes, I think so, for an increase in this activity would seem to indicate an activation of the inflammatory process; and this, other things being equal, would suggest that the optimal corticosteroid dosage is not being given.

Bent Harvald and Sten Madsen (Copenhagen). Long-Term Treatment of Cirrhosis of the Liver with Prednisone (Meticorten, Etc.). Acta med. scandinav. 169:381, 1961.

COLITIS

"It has seemed to me that an inadequate response of ulcerative colitis to the corticosteroids is a poor prognostic sign for the ultimate outcome in the patient. What has been the effect of the use of the corticosteroids on the surgical aspects of the disease?"

Reply: At the Mt. Sinai Hospital in New York, Korelitz and Lindner analyzed the results of this therapy in 238 patients with severe or moderately severe ulcerative colitis.

Their conclusion was that the incidence of surgical intervention has not lessened but that the indications for operation have been toward more elective and less emergency procedures; and the overall mortality rate has markedly diminished. Several years ago, J. V. Prohaska and associates (University of Chicago), looking at the matter from the surgeon's standpoint, found that the patient who has been on corticosteroids is not less able to tolerate surgical trauma than the nontreated patient, but they did find that in these individuals there is definite retardation of wound healing and that healing is also often followed by moderate keloid formation.

Burton I. Korelitz and Arthur E. Lindner. Influence of Corticotropin and Adrenal Steroids on Course of Ulcerative Colitis: Comparison with Presteroid Era. Gastroenterology 46:671, 1964. John V. Prohaska, Lester R. Dragstedt and Richard G. Thompson. Ulcerative Colitis: Surgical Problems in Corticosteroid-Treated Patients. Ann. Surg. 154:408, 1961.

"Has the topical use of corticosteroids favorably influenced therapy in ulcerative colitis?"

Reply: From a retrospective study of the 10 year experience with this type of therapy at the University of Texas, Patterson's group have concluded that it does improve the course of the disease, particularly when given early and in patients with restricted involvement, but they feel that more observation is necessary to confirm this opinion. They use the following techniques: (a) patients with acute or chronic disease limited to the rectum or rectosigmoid and without systemic symptoms: a hydrocortisone acetate suppository of 10 or 15 mg. inserted rectally four times daily; (b) patients with left-side involvement or with systemic symptoms who fail to respond to suppositories: a retention enema of hydrocortisone acetate (50 mg.) or prednisone (10 mg.) or methylprednisolone acetate (40–120 mg.) in 120 ml. of water twice daily; (c) patients with extensive disease or who could not retain the enema: proctoclysis daily of 50–100 mg. of hydrocortisone sodium succinate in 500 ml. of normal saline.

M. Patterson, J. McGivney, Helen Ong and A. Drake. Topical Steroid Therapy of Ulcerative Colitis. Gastroenterologia 103:141, 1965.

"I am sure that corticosteroids have reduced the number of my patients with ulcerative colitis who need an emergency operation when debilitated by massive bleeding or sepsis. But I have not been able to determine, in a rather limited experience, just when surgical help should be obtained for these patients. Is authoritative information available?"

Reply: In a study of 55 patients at the Peter Bent Brigham Hospital, Boston, John Brooks and Frank Veith concluded that patients with acute fulminating ulcerative colitis, whether it be de novo disease or an acute exacerbation of a chronic process, should be operated on if steroid therapy produces no apparent remission in 2 weeks. But they emphasized also the necessity for extreme vigilance during this time, since deterioration of the patient's condition (through bleeding, sepsis or toxicity) during a corticosteroid regime might make surgery necessary before 2 or even 1 week. They felt that if all patients requiring medical attention for ulcerative colitis are considered, more than 14% will need major surgical intervention.

John R. Brooks and Frank J. Veith. The Timing and Choice of Surgery for Ulcerative Colitis. J.A.M.A. 194:115, Oct. 11, 1965.

"I have a patient with ulcerative colitis to whom I have been giving salicylazosulfapyridine (Azulfidine) for some time, and he has now developed Heinz bodies in the erythrocytes. What is the significance of this?"

Reply: In most instances the production of these bodies during treatment with sulfonamides has had no clinical significance and anemia has not developed.

L. E. Böttiger, L. Engstedt, R. Lagercrantz and A. Nyberg (Karolinska Hosp., Stockholm). Occurrence of Heinz Bodies during Azulfidine Treatment of Ulcerative Colitis. Gastroenterologia 100:33, 1963.

"Has it been found efficacious to exclude milk from the diet of a patient with ulcerative colitis who is receiving the standard corticosteroid therapy?"

Reply: At the Radcliffe Infirmary, Oxford, Ralph Wright and S. C. Truelove used a milk-free, low-roughage diet excluding all milk and milk products whether in the form of dairy produce such as fresh milk and cheese or powdered milk, but permitting butter. There were 77 patients in the trial, which extended for 1 year. Their conclusion was that the milk-free diet is beneficial to about 1 in 5 patients, with a suggestion that the proportion may be higher in patients having their first attack of the disease.

Ralph Wright and S. C. Truelove. A Controlled Therapeutic Trial of Various Diets in Ulcerative Colitis. Brit. M. J. 2:138, 1965.

"In the gastrointestinal field, I find that my most notorious weight losers are patients with duodenal ulcer, hypertrophic gastritis, dumping syndrome, ulcerative colitis, regional ileitis, and cirrhosis of the liver if judged upon a nonascites basis. The anabolic hormones are sometimes helpful, but is there any 'best' among them?"

Reply: Anthony Kasich, in New York, has

preferred nandrolone phenpropionate (Durabolin) because of its low hepatotoxicity. He administers it intramuscularly once a week in dosage of 25–50 mg., in courses ranging from 12–15 weeks. In 39 of his 48 ambulatory patients there was appetite increase, weight gain and improved sense of well-being. There was no evidence of hepatotoxicity, androgenicity or fluid retention in any of the patients; and in 2 with cirrhosis, the liver function tests actually showed improvement. Of course this was only one man's experience and admittedly the number of cases was small, still it can be taken for what it is worth in answer to your question. I don't want to be disagreeable, but it does seem that the gastroenterologists are sometimes easily, shall one say desperately, pleased? However, it is nice to know that they and their patients can sometimes experience the warm glow of success.

Anthony M. Kasich. Clinical Evaluation of Nandrolone Phenpropionate (Durabolin) in Patients with Gastrointestinal Disease. Am. J. Gastroenterol. 40:628, 1963.

"Would the use of an antineoplastic agent be rational in the treatment of an intractable ulcerative colitis?"

Reply: How "rational" is difficult to say because the malady is certainly one of obscure etiology and I suppose the trial of almost any remedial agent could be rationalized in such a case. Actually, in Australia, R. H. D. Bean reported consistent improvement but no cures in 7 patients treated with 6-mercaptopurine (Purinethol). The antineoplastics are all very potent agents and likely to make the patient pretty sick. Be careful.

R. H. D. Bean. Treatment of Ulcerative Colitis with Antimetabolites. Brit. M. J. 1:1081, Apr. 30, 1966.

"I have a patient with ulcerative colitis, under treatment with the usual remedial agents, who has now developed hemolytic anemia. How might this be explained?"

Reply: Of course it is not at all unusual to see anemia of other sorts than hemolytic in chronic ulcerative colitis, usually ascribable to blood loss, nutritional factors, a decrease in bone marrow productivity or a shortening in the survival time of erythrocytes. But there have also been reported a few cases of hemolytic anemia associated with the use of salicylazosulfapyridine (Azulfidine), that is very much used in the treatment of this disorder. Had you been using this drug in your patient?

Morris D. Gardner and J. Arnold Bargen (Texas). Hemolytic Anemia Secondary to Salicylazosulfapyridine (Azulfidine) Therapy. J.A.M.A. 190:71, Oct. 5, 1964.

"In a case of colitis in which Actinomyces bovis

has been identified as the causative organism, what is the therapy?"*

Reply: H. Leonard Jones and Orville Nielsen, at the U.S. Naval Hospital, Philadelphia, say that the prognosis for permanent cure is now excellent if one uses penicillin either intramuscularly or intravenously in high dosage. They advocate 120,000 units initially and then 80,000 units every 4 hours for a total of 6–8 million units, or even more.

H. Leonard Jones, Jr., and Orville F. Nielsen. Colitis: Management Based on Pathogenic Mechanisms. M. Clin. North America 49:1271, 1965.

"In a case of colitis associated with recovery of Dientamoeba fragilis, or Trichomonas hominis (both only presumptively pathogenic), what is the therapy?"

Reply: 250 mg. of carbarsone orally twice daily for 10 days.

COLORADO TICK FEVER

"Every summer I see a few cases of Colorado tick fever. These people always recover but they feel pretty miserable for a while despite my symptomatic therapy. Is there any specific therapy likely to be soon available?"

Reply: I know of none.

COMA

"Are analeptic drugs indicated in the treatment of coma?"

Reply: This is a controversial subject, with perhaps most reports being adverse with regard to use of these agents in the unconscious barbiturate-poisoned patient. However, Robert Hoagland, of the U.S. Army, has recently published rather convincingly on the use of one of the drugs, methylphenidate (Ritalin) in the treatment of coma of diverse origin: mass brain lesions, trauma, metabolic disorders including uremia and liver disease, bacterial toxins, ingestion of nonsedative chemicals, depressant drugs and anoxia. I have seen no reports suggesting damage to the hematologic, hepatic or urinary systems with this drug, nor of any severe allergic reactions. It may occasionally cause gastrointestinal disturbances, palpitation, dizziness, slight blood pressure and pulse alterations up or down, dryness of the mouth and subjective numbness of the extremities, but none of these things is likely to be of importance in using the drug to combat a comatose state.

Robert J. Hoagland. Pharmacologic Treatment of Coma of Diverse Origin. Am. J. M. Sc. 35:623, 1965.

COMMON COLD

"Most of the over-the-counter preparations recommended by pharmacists for the common cold contain a rather routine mixture of ingredients: an antitussive, an antihistamine, an analgesic-antipyretic, a vasoconstricting nasal decongestant and sometimes a belladonna alkaloid and caffeine. Now I know that this is shotgun prescribing, and I am as much opposed to it as you are sure to be, but what is one to do? If one were to prescribe several of these ingredients separately — and often it appears desirable to attack the individual symptoms with drugs from the different categories — the experience would turn out to be more expensive for the patient than was his last common cold which his druggist treated for him with one of the aforementioned proprietary mixtures."

Reply: I am not as much opposed to these common cold mixtures as are some of my associates. To be sure when you use them you are attempting to strike at everything at once and you have no way of knowing which ingredient, if any, has been helpful or no way to lower or raise the dosages of the individual constituents. But do you have time to do much of this anyway in treating a common cold? As a matter of fact are you likely to see the patient more than once? And it is certainly debatable whether anything you do for him is really going to be more helpful than perhaps to take off the edge of some of his greater discomforts. The cold wears itself out in a few days and I can think of much more harmful placebos than these, some of which are used in more serious maladies. I do think, however, that you should by no means condone the use of common cold remedies that contain either an antibiotic or a sulfonamide, for to do so may be to court an anaphylactic or other type of hypersensitivity reaction.

"In my part of the country it has long been usual practice to prescribe or inject an antibiotic in treatment of the common cold. Is there really any justification for this?"

Reply: Oh! come now, I am not even going to cite the evidence. The antibiotics are *not* efficacious in treatment of the common cold.

CONGENITAL PYLORIC STENOSIS

"I have a case of congenital pyloric stenosis in which I have obtained excellent results through the use of methyl-scopolamine-nitrate (Skopolate) in dosage of 0.05 mg. subcutaneously 20 minutes before meals, changing to 0.1 mg. orally as the child improved. I am now wondering whether I should not give this therapy a considerable trial in all cases instead of recommending surgery as I have done habitually?"

Reply: At the Columbia-Presbyterian Medical Center, Gilbert Mellin's group studied this matter in 21 infants, of whom 11 were randomly chosen for surgery and the other 10 treated medically, much as you have done. Of the 11 patients treated by pyloromyotomy, 1 died. Of the 10 treated medically, 4 subsequently had pyloromyotomy and the remaining 6 had rather stormy careers before finally coming under control, and they required more intense nursing care while in hospital and more frequent follow-up than those treated surgically. But all cases, both medical and surgical, were asymptomatic at the 6 months follow-up period. The conclusion from this study was that the drug therapy is not a substitute for pyloromyotomy if competent surgical assistance is at hand.

Gilbert W. Mellin, Thomas V. Santulli and Harry S. Altman. Congenital Pyloric Stenosis. J. Pediat. 66:649, 1965.

CONGESTIVE HEART FAILURE

"Why is it that after all these years we still have so much digitalis toxicity?"

Reply: I shall quote to you a statement from Dubnow and Burchell's study of the matter at the Mayo Clinic: "The results confirm the view that, for each new patient being digitalized, dosage should be considered a bedside therapeutic experiment in which choice of drug is much less important than wise use of the one chosen." A few years ago, M. W. Shrager carefully studied 40 cases of digitalis intoxication and concluded that 80% of the instances could have been prevented and that 88% were attributable to errors in dosage.

Morton H. Dubnow and Howard B. Burchell. Comparison of Digitalis Intoxication in Two Separate Periods. Ann. Int. Med. 62:956, 1965. M. W. Shrager. Digitalis Intoxication: Review and Report of 40 Cases, with Emphasis on Etiology. Arch. Int. Med. 100:881, 1957.

"I am convinced that through the years I have lost a number of congestive heart failure patients on digitalis simply because their maintenance dosage was not properly adjusted. Have you anything to suggest?"

Reply: Nothing that is very likely to be helpful, unfortunately. Establishment of maintenance dosage is not easy because it seems to vary somewhat from day to day in individuals and considerably from person to person; it has therefore to be worked out for each individual patient and cannot be counted upon always to be satisfactory month after month in any individual. Of course the price to be paid for too high dosage is overaction and possibly a toxic death, but on the other hand if the dose is underestimated and the patient is not seen at frequent intervals he can easily slide into failure even though he is taking several doses daily. Several years ago, Blackard and Harrison advocated brief periods of augmented dosage in individuals on maintenance dosage to determine their true therapeutic status; the amount of the increase in dosage which will be tolerated before evidences of toxicity appear will provide the answer when this maneuver is employed.

E. H. Blackard and T. R. Harrison. Augmentation: Third Stage of Digitalis Therapy. Arch. Int. Med. 103:543, 1959.

"The revered but quite elderly leader in our group persists in the use of digitalis leaf despite the fact that all of us younger men are using the crystalline compounds. Can you supply a brief statement authoritatively supporting our position?"

Reply: Sorry, but I must side with the old man. The patient will not be any more efficiently or safely digitalized with the newer preparations than with the leaf, or any more satisfactorily maintained in a state of digitalization. If one is fully cognizant of what can be accomplished with the leaf preparation of a given manufacturer, it seems to me that switching to the crystalline or amorphous preparations, which are more expensive, would usually be undesirable except when the psychologic effect of the change promised to be rewarding. Defining the therapeutic range of digitalis dosage as the gap between the lowest dose that will produce adequate therapeutic effect and the maximum dose tolerated without excessive toxicity, it must be admitted that as the patient's heart disease progresses the therapeutic range becomes smaller until the gap between the therapeutic and toxic dosages is eliminated. At this point of course one will no longer achieve salutary effects and, if all other measures are failing also, the patient will die. But this point is reached just as rapidly with the newer preparations as with the leaf. Of course it is an admitted disadvantage of the leaf that it can be given only by mouth.

"Since thromboembolic episodes are frequent and dreaded complications of congestive failure it is important to know whether digitalis increases the coagulability of the blood as some animal experimentation suggests. Does it?"

Reply: Levin and Ruskin concluded that such is not the case, but it seems to me that the significance of their findings was lessened by the fact that they used patients who were without evidence of congestive failure. It is precisely with the patient in failure that we are concerned. The fluid losses accomplished now through lowsalt diets, potent diuretics and digitalis are much greater than formerly; the resulting hemoconcentration may provide increased thromboplastin and prothrombin concentrations and alter the concentration of antithrombin. The point that appears to demand more thorough investigation than it has had is whether there is an effect on coagulation time in proportion to the amount of diuresis that has been achieved. So you see I have not been able to give you a satisfactory reply.

W. C. Levin and A. Ruskin. Effects of Digitoxin on Heparin Tolerance, Coagulation Time and Prothrombin Activity. Texas J. Med. 48:590, 1952.

"In a patient with exertional dyspnea but no signs or history of congestive failure, what period of digitalis therapy may one feel is reasonable to determine whether the patient will be helped by this drug?"

Reply: This is a very important matter because the drug certainly has a high potentiality for toxic actions, and undoubtedly numerous individuals all over the world are being needlessly treated with it. In a thorough study a few years ago, Harry Gold and associates, at Cornell University, satisfied themselves that a 2–3 week trial of digitalis should suffice. If there is no effect, stop the drug; if the results are equivocal, try a placebo for a similar period. A similar trial may be made with a diuretic in a patient who does not respond to digitalis.

Harry Gold, Theodore Greiner, Nathaniel T. Kwit, Harold L. Otto and Leon Warshaw. Effect of Digitalis and Diuretics on Exertional Dyspnea: Study in Ambulant Patients with Chronic Heart Disease. J.A.M.A. 169:229, Jan. 17, 1959.

"Patients are sometimes referred to me because they are said to be in a 'refractory' stage of congestive heart failure, i.e., fully digitalized but not responding adequately to the drug. I am often doubtful that the patient is truly fully digitalized and inclined to believe that the referring physician has mistaken anorexia and nausea due to abdominal congestion for that due to digitalis, or that he has been frightened by premature contractions that might have been due to the underlying cardiac disorder. The temptation is great in these cases to add more digitalis to that which the patient is alleged to be under the influence of, but this is risky from the standpoint of liability. Can you support me with authoritative experience in this situation?"

Reply: Yes. In 18 patients in precisely this condition, Embree Blackard and Tinsley Harrison (Medical College of Alabama) found that 11 were able to retain at least 5 mg. gitalin, which is in the range of the initial digitalization dose, and all were able to retain 2.5 mg. or more. Fifteen of the group experienced subjective improvement with increased exercise tolerance, and 11 improved cardiac function. The patients were instructed to keep careful watch for sudden decrease in appetite, or nausea, vomiting or diarrhea when gitalin was given three or four times daily after meals in total daily doses of 1.5–4 mg., with each dose supplemented by 1 Gm. potassium chloride. They all became toxic, but the study certainly showed that "full digitalization" is not always what the term implies. The point made by these observers, as a result of the experience, was that periodic augmentation of digitalis dosage can be of advantage in patients still having symptoms when treated with current standard methods using average dosage. During such a period of augmentation the patient should be seen daily by his physician; potassium chloride should be given with each dose of digitalis during the supplementary period; anorexia and nausea due to digitalis should be distinguished from that due to abdominal congestion or concurrent disease or from other drugs; and it should be recognized that premature beats are often due to the underlying cardiac disorder and may be abolished by digitalis.

Embree H. Blackard and Tinsley R. Harrison. Augmentation: Third Stage of Digitalis Therapy. A.M.A. Arch. Int. Med. 103:543, 1959.

"Studies in recent years have apparently established the fact that potassium depletion sensitizes the atrium to the toxic action of digitalis, and that in selected instances the paroxysmal atrial tachycardia with block that is evidence of this sensitization should be terminated by administration of potassium salts. Is the latter usually considered a safe procedure?"

Reply: I think that one should certainly proceed with utmost caution in such a situation, including continuous electrocardiographic supervision, not only because this arrhythmia is seen almost exclusively in patients with advanced congestive heart failure, but because Brown and associates showed that potassium salts may produce toxic effects in patients with severe heart disease despite adequate urinary output. In fact, the studies of Fisch and associates convey the impression that intravenous administration in digitalis intoxication might be dangerous because of a suppositious "block" by digitalis of the intracellular transfer of the infused cation.

H. Brown, G. L. Tanner and H. H. Hecht. Effects of Potassium Salts in Subjects with Heart Disease. J. Lab. & Clin. Med. 37:506, 1951. C. Fisch, E. F. Steinmetz, A. F. Fasola and B. L. Martz. Effect of Potassium and "Toxic" Doses of Digitalis on the Myocardium. Circulation Res. 7:424, 1959.

"While not at all disparaging other drugs and ancillary measures in the treatment of congestive heart failure, it is only digitalis that I can count upon to strengthen the myocardium sufficiently to overcome the imbalance between the strength of the muscle and the load it must propel when there is failure. But it does not always increase output as one would wish it to do; why is this?"

Reply: Digitalis's primary action of strengthening the contractile power of the myocardium is manifested as increased cardiac output only in the group of heart failures in which there is decreased cardiac output, the so-called "low output" group. Fortunately these latter comprise the majority of the cases of congestive heart failure and in most of them digitalis can be counted upon to restore compensation (re-establish satisfactory cardiac output) whether the failure resulted from hypertensive, ischemic (coronary), arteriosclerotic or valvular disease and independently of the heart rate and the rhythm of the atria. But there are types of failure in which the drug is not effective. It has practically no value in instances of disability due to mere mechanical constriction within the heart, as in some cases of the type described by Lown and Levine as "tight mitral stenosis with pulmonary congestion and normal sinus rhythm"; it is ineffective when ventricular filling is interfered with by cardiac tamponade or constrictive pericarditis (unless there is also failure); it has limited value in cyanotic congenital heart disease and is also of no value if rheumatic carditis is actively present; and it affords practically no help in cases of failure with the "high output" demanded by such conditions as diminished oxygen-carrying power of the blood (anemia, emphysema), metabolic disturbances (beriberi, thyrotoxicosis), mechanical overload (arteriovenous aneurysm, osteitis deformans).

B. Lown and S. A. Levine. Current Concepts in Digitalis Therapy. New England J. Med. 250:771, 819 and 866, 1954.

"Has a chelating agent been effectively used to reduce calcium in cases of digitalis intoxication?"

Reply: Yes, Eliot and Blount (University of Colorado) used edathamil disodium (Endrate Disodium) successfully in relief of both the arrhythmias and subjective symptoms of digitalis intoxication in their 18 patients. *Dosage:* they gave an average of 3.25 Gm. in 12 minutes, the infusion solution containing 15 mg./ml. About 40% of the patients experienced arm pain, circumoral paresthesia and apprehension during the infusions.

Robert S. Eliot and S. Gilbert Blount, Jr. Calcium, Chelates and Digitalis: Clinical Study. Am. Heart J. 62:7, 1961.

"After the initial parenteral digitalization of a patient who needs to have the drug's action rapidly induced, should one institute full digitalization orally to maintain the advantage gained by the emergency measure, or is it satisfactory as well as safer to resume therapy with maintenance oral dosage?"

Reply: At Mount Zion Hospital, San Francisco, Harold Rosenblum undertook to obtain answer to this oft-recurring practical question through investigation of the problem in a controlled series of 39 hospitalized patients with auricular fibrillation, using gravimetrically standardized cardiac glycosides of chemical purity and consistent potency. His conclusion was that, while careful individualization is necessary for maximum benefit, the rapid redigitalization of patients in 24 hours after initial rapid intravenous digitalization did not provide added benefit but did produce toxic effects more often.

Harold Rosenblum. Maintenance of Digitalis Effects after Rapid Parenteral Digitalization. J.A.M.A. 182:192, Oct. 13, 1962.

"I find a bewildering difference among my digitalized patients in the speed and degree to which they manifest evidences of the drug's toxicity. What factors underlie these differences?"

Reply: I think that one may list the following safely as among the principal things influencing the response of the patient and of his heart: age, physical activity, mental status, type and stage of the cardiac malady, the underlying heart rhythm, electrolyte balance, concomitant administration of other drugs, individual rates of absorption and dissipation of the drug, and accompanying diseases. Church and associates, in Baltimore, also point out cogently that there are variables due to the observer, since it is not always easy to be sure that a sign or symptom is ascribable to the drug, and digitalis "toxicity" is not really precisely defined.

G. Church. L. Schamroth, Neil L. Schwartz and Henry J. L. Marriott. Deliberate Digitalis Intoxication. Comparison of Effects of Four Glycoside Preparations. Ann. Int. Med. 57:946, 1962.

"Is the sensitivity to digitalis of the patient with cirrhosis explainable on the basis of an alteration in metabolism of the drug?"

Reply: Actually one cannot legitimately speak of *digitalis* metabolism as an entity, because we find in animal experimentation that individual compounds are dealt with quite differently, and this appears to be true to some extent in man also. For example, St. George's group, using the embryonic duck heart method which is very delicate, found that whereas young subjects cannot excrete more than 5% of a given dose of digitoxin in

24 hours or more than 14% in 72 hours, they can excrete approximately 14 and 29%, respectively, of administered digoxin during the same time intervals. They also found that digoxin is not detectable in the urine after 8 days, but that digitoxin can still be found in most instances after 15 days. I can therefore answer your question only with regard to one of the digitalis preparations, namely digoxin. Studying the metabolism of this agent given in its triturated form in cirrhotic patients, Marcus and Kapadia, at Georgetown University, determined that the sensitivity of these patients to digoxin must be explained on a basis other than an alteration in metabolism of the drug.

Frank I. Marcus and Geeta G. Kapadia. Metabolism of Triturated Digoxin in Cirrhotic Patients. Gastroenterology 47:517, 1964. Shirley St. George, Meyer Friedman and Tadashi Ishida. The Renal Excretion of Digoxin in the Normal Young Subject. J. Clin. Invest. 37:836, 1958.

"How am I to determine whether I may dare institute digitalis therapy in a new patient who does not know whether he has had the drug recently?"

Reply: Tinsley Harrison has said that when one is in doubt regarding a patient's digitalis status, administration of a high carbohydrate meal, or of 25 Gm. of glucose intravenously, with ECG's made at intervals during the next 90 minutes, is likely to settle the question: frequent premature systoles may be precipitated in the individual who is on the verge of digitalis intoxication.

T. R. Harrison. Editorial Comment: Precipitation of Ventricular Arrhythmias Due to Digitalis by Carbohydrate Administration. Year Book of Medicine 1956–57, p. 415.

"How should one proceed when digitalis has produced heart block in a patient who badly needs the drug?"

Reply: Heart block may appear in three forms: first degree (delayed conduction time), second degree (partial block), or complete block. The first cannot readily be detected without an ECG. The second is easily recognized by noting an occasional dropped beat on auscultation. Complete digitalis heart block, which is rare, may offer some diagnostic difficulty; the ventricular rate in this block is not around 30, as in Adams-Stokes disease, but generally 60 or more and possibly over 80 or 100. The first two types of block are not harmful if they occur alone, and inasmuch as slowing of the ventricle results they may be beneficial. They serve merely as a signal that further dosage should be given cautiously. But it is well to consider that complete block requires discontinuance of the drug or, at the least, considerable curtailment in dosage. If electrocardiographic acid is not utilized, digitalis should be omitted when a heart, previously grossly irregular, becomes regular under the drug. The regularization may be due either to resumption of the normal rhythm or to the fact that the ventricles have begun to beat regularly while the atria are still fibrillating, which would mean complete block. In the first instance nothing will be lost by omitting digitalis for a few days; in the latter, harm might result from continuing its use.

"I have recently had a 79-year-old patient who developed severe digitalis toxicity on dosage of the rapidly excreted glycoside, digoxin, that should not have caused any trouble at all. Has such an experience often been had by others?"

Reply: In discussing his 24 cases of digitalis toxicity encountered during one year, Alfred Soffer (Rochester, New York, General Hospital) remarked on the particularly tragic paradox that those who most require the unique action of digitalis are the most intolerant of slight variations in dosage. The average age of his patients was 69.7 years, and in 20 of them (83%) digoxin in low dosage produced intoxication. It appears simply to be the fact that as the ratio between therapeutic and toxic dosage narrows, the point may be reached at which the aged heart is unable to tolerate any therapeutic amount of digitalis. This state of affairs, which does not seem to have been encountered in an earlier period, appears to mean that persons who would formerly have succumbed to infectious and other diseases at a relatively early age now survive into a period when their hearts can no longer cope with the amount of digitalis necessary to provide the most help from the drug.

Alfred Soffer. Changing Clinical Picture of Digitalis Intoxication. Arch. Int. Med. 107:681, 1961.

"I have recently made a false diagnosis of mesenteric thrombosis in a patient in whom at necropsy there was found to be no mesenteric arterial involvement at all but only venous engorgement with hemorrhage and edema of the wall—such changes, in fact, as one would be tempted to describe as gangrenous except that there was little or no inflammatory reaction and no massive infarction was present. Is it possible that this acute and fatal episode could have resulted from the large dosage of digitalis that the patient was taking?"

Reply: Yes it is. At the Medical College of South Carolina, Gazes and associates reported 10 necropsy cases in which this was precisely the situation. Explanation is merely speculative, the postulation being that digitalization causes constriction of the hepatic vein or sinusoidal sphincter, with the result that there is portal splanchnic venous congestion. Gazes' patients were all on high dosage of digitalis and several had the classic signs of digitalis toxicity when the episode began. I do not know that the picture has ever been seen in a conservatively digitalized patient.

Peter C. Gazes, Charles R. Holmes, Vince Moseley and H. Rawling Pratt-Thomas (Med. College of South Carolina). Acute Hemorrhage and Necrosis of Intestines Associated with Digitalization. Circulation 23:358, 1961.

"I have a patient who has been on various digitalis preparations for a recurrent and persistent congestive heart failure during the last 4 years. He has had no mental illness, but during a recent period in which he was on maintenance gitalin, 0.5 mg. daily, he developed short spells of confusion, visual hallucinations and some aggressiveness in behavior. I took him off of the drug and all of the symptoms disappeared in less than 3 days. Could this have been due to the digitalis?"

Reply: It is rare, but it does happen. In fact, delirium associated with digitalis therapy has been recognized in the law courts.

Gerald Church and Henry J. L. Marriott (University of Maryland). Digitalis Delirium: Report of Three Cases. Circulation 20:549, 1959.

"I have recently had a patient with atrial fibrillation in whom it was necessary to use astonishingly high dosage of digitalis to accomplish reversion. None of my close associates have ever had to use such high dosage; is this sort of thing extremely rare?"

Reply: I do not know how *extremely* rare such occurrences are, but they are certainly not often recorded. It is a fact, however, that the standardization of digitalis dosage usually employed for guidance is based exclusively on use of the drug in reducing an acute congestive heart failure. Perhaps a different type of dosage could be based upon the purely antiarrhythmic action of the drug? In Palo Alto, California, David Hunt has reported 2 cases of atrial fibrillation in which satisfactory digitalis effect was obtained only after establishing maintenance dosage of 1.0 Gm. of digitalis leaf daily.

David D. Hunt. Unusual Tolerance to Digitalis. Dis. Chest. (Am. College Chest Physicians) 46:474, 1964.

"Will wonders never cease? I have heard it rumored that digitalis toxicity can be successfully counteracted with antiepileptic drugs. Can this be true?"

Reply: Sounds unlikely, doesn't it? Nevertheless, at the Cedars of Lebanon Hospital, Los Angeles, Tzu-Wang Lang's group have actually reported the successful treatment of 4 patients with digitalis-induced arrhythmias through use of diphenylhydantoin (Dilantin). In a typical case, 100 mg. of the drug was diluted in 10 ml. of 5% dextrose in water and given intravenously during a 5 minute period. Considerable experimentation in dogs had justified the attempt in man. Some evidence has been adduced that diphenylhydantoin reduces the concentration of intracellular sodium, and thus by inference increases that of potassium. This is all that may be offered in explanation of the action so far.

Tzu-Wang Lang, Harold Bernstein, F. Fernandez Barbieri, Herbert Gold and Eliot Corday. Digitalis Toxicity. Arch. Int. Med. 116:573, 1965.

"Do changes in the thyroid state modify the effectiveness of digitalis; i.e., is a thyrotoxic patient who has congestive heart failure or atrial fibrillation relatively unresponsive to the usual doses of the drug?"

Reply: At the National Institutes of Health, Robert Frye and Eugene Braunwald undertook to obtain an answer to this question in the study of 7 patients with chronic heart disease, all of whom had chronic atrial fibrillation, none of them being in congestive heart failure at the time. In these patients the daily oral administration of 75–500 μg. liothyronine (Cytomel), in divided doses or by single intravenous injection, increased the digitalis requirement on the basis of alterations in ventricular rate. Induction of mild thyrotoxicosis in these patients resulted in a three- to fourfold increase in the dosage of digoxin required to maintain the ventricular rate at the level present during the euthyroid state. These investigators also determined the apparent advisability of administering syrosingopine (Singoserp) or reserpine (Serpasil, etc.) together with digitalis when treating heart disease in a thyrotoxic patient since the rauwolfia alkaloids and derivatives ameliorate the signs and symptoms, including hypermetabolism and tachycardia, of thyrotoxicosis. The intramuscular administration of syrosingopine was recommended rather than the oral because the bradycrotic effect of the drug is obtained much more promptly in this way. Patients so treated, however, still require specific antithyroid therapy. The subsequent studies of James Doherty and William Perkins, at the University of Arkansas, have supplied good evidence to support cutting down on digitalis dosage for *hypothyroid* and increasing for *hyperthyroid* patients.

Robert L. Frye and Eugene Braunwald. Studies on Digitalis: III. Influence of Triiodothyronine (Cytomel) on Digitalis Requirements. Circulation 23:376, 1961. James E. Doherty and William H. Perkins. Digitalis Metabolism in Hypo- and Hyperthyroidism. Ann. Int. Med. 64:489, 1966.

"A number of my associates consider that 'redigitalization' of a patient is possible through use of diuretic agents. What is your thought?"

Reply: If it were true that considerable amounts of digitalis accumulate in edema fluid and that the use of potent diuretic agents "liberates" these portions of the drug into the blood stream as the edema fluids are mobilized and excreted by the kidneys, there might ensue a "redigitalization" to the point of toxicity of an already adequately digitalized patient. It has seemed to me that the clinical impression of such a redigitalization has become more firmly entrenched in recent years with the combination of low salt dieting and liberal use of diuretics, but the observations of St. George and associates, using the embryonic duck heart technique, have aimed a sharp blow at this belief because they failed to find more than minute amounts of drug in the edema fluids of any of the digitalized patients they studied. It would appear that even extremely rapid diuresis could hardly deliver amounts of digitalis that were of significance if their findings are truly representative.

S. St. George, C. F. Naegele, F. S. French, R. H. Rosenman and M. Friedman. A Quantitative Study of the Digitoxin Content of Edema Fluids. J. Clin. Invest. 32:1222, 1953.

"We now have an abundance of fine diuretics; how is one to choose among them to get maximum effect without excessive overaction in congestive heart failure?"

Reply: Swartz's group (Hahnemann Medical College) studied the clinical pharmacology of 12 of them and seems to have found them equally effective and none more toxic than the others. It is difficult, of course, to extrapolate such findings to individual cases because the circumstances are never quite the same in two consecutive patients. The patients in Swartz's series, carefully chosen for the purposes of the study, were all free of renal disease and of derangement in water or electrolyte metabolism. The maximum effective dosage of the drugs they evaluated was as follows: (b.i.d.: twice daily; o.d.: once daily; i.m.: intramuscularly) chlorothiazide (Diuril), 1000 mg. b.i.d.; chlorthalidone (Hygroton), 200 mg. o.d.; quinethazone (Hydromox), 200 mg. o.d.; benzthiazide (Exna), 100 mg. b.i.d.; hydrochlorothiazide (Hydro-Diuril, Esidrix, Oretic), 100 mg. b.i.d.; hydroflumethiazide (Saluron), 100 mg. b.i.d.; benzydroflumethiazide (Naturetin, Benuron), 10 mg. o.d.; methyclothiazide (Enduron), 10 mg. o.d.; cyclothiazide (Anhydron),

4 mg. b.i.d.; trichlormethiazide (Metahydrin, Naqua), 4 mg. b.i.d.; polythiazide (Renese), 4 mg. b.i.d.; meralluride (Mercuhydrin), 2 ml. i.m.

Charles Swartz, Robert Seller, Morton Fuchs, Albert N. Brest and John H. Moyer. Five Years' Experience with Evaluation of Diuretic Agents. Circulation 28:1042, 1963.

"It is difficult to avoid the conviction that circulatory congestion does not necessarily indicate, or correlate with, the status of cardiac function because one can frequently obliterate the congestion and relieve the patient through use of a diuretic without altering cardiac function directly. Is such a conclusion really soundly based?"

Reply: I think all of us have felt this to be the case and it appears that Rader and associates (New York University) have shown it to be so in their careful study of 18 patients, in whom full mercurial diuresis alone sometimes improved cardiocirculatory function sufficiently so that no further improvement occurred upon subsequent digitalization. In other cases, subsequent digitalization did increase cardiac output and bring the arteriovenous oxygen difference toward normal, but these individuals usually had had one or more previous episodes of failure. Where there was persistent chronic congestive failure, the low cardiac output and high arteriovenous oxygen difference were not altered by either mercurial diuretics or digitalis. The important point was that removal of the edema and congestion by diuresis alone effected subjective improvement.

Bertha Rader, Warren W. Smith, Adolph R. Berger and Ludwig W. Eichna. Comparison of Hemodynamic Effects of Mercurial Diuretics and Digitalis in Congestive Heart Failure. Circulation 29:328, 1964.

"Has the use of the diuretic drugs nowadays in so many conditions in which there is no obvious need for diuresis been foisted upon us by the pharmaceutical manufacturers or is there some rationality in all of this?"

Reply: When the urine is retained in excessive quantities in the bladder we speak of urinary *retention*, and diuretics will not help us here. When it is not properly produced because of some fault of the kidneys, we say there is urinary *suppression*, and diuretics are of no help here either. But when it is not produced because of some unhealthy behavior in the body proximal to the kidneys, then the fluid that should be formed into urine is not made available for the purpose but collects in the tissues and body cavities instead, and we are concerned with the problem of *edema*. It is here that the diuretic agents come to our aid.

Actually, however, although in the main these drugs find the expression of their action at the kidney level, and although the measurable output of urinary salts and water under their influence is a tangible evidence of that action in many of the clinical situations in which they are used, the essence of their activity comprises a rejuggling of the electrolyte balances of the body as a whole. Thus it is that the "diuretic" drugs are not always used primarily for promotion of urinary output and that, in addition to their position of unchallenged importance in the therapy of cardiac edema, they have at least adjuvant usefulness in such diverse conditions as hepatic cirrhosis, eclampsia and pre-eclampsia, polyhydramnios, Ménière's syndrome, glaucoma, epilepsy, hypertension, migraine, premenstrual tension, several types of drug intoxication, nocturnal dyspnea, respiratory acidosis, post-alcoholic syndrome, obesity, renal stone, sickle cell anemia, alkalosis, nephrogenic diabetes insipidus and several other entities not definitely or at least not directly related to an edematous state.

"Since the sulfonamides and related diuretics sometimes produce hyperuricemia, would it not be advisable to use a uricosuric agent concomitantly with them?"

Reply: It seems to me that this would be going too far because the use of such a drug can be counted upon to reduce the hyperuricemia if it should occur. Admittedly the incidence of this reaction to drugs of this type is high; for example, hyperuricemia was induced or aggravated in 19 of 32 hypertensive patients treated with the oral sulfonamide diuretic quinethazone (Hydromox) by Brest and associates in Philadelphia, but probenecid (Benemid) administration reduced the serum uric acid levels in 18 of 19 patients, normal levels being achieved in 13. Actually, gouty symptoms have rarely been associated with the hyperuricemia induced by the diuretics.

Albert N. Brest, Charles Heider, Hassan Mehbod and Gaddo Onesti. Drug Control of Diuretic-Induced Hyperuricemia. J.A.M.A. 195:42, Jan. 3, 1966.

"If it is true that I am in danger of precipitating diabetes through prolonged use of a thiazide diuretic in my patient, how am I going to hedge?"

Reply: You simply cannot hedge. If regular routine urine tests – and they should be done at frequent intervals – in a patient on a thiazide diuretic for a long period reveal sugar, you have diabetes present. This may have been actually precipitated or merely uncovered, but it is diabetes nevertheless. The study of Samaan's group (Postgraduate Medical School,

London) suggested some effect of the drug on the function of the pancreatic islets, perhaps both a lowered rate of insulin secretion and a diminished reserve of insulin available for secretion in response to the normal stimulus. There is also some indication from the work of other investigators that potassium supplementation will oppose the diabetogenic action of the thiazides.

N. Samaan, C. T. Dollery and Russell Fraser. Diabetogenic Action of Benzo-thiadiazines: Serum Insulin-Like Activity in Diabetes Worsened or Precipitated by Thiazide Diuretics. Lancet 2:1244, Dec. 14, 1963. Morton I. Rapoport and H. F. Hurd (William Beaumont Gen'l. Hospital). Thiazide-Induced Glucose Intolerance Treated with Potassium. Arch. Int. Med. 113:405, 1964.

"I have a patient on thiazide diuretics who developed acute anuria. Fortunately, conservative management sufficed to bring him through the episode, but this complication was a very serious affair. Does it occur often?"

Reply: Fortunately, no. I have only seen the report of Gelfand's (New York) 2 cases, and both of these patients had underlying chronic, hypertensive renal disease. They, too, recovered. Of course, early recognition of an impending renal failure might prevent the development of irreversible changes, but routine urinary volume and serum electrolyte studies are hardly practicable under most circumstances in which the thiazides are prescribed.

Maxwell L. Gelfand, Mitchel G. Garren and Robert L. Rowan. Acute Anuria Associated with Chlorothiazide (Diuril) and Hydrochlorothiazide (Hydro-Diuril) Therapy: Recovery. New York J. Med. 64:1865, July 15, 1964.

"One of my associates has had a case of transient myopia occurring in an obstetrical patient while under diuretic therapy. Could this have been truly ascribable to the drug?"

Reply: Yes, it is possible. In Sweden, Ericson reported 2 cases of transient myopia in pregnant women after treatment with chlorthalidone (Hygroton). This drug, like the carbonic anhydrase inhibitors and the thiazide derivatives, is a sulfonamide derivative, although it has a chemical replacement designed to prolong its action and cause less potassium loss than the thiazides. Nevertheless, it seems to me advisable to expect that in its toxic potentialities it will pretty closely resemble the latter group.

Martin F. Jones and John R. Caldwell (Henry Ford Hosp.). Acute Hemorrhagic Pancreatitis Associated with the Administration of Chlorthalidone: Report of a Case. New England J. Med. 267:1029, 1962. J. Marion Bryant, Ts'ai Fan Yü, Lawrence Berger, Natalio Schvartz, Seta Torosdag, Lucian Fletcher, Jr., Harrison Fertig, M. Stephen Schwartz and Richard B. F. Quan (New York).

Hyperuricemia Induced by Administration of Chlorthalidone and Other Sulfonamide Diuretics. Am. J. Med. 33:408, 1962. Lennart A. Ericson (Central Hosp., Uddevalla, Sweden). Hygroton-Induced Myopia and Retinal Edema. Acta ophth. 41:538, 1963.

"Is it true that the administration of potassium chloride simultaneously with a thiazide diuretic causes lesions of the small bowel?"

Reply: Indeed no. The use of potassium chloride together with the thiazides dates practically from the beginning of the use of these new diuretics because it was early realized that they promoted potassium excretion. The potassium salt is either given alone or combined with the thiazide diuretic in a single tablet, and no harm has come of this. It was only when enteric-coated tablets of potassium chloride came to be used that a striking increase in the incidence of small-bowel ulcerative lesions began to be reported and ultimately traced to the ingestion of these enteric-coated preparations. It is now fully established, through both experimental and clinical evidence, that there is a specific form of small-intestinal ulcerative disease caused by ingestion of enteric-coated potassium chloride, and it appears from the work of Arthur Allen and associates, at the Jewish Hospital of Brooklyn, that the lesion is basically a segmental venous infarction. The enteric-coated tablets have been withdrawn from the market.

Scott J. Boley, Arthur C. Allen, Leon Schultz and Solomon Schwartz. Potassium-Induced Lesions of the Small Bowel. J.A.M.A. 193:12, Sept. 29, 1965. Arthur C. Allen, Scott J. Boley, Leon Schultz and Solomon Schwartz. Potassium-Induced Lesions of the Small Bowel. J.A.M.A. 193:997, Sept. 20, 1965.

"What is the effect on the electrolytes of the thiazide-derivative diuretics?"

Reply: The most frequent undesirable occurrence when these drugs are used is induced potassium deficiency. The signs of this hypokalemia are a bitter taste, thirst, gastrointestinal symptoms, weakness and malaise and perhaps even muscle paralysis. Some degree of this occurs in a very high proportion of patients even though potassium chloride is being taken concomitantly. There may also be a hypochloremic alkalosis if the loss of chlorides in relation to sodium has been excessive. The latter is combated by administration of ammonium chloride, but this should be avoided in the patient with liver involvement. One should be aware with regard to the hypokalemia that it will increase the sensitivity to digitalis, i.e., promote digitalis toxicity, and that it is likely to promote arrhythmias in the patient with coronary disease. It is actually possible with these drugs to produce a low salt syndrome of sufficient severity to require infusion of hypertonic saline solution.

When the drugs are used in the treatment of cirrhosis of the liver it is advisable to be on guard against precipitation of hepatic coma through the induced electrolyte imbalance; premonitory symptoms are flapping tremor, confusion and somnolence.

"A hypertensive patient who has been for some time on chlorthalidone (Hygroton) has now developed hyperuricemia though there is no history of a tendency to gout in himself or in his forebears. Could the drug have provoked this?"

Reply: Hyperuricemia is due to suppression of renal excretion of uric acid and may be due to a number of drugs, including ordinary analgesic dosage of aspirin, and the thiazide diuretics. In a study by one of the outstanding students of gout, Ts'ai Fan Yü and her associates, in New York, it was found that chlorthalidone may be added to the list.

J. Marion Bryant, Ts'ai Fan Yü, Lawrence Berger, Natalio Schvartz, Seta Torosdag, Lucian Fletcher, Jr., Harrison Fertig, M. Stephen Schwartz and Richard B. F. Quan. Hyperuricemia Induced by Administration of Chlorthalidone (Hygroton) and Other Sulfonamide Diuretics. Am. J. Med. 33:408, 1962.

"I have a patient with congestive heart failure who is obtaining a very satisfactory diuretic action from chlorthalidone (Hygroton), but he has developed hyperuricemia. Is it possible to overcome this development without discontinuing the diuretic drug?"

Reply: Yes, it appears to be. At the Bronx Veterans Administration Hospital, Robert Sperber's group effectively reduced the hyperuricemia induced by chlorthalidone through administration of 200 mg. of sulfinpyrazone (Anturane) daily despite continuation of the diuretic therapy.

Robert J. Sperber, Solomon Fisch, Arthur C. DeGraff and Roslyn R. Freudenthal. Correction of Diuretic-Induced Hypokalemia and Hyperuricemia. Am. J. Med. Sc. 249: 269, 1965.

"Most of my friends are so convinced of the diuretic superiority of the thiazide derivatives nowadays that they look askance at the mention of a mercurial. Is there nothing to be said on the other side?"

Reply: I can cite to you the authoritative report of Harry Gold and his associates, at Cornell University, who in a very careful study with their classic method of assessing diuretic efficiency, found that 2 Gm. of chlorothiazide (Diuril, etc.), given orally, exerted only 40% of the diuretic effect of 2 ml. of meralluride (Mercuhydrin), given intramuscularly. And in a later test they failed to obtain convincing assurance that polythiazide (Renese) is less efficacious than meralluride, both drugs being given intramuscularly in ceiling doses. Of course, there are things that may be said about the relative toxicity of the two groups and the ease of oral administration with the thiazides; but these are different matters.

Harry Gold, Nathaniel T. Kwit, Charles R. Messeloff, Milton L. Kramer, Argyrios J. Golfins, Theodore H. Greiner, Elizabeth A. Goessel, John H. Hughes and Leon Warshaw. Comparison of Chlorothiazide and Meralluride: New Rapid Method for Quantitative Evaluation of Diuretics in Bed Patients in Congestive Heart Failure. J.A.M.A. 173: 745, June 18, 1960. Harry Gold, Nathaniel T. Kwit and Dilip Mehta. Diuretic Effect of Polythiazide (Renese) and Sodium Meralluride (Mercuhydrin): Comparison in Bedfast Patients with Edema. J.A.M.A. 190:571, Nov. 16, 1964.

"When an organomercurial diuretic compound is administered is there danger that the kidney may be injured by inorganic mercury split off from the drug?"

Reply: John Moyer's group has shown conclusively that practically all of the mercury is excreted in a form closely resembling the administered organomercurial compound, which disposes of the claim that the kidney is damaged by inorganic mercury liberated during metabolic processes.

J. H. Moyer, R. A. Seibert and C. A. Handley. Chromatography Studies of the Excretion Products After Meralluride Administration in Normal Subjects and Cardiac Patients. Circulation Res. 5:493, 1957.

"How are the electrolytes affected by the mercurial diuretics?"

Reply: Both sodium and chloride excretion are increased, but sodium not as much as chloride, so that the potentiality of hypochloremic alkalosis is established. Calcium excretion is moderately increased, potassium may or may not be; phosphates, sulfates, ammonia, titratable acids and total nitrogen are not affected. There is less effect on water than on electrolyte reabsorption.

The possibility of disastrous effects from excessive restriction of salt accompanied by overtreatment with organomercurials must always be borne in mind. Weakness, lassitude, anorexia, nausea, vomiting, restlessness, thirst not relieved by plain water, apathy, mental confusion, fall in blood pressure, acceleration of pulse rate and diminution of pulse volume, clammy skin, shock and coma are all symptoms or signs pointing to hyponatremia, though any of them may be due to other causes.

"I have found to my surprise that one of my associates is still using organomercurial diuretics in combination with ammonium chloride in treating edematous states. Is this not completely archaic therapy?"

Reply: By no means. Principal utilization of these drugs in combination is made in treating congestive heart failure, but sometimes ammonium chloride alone is effectively diuretic when its use is persisted in after the organomercurial has been stopped. Sometimes this drug, used without the organomercurial, is helpful in moving the fluid in portal cirrhosis and in the edemas of chronic nephritis and nephrosis, pre-eclampsia and overdosage with testosterone, and the excessive fluid accumulation in hydramnios. Premenstrual tension, which may be approached as an aberration in electrolyte and water balance, is sometimes effectively treated with ammonium chloride to prevent retention of sodium in the tissues.

"When using ammonium chloride for diuretic or other purposes what precautions should be taken?"

Reply: Ammonium chloride must be given intravenously with great caution because the ammonium is toxic when delivered directly into the blood stream more rapidly than its conversion can take place. Even when the drug is given orally it may be dangerous in individuals, especially elderly persons, in whom the kidneys' ability to excrete a maximally acid urine and produce ammonia may be diminished. In such cases there will be a tremendous loss of sodium and occurrence of acidosis requiring not only cessation of the medication but perhaps even intravenous administration of 1000 ml. or more of sixth-molar sodium lactate solution as antidote. The symptoms are weakness, nausea and vomiting, progressive stupor, perhaps Kussmaul breathing. The high level of plasma chlorides, reflecting increased chloride reabsorption and excessive water loss, differentiates from the low salt "hyponatremia" syndrome. Ammonium chloride poisoning of this sort is very unlikely to be seen if the drug is used only in courses of a few consecutive days, but one should use it cautiously in any patient with cardiac failure presenting cerebral manifestations or severe impairment of liver function.

"A patient on spironolactone (Aldactone-A) therapy has recently developed gynecomastia. I have also had this occur with digitalis therapy in

the past. Is there any connection between these two occurrences, and is the appearance of the gynecomastia a signal for discontinuance of the therapy?"*

Reply: There is a structural similarity between the cardiotonic glycosides and spironolactone and it may therefore well be that the effect on the breasts is related to this chemical similarity. It should be recalled, however, that enlargement of the male breast occurs in several clinical conditions that have no apparent common ground and also that no convincing relationship has been found between gynecomastia and estrogen imbalance. As for discontinuance of the therapy, I think the appearance of gynecomastia does not make this mandatory unless it be for psychic or cosmetic effects. At the Lenox Hill Hospital, New York, Eugene Clark observed gynecomastia in 4 of 7 men but in none of 5 women treated with spironolactones, a small series but sufficient to indicate that the incidence of this occurrence may be greater than has been suspected. The mechanism of this breast enlargement has not been determined.

Eugene Clark. Spironolactone Therapy and Gynecomastia. J.A.M.A. 193:163, July 12, 1965.

"I am aware that in using spironolactone (Aldactone) as a supplemental diuretic agent there is some danger of causing a rise of serum potassium to toxic levels. Are there peculiarities in the individual patient that make him more prone to the development of this serious side action?"

Reply: Bayley and associates (Toronto) found that the effect does not appear to be necessarily related to renal insufficiency and a rise in the blood urea nitrogen. Bondy (Yale University) has pointed out that the severe Na retention makes the patient particularly prone to develop hyperkalemia because when the Na in the urine is low there is difficulty in excreting K. He also made the point that hyperkalemia is likely in the patient with renal insufficiency, somewhat in contradiction of the findings of Bayley's group, if his tubular exchange of K for Na is depressed by spironolactone since the normal excretion of dietary potassium is increased through its tubular secretion.

T. A. Bayley, P. G. Forbath, J. K. Wilson and H. P. Higgins. Metabolic Studies on Patients with Resistant Heart Failure Treated by Spironolactone (Aldactone). Canad. M. A. J. 87:1263, Dec. 15, 1962. P. K. Bondy. Hyperkalemia and Sudden Death During Spironolactone Therapy. (Editorial Comment in 1963–1964 Year Book of Medicine, p. 673.)

"A preparation known as Aldactazide-A, which contains 75 mg. of spironolactone and 25 mg.

of hydrochlorothiazide, is considerably used in our area in the treatment of refractory cardiac edema. What do you think of this preparation?"

Reply: I have no reason to doubt that the two ingredients of this preparation nicely complement each other in their actions, as is claimed: i.e., that spironolactone acts at the distal convoluted tubule and hydrochlorothiazide at the proximal convoluted tubule; that both drugs enhance sodium excretion, while the thiazide also promotes potassium excretion and the spironolactone favors its retention; that the drugs in combination enhance salt and water excretion in a synergistic manner; and that the potassium balance is relatively easily maintained with the preparation. There is but one objection to prefabricated medication of this sort (and my associates are very tired of hearing me reiterate it), namely, that if your patient exhibits signs of serious electrolyte imbalance under the influence of the preparation, you have no way of determining which of the ingredients is responsible and are therefore incapable of adjusting dosage of the individual ingredients in accordance.

Edward Settel (Brooklyn). Further Experience with Spirono-lactone-Hydrochlorothiazide (Aldactazide-A) in Long-Term Treatment of Refractory Cardiac Edema. J. Am. Geriatrics Soc. 13:655, 1965.

"I have heard something of the use of mepyra-pone (Metopirone) as aldosterone antagonist. Has it been shown to have any advantage over spironolactone (Aldactone)?"

Reply: M. S. Davies and associates used it, together with prednisolone to suppress release of corticotropin, and did not produce evidence that seemed to me very convincing of its usefulness.

M. S. Davies, B. S. Hetzel, G. M. E. Kearney and G. M. Wilson. Use of Metyrapone (Metopirone) as Aldosterone Antagonist. Clin. Pharmacol. & Therap. 5:296, 1964.

"I have been using the new drug, triamterene (Dyrenium), cautiously in a few cases of congestive heart failure and have been much pleased with the diuretic effect I have gotten when combining the drug with hydrochlorothiazide. Best results seem to be obtained with 100–200 mg. of tri-amterene daily in two divided doses with the addition of 50 mg. of hydrochlorothiazide (Hydro-Diuril, etc.) daily. What may I expect the effect of this combination to be on the serum potassium level?"

Reply: At the Jewish General Hospital, Montreal, J. Wener and associates studied this matter and found that the addition of tri-amterene always corrected any hypokalemia which may have been present when hydro-chlorothiazide was given alone without a generous potassium supplement. This was verified many times in their study by substituting a thiazide for triamterene in the patients' therapy and observing a prompt fall in serum potassium levels and a quick return of these levels to normal when triamterene was given and the thiazide stopped.

J. Wener, R. Schucher and R. Friedman. Treatment of Congestive Heart Failure with Triamterene. Canad. M. A. J. 92:452, Feb. 27, 1965.

"I have found a new diuretic, triamterene (Dyrenium), very effective when combined with hydro-chlorothiazide (Hydro-Diuril) in the prolonged treatment of chronic congestive heart failure, and some of my associates have used it to good advantage in cirrhotic individuals with ascites. Some nausea, headache, weakness, dizziness and diarrhea have occurred in the experience of all of us, but these things have receded nicely under dosage adjustment. I understand that there have also been a few reported instances of leukopenia, but have not encountered this complication myself. Is there any special precaution I should take in using this drug?"

Reply: I think that you should cease using potassium supplementation when employing triamterene and hydrochlorothiazide together since the new drug does not promote potassium excretion.

"I have not found ethacrynic acid always the superior diuretic that the promotion has indicated it would be; what has been the usual experience?"

Reply: The drug is extremely variable in its action. Denis Daley and Byron Evans (Cardiff, Wales) compared the diuretic effect with that obtained with mersalyl. Ethacrynic acid, 150 mg. orally, and mersalyl, 2 ml. intramuscularly, were given alternately, and the efficacy of each estimated from weight loss. With the efficacy of mersalyl assumed to be 100%, that of ethacrynic acid varied from zero to 680%. However, some patients respond to this drug when they have previously resisted other diuretics. Particularly gratifying have been the responses in acute pulmonary edema, but there are some unpleasant side effects, too. In the 67 patients plus 15 normal volunteers studied by Paul Cannon's group at Columbia-Presbyterian Medical Center, anorexia occurred in 8, transient azotemia in 5 with renal disease, hyperuricemia in 8, orthostatic hypotension in 1 cardiac, and massive diuresis in 2 cirrhotic patients, which induced hepatic coma. And I have seen the report of transient hearing loss in 5 instances.

Denis Daley and Byron Evans. Diuretic Action of Ethacrynic Acid in Congestive Heart Failure. Brit. M. J. 2:1169, Nov. 9, 1963. George V. Irons, Jr., Yi-Hong Kong, William M. Ginn, Jr. and Edward S. Orgain. Clinical Experience with Intravenous Administration of Ethacrynic Acid. J.A.M.A. 194:1348, Dec. 27, 1965. Paul J. Cannon, Henry J. Heinemann, William B. Stason and John H. Laragh. Ethacrynic Acid: Effectiveness and Mode of Diuretic Action in Man. Circulation 31:5, Jan. 1965. William J. Schneider and E. Lovell Becker. Acute Transient Hearing Loss After Ethacrynic Acid Therapy. Arch. Int. Med. 117:715, 1966.

"My associates and I have had fairly extensive experience with the oral administration of the new diuretic, ethacrynic acid, and are now wondering whether the drug may be used effectively intravenously?"

Reply: The observations are limited so far, but I can cite the experience of George Irons' group at Duke University, who gave the drug intravenously on 61 occasions to 31 edematous subjects. Maximal water, sodium, chloride and potassium diuresis occurred within the first hour, and potassium diuresis continued into the following day. No significant electrolyte alterations occurred after a single intravenous injection, and effective diuresis was achieved in spite of azotemia, hypochloremia, hyponatremia and hypokalemia. The drug was found to be particularly effective when administered to 8 patients manifesting pulmonary edema on 12 occasions. There were no significant side effects. The powdered drug was diluted in 5% glucose in water immediately prior to administration and a dose of 0.5 mg./kg. was diluted in a 20 ml. volume and given slowly intravenously over a 3–5 minute period.

George V. Irons, Jr., Yi-Hong Kong, William M. Ginn, Jr. and Edward S. Orgain. Clinical Experience With Intravenous Administration of Ethacrynic Acid. J.A.M.A. 194: 1348, Dec. 27, 1965.

"I have a patient with anemia complicated by fluid retention; can I reduce the risk of precipitating pulmonary edema, when transfusing, by adding ethacrynic acid to the blood?"

Reply: J. G. G. Ledingham (Westminster Hospital, London) did so successfully in 7 patients. The dose of ethacrynic acid added to the bottle of blood varied from 12.5 to 50 mg. No problems ensued.

J. G. G. Ledingham. Ethacrynic Acid Parenterally in Treatment and Prevention of Pulmonary Edema. Lancet 1: 952, May 2, 1964.

"In a patient with cardiac edema who is not responsive to the thiazide derivatives or the mercurials even when ammonium chloride is used with the latter, what would you suggest that one might turn to?"

Reply: Try aminophylline. In Birmingham, England, a few years ago, Domenet and associates gave such patients mercaptomerin (Thiomerin) intramuscularly and after 2 hours aminophylline intravenously. Of 35 patients, 28 responded with sustained diuresis and clinical improvement, 21 showing a maximum rate of weight loss.

J. G. Domenet, D. W. Evans and O. Brenner. Value of Mercaptomerin (Thiomerin) and Intravenous Aminophylline in Cardiac Edema Resistant to Other Diuretics. Brit. M. J. 1:1130, Apr. 22, 1961.

"Does urea as an osmotic diuretic have any place today in the therapy of the patient with chronic heart failure with edema?"

Reply: Yes, I think it does. At worst the drug seems rarely to be harmful, though it may have to be discontinued on account of the patient's distaste or because of nausea and vomiting. At best it may be the means of maintaining in non-strenuous occupation for several years a patient in whom this result is unattainable by other medications singly or in combination. Between such extremes are patients in chronic congestive failure who may receive many months of benefit, at first by prolongation of quiet activity free from edema, and later by mitigation or abolition of distressing edema and effusions until the last days of the illness. It may certainly be said that urea has one great advantage, shared with few of the other diuretics, of continuing to exert its effect as long as its administration is continued, though of course not irrespective of the advancing pathologic process. In the presence of reduced renal function it may contribute to the picture of nitrogen retention.

Usual dosage of urea is 30–40 ml. of a 50% solution, stirred in water or fruit juice, three or four times daily. Grape juice seems a particularly acceptable vehicle. Or it may be prescribed in suspension in a flavored vehicle.

"I have recently had a patient with congestive heart failure who responded very well to corticosteroid therapy after becoming resistant to traditional therapy alone. Why is there a general feeling that the corticosteroids should not be used in most instances in this malady?"

Reply: In 1959, Mickerson and Swale (Charing Cross Hospital, London) reported the supplementation of existing digitalis and diuretic therapy by prednisolone (Hydeltra, etc.), 5 mg. three times daily for 1–2 days and then 2.5 mg. two or three times daily, in 13 patients whose congestive failure had become resistant to traditional therapy. In all, there were symptoms suggestive of adrenocortical deficiency, however. There was rapid improvement, within 3–4 days: symptoms relieved, diuresis established, disappearance of edema and congestive failure in 2–4 weeks. These investigators reasoned that in elderly patients with poor pituitary reserves, the anterior pituitary may be unable to meet the demands imposed by the congestive failure, and the result is adrenocortical deficiency. Again, in 1960, Mickerson reported a small group of patients, this time with congestive failure in chronic pulmonary heart disease, who had responded well to corticosteroid therapy. However, I believe that most men are refraining from the use of these drugs because of the thoroughly documented study of the clinical and cardiodynamic effects of corticosteroid therapy in 9 patients with congestive heart failure, that was made by Green and associates, in 1960. The patients in this group had responded as follows: in 5, there was an increase in the failure; in 3, there was no significant change in the clinical state; and in only 1 was there an improvement in cardiodynamics as well as in clinical state. This one record at least appears to indicate a more detrimental than beneficial effect from corticosteroids in most instances of congestive heart failure.

J. N. Mickerson and J. Swale. Diuretic Effect of Steroid Therapy in Obstinate Heart Failure. Brit. M. J. 1:876, Apr. 4, 1959. J. N. Mickerson. Prednisolone Maintenance Therapy in Chronic Pulmonary Heart Disease. Brit. Heart J. 22:220, 1960. M. A. Greene, A. Gordon and A. J. Boltax. Circulation 21:661, 1960.

"Since decompensation in a patient with heart disease is often precipitated by pulmonary infection, and differentiation of such an infection from pulmonary congestion is difficult by physical examination or roentgenography, is it advisable to administer antibiotics routinely to all patients with acute decompensation?"

Reply: Petersdorf and Merchant put this matter to the test at the Yale–New Haven Medical Center through examining the course and frequency of pulmonary infections in 150 patients with acute heart failure, half of whom received 0.5 Gm. chloramphenicol (Chloromycetin) orally every 6 hours for 7 days and the others a placebo. All patients were treated routinely for the failure. The findings did not indicate in any respect that antibiotic prophylaxis was of value. As for the detection of pneumonia in patients with pulmonary congestion, the radiologic examination was found to be quite reliable; pneumonia was present in 10 of 28 patients in whom it was suspected by the x-ray film of the chest and was missed by their radiologist only twice in 112 patients.

Robert G. Petersdorf and Richard K. Merchant. Study of Antibiotic Prophylaxis in Patients with Acute Heart Failure. New England J. Med. 260:565, Mar. 19, 1959.

"If an emergency situation appears to necessitate the use of metaraminol (Aramine) in an individual with chronic mitral valvular disease of considerable severity, what is to be expected?"

Reply: Harald Eliasch and associates (Karolinska Institutet, Stockholm) did not have the emergency situation but they did study the effect of the drug in individuals with mitral valvular disease and found that there occurs in this situation a rise in systemic arterial pressure and an increase in cardiac output and myocardial contractility.

Harald Eliasch, Robert O. Malmborg, Bengt Pernow and Staffan Zetterquist. Effects of Aramine (Metaraminol) on Splanchnic, Cardiopulmonary and Systemic Circulation in Patients with Mitral Valvular Disease. Acta med. scandinav. 175:167, 1964.

"Can you suggest anything to break the vicious circle established in low output heart failure when the diminished cardiac output adds additionally to the load of the failing heart by increasing reflex peripheral resistance and central venous congestion?"

Reply: Presumably in your hypothetical case you have already accomplished all that is possible with digitalis and diuretics. In such a situation R. T. Kelley's group felt that their use of hexamethonium chloride (Esomid, Hiohex, Methium) was successful since all 19 patients had significant reduction in venous pressure, and there were gratifying improvements in the other parameters of the state. R. R. Burch confirmed this finding independently. Oral dosage of the drug usually begins at 125–250 mg. three or four times daily but not to exceed 3 Gm. total in most instances; intramuscular or subcutaneous doses of 50–100 mg. may be repeated at 6 hour intervals.

R. T. Kelley, E. D. Freis and T. F. Higgins. Effects of Hexamethonium on Certain Manifestations of Congestive Heart Failure. Circulation 7:169, 1953. R. R. Burch. The Effects of Intravenous Hexamethonium on Venous Pressure of Normotensive and Hypertensive Patients with and without Congestive Heart Failure. Circulation 11:271, 1955.

"Sometimes a patient in heart failure will be wheezing without rales. Would the use of epinephrine be rational under such circumstances?"

Reply: Because wheezing may occur without moist basal rales in heart failure, it is sometimes postulated that edema of the bronchioles can be present without free fluid in the alveolar spaces. Epinephrine would of course dilate these bronchioles but it is probable that the constriction of the vessels that would also be desirable would require the use of higher dosage than might ordinarily seem advisable.

"I have not often been under the necessity of digitalizing an infant, but in doing so recently was again surprised as I had been earlier at the large amount of the drug that was required. Has this been general experience?"

Reply: Many pediatricians have come to the conclusion that children require as large doses of digitalis as adults, body weight apparently being of no importance with respect to the therapeutic activity of the drug. Hauck and associates reported that, in a series of 86 infants and children treated with digoxin (Lanoxin), 0.03–0.04 mg./pound was the oral dose most often required during the first 24 hours for digitalization of children up to 2 years; in those 2 years or older. 0.02–0.03 mg./pound was needed. They felt that half of the digitalizing dose should be given initially and the remainder in equal portions at 6–8 hour intervals, continuing the latter dosage until there has been a satisfactory response or until toxic signs appear. In this study the correlation between age and dosage was real and not simply due to different types of heart disease in the two groups. Maintenance dosage 1/10 that of the digitalizing dose was usually satisfactory.

A. J. Hauck. P. A. Ongley and A. S. Nadas. The Use of Digoxin in Infants and Children. Am. Heart J. 56:443, 1958.

"One has occasionally to give a diuretic drug in the treatment of congestive heart failure in the small infant. Has the response of the infant kidney to these drugs been closely studied, and what is recommended dosage?"

Reply: At the Children's Hospital of Winnipeg, Robert Walker and Gordon Cumming studied the diuretic response of infants, 6–47 days of age, to mercaptomerin (Thiomerin), chlorothiazide (Diuril), acetazolamide (Diamox) and triamterene (Dyrenium) and found it qualitatively similar to that of adults. Recommended doses of mercaptomerin have been from 0.1 to 0.5 ml., but these investigators pointed out that the higher doses exceed the safe limit suggested by Pitts, and they felt that in the small infant such dosage would appear to be unnecessary. Suggested chlorothiazide dosage has ranged from 2–15 mg./kg./day, and these investigators felt that doses under 5 mg./kg./day were unlikely to be effective. Suggested dosage of acetazolamide has been 5 mg./kg./day, but it appears that larger doses are required for adequate diuresis. Triamterene dosage of 20 mg. was used in this study.

Robert D. Walker and Gordon R. Cumming. Response of the Infant Kidney to Diuretic Drugs. Canad. M. A. J. 91: 1149, November 28, 1964.

"Upon numerous occasions I have succeeded in abolishing Cheyne-Stokes respiration in individuals with congestive heart failure and/or uremia through intravenous administration of 250 mg. of aminophylline, but I have never understood the action of the drug. Has it been explained?"

Reply: At Duke University, A. R. Dowell and associates measured the respiratory responses to the drug in 8 patients with Cheyne-Stokes respiration and in 6 with emphysema. It was found to abolish periodic breathing, increase ventilation, lower the arterial carbon dioxide tension and increase arterial blood pH significantly in the patients with Cheyne-Stokes respiration. Apparently the respiratory threshold to carbon dioxide was lowered in both groups of patients, but the carbon dioxide sensitivity was not altered in either. It appeared that Cheyne-Stokes respiration is abolished through lowering of the threshold of carbon dioxide tension so that the respiratory response occurs more promptly when the blood carbon dioxide tension rises.

A. R. Dowell, A. Heyman, H. O. Sieker and K. Tripathy. Effect of Aminophylline on Respiratory Center Sensitivity in Cheyne-Stokes Respiration and in Pulmonary Emphysema. New England J. Med. 273:1447, Dec. 30, 1965.

CONSTIPATION

"What suppository would you recommend for rapid evacuation?"

Reply: The U.S.P. glycerin suppository has been in use for this purpose for a great many years. There is also a Dulcolax suppository that will usually produce evacuation within an hour. It has been reported that if rapid evacuation of the rectum and colon is desired, a 300 mg. quinine dihydrochloride suppository will promptly accomplish it.

"In our geriatric patients in nursing homes it is frequently necessary to resort to enemas for satisfactory evacuation of the lower bowel, but this is an unpleasant procedure from the standpoint of every one concerned. Have any of the evacuant suppositories, less drastic than the U.S.P. glycerin suppository, had convincing trials?"

Reply: Yes, there have been several favorable reports of the use of the bisacodyl (Dulcolax) suppository. The most recent to come to my attention was that of Roswell Phillips of the VA Hospital, Spokane, Washington, who used the commercially available 10 mg. suppository in 100 consecutive geriatric patients, most of whom spent much of the day in bed, had poor muscle tone, and often had cerebral dysfunction. Ninety-three patients had a satisfactory bowel evacuation, failure occurring only when there was fecal impaction. Evacuation occurred in an average time of 24 minutes, but as much as 2 hours was required in a few instances. Three of the patients experienced some rectal burning and loose stools, but these symptoms were mild and lasted less than a day.

Roswell W. Phillips. Bisacodyl Suppository as an Enema Substitute. J. Am. Geriatrics Soc. 13:78, 1965.

"What laxatives would you recommend that may be given at night to a chronically constipated individual to produce a single formed, though perhaps slightly soft, stool in the morning?"

Reply: Cascara sagrada fluid extract is used in dosage of up to 12 ml. or perhaps even more for the adult; tolerance to this preparation seems very rarely to develop and griping is quite unusual. Dulcolax is used in dosage of 1 or 2 of the 5 mg. enteric-coated tablets. Senokot is given in average dose of 1 teaspoonful of the granules or 2 tablets. Phenolphthalein, in a proprietary preparation such as Phenolax Wafer, is upon the whole a very reliable laxative in this class, though sometimes a small dose acts excessively whereas a large dose may fail to act at all.

"Would you kindly suggest a saline cathartic or two that is not excessively nasty to take?"

Reply: Perhaps the two that are least offensive are the milk of magnesia (an 8% aqueous suspension of magnesium hydroxide that is palatable and easy to give to children and also acts as an antacid) and magnesium citrate, principally used as the solution available in effervescent form in 12 ounce bottles. The laxative dose of milk of magnesia is 8–16 ml. (2–4 teaspoonfuls) taken from a spoon or stirred in cold water. Addition of fruit juice converts this drug in part to magnesium citrate, which is more active. The dose of the magnesium citrate effervescent preparation is one bottle or less, but in fact this is often nauseating and sometimes quite violent in action. Then there is effervescent sodium phosphate, which is mild and fairly pleasant to take in dosage of 8–12 grams (2–3 teaspoonfuls) in water.

"Were the serious charges that were brought against liquid petrolatum a number of years ago ever satisfactorily refuted?"

Reply: Not to my knowledge. These charges were the following: (a) the rectum, being kept partially filled most of the time, is thus abnormally converted into a receptacle for fecal material; (b) complete evacuation is impossible for there is always a tenacious layer of a dirty mixture of oil and feces covering the rectal mucosa; (c) absorption of carotene and, to a lesser extent, of vitamins A and D, is seriously interfered with; (d) digestion is incomplete because the passage of the contents through the bowel is hastened; (e) the healing of postoperative wounds in the ano-rectal region is delayed; (f) leakage from the anus may give rise to pruritus ani; (g) mineral oil may be absorbed and cause pathologic changes in the abdominal viscera. In addition it should be noted that benign pneumonitis, due to inhalation of minute amounts of the oil by persons taking it habitually, has occurred and, when unilateral, been mistaken for a malignant neoplasm.

"What would you suggest for use merely to soften the stool to facilitate elimination in an individual with painful anal lesions?"

Reply: Doxinate, Colace, Polykol, among others in their class, are inert surface-acting compounds that perform in the bowel as detergents to permit water and fatty material to be better mixed with the fecal material, thus softening it. Dosage of the first two of these agents is 10–20 mg. daily for infants and children, up to 60 or even 100 mg. daily in divided doses for adults; of the last of the three agents, 200 mg. one to three times daily for children of 3–12 years, 100–200 mg. once or twice daily for adults.

"When I want a bulk-providing laxative in the treatment of constipation, what are the better preparations?"

Reply: Konsyl is a powder prepared from the outer layers of the psyllium seed; it is used in 1 or 2 teaspoonful doses stirred in milk or three times daily before meals. Metamucil is a 50% mixture of glucose and a psyllium extract; a rounded teaspoonful is stirred into a glass of water, milk or fruit juice three times daily and followed by a large glass of water. Cellothyl is a methylcellulose that is said to be effective in some very recalcitrant forms of constipation. Usually satisfactory dosage appears to be 4 of the 0.5 Gm. tablets dissolved in about a half-tumblerful of lukewarm water, to be taken during or between meals as seems indicated for best results; or the liquid preparations, Cologel and Hydrolose, may be used in tablespoonful dosage. Bran, barium and beet pulp: some individuals obtain a satisfactory effect from bran in the form of cookies, muffins, bread or cakes, or through taking it with sugar and cream to replace the morning cereal. Bran should not be used on the principle that if a little is good a lot is better, for there are actually on record one or two instances in which chuckleheads had stuffed themselves with this dry material until they produced obstruction. Bulk can be satisfactorily provided without irritation through use of 1 or 2 tablespoonfuls of ordinary x-ray barium in water two or three times daily. Beet pulp in the same dosage has also given satisfaction. Sometimes any of the cellulose materials may produce a large amount of gas.

CONTRACEPTION

"Admittedly in using the contraceptive pill some dropouts are due to edema of the lower legs, weight increase, abdominal distention and nausea and vomiting, mastalgia and breast engorgement, acne, dizziness, headache, fatigue, breakthrough bleeding and rarely chloasma. In most instances, however, I can handle these things if the patient is willing to cooperate through dosage adjustment or a switching about among the several preparations now available. But there are practitioners in this area who for reasons of their own are making charges against the pill which I do not believe but have nevertheless to discuss with my patients; such as that the pill may cause masculinization of the female fetus, that it may postpone the menopause, that it may re-establish fertility in a menopausal woman, that it is carcinogenetic, that it causes diabetes and thrombophlebitis. Can you answer these things?"

Reply: Elsewhere I have discussed some of these matters but shall now try to put some brief answers together in a single package. Regarding fetal masculinization resulting from use of the pill during the early stages of an unrecognized pregnancy, it is the belief of many investigators in this field that such instances as have occurred can be explained fully by random coincidence. In any case, according to John Rock, it is very likely that a woman would have to take the preparation fairly constantly during the first 2 or 3 months of her pregnancy in order to bring about such an effect, if it is really possible. There is simply no evidence whatsoever that the menopause can be postponed or fertility re-established after menopause through use of the pill. The only evidence so far uncovered with regard to relationship of the pill to cancer is that, if anything, the incidence seems to be lower in the users of the pill than in nonusers. Obviously, however, no estrogen-containing

preparations should be given to patients with hormone-sensitive malignancies such as carcinoma of the breast any more than, as pointed out by Joseph Goldzieher, one would want to risk the aggravation of conditions influenced by water retention (epilepsy, asthma, migraine), though admittedly the possibility of such aggravation is presently purely speculative. Speculative also is the possibility that a uterine fibromyoma might undergo degeneration (I have seen report of one relevant case) as in normal pregnancy. It is true that normal pregnancy is so fully simulated under the influence of the pill as sometimes to uncover a case of latent diabetes. But as such a discovery would almost certainly come in later years without the use of the pill, the patient in whom this early uncovering occurs is really lucky. And as for thrombophlebitis, it has not been demonstrated, though some people have tried very hard to do so, that there has been a significant increase in the risk of thrombo-embolic death among the users of the pill. Again, as in the case of the diabetic, women who have had trouble from varicose veins may be more prone to development of thrombophlebitis, as they would be with a normal pregnancy, and perhaps such an individual might do well not to use the pill.

John Rock. Let's Be Honest About the Pill! J.A.M.A. 192: 401, May 3, 1965. Joseph W. Goldzieher. Newer Drugs in Oral Contraception. M. Clin. North America 48:529, 1964. I. C. Winter. The Incidence of Thromboembolism in Enovid Users. Metabolism 14 (Part 2):422, 1965. José Donayre and Gregory Pincus. Effects of Enovid on Blood-Clotting Factors. Metabolism 14 (Part 2):418, 1965. Cecil Hougie, Robert N. Rutherford, A. Lawrence Banks and W. A. Coburn. Effect of Progestin-Estrogen Oral Contraceptive on Blood-Clotting Factors. Metabolism 14 (Part 2):411, 1965. G. L. Wied, M. E. Davis, R. Frank, P. B. Segal, P. Meier and E. Rosenthal. Statistical Evaluation of the Effect of Hormonal Contraceptives on the Cytologic Smear Pattern. Obst. & Gynec. 27:327, 1966.

"Is it true that hepatic impairment has resulted from the use of the contraceptive pill?"

Reply: I have seen two reports indicating that there have been such occurrences when estrogen-progestin combinations of this sort have been used in postmenopausal women. Attracted by the possibility that liver impairment may be found only in menopausal women, John Bakke (Seattle) performed liver function tests in 36 menopausal women who had been treated with Enovid for from 1 to 24 months. He found no evidences of hepatic impairment other than in the few instances in which the marginal abnormalities on test probably merely revealed the incidence that might be expected in a control group of the same age. Since the two reports of definite liver dysfunction in a high proportion of post-menopausal women emanated from the single city of Helsinki, Finland, there is the suggestion that differences in climate, nutrition, or endemic hepatitis virus might explain these findings. A case of Enovid-induced cholestatic jaundice has been reported by William Boake and associates (University of Wisconsin) in a 28-year-old woman, but she had had jaundice of a similar type in each of her three successive pregnancies; similarly, there was definite history of previous jaundice in 2 of Thulin and Nermark's 7 cases in Sweden.

John L. Bakke. Hepatic Impairment During Intake of Contraceptive Pills: Observations in Post-menopausal Women. Brit. M. J. 1:631, Mar. 6, 1965. William C. Boake, Stanley G. Schade, John F. Morrissey and Fenton Schaffner. Intrahepatic Cholestatic Jaundice of Pregnancy Followed by Enovid-Induced Cholestatic Jaundice. Ann. Int. Med. 63:302, 1965. G. I. M. Swyer and Valerie Little. Absence of Hepatic Impairment in Long-Term Oral-Contraceptive Users. Brit. M. J. 1:1412, 1965. K. E. Thulin and Jerker Nermark. Seven Cases of Jaundice in Women Taking an Oral Contraceptive, Anovlar. Brit. M. J. 1:584, Mar. 5, 1966.

"Since the use of estrogens alone for preventing conception by the hormonal suppression of ovulation was not unknown long before the present 'pill' became popular, and since estrogen alone would be much less expensive than estrogen-progestin, might it not be advisable to give the older treatment a new trial?"

Reply: This was done in fact by Edmund Middleton, in Baltimore, who concluded after a 2 year study of stilbestrol use alone that unopposed estrogen is not as suitable for conception control as are the preparations that contain a progestin; endometrial hyperplasia and more frequent breakthrough bleeding are the significant disadvantages.

Edmund B. Middleton. Ovulation Control with Stilbestrol. Obst. & Gynec. 26:253, 1965.

"What is the position of the new sequential oral contraceptives, C-Quens and Oracon, vis-à-vis the older preparations, Enovid-E, Ortho-Novum, Norinyl, Norlestrin, Provest?"

Reply: At the time of this writing, I have not seen published evidence of their superiority.

Gregorio Oclander. Sequential Therapy to Achieve Anovulatory Cycles. Canad. M. A. J. 94:216, 1966. John A. Board. Sequential Mestranol-Norethindrone for Oral Contraception. Obst. & Gynec. 27:217, 1966.

"Like many of my associates, I have been using the contraceptive 'pill' with complete satisfaction, but still there are the little annoying worries. What precisely is the position regarding thrombophlebitis, induction of cancer, effects on the infant, psychologic effect on the patient, fertility following termination of the therapy?"

Reply: Regarding thrombophlebitis, there have certainly been individual case reports casting suspicion on these drugs, but in the larger-scale studies justification for the fear seems to disappear. For example, Eleanor Mears, who has studied this matter very carefully in London's 370 Family Planning Association Clinics, reports that 4 cases of thrombophlebitis have occurred among 1200 patients and that the normal incidence of this malady among nonpregnant women of this age group in Britain is 2–4/1000. And there is also the report of the Ad Hoc Advisory Committee, established by the Food and Drug Administration for the evaluation of a possible etiologic relation of Enovid with thromboembolic conditions, in which it was concluded (J.A.M.A. 185:776, 1963) that available data did not reveal a significant increase in the risk of thromboembolic death from use of the drug. As for the induction of cancer, Mears found 4 positive or suspicious cancer smears in her 1200 patients, with an expectation of 4/1000. Both masculinization and feminization of the infant have been reported, but these have been extremely rare occurrences. As for the effect on the psyche of the woman taking the pill, Zell and Crisp (Phoenix, Arizona) found numerous fears in women under intensive psychotherapy while taking the pill; but do you not expect to find fears of all sorts if you probe for them under practically all circumstances? Fertility subsequent to discontinuing use of the pill is not disturbed; that is thoroughly established.

Eleanor Mears. Ovulation Inhibitors: Large-Scale Clinical Trials. Internat. J. Fertil. 9:1, 1964. Earnest M. Curtis (Emory University). Oral-Contraceptive Feminization of Normal Male Infant: Report of Case. Obst. & Gynec. 23:295, 1964. John R. Zell and William E. Crisp. Psychiatric Evaluation of Use of Oral Contraceptives: Study of 250 Private Patients. Obst. & Gynec. 23:657, 1964. Joseph W. Goldzieher, Edris Rice-Wray, Miguel Schulz-Contreras and Alberto Aranda-Rosell (San Antonio, Texas). Fertility Following Termination of Contraception with Norethindrone (Ortho-Novum): Endometrial Morphology and Conception Rate. Am. J. Obst. & Gynec. 84:1474, 1962. E. Fine, H. M. Levin and E. L. McConnell, Jr. Masculinization of Female Infants Associated with Norethindrone Acetate. Obstet. & Gynec. 22:210, 1963. A. Lawrence Banks, Robert N. Rutherford and W. A. Coburn. Pregnancy and Progeny After Use of Progestin-like Substances for Contraception. Obst. & Gynec. 26:760, 1965.

"Has any record been made of the acceptance of an oral contraceptive in a very large population?"

Reply: The acceptability of Enovid used in the established cyclic manner over periods of up to 37 months in more than 14,000 patients for a total of approximately 160,000 cycles, was shown by Richard Frank and Christopher Tietze in the large metropolitan area to which the centers of the Planned

Parenthood Association, Chicago Area, have access, to be excellent inasmuch as approximately three-fourths of all patients who began using the pill were still using it after 30 months.

Richard Frank and Christopher Tietze. Acceptance of an Oral Contraceptive Program in a Large Metropolitan Area. Am. J. Obst. & Gynec. 93:112, 1965.

"I have had excellent acceptance of the contraceptive pill in my private middle-class practice, but now there is talk of extending the use of this method of contraception to the very poor in public clinics in our area. Has there been good acceptance of this method by people of this social class?"

Reply: Indeed, yes. Edris Rice-Wray and her associates in Mexico City have found acceptability of the pill very high in women of all classes of society including the 78.7% of very poor patients who come to their clinic specifically requesting the pill. Incidentally, 98% of these women are Catholic.

Edris Rice-Wray, Ofelia González, Susana Ferrer, Alberto Aranda-Rosell, Manuel Mazueo, Hector Munguía. Clinical Evaluation of Norethindrone Acetate in Fertility Control. Am. J. Obst. & Gynec. 93:115, 1965.

CORONARY DISEASE

"Is it possible to maintain patients on prolonged oral anticoagulant therapy so that the prothrombin values remain within the desired range at least 95% of the time?"

Reply: I suppose it is *possible*, at least Charles Moore considered that it is when concluding his study of the matter at the Ochsner Clinic in New Orleans, but in fact only 23 of his 62 patients did remain within this desirable range during the entire year, though the study appears to have been performed under most careful conditions.

Charles B. Moore. Feasibility of Prolonged Anticoagulation Therapy. J. Louisiana M. Soc. 117:230, 1965.

"One of our group gave an anabolic preparation to a patient on long-time anticoagulant therapy and promptly had a bleeding situation on his hands. Was this more than coincidence?"

Reply: Decidedly more. Pyörälä and Kekki (University of Helsinki) gave a 10 mg. dose of methandrostenolone (Dianabol) to 7 patients who were well stabilized on maintenance warfarin therapy and obtained an increased sensitivity to warfarin in all of them during the first week, the anticoagulant requirements rising within a week after cessation of the anabolic administration.

K. Pyörälä and M. Kekki. Decreased Anticoagulant Tolerance during Methandrostenolone Therapy. Scandinav. J. Clin. & Lab. Invest. 15:367, 1963.

"In a recent patient with an excessively reduced prothrombin activity while on a coumarin anticoagulant, I did not have the success with the antidotal vitamin K_1 compound, phytonadione (Mephyton, Mono-Kay), that had been my earlier experience. What do you suppose might have been at fault?"

Reply: It was probably a matter of incorrect dosage for the particular situation. The norm for the use of the drug was established by the Mayo Clinic group several years ago. They found that 2.5 mg. or less of phytonadione, given orally, significantly shortened the prothrombin time toward normal in 15 of 16 patients whose prothrombin time in seconds varied from 26 to 90; but in 14 others with a prothrombin time from 33 to 103 seconds, a dosage of 5 or 10 mg. resulted in the return of the prothrombin activity only toward but not completely to normal. They also found that the response depends partly on the length of time the anticoagulant has been administered, higher doses, perhaps 5–10 mg., being advisable when the anticoagulant has been given for 10 days or more or when plasma prothrombin activity is reduced to below 5% of normal. Of course severe hepatic disease may make the response to vitamin K_1 less predictable. I would add that when phytonadione is given intravenously, the emulsion should be diluted 1 : 5 with 5% glucose solution and injected no more rapidly than 10 mg./minute. In about 15 minutes there should be a response, and bleeding should stop in 2–4 hours, with return of prothrombin to normal in 8–14 hours. It is well to notice also that the addition for a while of heparin to the subsequent anticoagulant regimen may be advisable because a period of relative resistance to the action of anticoagulants of the coumarin and indandione derivative types follows administration of vitamin K in high dosage.

Alexander Schirger, John A. Spittel, Jr. and Patrick A. Ragen. Small Doses of Vitamin K_1 for Correction of Reduced Prothrombin Activity. Proc. Staff Meet. Mayo Clin. 34:453, Sept. 16, 1959.

"I am not sure that initial heparin therapy in acute myocardial infarction has really been helpful in my practice. What has been the consensus?"

Reply: I do not think that definitive conclusion has been reached. Among recent studies, that of Brown and MacMillan (Toronto General Hospital) produced findings that did not support this early use of heparin either in the attempt to prevent infarction in "acute coronary insufficiency" or in the early treatment in an acute infarction. They gave 100 mg. heparin intravenously immediately and at 8 hour intervals for the first 48 hours, and the number of individuals in both the treated and control groups was large. Harden (Western Infirmary, Glasgow) found injections at every 6 hours rather than 8 hours also unsatisfactory because the clotting time fluctuated greatly, rising to over 90 minutes within 5 minutes of the injection of 10,000 units and falling to normal within 6 hours in most patients. However, when this latter observer gave continuous infusions of 20,000 units of heparin in 500 ml. of 5% glucose every 12 hours, at a rate of about 15 drops/minute, the clotting time was maintained within the therapeutic range. He actually treated over 150 patients by continuous infusion of 40,000 units daily for 2 days without making any measurements of the blood clotting time. There were no signs of heparin overdosage or serious complications. Convincing evidence of a salutary effect of this therapy on mortality was not offered in Harden's article, as I recall. Definite criteria for exclusion of the patients from their study, and therefore presumably from use of initial heparin in routine practice, were developed by Brown and MacMillan: age over 75 years; acute attack longer than 48 hours before admission; patient currently receiving oral anticoagulants; hypertension (diastolic pressure above 120 mm. Hg); presence of a lesion predisposing to hemorrhage, i.e., history of peptic ulcer. So it would appear that we are really not sure whether starting off the anticoagulant therapy of an acute myocardial episode with heparin is worthwhile or not.

K. W. G. Brown and R. L. MacMillan. Initial Heparin Therapy in Acute Myocardial Infarction. Canad. M. A. J. 90: 1345, June 13, 1964. R. McG. Harden. Method for Intravenous Administration of Heparin in Myocardial Infarction. Brit. M. J. 2:1106, Nov. 2, 1963.

"I have put my first patient on long-term anticoagulant therapy after recovery from an acute myocardial infarction. But now I wish that I hadn't, because I do not know how to get him off the drugs safely. Must he continue taking them for the rest of his time?"

Reply: There have been some discouraging occurrences when these patients are taken off their drug. Certainly anticoagulant therapy does not arrest the underlying disease process, and so when it is discontinued the thrombotic tendency becomes manifest again; Thomes and his associates, at the University of Minnesota, even felt as a result of their large-scale study that it really tends to "catch up." At the end of 5 years, 82% of their patients receiving continuous treatment would have had no recurrence, compared to only 39.6% of those who had discontinued treatment. One can easily agree with J. A. Fuller (General Hospital, Newcastle-upon-Tyne), who feels that prolonged anticoagulant therapy should be reserved for intelligent patients who will understand the undesirability of taking themselves off the drug on a whim. It seems to me only rational, when withdrawing a patient from this prolonged therapy, to taper off the dosage very gradually, say during 6–8 weeks; but I do not know any control study to support this view.

A. Boyd Thomes, Raymond W. Scallen and I. Richard Savage. Prophylactic Value of Long-Term Anticoagulant Therapy. Circulation 21:354, 1960. J. A. Fuller. Experiences with Long-Term Anticoagulant Treatment. Lancet 2:489, Oct. 3, 1959.

"In our group we perform daily prothrombin time studies on our warfarin (Coumadin)-treated patients during an acute coronary episode. But I have heard that at some centers these studies are being done at only 3 day intervals. Is this safe?"

Reply: Even Ovid Meyer at the University of Wisconsin, who has had enviable experience in use of anticoagulant drugs and reported the 3 day method a number of years ago, was not willing to advocate that all patients be treated in this way from the onset of the therapy. He excluded those who were less than 14 days postpartum or postoperative, those given heparin as well as warfarin, those showing a sensitive or resistant response to an initial 50 mg. warfarin sodium, those with pretreatment prothrombin levels below 100%, those taking neither liquids nor food by mouth, those already on anticoagulant therapy, and those critically ill. He also stated most explicitly that a high degree of laboratory accuracy is essential to success with this method.

William H. Atwood, Jr., and Ovid O. Meyer. Management of Patients Receiving Warfarin Sodium (Coumadin) Therapy with Prothrombin Time Determinations at Three-Day Intervals. Am. J. M. Sc. 238:720, 1959.

"In using heparin to initiate anticoagulant therapy in acute myocardial infarction, both the patients and I are disturbed by the ecchymoses and pain at the site of injections. Can this be reduced or obviated in any way?"

Reply: George Griffith and associates (Los Angeles) found that both of these things were sharply reduced when injection was made slowly into the subcutaneous fat tissue above the iliac crest, with a small-bore needle (No. 25 or 26).

George C. Griffith, Willard J. Zinn, Hyman Engelberg, James V. Dooley and Richard Anderson. J.A.M.A. 174: 1157, Oct. 29, 1960.

"Let us assume that a patient comes to me with a history of an anginal attack or attacks. I can find no grossly abnormal electrocardiographic changes at rest, but can provoke some by an exercise test. These yield pretty well to nitroglycerin. But it is very probable that the pain reflects ischemia from the gradual atherosclerotic closure of a coronary vessel; possibly there are already some small transmural or subendocardial clusters of dead cells. But there is not yet leucocytosis, accelerated sedimentation rate or increase in the C-reactive protein or serum transaminase. Will it be of advantage to the patient to have anticoagulant drugs in the blood stream when the eventual infarction occurs? In other words, shall I anticoagulate the angina patient in whom gross infarction has not yet been diagnosed? I am aware of course that the drugs sometimes have an alleviating effect on angina itself, but this is not presently my main concern."

Reply: The reply to this question cannot be a simple one. Of course one may hope that with the anticoagulants the propagation of the thrombus may be slowed and the likelihood of new thrombus development lessened; indeed there are some who feel that one may even dissolve unorganized clots to some extent. So ideally it would be advantageous to have the blood in a relatively noncoagulable state. But to accomplish this requires recognition of the fact that two absolutely essential conditions to be met are that the patient must be completely cooperative and there must be available technical competence to perform the determinations that condition dosage. An additional consideration is that of the definite contraindications to the use of these drugs: ulcerative lesions anywhere in the gastrointestinal tract; severe hypertension; pregnancy (danger to the fetus or of hemorrhage at term or during abortion); surgical procedures; renal insufficiency; and possibly hepatic insufficiency. Furthermore, there is the undeniable fact that progression of the lesion and of the malady in an individual case is not really predictable. Nor can we really say with assurance that this or that environmental alteration will propel the patient into the feared episode. Pell and D'Alonzo studied 653 patients in all employment categories in a large industrial corporation, and found that the incidence of a coronary episode in these people was essentially the same whether they were at work, on vacation, at home or at other places; only 5.4% of the attacks occurred while the individual was strenuously active, about half of them while he was asleep or at rest. And in only one fourth of these patients had there been electrocardiographic abnormalities on examination before the attack. Sprague also brought together some evidence indicating the unlikely association of emotional factors and coronary episodes. It has been found also that overweight, despite the great emphasis placed upon it nowadays, predisposes to the full attack only in individuals under 45 years of age. Does one have no guideposts, then, in this situation? My answer would be: do not routinely anticoagulate all anginal patients but only those whose *worsening* state raises suspicion of impending infarction. Here's a list of the criteria of impending infarction, as compiled by numerous observers: angina that was not readily controlled by rest and nitrites from its very inception; increasing provocative effect of exertion and necessity for considerable increase in nitrite dosage; the beginning of radiation of pain to areas not earlier involved, and accompanying occurrences of nausea, sweating and extreme fear of death; angina that occurs more than once in a single night or that begins to occur at night when it had not previously done so; the occurrence of bizarre symptoms of any kind, which may actually signalize "silent" infarction.

Sidney Pell and C. A. D'Alonzo. A Three Year Study of Myocardial Infarction in a Large Employed Population. J.A.M.A. 175:463, 1961. Howard B. Sprague. Emotional Factors in Coronary Heart Disease. Circulation 23:648, 1961.

"In our outpatient anticoagulant therapy it has seemed to us that alterations in dosage could oftentimes be profitably made for abrupt changes in barometric pressure or temperature, but of course this is extremely difficult to do. What other environmental changes may affect this therapy?"

Reply: Perhaps one could not precisely call it an environmental alteration, but the dependence of the patient on his physician and on the medication can certainly be a factor that importantly enters into the fluctuations in response in some instances. Some patients are also considerably affected emotionally by daily reminders, or the lack of same, that they are "crippled," and this may possibly be reflected in the response to fixed dosage of the anticoagulant. The necessity for maintaining the regular dosage daily is also a disturbing thing for some individuals. In discussing the pitfalls in anticoagulant therapy, Charles Moore (Ochsner Clinic, New Orleans) has listed the following factors which he finds frequently involved in fluctuations in prothrombin time in outpatients: weather changes, alcoholic ingestion, febrile illnesses, exposure to organic solvents, "lost weekends," change in bowel habits, dietary indiscretions, concomitant use of other drugs (phenylbutazone, sulfonamides, antibiotics, narcotics possibly, vitamin K in foods and in polyvitamin mixtures, salicylates more than 1 Gm./day).

Charles B. Moore. Pitfalls in Anticoagulant Therapy for Myocardial Infarction. Angiology 15:27, 1964.

"Will you please supply a list of drugs that will increase the danger of hemorrhage in a patient on anticoagulant therapy: i.e., drugs that will decrease prothrombin concentration?"

Reply: The drugs in the following list, which is probably not complete, *may* cause a decrease in prothrombin concentration: PAS, quinine (occasionally), theophylline, thiouracils, skeletal muscle relaxants (?), anabolic steroids, any drug interfering with vitamin K absorption (such bowel sterilizing antibiotics as chloramphenicol, neomycin, the tetracyclines; drastic cathartics; sulfonamides), and theoretically any drug that depresses liver function. I append here a list of liver function depressing agents, some of which have much greater potentiality for causing liver damage than others: amethopterin (methotrexate), amodiaquin (Camoquin) high dosage, anabolic steroids, antimonials, chlorpropamide (Diabinese), cinchophens, cyclophosphamide (Cytoxan), erythromycin (?), gold salts, isoniazid (I.N.H.), methsuximide (Celontin), methyldopa (Aldomet), oleandomycin (Matromycin) and triacetyloleandomycin (Tao) (?), organic arsenicals, oxyphenbutazone (Tandearil), phenacemide (Phenurone), phenothiazine substitute tranquilizers, phenylbutazone (Butazolidin), pyrazinamide (Aldinamide), probenecid (Benemid), sulfonamides, testosterone and substitutes, tetracyclines (?), thiouracils, and urethane.

"Continuous anticoagulant therapy following the patient's recovery from acute myocardial infarction is a very cumbersome business and I sometimes think that perhaps we are not really accomplishing what we attempt anyway. What is your reaction?"

Reply: How is one to give categorical answer in such a controversial subject? One thing is certain, namely, that the volume of literature in this field is notably diminishing recently. Why is this? Is it because fewer men are concerning themselves with the subject, or is it because (and this I believe to be the case) the subject has been so popularized that lay demand in many metropolitan centers has made the regimen almost mandatory "or else." If the latter supposition truly represents the state of affairs, then I suppose it can be reasoned that further deep concern with the matter might be construed as mere timewasting. But the men who are still coming into the literature to advocate this modality certainly do not seem to be entirely convinced themselves. They disagree somewhat as to what the real aim is; some of them want only "moderate" control and others "rigid" control; they are all concerned with enumeration of factors that might detrimentally affect the record; and to some extent they are still vacillating regarding the drug group of choice. Of course, there is the classic study of Benjamin Manchester (George Washington University), on which he very properly continues to give us progress reports. In the latest of these reports, after 5–15 years of study, he finds a subsequent infarction rate of 47% in treated patients (mortality 22%), and reinfarction of 56% (mortality 36.5%) in the control placebo group. In the first 10 years of the study, only 9.9% of treated patients could not be employed because of severity of illness, whereas there were 25% unemployable in the placebo group and 34.4% in the untreated group. Of course, this all looks very good, but Manchester has devoted himself intensively to this subject, and I think it legitimate to doubt whether his results are truly representative of those being achieved in routine practice throughout the country. Manchester himself stresses the necessity to individualize the therapy and insists that it can be successful only in the completely cooperative patient. Furthermore, he requires a meticulousness about details that is surely difficult to achieve in most practices, and he seems to feel that the continuous regimen will be dangerous and less effective than other types of therapy in the hands of any physician who lacks understanding of the significance of thromboplastin times, the kinetics of hemostasis, and the pharmacology of oral anticoagulant drugs. In fairness, I think that the recently reported study of Seaman's group (Portland, Ore.) should also be briefly mentioned. These people presented a progress report on 196 patients who had entered the study either immediately or on the eighth week after an acute infarction or who presented unequivocal evidence of an earlier infarction. No reduction in mortality of patients receiving continuous prophylactic anticoagulant therapy was seen at either 1 or at 7 years in comparison with the placebo treated group. They expressed the intention of continuing the study for another 7 years; of course mere persistence can be in itself a source of pride and satisfaction in a subject of such serious import as is this one.

A thing that troubles me with regard to the favorable reports is the extent to which rather nonrepresentative groups are studied. Let us take, for example, a typical study, that of Loyal Conrad's group in Oklahoma City. Patients were rejected for participation in this study for the following reasons: died in first month, 15%; date of infarct or ECG changes indefinite, 21%; renal disease and/or hypertension 1 month after the infarct, 15%; diabetes mellitus, 6%; malignancy, 6%; gastrointestinal bleeding, 8%; and other (unreliable, distance, refuse), 29%. Thus a very homogeneous group was provided, but how representative would such a group be of the population in a private practice?

In summary, then, I shall say I do not find the evidence convincing that long-term anticoagulant therapy following myocardial infarction is effectively preventive of reinfarction. The thing most urgently needed in this field is a test that will reveal the patient who is imminently threatened with thrombosis, for in him we would have a good chance of preventing pulmonary and arterial embolism through prophylactic use of anticoagulants.

Benjamin Manchester. Continuous Anticoagulant Therapy Following Myocardial Infarction. Angiology 15:19, 1964. Arthur J. Seaman, Herbert E. Griswold, Ralph B. Reaume and Leonard W. Ritzman. Prophylactic Anticoagulant Therapy for Coronary Artery Disease: Seven-Year Controlled Study. J.A.M.A. 189:183, July 20, 1964. Lloyd L. Conrad, John D. Kyriacopoulos, Carryl W. Wiggins and Gerald L. Honick. Prevention of Recurrences of Myocardial Infarction: Double-Blind Study of Effectiveness of Long-Term Oral Anticoagulant Therapy. Arch. Int. Med. 114:348, 1964.

"Is it mandatory to discontinue use of the oral anticoagulants when the patient is to undergo surgery?"

Reply: I think most men feel it prudent, if the procedure is to be an elective one, to discontinue the drugs slowly during the preceding week or 10 days and then resume their use about 48 hours after the operation. However, numerous operations have been performed without dire results on patients in whom the dosage of anticoagulants has not been altered at all even though there had been sufficient time in which this might have been done. If a patient on oral anticoagulants comes up for emergency surgery it is the practice of many men to give an intravenous injection of 20 mg. of vitamin K_1 (Konakion, AquaMephyton, Mono-Kay) to bring down the prothrombin time somewhat.

"In our hospital we have not reached a consensus regarding anticoagulant therapy of acute myocardial infarction. The question at issue is whether heparin or anticoagulants of the oral group are preferable. The heparin proponents argue the fast action, high margin of safety and low toxicity, and multiple effects on the clotting mechanism, in favor of their drug. They say, too, that there is less need for careful laboratory control when using heparin rather than the oral drugs and that one should also take into account the drug's actions in decreasing blood viscosity, inhibiting experimental pulmonary edema, and altering the partition of serum lipoproteins towards normal. Has a comparison of the two drug types been made in a sufficiently large number of cases to give the findings true significance?"

Reply: Of course you are aware that there are some investigators who favor the use of no anticoagulants at all, but leaving that aside, one must say that the picture remains still confusing because a number of studies have appeared in recent years with findings in favor of both drugs. However, the most recent large scale study that has come to my attention definitely yielded findings in favor of the oral anticoagulants. This was the investigation by a large group of individuals who based their conclusions on study of 798 cases of acute myocardial infarction at 13 hospitals widely scattered throughout the country. A schedule of strict randomization was adhered to in allocating patients into two groups, to receive alone either sodium heparin or sodium warfarin (Coumadin, Panwarfin). The agents were administered for a minimum of 21 days and the effort was made to continue through a full 4 weeks of convalescence. The results indicated no justification for preferring heparin over warfarin, since complications such as thromboembolism, additional infarctions, shock and cardiac decompensation were significantly lower in patients treated with the latter drug. Death rates in the first 2 days were identical for the two groups, but the 28 day mortality was significantly higher in the heparin than in the warfarin group. Nevertheless, an entirely clear picture was not presented by the findings, for there were 28 deaths during the first 2 days after infarction on the warfarin-supplemented-by-heparin regimen but only 15 deaths when the patients received only heparin; furthermore, among the patients who had the most severe symptoms at the time of admission, the pronounced overall tendency toward a lower death rate in the heparin group was not evident. Thus it is obvious that still further study is required to supply a fully satisfactory answer to your question.

Sodium Heparin vs. Sodium Warfarin in Acute Myocardial Infarction. J.A.M.A. 189:555, Aug. 17, 1964.

"While admittedly the major risk in long-term anticoagulant therapy is hemorrhage, it is nevertheless difficult to know precisely what this risk is since all the published studies, giving an incidence range between 1.5% and 10%, have been done in large medical centers. Has there been any report of comparable experience in private practice?"

Reply: I've seen only one such report, that of Reinberg and Lipson published at the end of 1965. They followed 188 patients receiving long-term anticoagulant therapy and reported an incidence of serious hemorrhage of 7.5%, with no hemorrhagic deaths. Unfortunately, it was not specifically stated in the report just how long the drugs had been used in these patients.

Martin H. Reinberg and Morris Lipson. Long-Term Use of Anticoagulants in Private Practice. J.A.M.A. 194:13, Dec. 27, 1965.

"The patient has an acute coronary episode and is placed at once on anticoagulant therapy. Shortly, the condition worsens and we say that there has been an 'extension' of the infarct. How often is this really an unrecognized intramural or subendocardial hemorrhage resulting from the use of the anticoagulants?"

Reply: That this occurs is undoubted, but I do not believe that the actual incidence is a matter of record. Perhaps it is much greater than ordinarily believed?

"Is there any way for the ambulatory post-infarction patient who is on anticoagulants to hedge against hemorrhage?"

Reply: If he will carry with him 5 mg. tablets of phytonadione (Mephyton, Mono-Kay), and will take 1 of these upon the appearance of slight bleeding, his prothrombin time will likely be returned to normal within 12 hours, at which time he can usually safely resume anticoagulant therapy. But if the bleeding is considerable, he should take 3 or even 4 of the tablets and hustle to his physician's office or an outpatient clinic, where Mephyton (Emulsion) may be administered or a blood transfusion given, according to indications.

"In the long-term anticoagulation treatment of coronary disease, what degree of control should one attempt?"

Reply: This matter was studied at the Boston City Hospital by Christos Moschos and associates, who obtained results suggesting that moderate treatment aimed at a Factor II (prothrombin) level of 30–50%, Quick test time of 15–20 seconds, P-P test results of 20–60%, and thrombotest results of 8–25% gives approximately the optimal therapeutic range. With these gauges, the risk of hemorrhage is said to be negligible and protection from thromboembolic complications adequate, although not complete.

Christos B. Moschos, Peter C. Y. Wong and Herbert S. Sise. Controlled Study of the Effective Level of Long-Term Anticoagulation. J.A.M.A. 190:799, Nov. 30, 1964.

"I understand that in England the indandione compounds — such agents as anisindione (Miradon), diphenadione (Dipaxin), phenindione (Danilone, Hedulin, Indon, Dindevan, Eridione) and bromindione (Halinone) — are preferred to the coumarin type of anticoagulants, but in our region here in the United States we hardly hear of these drugs at all. Why is this?"

Reply: Actually there are quite a number of men here in the United States who still use

these drugs, but perhaps most practitioners look upon them as being more provocative of serious side actions than the coumarin type of compound. A number of cases of agranulocytosis have been reported, as well as purpura, rashes, drug fever, severe diarrhea, and liver and renal damage. To be sure, some of these things seem to have appeared only with excessively high dosage, but nevertheless the American profession appears to feel more at ease with the coumarins. Many British physicians, however, feel that they not only get a quicker effect with the indandiones but that prothrombin time is easier to control with them.

"If a patient suspected of having had a recent myocardial infarction is given an opiate before determining transaminase activity, will the drug interfere with the findings?"

Reply: Not all observers have been in agreement, but the conclusion from the latest report I have seen, that of Frederick Shuster and associates (University of Michigan) was that administration of codeine, meperidine (Demerol) and morphine should not interfere with the determination of transaminase activity unless the patient has concomitant biliary tract disease or has had cholecystectomy.

Frederick Shuster, Edward A. Napier, Jr., and Keith S. Henley. Am. J. M. Sc. 246:714, 1963.

"I am aware that drugs of the epinephrine class are very likely to provoke anginal symptoms in a patient with coronary disease, but what of drugs that act in the opposite direction?"

Reply: Your suspicion is fully justified; vasodilator agents are likewise prone to cause such symptoms in a patient of this sort.

"What is your opinion regarding the use of the antidepressant drugs in the treatment of angina pectoris?"

Reply: Since you ask only for an "opinion" I shall give you just that. I do not believe that these drugs have been shown convincingly to effect relief in angina pectoris on any organic basis; i.e., through effecting dilatation of the coronary vessels or otherwise improving coronary or myocardial performance through direct action. There is some extant evidence that they sometimes have an apparently salutary subjective effect through their ability to improve the patient's mood in selected cases. But such an effect might introduce a hazard of its own through stimulating the patient to the performance of physical tasks that are beyond his cardiac capacity. I should not use these drugs for this purpose.

"One of the men in our area, being dissatisfied as we all are with our inability to bring all of our patients through the acute phase of a myocardial infarction, has told me that he is thinking of resorting to the use of atropine. What would be the rationale of such therapy?"

Reply: The aim of this therapy is to counteract the allegedly vagus-mediated reflex coronary vasoconstriction which would decrease the blood supply not only to the uninfarcted tissue but also, through the anastomosing vessels, to the infarcted area. There is actually reason to doubt, however, that this vasoconstriction occurs. Upon the other hand, it has been shown that in coronary disease the coronary bed is usually near maximal vasodilation, and further that an increase in heart rate, such as atropine might impose, could demand an increase in oxygen supply to the myocardium that might not be possible under the circumstances. Scott and Balourdas found that removal of cardiac vagal controls through atropinization decreases ventricular efficiency. Doubt is therefore cast upon the rationale of giving atropine in coronary occlusion. Perhaps the ability of the drug to lower mortality in experimental coronary artery ligation, and allegedly in human coronary disease also, is due to its opposition to epinephrine's tendency to produce ventricular tachycardia, such opposition consisting in raising the rate of the sinus pacemaker to exceed the rate of the ectopic pacemaker set off by epinephrine. But this it will do only in high dosage; in low dosage atropine may actually slow the heart rate, probably through central vagus stimulation.

J. C. Scott and T. A. Balourdas. An Analysis of Coronary Flow and Related Factors Following Vagotomy, Atropine, and Sympathectomy. Circulation Res. 7:162, 1959.

"In addition to being the sheet-anchor drugs for treatment of angina pectoris, what are the other uses of the nitrites and nitrates?"

Reply: In an individual in the pulmonary crisis of *paroxysmal cardiac dyspnea*, the quick-acting nitrites are sometimes helpful because through their generalized relaxing effect on vessels they pool blood in the splanchnic area and reduce the return flow to the heart, thus indirectly affecting myocardial improvement in the handicapped heart; Johnson and associates demonstrated prompt reduction in the pulmonary artery hypertension associated with failure of this sort. The longer-acting nitrates will sometimes sustain lowering of blood pressure for 3–6 hours in *hypertensive* individuals, but unfortunately the necessary dosage is often associated with intolerable nitrite side effects and tolerance for the slower-acting compounds

that are necessarily used in this therapy develops in a week or two. The nitrites do not effectively influence circulation in the hands and feet sufficiently to be helpful in the *peripheral vascular diseases* unless used in dosage that is intolerable. It has been alleged that relief can be obtained in *Raynaud's disease* from application of a nitroglycerin ointment, but most men of my acquaintance who have tried this treatment have not succeeded with it. The nitrites have a relaxing effect on the sphincter of Oddi, but it must be admitted that the effect of the quick-acting members of the group is too fleeting to be of much use, and the blood pressure–lowering feature of their action may be objectionable. However, they are occasionally effectively used not only in *gallstone colic* and *biliary dyskinesia* but also in acute and chronic *pancreatitis*. In an exhaustive study of the physiology of the intact human *ureter* some years ago, Lapides found that the nitrites had no effect on the tonus or rhythmic contractions of the structure. Relief is occasionally afforded by the nitrites in cases of generalized *pruritus* that have resisted all other measures. There is also a miscellany of uses to which the nitrites have been put for the purpose of relieving symptoms through the relaxation of smooth muscle, but I cannot list them all.

An employment of the nitrites that is entirely unrelated to the smooth muscle–relaxing action is in the combating of cyanide poisoning. No other therapy is so effective in this type of poisoning.

J. B. Johnson, J. F. Gross and E. Hale. Effects of Sublingual Administration of Nitroglycerin on Pulmonary-Artery Pressure in Patients with Failure of the Left Ventricle. New England J. Med. 257:1114, 1957. J. Lapides. The Physiology of the Intact Human Ureter. J. Urol. 59:501, 1948. K. K. Chen and C. L. Rose. Treatment of Acute Cyanide Poisoning. J.A.M.A. 162:1154, 1956.

"I have an anginal patient, accustomed to using nitroglycerin, who recently had an episode of reversible, but very frightening, symptoms of cerebral ischemia following taking of the drug sublingually while in the standing position. Could the drug have caused this?"

Reply: Absolutely. Vagn Rønnov-Jessen (Aarhus, Denmark) has recently reported three such instances. Elsewhere I have said, "The desirability of meticulous individualization of nitrite dosage is too often overlooked. Ordinary dosage for most individuals may be overdosage for some. It is an easy routine in the office to try 1/400–1/200 nitroglycerine in each new case to detect the occasional person who is hypersusceptible to the drug's action. Christian advised, many years ago, that every patient be urged to remove the undissolved portion of the tablet as soon as relief is obtained."

Vagn Rønnov-Jessen. Cerebral Complications in Nitro-glycerin Treatment of Angina Pectoris. Acta med. scandinav. 174:523, 1963. Harry Beckman. Editorial Comment, 1964–65 Year Book of Drug Therapy, p. 102.

"There have been some claims in recent years that the nitrites are without value in angina pectoris. What of this?"

Reply: Henry I. Russek and J. Campbell Howard, Jr. (Brooklyn) put the matter to the test with a Master two-step test begun 5 minutes after sublingual administration of a tablet that contained either glyceryl trinitrate (nitroglycerin) disguised as to taste in two different ways or else was merely a placebo; when pain occurred an ECG was recorded. Of the 15 patients, 14 performed more exercise on the nitrite than on the placebo. No patient recognized the nitroglycerin tablets, but 4 of the 10 accustomed to their use thought the effect resembled closely that of nitroglycerin. There was also a marked correlation between increase in exercise tolerance and improvement in ECG response to the measured exercise. I have not found it easy to accept the adverse claims of which you have spoken.

Henry I. Russek and J. Campbell Howard, Jr. Glyceryl Trinitrate in Angina Pectoris: Test of Efficacy. J.A.M.A. 189:108, July 13, 1964.

"I am unimpressed by the reported 'evidence' that nitrites are ineffective in the prophylaxis of anginal symptoms because my experience assures me that the opposite is true. But I would like to know how best to use the drugs, i.e., how to space dosage throughout the day for best protection."

Reply: Henry Russek feels that the best possible prophylactic management with the drugs currently available comprises administration of pentaerythritol tetranitrate (Peritrate, etc.) three times daily shortly before meals, together with erythrol tetranitrate (Cardilate, Erythrol Tetranitrate) sublingually on arising and at 5:00 p.m. on leaving work. He makes the point that giving the drug only three times daily before meals leaves the patient unprotected during several of the most crucial portions of the day, i.e., on arising, while traveling to work, while returning from work, and for some time after taking the evening dose.

Henry I. Russek. Evaluation of Nitrites in Treatment of Angina Pectoris: Erythrol Tetranitrate (ETN) and Penta-erythritol Tetranitrate (PETN) as Therapeutic Agents. Am. J. M. Sc. 239:478, 1960.

"What is your opinion of the use of a preparation containing a tranquilizing agent and a nitrite in combination in the treatment of angina pectoris?"

Reply: There is no doubt about the efficacy of the nitrites in effecting relief in angina pectoris, and I think that the usefulness of tranquilizers, in some individuals at least, is also pretty well established; therefore the use of an agent from each of these groups in combination would certainly be rational. But I would be opposed to the use of such a preparation routinely because not all patients will require both ingredients, and one furthermore loses the opportunity of adjusting dosage of the components independently.

"In our community there are men who use quinidine routinely in myocardial infarction. Is this justified?"

Reply: The drug certainly has its place when used specifically to restore normal cardiac rhythm in selected cases. Regarding routine employment, the most recent study to come to my attention was that of T. B. Begg (Royal Victoria Infirmary, Newcastle-upon-Tyne), who again found, as others had, no evidence of an influence on mortality rate as a result of use of quinidine in 26 patients with recent myocardial infarction; there were 44 controls. When the measure was declining in popularity some years ago, it seemed to me that the coup de grâce was given by Gold, who said he thought this therapy impractical because if the dose of the drug is fairly large it is dangerous, and if it is small it will fail in most instances to prevent the disorders of rhythm.

T. B. Begg. Prophylactic Quinidine after Myocardial Infarction. Brit. Heart J. 23:415, 1961.

"I have a patient with intractable angina pectoris, in whom I am thinking of inducing hypothyroidism with I[131] since I do not wish to subject him to surgical procedures. Has the recent experience been favorable?"

Reply: I have not been particularly impressed. For example, of the 21 patients of Strong and Turner (Edinburgh) only 9 had a good response (though it did last for an average of 21 months), 7 a fair response (average 30 months), and 2 a poor response.

J. A. Strong and R. W. D. Turner. Radioiodine in Management of Refractory Cardiac Pain. Quart. J. Med. 31:221, 1962.

"Have the corticosteroids found a firm place in therapy of acute myocardial infarction?"

Reply: I should say, with some reservation, that they have not. There have been some reports favorable to their use but the numbers of cases involved have not been sufficient, in my opinion, to provide firm assurance of the value of the measure.

Naseeb B. Baroody and Waddy G. Baroody. Adrenocorticosteroids in Acute Myocardial Infarction. Am. J. M. Sc. 250:402, 1965.

"Occasionally in a myocardial infarction the patient will suffer severely from nausea and vomiting. Some of this is undoubtedly due to the analgesics but it is not unlikely that it is also elicited by reflexes from the heart itself. In any case, vomiting is accompanied by bradycardia and vasodilatation, and I have always been concerned over it as possibly contributing severely to the debacle. Can one safely use the newer antiemetic drugs in this situation?"

Reply: Bjerkelund and associates studied this matter in Oslo and found that the use of one of these drugs, perphenazine (Trilafon), reduced both nausea and vomiting quite effectively and also reduced the need for analgesics. The study was carefully planned and controlled on a double-blind basis and there were no significant differences in mortality in the treated and untreated groups.

Christopher Bjerkelund, Sigurd Nitter-Hauge and Erling Jakobsen. Perphenazine (Trilafon) in the Prophylaxis of Nausea and Vomiting Following Acute Myocardial Infarct. Acta med. scandinav. 177:729, 1965.

"I am tempted to try a uricosuric agent in one of my myocardial infarction patients because there are patent relationships between high levels of uric acid in gout and often in atherosclerosis. Should I do this?"

Reply: I do not think so. Jerry Edelman and associates (Philadelphia General Hospital) tried it with results that were not of significant benefit.

Jerry Edelman, Alfred Kershbaum, Herschel Sandberg and Samuel Bellet. Effect of Probenecid (Benemid) Administration on Blood Lipids and Lipid Tolerance Curves in Subjects with Myocardial Infarction. Am. J. M. Sc. 241: 96, 1961.

"I suppose that oxygen is not a drug—or is it? At any rate, I should much like to know under what circumstances we can do harm through the administration of oxygen."

Reply: A type of oxygen "poisoning" is that occasionally seen when a patient under the influence of a general anesthetic (ether is the principal exception for it establishes vagal reflexes through stimulation of sensory endings in the respiratory tract) stops breathing after a few inhalations of 100% oxygen. This is explained by the fact that in such a patient the sensitivity of the medullary centers to carbon dioxide may have become sufficiently depressed that respiration is being maintained largely by the reflex response to the hypoxic state of the blood in the carotid sinus and aortic arch; elimination of this hypoxia through administration of oxygen removes this last stimulus, and respiration ceases.

A patient with chronic emphysema may become comatose under 100% oxygen because the prolonged elevation of arterial carbon dioxide tension may have made the respiratory center insensitive to carbon dioxide and the latter may accumulate to a point sufficient to depress the cerebral cortex when administration of oxygen removes one of the two mechanisms (carotid sinus hypoxia and vagal reflexes) that are keeping respiration going. In addition, Schmidt and Comroe have shown that strong carotid stimulation (by the hypoxia in this case) may result in stimulation of the cerebral cortex as well as of the medullary centers.

A remote but nevertheless real danger when 100% oxygen is being used is that sudden obstruction of the airway, as by a mucous plug, may cause atelectasis when the alveoli collapse as their contained oxygen is absorbed.

Another type of oxygen "poisoning" is that which is seen when oxygen is delivered at greater than atmospheric pressure for more than a brief period. The symptoms comprise diverse evidences of damage to the central nervous systems and the underlying mechanisms are unknown although there are interesting suggestions in the work of Dickens of a toxic effect on cerebral enzyme systems.

Excessive administration of oxygen appears to have been almost solely responsible for a type of blindness, known as retrolental fibroplasia, that made its appearance mysteriously among premature infants a few years ago and has now practically disappeared again. The cause was shown to be the use of high concentrations of oxygen in incubators in the attempt to prevent the irregular breathing that is common in prematures. As demonstrated in the studies of Patz and his group, Ashton and Cook and others, during the mid-1950's, the effects of oxygen on the retina with an immature vasculature are observed in two stages: (1) an initial vasoconstriction, which favors accumulation of metabolic end-products in the inner layers of the retina; and (2) a secondary proliferative reaction, with dilatation, tortuosity and overgrowth of retinal vessels into the vitreous, plus retinal detachment and the production of a grayish, fibrous formation behind the lens. When the concerted attack upon the problem by a number of keen investigators in several countries revealed that maintenance of oxygen concentrations above 40% in the incubators of prematures, and the sudden transference to atmospheric oxygen at the termination of incubation, were the principal causative factors, the disease practically ceased to exist except in rare sporadic instances.

N. Ashton and C. Cook. Direct Observation of Effect of Oxygen on Developing Vessels: Preliminary Report. Brit. J. Ophth. 38:433, 1954. F. Dickens. The Toxic Effects of Oxygen on Brain Metabolism and Tissue Enzymes. I. Brain Metabolism. Biochem. J. 40:145, 1946. II. Tissue Enzymes. Ibid. 40:171, 1946. A. Patz. Oxygen Studies in Retrolental Fibroplasia. IV. Clinical and Experimental Observations. Am. J. Ophth. 38:291, 1954. C. F. Schmidt and J. H. Comroe, Jr. The Role of the Carotid and Aortic Bodies in the Defense of the Mammalian Organism Against Oxygen Lack. Science, 92:510, 1940.

"Although I am aware that the manufacturers do not recommend it, I have nevertheless used angiotensin (Hypertensin) with good effect in a few instances of acute myocardial infarction with shock. Am I being too bold?"

Reply: I should not be entirely at ease with such therapy myself, although this use of the drug has been favorably reported by Belle and Jaffee, in Miami, who liked the drug because it could be used in small amounts of fluid, infiltration with it did not cause necrosis, and tachyphylaxis did not occur. But what about the risk of using an agent in myocardial infarction that raises peripheral resistance without simultaneously having a cardiac stimulating action?

Martin S. Belle and Robert J. Jaffee. Use of Large Doses of Angiotensin in Acute Myocardial Infarction with Shock. Journal-Lancet 85:193, 1965.

"I have recently had a patient in whom very prolonged administration of metaraminol (Aramine) was necessary in order to bolster the peripheral vascular system. In some cases, however, the hypotension seems rather directly to reflect diminished cardiac output; might the drug be indicated in such circumstances also?"

Reply: Malmcrona and associates (University of Göteborg) studied this matter very carefully in 11 patients. In all of them the heart rate was lowered, and the stroke volume increased during the infusion, and the arterial pressure rose. In some instances there was a rise in cardiac output, in others a rise in peripheral resistance, but in most patients there were small rises in both output and resistance. They found that the type of reaction was not directly correlated to the factor apparently responsible for the low blood pressure in a given instance. Probably, therefore, one is justified in considering the drug to be indicated, other things being equal, in an infarction with low pressure regardless of the altered mechanisms immediately responsible

for the hypotension. This is, however, only tentative opinion; much more study needs to be done.

Raoul Malmcrona, Gustav Schröder and Lars Werkö. Hemodynamic Effects of Metaraminol (Aramine): II. Patients with Acute Myocardial Infarction. Am. J. Cardiol. 13:15, 1964. Richard T. Chamberlin and Willard S. Putnam (Boston VA Hosp.). Prolonged Cardiogenic Shock. Am. J. Med. 35:396, 1963.

"Not infrequently when sustaining the blood pressure of a patient in cardiogenic shock through intravenous infusion of metaraminol (Aramine) the pressure will fall precipitously time after time when one attempts to withdraw the drug. Sometimes this state of affairs continues for many days and occasionally even for a number of weeks. Has any method been devised for terminating dependence on this drug?"

Reply: At the Rancocas Valley Hospital, Willingboro, New Jersey, Jonas Brachfeld and Ralph Myerson appear to have terminated dependence on metaraminol (Aramine) or levarterenol (Levophed) through intravenous injection of 20 mg. of methylphenidate (Ritalin) and immediate discontinuance of the pressor drug. The methylphenidate was given in 200 ml. of 5% glucose in water during a 45 minute period. Previously I had seen a report of the use of this drug successfully to potentiate the pressor action of levarterenol in a patient whose hypotension resulted from attempted suicide with sedatives, but there had been some animal experimentation suggesting potentiating action of this sort.

At the University of Pennsylvania, Edeiken and Bass appeared to terminate dependence on vasopressors through use of corticosteroids, but in other reports the effectiveness of these agents has been questionable.

Jonas Brachfeld and Ralph M. Myerson. Treatment of Cardiogenic Shock and Vasopressor Dependency with Intravenous Methylphenidate (Ritalin). Am. J. Cardiol. 15:665, 1965. Joseph Edeiken and Harry Bass. Prolonged Shock After Myocardial Infarction Relieved by ACTH and Cortisone. Am. Heart J. 68:686, 1964.

"In the therapy of cardiogenic shock during an acute myocardial infarction is it preferable to use epinephrine or one of the newer substitutes, such as mephentermine (Wyamine) or metaraminol (Aramine)?"

Reply: The newer drugs are preferred because of their greater peripheral constrictor action coupled with a lower tendency to produce arrhythmias. One should never forget, however, that there is always the lurking danger of arrhythmias even with these compounds, and also bear in mind the possibility, despite the increase in mean systemic arterial pressure, of a striking increase in cerebrovascular resistance and consequent decrease in cerebral blood flow.

"Since orally administered procaine amide (Pronestyl) may reverse abnormal ventricular rhythms, should one not use it prophylactically in patients with recent myocardial infarction?"

Reply: Your idea is a rational and good one, but apparently the thing does not work. At least P. C. Reynell, in England, did not find it reducing mortality or protecting against ventricular fibrillation in his 51 patients who received the drug against 55 controls.

P. C. Reynell. Prophylactic Procaine Amide in Myocardial Infarction. Brit. Heart J. 23:421, 1961.

"Some years ago I heard it rumored that the sludging of the blood, allegedly demonstrated to occur in patients with coronary disease, could be abolished by treatment with antimalarial compounds. Has anything come of this?"

Reply: William McCrae and associates (Western Infirmary, Glasgow) put it to the test with hydroxychloroquine (Plaquenil) and failed to observe any therapeutic benefit.

William M. McCrae, Robert Hume and John B. McGuiness. Hydroxychloroquine Sulfate (Plaquenil) in Angina Pectoris. J.A.M.A. 187:53, Jan. 4, 1964.

"I have recently tried a drug that has been around for several years, dipyridamole (Persantin), in a small group of patients with angina pectoris. Except in two instances, in which some relief seemed to be obtained after more than a month of therapy, I was not impressed with the efficacy of the agent. Since there have been favorable reports, I believe, what is one to think of such an experience?"

Reply: Yes, Arthur Griep (Evansville, Ind.) reported benefit in 70% of a group of 200 patients, in 1964. In most instances, however, the relief was experienced only after protracted administration, and it is a bit difficult to understand why this would be the case if the relief were truly ascribable to the drug, whose action is allegedly that of improving coronary blood flow through selective action on the coronary vessels with an additional salutary effect on the metabolism of the hypoxic myocardial cell. Evidence of the salutary effect of the drug in earlier studies has been quite conflicting. It seems to me that in cases of this sort in which there has not been fairly consistent report of good results with an agent, one is justified in remaining somewhat skeptical unless the latest favorable report is based upon a method of employment not previously used.

Arthur H. Griep. Approach to Long-Term Therapy of Ischemic Heart Disease. Vasc. Dis. 1:299, 1964. D. Kimsella, W. Troup and M. McGregor (Montreal). Studies with a New Coronary Vasodilator Drug, Persantin. Am. Heart J. 63:146, 1962.

"A number of men in our area are using piminodine (Alvodine) for analgesic purposes in cases of acute myocardial infarction. What is the record of this drug?"

Reply: I shall cite two reports. At the VA Hospital, in the Bronx, Hoff and associates found the drug to be a potent analgesic in the situation mentioned and felt it to be particularly useful when concomitant sedation is undesirable. In Chicago, Sadove and associates also obtained effective analgesia without serious narcotic side effects with the drug, but they found that both respiratory depression and sleep may be induced by it when it is used in combination with barbiturates, general anesthesia or potentiating drugs of the phenothiazine group.

H. Richard Hoff, Margaret M. Hotz, Robert J. Sperber, Solomon Fisch and Arthur C. DeGraff. Analgesia in Myocardial Infarction: Double-Blind Comparison of Piminodine (Alvodine) and Morphine. Am. J. M. Sc. 249:495, 1965. Max S. Sadove, José D. Sanchez and Myron J. Levin. Piminodine as an Adjunct to Anesthesia. Illinois M. J. 121:261, 1962.

"It seems to me that papaverine has all the attributes that would be desirable for coronary vessel dilatation in an individual who has suffered a myocardial infarction, but the drug has not been clinically successful. Why is this?"

Reply: The usual oral dosage of papaverine in attempting to relieve the pain of acute myocardial infarction is 100–200 mg. every 2–3 hours, but it seems unreasonable to expect very much effect from the drug no matter what dosage is given by mouth, or even intravenously unless by the continuous drip method, for although rapidly absorbed it is just as rapidly inactivated through protein binding. For years, therefore, I have been proposing to my cardiologist friends that they have papaverine incorporated in rectal suppositories and prescribe one of these for use at regular intervals around the clock, thus allowing the rectal mucosa to supply the drug steadily to the blood stream. Of the few who have given the method a trial (the drug is unfortunately expensive and comes under narcotic restrictions), most have found that when papaverine administration is started rectally as early in the myocardial episode as possible it is rarely necessary to give a dose of morphine after the first few hours. Conditions permitting, a suppository containing 200 mg. should be given at 3 hour intervals throughout the day and one of

600 mg. the last thing at night. I wish that someone would perform a double-blind study of this method of using papaverine in coronary disease or in one of the other maladies in which maintained smooth muscle relaxation is desirable.

"The allegation has been made that there is a high incidence of thromboembolism after cessation of long-term anticoagulant therapy, but so far as I am aware the "findings" have all been based upon retrospective reviews. Has a prospective study of the matter ever been made?"

Reply: Yes, at the San Diego Naval Hospital, Robert Van Cleve gradually tapered long-term anticoagulant therapy with warfarin (Coumadin) over a 6 week period in 63 patients, and stopped the therapy abruptly in an additional 71, all of the patients having been on the drug following myocardial infarction. A careful follow-up showed that there was no difference in the incidence of thrombotic events in the first 6 weeks after discontinuation of therapy, whether this was stopped abruptly or gradually. Thus it seems that there is no hazard inherent in stopping long-term anticoagulant therapy, but it is possible that such a conclusion should be qualified by saying that if the sudden discontinuation of the drug was due to a bleeding episode, the observation of H. S. Sise and associates several years ago indicated that this might provoke a rebound hypercoagulable state.

Robert Van Cleve. The Rebound Phenomenon — Fact or Fancy? Experience with Discontinuation of Long-Term Anticoagulation Therapy After Myocardial Infarction. Circulation 32:878, 1965. H. S. Sise, C. B. Moschos, J. Gaethier and R. Becker. The Risk of Interrupting Long-Term Anticoagulant Therapy. A Rebound Hypercoagulable State Following Hemorrhage. Circulation 24:1137, 1961.

"Like all of my colleagues in our hospital, I routinely anticoagulate all of my acute myocardial infarction cases as soon as is feasible after diagnosis, but this is a difficult, troublesome and potentially dangerous procedure and I do not know that it is justified. Is it?"

Reply: Following the early studies of Wright and his associates there was almost universal acceptance of this therapy until the observations of Hilden and his group, in Copenhagen, provoked serious doubts of its efficacy. Hilden reported on a 4-year program involving 800 patients with acute myocardial infarction, 371 of whom were treated with anticoagulants and 429 not. Total mortality in the anticoagulated patients was 22.0% and in the nonanticoagulated patients 25.4%, a difference that was not statistically significant. In a subsequent review, Iversen and Hilden

adversely criticized most of the previously published favorable studies and were particularly critical of the large study of Wright, Marple and Beck, in which they felt that bias in the selection of patients might have accounted for some of the differences in mortality between the anticoagulated and coagulated groups. More recently, Albert Wasserman and associates, at the Medical College of Virginia, have reported a study which suggests that factors other than those affected by anticoagulants must influence the prognosis in the first weeks of acute myocardial infarction. Their 147 consecutive male patients with acute myocardial infarction were divided into three groups: those adequately anticoagulated, those inadequately anticoagulated, and those not anticoagulated. The patients were randomly assigned, and the groups were shown to be comparable, except for an increased incidence of a history of previous heart failure in the untreated group. There was no significant reduction in mortality in the anticoagulated groups when compared to the control group. As the matter stands at present, it appears admissible to conclude that the preponderance of acceptable evidence in recent times does not support the use of anticoagulants as a routine measure in the acute episode in this malady.

Albert J. Wasserman, Lorence A. Gutterman, Klara E. Yoe, V. Eric Kemp, Jr., and David W. Richardson. Anticoagulants in Acute Myocardial Infarction: The Failure of Anticoagulants to Alter Mortality in a Randomized Series. Am. Heart J. 71:43, 1966. I. S. Wright, C. D. Marple and D. F. Beck. Anticoagulant Therapy of Coronary Thrombosis with Myocardial Infarction. J.A.M.A. 138:1074, 1948. T. Hilden, K. Iversen, F. Raaschou and M. Schwartz. Anticoagulants in Acute Myocardial Infarction. Lancet 2:327, 1961. K. Iversen and T. Hilden. The Use of Anticoagulants in Coronary Heart Disease. M. Clin. North America 46:1613, 1962.

CORTICOSTEROIDS

"Would you kindly distinguish between the principal adrenal corticosteroids as to the purposes for which they are used and their dosages?"

Reply

CORTISONE ACETATE (CORTONE, CORTOGEN). Used orally and intramuscularly for all generalized types of systemic glucocorticoid action. The first compound introduced; now known not to be a natural body constituent and to act when administered only after conversion to hydrocortisone. The least expensive of all.

Dosage: Severe disorders, 300 mg. first day, 200 mg. second day, 100 mg. or less daily thereafter, divided into three to four doses if given orally.

PREDNISONE (DELTRA, DELTASONE, METI-CORTEN, PARACORT). Less retention of electrolytes than cortisone, equally effective but just as likely to produce objectionable side actions. Sufficiently soluble to be nebulized.

Dosage: Orally, severe disorders, 30–50 mg. daily in four divided doses for 2–7 days; decrease every 4 or 5 days to determine maintenance dose.

HYDROCORTISONE (CORTEF, CORTRIL, CORTIFAN, HYCORTOLE, HYDROCORTONE). Used orally, intramuscularly, intravenously for about the same effects, including adrenal cortical replacement, achievable with cortisone. Also used topically.

Dosage: Severe disorders, 40–80 mg. daily, orally, in four divided doses for not over 2 weeks usually, then reduce less than 10 mg. at a time every few days to determine maintenance; intravenously, 4 mg./hr., for 24 hours, yields effects of daily dose of 200 mg. of cortisone, 10–12 mg./hr., for 8 hours, equivalent to daily dose of 400–500 mg. cortisone; topical dosage, 10–20 mg. daily.

-ACETATE (CORTEF-ACETATE, CORTRIL ACETATE, ETC.). Much used for intrasynovial injection and into aponeurotic or tendon cysts to promote resolution without causing systemic effects; also topically. Intrasynovial injection, 5–10 mg. for small joints or bursae, up to 37.5 mg. for large joints. Topically in ointment, ophthalmologically in ointment or suspension.

-CYCLOPENTANEPROPIONATE (CORTEF FLUID). Used as oral suspension. More slowly absorbed than hydrocortisone but more palatable; dosage as for hydrocortisone.

-SODIUM SUCCINATE (SOLU-CORTEF). So soluble that it may be given in very small amounts of fluid, intramuscularly or intravenously in an emergency; equivalent of 100 mg. of hydrocortisone may be placed in 2 ml. of water or saline and given during 30–60 seconds.

PREDNISOLONE (DELTA-CORTEF, HYDELTRA, STEROLONE, METICORTELONE, METI-DERM, PARACORTOL). When given orally has about the same effectiveness as prednisone; used topically in treating dermatoses without evidence of systemic effects; sufficiently soluble to be nebulized.

Dosage: Oral, as for prednisone.

-ACETATE (STERANE, NISOLONE). Suitable for intramuscular injection.

-BUTYLACETATE (HYDELTRA-T.B.A.). Suitable for intrasynovial and soft tissue injection; relief may be delayed for 24–48 hours because of poor solubility but then will last for 2–3 weeks or more.

-PHOSPHATE SODIUM (HYDELTRASOL). More soluble than the other prednisolone esters, used by intramuscular and intravenous injection for full systemic effects, by intrasynovial, intrabursal and soft tissue injection for local effects, and topically on the skin and in the eye and ear.

Dosage: Parenteral injection, 10–100 mg. according to circumstances, usually not more than 400 mg. daily; locally, 10–30 mg. by injection.

METHYLPREDNISOLONE (MEDROL, DEPO-MEDROL, WYACORT, ETC.). Much like prednisolone in its effects but less retentive of electrolytes.

Dosage: About two-thirds that of prednisolone.

-ACETATE (DEPO-MEDROL, MEDROL ACETATE). May be used topically by injection in certain dermatoses; may be injected intrasynovially and into soft tissues as well as injected intramuscularly for parenteral effects.

-SODIUM SUCCINATE (SOLU-MEDROL). Solubility permits intramuscular or intravenous injection in small volume of fluid in emergencies; also used locally in rectum in treating ulcerative colitis.

Dosage: Parenterally, 40 mg. at once or in greater dilution by slow intravenous drip; rectally, 40–80 mg. as retention enema several times weekly.

HYDROCORTAMATE HYDROCHLORIDE (MAGNACORT). Used topically for anti-inflammatory action in the dermatoses, with little evidence of systemic action.

DEXAMETHASONE (DECADRON, DEXAMETH, HEXADROL, DERONIL, GAMMACORTEN). Effects probably about the same as achievable with other agents of the group that lack much electrolyte retaining property, such as prednisone, prednisolone, methylprednisolone and triamcinolone.

Dosage: Orally, for prolonged therapy, 1.5–3.0 mg. daily initially, then decreasing to determine maintenance, or may start with 0.75 mg. and build up to effect; for potentially fatal conditions such as pemphigus or disseminated lupus erythematosus, 2–4.5 mg.; for acute rheumatic fever and various viruses, 7.5–10 mg. or more.

BETAMETHASONE (CELESTONE). About the same anti-inflammatory properties as dexamethasone but is also used topically by inunction or under occlusive dressings.

Dosage: Initially 0.6–8.4 mg., then decreasing gradually during 2–3 weeks to determine maintenance. Topically applied as the commercially available 0.2% cream.

TRIAMCINOLONE (ARISTOCORT, KENACORT). Probably the least electrolyte-retaining compound of the group, in fact may even provoke diuresis and slight sodium loss in beginning of its use; otherwise equivalent to the others in systemic effects though perhaps less inclined to cause psychic stimulation; sometimes causes anorexia, weight loss, muscular weakness, hypoproteinemia, cutaneous erythema, headache, dizziness and sleepiness.

Dosage: Orally, initially 8–20 mg. daily in divided doses, with gradual decrements of 2 mg. every 2–3 days to reach maintenance.

FLUDROCORTISONE ACETATE (ALFLORONE, F-CORTEF, FLORINEF). Used almost exclusively topically in treatment of dermatoses; highly electrolyte-retaining when absorbed, and it is occasionally.

Dosage: Probably advisable not to apply more than 2–6 mg. daily in lotion form or twice this amount in ointment; there appears to be no rational use for the tablets except in replacement therapy of adrenocortical deficiency.

FLUOROMETHOLONE (OXYLONE). Used exclusively for anti-inflammatory action on the skin; the usual type of systemic action expected of the glucocorticoids is so little developed in this compound that little evidence of action is to be expected if some absorption occurs at the site of application.

FLUOCINOLONE ACETONIDE (SYNALAR). Used topically in the treatment of dermatoses and pruritus vulvae, ani, scroti.

Dosage: Applied by inunction of the commercially available cream or ointment or used with occlusive dressings.

FLUPREDNISOLONE (ALPHADROL). There is not yet sufficient evidence regarding the usefulness of this preparation to justify a more positive statement than that it is used orally as an anti-inflammatory agent in substitution for one or more of the others.

Dosage: Initial adult dosage appears to range from 2 to 15 mg. daily, with gradual reduction during 2–3 weeks to determine maintenace.

FLURANDRENOLONE (CORDRAN). Used topically in treatment of the dermatoses, pruritus vulvae, ani and scroti, and with occlusive dressings. Commercially available in a cream and an ointment.

PARAMETHASONE ACETATE (HALDRONE). Used orally as an anti-inflammatory agent in competition with the numerous others in this category.

Dosage: Initial adult dosage is 6–12 mg. daily in divided doses, but it appears that twice this dosage is sometimes needed; gradual reduction during 2–3 weeks may establish a maintenance dosage of 1–8 mg.

"Has anyone devised a method for gaining some inkling of which corticosteroid an individual patient is most likely to respond to?"

Reply: Unfortunately, no.

"What are the effects of corticosteroids on protein metabolism?"

Reply: The increased protein catabolism and negative nitrogen balance which sometimes, but not invariably, occur with use of these drugs may be reflected in some degree of muscle wasting, which will sometimes be manifested as purplish abdominal striae. An additional and potentially serious result of protein depletion is a weakening of the connective tissue stroma on which calcium and phosphorus are deposited; this may result in osteoporosis and spontaneous fractures, the latter chiefly in postmenopausal women and elderly individuals of both sexes.

"I am unable to reconcile the fact that some of my patients on corticosteroids increase in strength and weight during this therapy with the frequent allegation that these drugs are protein catabolic or protein antianabolic in their action."

Reply: Some years ago, H. F. West (University of Sheffield) presented evidence, through determination of urinary excretion of creatinine as reflector of muscle mass in rheumatoid arthritis patients under prolonged treatment with corticosteroids, that this therapy may be accompanied by a gain in protein stores provided the patients eat normally and exercise enough to prevent muscle involution from disuse.

H. F. West. Protein Metabolism during Corticosteroid Therapy. Lancet 2:877, Oct. 25, 1958.

"What are the electrolyte disturbances that may be induced by the corticosteroids?"

Reply: These drugs promote sodium retention and potassium loss through actions that have not been completely explained but which probably consist in an ionic redistribution in the fluid compartments of the body as well as an effect on renal function. The effect is not likely to be a sustained one, however, and rarely necessitates abandonment of therapy in individuals with a normal cardiovascular system. If there is any degree of congestive heart failure, of course, the fluid retention consequent to the piling up of sodium may be a serious matter and may quickly lead to, or aggravate, edema. The potassium loss may be important, too, in the cardiac patient since it will contribute to a lowering of blood pressure, muscular weakness and electrocardiographic alterations; potassium salts may have to be administered if corticosteroid therapy must be continued in such cases. Prednisone and prednisolone and their derivative compounds are much less likely to cause significant electrolyte disturbances than are cortisone and hydrocortisone. A hypochloremic-hypopotassemic alkalosis may occur independently of water and salt retention.

"What are the effects of the corticosteroids on blood coagulation?"

Reply: Within 1 or 2 days of instituting therapy the blood becomes much more coagulable through the operation of mechanisms that are unknown. This may predispose to thromboembolic complications. Adlersberg and associates found that individuals with hypercholesterolemia are particularly prone to have such accidents while under these drugs. Chatterjea and Salomon found that when anticoagulant drugs were being used in cortisone-treated patients higher dosage of the anticoagulants was necessary.

Denko and Schroeder noted purpura, ecchymotic skin lesions and easy bruising in 20% of a group of 75 patients receiving prednisone for a variety of rheumatic disorders, suggesting action upon either platelets or capillary walls, or both.

D. Adlersberg, J. Stricker and H. Himes. Hazard of Corticotropin and Cortisone Therapy in Patients with Hypercholesteremia. J.A.M.A. 159:1731, 1955. J. B. Chatterjea and L. Salomon. Antagonistic Effect of ACTH and Cortisone on the Anticoagulant Activity of Ethyl Biscoumacetate. Brit. M. J. 2:790, 1954. C. W. Denko and L. R. Schroeder: Ecchymotic Skin Lesions in Patients Receiving Prednisone. J.A.M.A. 164:41, 1957.

"What are the neuropsychiatric reactions to the corticosteroids?"

Reply: These agents very frequently cause euphoria associated with slow wave changes in the elctroencephalogram, occasionally depression. The euphoria, though sometimes in part reflecting the relief from symptoms, is principally due to direct action on the central nervous system and may occur in a patient who is not otherwise clinically benefited. Sometimes there are distortions of personality, but frank psychoses have been rare. Despite statements to the contrary in the literature, I think that one should hesitate to give these drugs to patients with unstable personalities. Convulsions have been reported in association with administration of the corticosteroids, in some instances taking the form of status epilepticus in persons not previously epileptic.

"What alterations do the corticosteroids effect in carbohydrate metabolism?"

Reply: They promote hepatic gluconeogenesis (i.e., synthesis of carbohydrate from proteins through deamination of amino acids and combination into 6-carbon chains to form glucose), and they also promote storage of glycogen. Thus in making large amounts of glucose immediately available they impose the necessity for increased production of insulin. If this demand cannot be met, the patient develops a state of induced diabetes mellitus, but this is relatively unusual. The condition is usually completely reversible, though persistence after the cessation of therapy is on record. There are indications that perhaps some of the newer agents have a greater diabetogenic tendency than the two original cortisones. After use of the drugs is stopped there may be a brief period of hypoglycemia, the result of persistence for a while of insulin overproduction.

"What are the effects of the corticosteroids on the gastrointestinal tract?"

Reply: The drugs are undoubtedly ulcerogenic. Patients may in fact develop perforated peptic or colonic ulcers without antecedent symptoms, and those with a history of peptic ulcer or ulcerative colitis are very likely to have their gastrointestinal condition worsened by the drugs, particularly if they have rheumatoid arthritis, for this appears to predispose. It seems that some of the newer compounds are considerably worse offenders in this regard than the older cortisone and hydrocortisone. Other gastrointestinal involvements that have been reported in suspicious association with use of glucocorticoids are ulcerative esophagitis, acute pancreatis, peripancreatic fat necrosis, perforation of the cecum and perforation of the gallbladder. Some men have felt that when patients are taking more than minimal dosage of some of the newer drugs they should be placed on an ulcer regimen including frequent feedings, antacids and cholinergic blocking agents. Carbone's group found that use of a cholinergic blocking agent suppressed the increase in gastric hydrochloric acid and uropepsin production otherwise experienced by normal volunteers who ingested prednisone.

J. V. Carbone, D. Liebowitz and P. H. Forsham. Suppression of Prednisone-Induced Gastric Hypersecretion by an Anticholinergic Drug. Proc. Soc. Exper. Biol. & Med. 94, 293, 1957.

"What is the danger of causing peptic ulcer with corticosteroid therapy in low dosage over a prolonged period?"

Reply: I do not think that a firm answer can be given to this question at the present time. To be sure, Henry Sherwood and associates, at the Roosevelt Hospital in New York, have reported using triamcinolone (Aristocort) in dosage of 2–8 mg. daily in 100 allergy patients for 1½–5¼ years, without causing significant damage. Actually, 4 patients had healing of their ulcers, none with a healed ulcer had a recrudescence, and only 1 without proof of ulcer before the study had an active ulcer at the end. However, it is well to recall that a few years ago E. L. Dubois, at the University of Southern California, reported a 22% incidence of peptic ulcer while using dexamethasone (Decadron, etc.) in the treatment of 400 patients with systemic lupus erythematosus during a 10 year period. The manufacturers of rival corticosteroid preparations do not press very firmly the alleged differences in provocation of peptic ulceration of the respective compounds, and I do not think that anyone can show with statistical significance that the recurrence of this complication is particularly associated with the specific malady in which the drug is being used.

Henry Sherwood, Joseph I. Epstein and Harry Kaplan. Incidence of Peptic Ulcer in 100 Allergic Patients During Long-Term Corticosteroid Therapy. Connecticut Med. 28:801, 1964. Edmund L. Dubois. Current Therapy of Systemic Lupus Erythematosus: Comparative Evaluation of Corticosteroids and Their Side Effects with Emphasis on 50 Patients Treated with Dexamethasone (Decadron, etc.). J.A.M.A. 173:1633, Aug. 13, 1960.

"An increase in acid and pepsin production in an individual on corticosteroid therapy could account for the gastric lesions that sometimes appear, but I have a patient in whom there occurred an ulceration and perforation in a segment of the bowel that was not exposed to these secretions. Is some factor that fosters resistance to mucosal damage in the tract suppressed in some manner by the corticosteroids?"

Reply: I do not know. However, several years ago, Parker and Thomas (Stanford University) felt that in patients with rheumatoid arthritis there may be a slight tendency to widespread acute arterial lesions, which could be accentuated by treatment with corticosteroids.

R. A. Parker and Phyllis M. Thomas. Brit. M. J. 1:540, Feb. 28, 1959.

"Is the clinical course and pathology of the gastric ulcer developing during corticosteroid therapy different from that of other gastric ulcers?"

Reply: In a study of this matter at the Mayo Clinic, Allan Garb and associates determined that the corticosteroid gastric ulcer occurs at the same site and has the same configuration as the non-steroid ulcer and that its histology is not consistently different from that of the non-steroid ulcer. As I read the report it seemed that the only difference between the two was that the duration of gastrointestinal symptoms was short in the corticosteroid-treated patients.

Allan E. Garb, Edward H. Soule, Lloyd G. Bartholomew and James C. Cain. Steroid-Induced Gastric Ulcer. Arch. Int. Med. 116:899, 1965.

"What are the effects of the corticosteroids on gonadal function?"

Reply: These agents depress gonadal function, perhaps through partial inhibition of the secretion of pituitary gonadotropin. The reflections of this are the frequent inhibition of menstruation and, in the male, diminution of libido. Androgenic effects in the female are manifested in hirsutism and acne. Administration of estrogens is admissible in these patients.

"I am constantly fearful that one of my patients on corticosteroid therapy will develop a fatal infection without having provided any signs or symptoms that the process had begun. Is there any way in which one may detect the beginning of this thing?"

Reply: Certainly you have reason to be fearful, for this is the most serious of the deleterious effects of the corticosteroids. With the inflammatory reactions held in abeyance the individual can neither fight infection effectively nor manifest signs of an infective process going on anywhere in the body. I know of only two warning signs which, if heeded, may ward off disaster: if the temperature of a patient taking one of these drugs rises even a little, or if he begins to complain of even a small amount of new pain in an area in which serious diseases are normally manifested by severe pain, you should stop administration of the drug at once and study the situation with utmost care.

"In our practice we have an adolescent patient in whom intracranial hypertension appears to be associated with corticosteroid therapy. Has anything of this sort ever been recorded?"

Reply: Yes. In 1959, Dees and McKay said they had observed 3 young boys with long-standing severe asthma who developed benign intracranial hypertension when the dosage of the corticosteroid was being, or had been, decreased to low levels.

S. C. Dees and H. W. McKay. Pediatrics 23:1143, 1959.

"What are the principal features of the state sometimes referred to as 'shock' that supervenes when a patient is suddenly deprived of the corticosteroids that he has been taking for a protracted period?"

Reply: The syndrome that developed in a series of 19 patients from whom the drugs were suddenly withdrawn was described by Henneman and associates as having the following features: (a) rapidly worsening headache within 24–48 hours; (b) nausea, retching and sharp limitation of spontaneous food and fluid intake; (c) weight loss of 4–6 lbs. in 3–5 days; (d) malaise, tender muscles and arthralgia; (e) restlessness, fatigue, fitful sleep; (f) alarming appearance, but no major changes in temperature, pulse rate, respiratory rate or blood pressure; (g) increase in severity of symptoms during several days and then rather prompt recession and disappearance without therapy, though 1 patient had a recurrence after 7 days and another complained of weakness, fatigue and malaise for 2 months.

In view of the above, it is probably highly advisable to taper off dosage when it is desired to discontinue use of the drug in an individual who has been receiving it for a long time; reductions in daily dosage at intervals of 2–7 days are usually safe. And during the last 5 days it is well to administer corticotropin in moderate dosage.

P. H. Henneman, D. M. K. Wang, J. W. Irwin and W. S. Burrage. Syndrome Following Abrupt Cessation of Prolonged Cortisone Therapy. J.A.M.A. 158:384, 1955.

"We have just had the misfortune to have in our practice a case of pancreatitis, diagnosed only at necropsy, that was apparently associated with the administration of corticosteroids. Were we terribly remiss in not having made the clinical diagnosis before death?"

Reply: I do not think so. In reporting a case of their own, Robert Schrier and Roger Bulger (University of Washington) said that there had been only 15 reported cases of clinically apparent acute pancreatitis associated with this therapy and that, to their knowledge, their own was only the third case that had been diagnosed prior to exploratory surgery or necropsy.

Robert W. Schrier and Roger J. Bulger. Steroid-Induced Pancreatitis. J.A.M.A. 194:564, Nov. 1, 1965.

"I have a patient who has been on corticosteroids for a fairly long time and is now complaining of pain in the hip and beginning to limp a little. This worries me because I seem to remember hearing of a case of serious bone damage in the hip region associated with long administration of these drugs. Is this correct?"

Reply: Yes, you should certainly regard this development with greatest suspicion because there have been a few cases reported of aseptic necrosis of the femoral head associated with corticosteroid therapy. Both of Mervin Boksenbaum and Charles Mendelson's patients at the Henry Ford Hospital, Detroit, had received intensive corticosteroid therapy, one for pemphigus vulgaris and the other for exfoliative dermatitis. Early detection of the lesion, and discontinuation of the corticosteroid therapy, may prevent permanent destructive changes. In reporting their 11 cases of this arthropathy (joints other than the hip may be involved), Edward Velayos's group, in

Denver, proposed the title "avascular bone necrosis" for the lesion.

Mervin Boksenbaum and Charles G. Mendelson. Aseptic Necrosis of Femoral Head Associated with Steroid Therapy. J.A.M.A. 184:262, Apr. 27, 1963. F. G. O. Burrows. Avascular Necrosis of Bone Complicating Steroid Therapy. Brit. J. Radiol. 38:309, 1965. Edward E. Velayos, John D. Leidholt, Charley J. Smyth and Robert Priest. Arthropathy Associated with Steroid Therapy. Ann. Int. Med. 64:759, 1966.

"I have a patient on corticosteroids who has developed thyrotoxicosis; is there any connection?"

Reply: I have seen one report, that of Brown and Lowman (University of Minnesota), in which 2 patients *became* thyrotoxic after having received long-term ACTH and cortisone therapy for unrelated diseases. The *suppressive* effect of these drugs on thyroid activity is established in man as well as in the experimental animal.

David M. Brown and James T. Lowman. Thyrotoxicosis Occurring in Two Patients on Prolonged High Doses of Steroids. New England J. Med. 270:278, Feb. 6, 1964.

"The rumor has reached us here in our Western community that corticosteroid therapy may predispose to cryptococcal infection. Is this true?"

Reply: This may have started with the report that went the rounds a few years ago of an elderly man who died of fulminating cryptococcic meningitis after a year on corticosteroid therapy for asthma. Actually, this was a case seen by Bennington and associates, at the University of Chicago, in which they elicited the information that this 84-year-old man had felt so good on 10 mg. prednisone daily that he had doubled and finally tripled the dose in the attempt to gain even further improvement. These investigators then went on and reviewed the cases of cryptococcosis in their hospitals since 1950 and found that patients with the disease had had a significantly higher incidence of prolonged corticosteroid use than patients in the hospitals' total necropsy population during the same period.

James L. Bennington, Seth L. Haber and N. L. Morgenstern. Increased Susceptibility to Cryptococcosis Following Steroid Therapy. Dis. Chest 45:262, 1964.

"In an individual in whom it appears advisable to maintain corticosteroid therapy for a prolonged period is there any way to hedge against the occurrence of osteoporosis?"

Reply: In a study in which he maintained 47 patients on corticosteroids for 5–8 years, Harry Shubin (Philadelphia) gave anabolic steroids to 27 individuals and allowed the other 20 to remain as controls. Twelve of the 20 controls developed clinical and/or x-ray evidence of osteoporosis while only 1 of the 27 receiving anabolic steroids had evidence of this complication.

Harry Shubin. Long Term (Five or More Years) Administration of Corticosteroids in Pulmonary Diseases. Dis. Chest 48:287, 1965.

"Do severe side effects occur more often in patients on corticosteroids than on corticotropin (ACTH), and is there any difference in incidence between the sexes?"

Reply: Mild or moderately severe side effects are commoner with corticotropin but the more severe effects are experienced with corticosteroids. It appears that women are more prone than men to get into trouble with either type of therapy.

B. L. J. Tradwell, E. D. Sever, Oswald Savage and W. S. C. Copeman (West London Hosp.). Side Effects of Long-Term Treatment with Corticosteroids and Corticotropin. Lancet 1:1121, May 23, 1964.

"I see that some of my friends are switching patients on daily corticosteroid therapy to every-other-day regimens. Is this a rational procedure, and what are the limitations?"

Reply: This method of corticosteroid therapy was introduced by Harter and associates (Harvard Medical School) on the perfectly reasonable assumption that since the therapeutic effects of the corticosteroids appear to persist longer than the metabolic effects, intermittent dosage schedules might avoid cumulative effects by allowing rest periods long enough to re-establish metabolic equilibrium and yet short enough to maintain the antiallergic and anti-inflammatory actions of the drugs. In actual practice the every-other-day dosage schedule seems often to be equally as effective as the conventional four-times-a-day therapy, with a substantially lower incidence of side effects. When the new method is less effective therapeutically than the older, one has simply to weigh the advantages of lessening of the side effects against the disadvantages of the decreased therapeutic effect. It is of course going to require a long period of time to determine just how often the one side of the scale out-balances the other.

John G. Harter, William J. Reddy and George W. Thorn. Studies on Intermittent Corticosteroid Dosage Regimen. New England J. Med. 269:591, Sept. 19, 1963.

"How does one switch a patient who is taking corticosteroids on the conventional daily regimen to the every-other-day type of dosage?"

Reply: Harter and associates (Harvard Medical School), who introduced the every-other-day method, in general began corti-costeroid therapy with 10 mg. prednisone (Meticorten, etc.), or the equivalent dosage in triamcinolone (Aristocort, Kenacort) or dexamethasone (Decadron, etc.), four times daily for 4–10 days. Dosage was then decreased to 5–7.5 mg. four times daily for another 4–10 days, and then 20–40 mg. was given every other day with breakfast (i.e., the sum of 48 hour four-times-a-day dosage was given as a single dose with breakfast every other day). The attempt, in long-term maintenance therapy, was then made to cut by 5–10 mg. each dose every month.

John G. Harter, William J. Reddy and George W. Thorn. Studies on Intermittent Corticosteroid Dosage Regimen. New England J. Med. 269:591, Sept. 19, 1963.

"If a patient has been on every-other-day therapy with corticosteroids for many weeks or months, may one safely stop the drug without further tapering?"

Reply: I should prefer tapering off 10% at every third dose for several weeks.

John G. Harter, William J. Reddy and George W. Thorn (Harvard Med. School). Studies on Intermittent Corticosteroid Dosage Regimen. New England J. Med. 269: 591, Sept. 19, 1963. Donald A. Adams, Ernst M. Gold, Harvey C. Gonick and Morton H. Maxwell. Adrenocortical Function During Intermittent Corticosteroid Therapy. Ann. Int. Med. 64:542, 1966.

"I have used a long-acting intramuscular corticosteroid, prednisolone acetate (Depo-Medrol), in a number of diverse dermatoses with pretty good effect, but always with the occurrence of moon facies and sometimes boils before the result was achieved. Has this been the universal experience?"

Reply: That's it, always some degree of a Cushing reaction. A rather high price to pay for relief of relatively benign maladies, no?

"I have been applying corticosteroids topically in a number of dermatoses without evidences of systemic absorption; have I simply been lucky?"

Reply: No, I think not. This has in fact been the usual experience. For example, Charles Howell (Winston-Salem, North Carolina) reported such therapy in 211 cases, employing ointments, lotions and creams, without untoward effects or complications. But absorption of the compounds from the sites of application is documented, and you should be alert to the possibilities of systemic effects even though they have occurred very rarely.

Raul Fleischmajer (New York University Post-Grad. Med. School and Skin and Cancer Unit). Lack of Systemic Hydrocortisone Effects after Massive and Prolonged External Applications. J. Invest. Dermat. 36:11, 1961. Charles M. Howell, Jr. Simple and Effective Program for Use of Topical Fludrocortisone and Fludrocortisone-Antibiotic Combinations. Am. Pract. & Digest Treat. 10:1189,

1959. Randolph Philip Whitehead (Toledo, Ohio). Marked Hypokalemia Resulting from Percutaneous Absorption. Ohio M. J. 56:196, 1960.

"In a child who is receiving corticosteroids is there any reason to suspect that intercurrent leukocytosis is attributable to the drug?"

Reply: Eosinopenia and lymphopenia and moderate neutrophilic leukocytosis have been seen in adults when on these drugs, but I have seen only one report of the effect of large doses of these agents on the circulating white blood cells in children. In Denver, T. Jacob John gave large doses of corticosteroids to 10 children suffering from nonhematological disorders and studied them by serial white cell counts, none of the children presenting evidence of clinical infection during the period of study. All 10 of these patients manifested a striking and sustained leukocytosis, mainly neutrophilic and partly monocytic, while on the drugs.

T. Jacob John. Leukocytosis During Steroid Therapy. Am. J. Dis. Child. 111:68, 1966.

"I have heard that corticosteroid therapy makes a patient very susceptible to the development of herpes zoster. Is this true?"

Reply: I do not think that this is true. However, a group of observers in Budapest have reported a very interesting epidemic-like outbreak of herpes zoster that affected 6 patients among 56 in a ward, 4 of the patients having been treated with corticosteroids. Of the 10 patients who had been treated with corticosteroids, 4 developed herpes zoster, whereas the 46 patients who had not been so treated only 2 developed the disease. This is certainly an entertaining observation but a far cry from a statement that corticosteroid therapy makes an individual liable to the development of herpes zoster.

J. P. Rado, J. Tako, L. Geder and E. Jeney. Herpes Zoster House Epidemic in Steroid-Treated Patients. Arch. Int. Med. 116:329, 1965. J. Tako and J. P. Rado. Zoster Meningoencephalitis in a Steroid-Treated Patient. Arch. Neurol. 12:610, 1965.

"I have a case of local cutaneous atrophy at the site of a corticosteroid injection that much resembles that which I have seen occasionally at the site of insulin injection. What am I to expect?"

Reply: These cases, of which only relatively few have been reported, have been associated with the use of the slightly soluble compounds, as I presume yours was. A biopsy specimen obtained in 1 of the 2 cases reported by Iuel and Kryger, in Copenhagen, revealed crystals still present in the tissues 2 years after the injection. In some instances spontaneous healing is stated to have occurred at the site of these atrophies, but this was not the case in a follow-up 18 months later in the cases reported by the observers just mentioned.

Jørgen Iuel and Jørgen Kryger. Local Cutaneous Atrophy Following Corticosteroid Injection. Acta Rheum. Scand. 11:137, 1965.

"I have a patient who has presented acute neurological symptoms upon the sudden withdrawal of corticosteroid therapy. Is there any connection here?"

Reply: You do not state the precise nature of these neurological symptoms, but I can cite the interesting report of Crompton and Teare, in London, of 2 cases of acute necrotizing encephalitis after abrupt and massive reduction of corticosteroid therapy. The complication, which was felt to be almost certainly due to herpes simplex virus, developed in 1 case 7 weeks and in the other case 4 days after the withdrawal. Neither of the patients was known to have recurrent mucocutaneous herpes, but they may have had. These observers also mentioned a similar occurrence in relation to herpes zoster virus that was reported by other investigators, but I have not seen this report.

M. R. Crompton and R. D. Teare. Encephalitis After the Reduction of Steroid Maintenance Therapy. Lancet 2: 1318, Dec. 25, 1965.

COUGH

"Would you kindly list with their dosages the principal drugs used in the treatment of cough?"

Reply: Since almost any pharmacist stocks 50 or more preparations containing a congeries of cough remedies, one cannot easily denominate certain of these as the "principal" ones. However, I believe that the following listings and remarks may be considered as providing a satisfactory armamentarium for treatment of cough. Of course cough is itself only a symptom and I am sure you are aware that many other remedial measures must often be given pride of place in its therapy.

CODEINE is the old-reliable against which all of the newer compounds are actually titrated. I like to use it in the following prescription that has been the work-horse of many physicians through the years:

R̷ Codeine phosphate 0.45
  Ammonium chloride 15.00
  Syrup of citric acid 30.00
  Water to make 120.00
  Label: 1 teaspoonful every 3–4 hours.

DIHYDROCODEINONE (HYCODAN, DICODID,

TUSSIONEX) is thought to be less constipating than codeine but certainly is more addictive. It is used in 10 mg. dosage by mouth; children under 2 years, one-fourth the adult dose; over 2 years, one-half.

DEXTROMETHORPHAN (ROMILAR), another synthetic morphine derivative, appears to have about the same antitussive efficacy as codeine and to be associated with practically no side actions; it is non-addictive. Adult dosage is 10–20 mg. three or four times daily, with half dosage for children over 4 and one-quarter dosage for younger children.

BENZONATATE (TESSALON) is given in usual adult dosage of 100 mg. three to six times daily. The capsules will exert a local anesthetic effect if chewed or allowed to dissolve in the mouth. The efficacy of this agent appears to be somewhat less than that of codeine.

DIMETHOXANATE (COTHERA) may be about as effective as codeine but with a shorter duration of action. Adult dosage is 25–50 mg. three or four times daily, but it appears that dosage for children has not been definitely established.

LEVOPROPOXYPHENE (NOVRAD) is quite popular nowadays but I am not sure that its clinical efficacy has been convincingly shown to be equal to that in cough induced under experimental conditions. Adult dosage is 50–100 mg. every 4 hours, for children 1 mg./kg. at the same intervals.

PIPAZETHATE (THERATUSS) appears to be somewhat less effective than codeine, though it is non-addictive and does not cause constipation. Usual adult dosage is 20–40 mg. four times daily, 10 mg. for children over 7 years.

CHLOPHEDIANOL (ULO) appears to be about as effective as codeine, but it should be used cautiously in patients who are on either central nervous system depressants or stimulants because the drug has manifested some effects of its own on the central nervous system. Adult dosage is 25 mg. three or four times daily, 12.5–25 mg. for children 6–12 years of age and the lower range of this dosage for younger children.

EXPECTORANTS. As I have already mentioned *ammonium chloride* in connection with the use of codeine in prescription, something should be said of other expectorant agents. *Potassium or sodium iodide* is used in saturated solution in dosage of 2–3 drops in water every 2 or 3 hours, or the *syrup of hydriodic acid* in 5 ml. (1 teaspoonful) dosage or less in water, according to size and age of the patient. *Ipecac* is often preferred by pediatricians to any other expectorant, finding it more reliable and less objectionable in taste than ammonium chloride and not in itself harmful. Dosage of the *syrup* of ipecac (*not* the fluid extract!) is 1 or 2 drops every 3 hours for in-

fants and up to 8 drops for older children. *Carbon dioxide.* Many years ago Banyai and Cadden showed that carbon dioxide by inhalation not only stimulates the myoelastic structures of the lung and leads to forceful peristaltic movement of the bronchi, but also has a directly exerted expectorant action through liquifying the mucopurulent inflammatory exudate that stagnates in the bronchial tract. *Cough syrups.* And finally a word about these preparations. Vehicles liked by children to flavor iodides or the syrup of ipecac are syrup of raspberry, syrup of tolu balsam (which has a vanilla-like flavor and some expectorant action of its own through the tolu), syrup of cacao (chocolate flavor) and syrup of cinnamon. In Boyd's studies some years ago he learned that no truly expectorant action could be demonstrated for these syrups themselves unless they contained an expectorant such as tolu or possibly licorice; but they do have a buccopharyngeal demulcent and sialogogue (stimulation of salivary flow) effect.

E. M. Boyd. The Cough Syrup. Brit. M. J. 2:735, 1946. A. L. Banyai and A. V. Cadden. Carbon Dioxide by Inhalation as an Expectorant. Am. J. Med. Sc. 206:479, 1943.

"I have been getting fairly satisfactory results in the treatment of cough with the rather new compound, levopropoxyphene (Novrad), using 50–100 mg. orally every 4 hours in adults. I have heard that this drug is related to Darvon; if this is so, what are the implications?"

Reply: The dextrorotatory stereoisomer of levopropoxyphene (Novrad) is dextropropoxyphene (Darvon). Novrad is antitussive but not analgesic, while Darvon is just the reverse. Neither is addictive. With Novrad, serious reactions seem unlikely so far, but if the patient becomes drowsy under the drug he should certainly be warned against operating his car or other machinery.

"What drug would you recommend for rectal administration in a patient whose vomiting, associated with the paroxysms of coughing, precludes use of the oral route?"

Reply: Pipazethate (Theratuss) has been used effectively by rectum in these circumstances. Gerald Beckloff and Mark Hewitt (New Brunswick, N. J.) summarized the experience of five investigators in 172 pediatric patients. The drug was used in either suppository form (10 or 20 mg.) or as pediatric rectal applicator (20 mg.). Dosage ranged from 10 to 100 mg., either several times daily or singly as a night-time dose.

Gerald L. Beckloff and Mark I. Hewitt. Clinical Evaluation of Pipazethate (Theratuss) Administered Rectally in 172 Pediatric Patients. Am. J. M. Sc. 246:285, 1963.

"One of the bright young residents in our hospital has advocated the abandonment of expectorant medication because he has measured sputum viscosity before and after administration of these drugs and found no significant changes. Of course we are not responding as he would like because the clinical evidence of effectiveness of these drugs appears to be well established in our experience. What is the truth?"

Reply: The young man is both right and wrong. His error is attributable to the fact that drugs which increase respiratory tract fluid have come to be called "expectorants," which has naturally led to attempts to measure their efficacy in terms of the effects on *sputum* viscosity. Actually, when Holinger and associates a number of years ago collected respiratory tract fluid *through postural drainage and bronchoscopic suction*, they found that quite considerable liquifaction was effected by expectorant drugs.

P. Holinger, F. P. Basch and H. G. Poncher. The Influence of Expectorants and Gases on Sputum and on the Mucous Membrane of the Tracheobronchial Tree. J.A.M.A. 117: 675, 1941.

CRANIOCEREBRAL TRAUMA

"Is anything to be gained by the administration of a corticosteroid to a patient with acute craniocerebral trauma?"

Reply: This matter has been studied by Robert Sparacio and associates, in Brooklyn, who have concluded that if there is an associated lesion such as an intracranial blood clot, even though this is adequately removed, the usefulness of a corticosteroid is very slight; but in patients with severe brain injury without associated intracranial blood clot they found that the administration of a corticosteroid had a strikingly beneficial effect. The drug they used was methylprednisolone sodium succinate (Solu-Medrol), 40 mg. of which were given intravenously immediately upon admission of the patient and subsequently in similar dosage intramuscularly every 4 hours for 7 days, then half the dose was given at the same intervals for 2 days, then again for 2 days at 8 hour intervals and finally for 2 days at 12 hour intervals.

Robert R. Sparacio, Tung-Hui Lin and Albert W. Cook. Methylprednisolone Sodium Succinate in Acute Craniocerebral Trauma. Surg. Gynec. & Obst. 121:513, 1965.

CREEPING ERUPTION

"I have heard that down in Texas they are using thiabendazole (Mintezol) effectively in creeping eruption. We are not that far South but still we do occasionally see one of these cases. What dosage have they been using?"

Reply: Orville Stone and J. Fred Mullins, in Galveston, have reported the following dosage schedules: (1) 50 mg./kg. every 12 hours times three doses, used in 1 patient on bed rest with no side effects; (2) 50 mg./kg. in two successive doses in 8 patients, with 5 cases of dizziness, 4 accompanied by nausea: (3) 50 mg./kg. as a single dose in 2 patients, with mild dizziness in one; and (4) 25 mg./kg. twice a day for four doses in 6 patients, 2 of whom had dizziness and nausea.

Orville J. Stone and J. Fred Mullins. Thiabendazole (Mintezol) Effectiveness in Creeping Eruption. Arch. Dermat. 91:427, 1965.

CROUP

"Long ago my professor of pediatrics told me that ½–2 teaspoonful of the syrup of ipecac will often relieve the glottic spasm in croup, and I have found this to be true. How would you rationalize such therapy?"

Reply: The action appears to come about through an increase of vagal influence simply because central vagal stimulation is an accompaniment of the act of vomiting.

CRYOGLOBULINEMIA

"I have a patient in whom the diagnosis of cryoglobulinemia has been made by exclusion, so that I am unable to approach the therapy through treatment of any of the numerous diseases that usually underly this malady. Are there any drugs that have been found helpful in the simon-pure cases?"

Reply: I do not know of any, although of course the corticosteroids have been used.

CUSHING'S SYNDROME

"Just how should the corticosteroids be used before, during and after operation in a patient with Cushing's syndrome?"

Reply: George W. Thorn, at Harvard University, recommends the following schedule. Preoperatively: cortisone acetate, 100 mg. intramuscularly at 12 hours and 2 hours. During operation: hydrocortisone, 100 mg. intravenously, to be repeated at 6 and 12 hours, and then cortisone acetate, 50 mg. intramuscularly every 6 hours. Second and third days: cortisone acetate, 50 mg. intramuscularly every 8 hours; days 4, 5, 6 and 7, 50 mg. orally every 12 hours; days 8, 9 and 10, 25 mg. orally every 8 hours; and thereafter reduced slowly to determine maintenance needs. After the seventh day, it may be necessary to administer desoxycorticosterone for its salt-retaining properties, or fluorohydrocortisone may be used.

G. W. Thorn, D. Jenkins, J. C. Laidlaw, F. C. Gaetz, J. Bingman, W. L. Arons, D. H. P. Streeten and B. H. McCracken. Pharmacologic Aspects of Adrenocorticosteroids and ACTH in Man. New England J. Med. 248:232, 284, 323, 369, 414, 588, 632, 1953.

CYCLIC NEUTROPENIA

"A patient has just entered my practice with the rare malady, cyclic neutropenia. I am aware that splenectomy and the corticosteroids have each at times lessened the severity of the symptoms without influencing the periodic bouts of neutropenia or agranulocytosis that characterize the disorder. Has any newer treatment become available?"

Reply: In Philadelphia, Isadore Brodsky and associates have reported the case of a man whom they treated with large doses of testosterone. Testosterone therapy before splenectomy caused subjective and objective improvement. Splenectomy alone failed to alleviate the patient's symptoms or to alter the cyclic neutropenia, but retreatment with testosterone again abolished the symptoms and ameliorated the cyclic phenomena. Testosterone was given in the form of testosterone enanthate (Delatestryl), 600 mg. intramuscularly weekly.

Isadore Brodsky, Hobart A. Reimann and Lewis H. Dennis. Treatment of Cyclic Neutropenia with Testosterone. Am. J. Med. 38:802, 1965.

CYSTIC FIBROSIS

"I have a case of cystic fibrosis in my practice in which the safer antibiotics have failed to control the complicating infection. Is there a record of prolonged use of chloramphenicol (Chloromycetin) in this malady without undue bone marrow damage?"

Reply: In Boston, Anne V. C. Lloyd and associates reviewed their experience with chloramphenicol in 50 cases of cystic fibrosis treated during a period of 7 years. In most instances another antibiotic, usually erythromycin, was given at the same time as the chloramphenicol. Most children received a chloramphenicol dosage of 25–30 mg./kg. daily, the younger ones being given 150 mg. per teaspoonful. There was no evidence of chloramphenicol toxicity in these patients, and it was said that in the preceding 12 years about 400 other children with cystic fibrosis had received the drug for shorter periods, only 1 patient having a temporary hypoplastic anemia attributable to it. Thus it seems that most patients can be given the drug without adverse effects; certainly this appears to be true if the period of administration is short, but I should nevertheless be on the alert for possible bone marrow damage. And unfortunately there is recent report of serious visual disturbance under this therapy.

Anne V. C. Lloyd, Gilbert Grimes, Kon-Taik Khaw and Harry Shwachman. Chloramphenicol (Chloromycetin) for Long-Term Therapy of Cystic Fibrosis. J.A.M.A. 184: 1001, June 29, 1963. N. N. Huang, R. D. Harley, V. Promedhattavedi and A. Sproul. Visual Disturbances in Cystic Fibrosis Following Chloramphenicol Administration. J. Pediat. 68:32, 1966.

"What solutions for aerosol therapy have given best results in treating the obstructive pulmonary aspects of cystic fibrosis?"

Reply: Since you have a patient with this disease on your hands I need not say to you what a many-faceted malady this is. The report of LeRoy Matthews and associates, at Western Reserve University, is an exhaustive treatise on the most rewarding measures that are being currently used in therapy. In reply to your specific question I will say that these investigators use the following solutions for aerosol therapy:

(A) Propylene glycol U.S.P. 10 ml.
0.125% phenylephrine
HCl q.s. to 100 ml.
Give 2 ml. by aerosol
t.i.d. or q.i.d.
(B) Solution 1
Propylene glycol U.S.P. 10 ml.
0.125% phenylephrine
HCl q.s. to 100 ml.
Solution 2
Isoproterenol HCl 1:200 10 ml. bottle
Mix 1.8 ml. of solution
1 with 0.2 ml. of
solution 2 and give by
aerosol t.i.d. or q.i.d.
(C) Neomycin sulfate 10 Gm.
Propylene glycol U.S.P. 20 ml.
0.125% phenylephrine
HCl q.s. to 200 ml.
Give 2 ml. by aerosol t.i.d.
or q.i.d.

At Washington University, Herman Reas obtained improvement with N-acetylcysteine (Mucomyst) that correlated well with the amount of obstructive material present in the tracheobronchial tree, and was limited by the extent of pulmonary fibrosis, pneumonitis and bronchiectasis present. He gave 5 ml. of a 20% solution of N-acetylcysteine by aerosol twice daily. Sodium chloride, 3%, was nebulized for 2 weeks before active treatment was begun, and for 2 weeks a 7.1% sodium chloride–0.05% NaEDTA aerosol was used. The same volume of each solution was nebulized from a DeVilbiss No. 42 nebulizer into a small plastic face mask, distilled water, 2 ml., being given after the 5 ml. dose twice daily.

LeRoy W. Matthews, Carl F. Doershuk, Melvin Wise, George Eddy, Harry Nudelman and Samuel Spector. Therapeutic Regimen for Patients with Cystic Fibrosis. J. Pediat. 65:558, 1964. Herman W. Reas. Use of N-Acetylcysteine (Mucomyst) in Treatment of Cystic Fibrosis. J. Pediat. 65:542, 1964.

CYTOMEGALIC INCLUSION DISEASE

"I have in my practice a 4-year-old child with gastrointestinal manifestations of cytomegalic inclusion disease, in which I understand the prognosis to be very poor. Is there no systemic drug therapy from which help may be expected?"

Reply: None that I am aware of.

DEHYDRATION

"I know that one is probably unwarranted in looking upon electrolytes as drugs, but since they are often administered for therapeutic purposes it would be very helpful if you would propose a choice of solutions in specific instances."

Reply: VOMITING IN PYLORIC OBSTRUCTION. The adult patient will usually have obstruction from an old duodenal ulcer or gastric carcinoma, the infant from congenital pyloric stenosis. Unless there is achlorhydria, acid will be lost and alkalosis will be present. Isotonic sodium chloride usually suffices, but the use of Ringer's solution or even of the potassium mixture of Darrow and Pratt (half-normal saline and 40 mM. of potassium chloride [3 Gm.]/L. in a 2.5% glucose solution) may be advisable. Ammonium chloride would correct excessive alkalosis.

VOMITING IN DUODENAL, JEJUNAL OR UPPER ILEAL OBSTRUCTION. There is a fairly good balance of the acid and base elements in the mixture of gastric and pancreatic juices, bile succus entericus and saliva regurgitated in these cases. Isotonic or hypotonic sodium chloride or Ringer's solution is usually suitable.

BILE OR PANCREATIC FISTULA DRAINAGE. Acidosis can develop in either of these situations because both juices have more basic than chloride ions. Lactated Ringer's solution should be used.

ILEOSTOMY DRAINAGE. The situation is about the same as when bile or pancreatic juices are lost. Use lactated Ringer's solution.

DIARRHEA. The same as the above. Use lactated Ringer's solution.

CONTINUOUS GASTROINTESTINAL ASPIRA-TION. The situation is comparable with that of the vomiting in pyloric obstruction. Use isotonic sodium chloride but be alert for the necessity to use ammonium chloride.

SEVERE BURNS. There is a tremendous loss of fluid from the blood into the tissues beneath the burned area and in the exudate from the burned surface. This fluid is physiologic electrolyte solution; it should be replaced with isotonic sodium chloride solution.

HYPERNATREMIA. This situation, in which there is a serum sodium level above 150 mEq./L., is seen principally in instances of acute brain injury; in infants or very elderly individuals physically unable to recoup, by voluntary ingestion of water, excessive fluid lost in insensible perspiration during a febrile illness; and in some cases of diabetic acidosis. Glucose solution without saline is required here.

OLIGURIA. The cardinal signs of the lower nephron nephrosis syndrome are azotemia, excretion of heme pigment, hypertension, oliguria and finally anuria. Many cases resolve themselves spontaneously in 5 to 7 days and are succeeded by a period of excessively high urinary output, but alert watchfulness may reveal indications for fluid administration during the waiting period. Fluid should be given by mouth to replace that lost in insensible perspiration and otherwise; i.e., 1000 ml. plus the fluids in vomitus, stool and urine. Watch closely the chloride and carbon dioxide contents of the blood and give sodium chloride and sodium bicarbonate orally or intravenously, as indicated. Patients treated in this way sometimes remain comfortable and free of edema and heart strain despite persistant oliguria or anuria and progressive rise in blood urea nitrogen. An increased potassium concentration in the blood and the characteristic cardiographic pattern may substantiate a diagnosis of potassium intoxication in some instances. There is the threat of toxic action on the heart in this situation, but calcium gluconate and glucose in saline solution intravenously, and whole blood transfusion, will handle it. Calcium promotes ventricular contraction and is thus protective; glucose is stored as glycogen and carries potassium into storage with it. When the patient is recovering he may lose prodigious amounts of sodium chloride in the urine; one should be prepared to replace this with intravenous physiologic saline or the patient may be lost through dehydration and hypochloremia and hyponatremia.

I think it unfortunate that practitioners tend to overlook the great practical value of oral saline therapy under emergency conditions; patients can often be got to take very large amounts of fluid and electrolytes by this route. Bocanegra's group used an oral solution of 5.5 Gm. of sodium chloride and 4 Gm. of sodium bicarbonate in 1 liter of distilled water (140 mEq. of sodium, 93 mEq. of chloride and 47 mEq. of bicarbonate/liter).

D. C. Darrow and E. L. Pratt. Fluid Therapy: Relation to Tissue Composition and the Expenditure of Water and Electrolyte. J.A.M.A. 143:365 and 432, 1950. Manuel Bocanegra, Fidel Hinostroza, Nicholas A. Kefalides, Kehl Markley and Sanford M. Rosenthal. A Long-Term Study of Early Fluid Therapy in Severely Burned Adults. J.A.M.A. 195:268, Jan. 24, 1966.

"One of our surgical residents is maintaining a vigorous campaign for the institution of continuous Ringer's lactate solution infusion during all operations. Would this really be an advantageous maneuver?"

Reply: The matter was reported upon by Raymond Trudnowski, of the Roswell Park Memorial Institute, who says that in a study covering a period of 3 years during which there were 24,176 recovery-room admissions over 15 years of age covering all types of surgery, the conclusion was reached that under modern conditions of light general anesthesia, with normal kidney function, the use of Ringer's lactate (Hartmann's solution) is beneficial. He said that with moderate blood loss, blood pressure can be maintained by giving the solution intravenously at the rate of 500–1000 ml./hour as a supplement to minimal necessary blood transfusion. If the blood loss is equal to or greater than 700 ml., there was evidence in the study that administering the solution at rates greater than 1 liter/hour may be more effective.

Raymond J. Trudnowski. Hydration with Ringer's Lactate Solution. J.A.M.A. 195:545, Feb. 14, 1966.

"In replacing body fluids how much should actually be given?"

Reply: A fair assumption is that the average adult, dehydrated through gastrointestinal fluid loss, will require in 24 hours 1500 ml. for evaporation from lungs and skin, 1500 ml. for urine and 2600 ml. to make up his pathologic loss. This is a total of 5600 ml. but not all of this need be electrolyte solution because only water was evaporated. He should be given 2600 ml. of electrolyte solution and 3000 ml. of glucose solution, with modifications of course for circumstances. Fever, thyrotoxicosis or a humid environment will raise the water requirement, and poor renal concentrating power or acidosis will raise it even more.

One must be guided by the symptoms. The moderately dehydrated individual is weak and apathetic, has no appetite and is likely to be nauseated. As he approaches a severe state his blood pressure begins to fall, the skin and muscles lose their normal feel, the tongue looks very dry. He is far gone when the eyeballs feel soft.

During intravenous administration of sodium chloride some of it may spill into the urine even though the patient is still grossly salt deficient. When the urine test shows chloride for the first time, one should switch to glucose alone and have the patient void at half an hour and 1½ hours, discarding the 30 minute specimen and testing the 90 minute specimen for chlorides.

In handling the burn cases in the severe U.S.S. Bennington naval disaster a few years ago, Enyart and Miller administered blood and electrolyte in accordance with their modification of the Evans formula. During the first 24 hours an amount of physiologic saline was given that was equal to the body weight in kilograms times the per cent of the body burn, 50% being used as the maximum figure for the latter. For example, a man of 154 pounds (70 kg.) with a 40% burn, received 70 times 40 or 2800 ml. of physiologic saline; if he had a 70% burn, he received 70 times 50, or 3500 ml. An equivalent amount of plasma expander was also given during the first 24 hours. During the second 24 hours, administration of both the normal saline and the expander was continued, but in half amounts, and in addition half-normal saline, or a half-normal solution of sodium bicarbonate, sodium citrate and saline, was given orally to those who could take it. After the forty-eighth hour the saline was replaced by glucose in water in amounts sufficient to maintain hydration until the period of diuresis was completed. During the period of intravenous therapy the rate of administration was fast enough to keep the urinary output at approximately 50 ml. per hour.

It has become apparent from the study of Markley and associates that the oral administration of isotonic saline solution is effective and could be useful in mass catastrophes when intravenous administration is not feasible. Unfortunately, many individuals cannot easily swallow such a salty solution; this can be got around, however, by having the patient take a 320 mg. (5 grains) sodium chloride tablet with an ordinary (250 ml.) tumbler of water at frequent intervals, omitting the tablet with each fourth tumblerful.

Intraperitoneal administration of isotonic saline is perfectly admissible if other routes are not feasible, provided only that it is more than 12 hours postlaparotomy and that the patient does not have peritonitis or abdominal distention from other causes and does not have dyspnea from pneumonia. Dehydrated infants and children will quickly absorb 60–100 ml. given during 15–20 minutes.

In infantile diarrhea of moderate or severe degree, Stevenson, considering half the estimated weight loss due not to cellular disintegration but to actual loss of fluids, replaces it during the first day of therapy by hypodermoclysis or slow intravenous drip of a mixture of one part M/6 sodium lactate to two parts normal saline in 5% glucose; blood transfusion is given in addition, if indicated, at the rate of 10 ml./pound. An example of the calculation: A 20 pound (10 kg.) infant loses 20%, or 2000 Gm. body weight; he should be given 1000 ml. of lactate-saline and 200 ml. of whole blood. In addition to the replacement fluid there should be calculated, and given at the same time, an amount for maintenance that will be 50–150 ml. lactate-saline according to the infant's size, plus 5% glucose to make the total 24 hour fluid intake 150 ml./kg. (75 ml./pound). On the second day, if the baby is better, the maintenance therapy only is given with the addition of 4 mEq. of potassium/kg. (2 mEq./pound) to the glucose solution; potassium is withheld until this time because the infant must be urinating to excrete a possible excess and avoid hyperpotassemia (potassium chloride has 13.5 mEq./Gm.).

J. L. Enyart and D. W. Miller. Treatment of Burns Resulting from Disaster. J.A.M.A. 158:95, 1955. K. Markley, M. Bocanegra, A. Bazan, R. Temple, M. Chiapori, G. Morales and A. Carrion. Clinical Evaluation of Saline Solution Therapy in Burn Shock. J.A.M.A. 161:1465, 1956. E. I. Evans. The Early Management of the Severely Burned Patient. Surg. Gynec. & Obst. 94:273, 1952. S. S. Stevenson. Diarrhea in Infancy. Connecticut M. J. 16:671, 1952.

DELIRIUM

"Delirium of various causations is not rare currently in some types of practice. In addition to activities for possible correction of the underlying causative factors, what does one do for the immediate situation itself?"

Reply: I presume that you have in mind not that calm, cover-plucking delirium that was often a terminal event in typhoid fever in bygone times ("for after I saw him fumble with the sheets, and play with flowers, and smile upon his finger's end, I knew there was but one way: for his nose was as sharp as a pen, and a' babbled of green fields."—Shakespeare: Henry V), but rather the violent sort that demands that something be done. Before embarking upon the use of any drugs in such a situation, however, you should bear in mind that you may only worsen affairs if you introduce any type of potentially toxic agent into a patient who may have a severely handicapped cardiovascular system or be suffering from uremia. Otherwise, the use of such a sedative as the old-fashioned paraldehyde, that is so

little toxic, and the sedulous avoidance of barbiturates that may not only add to the patient's disorientation but later deepen a threatening coma, would be in order. Or for quieting effect I should use one of the true tranquilizing agents, such as meprobamate (Miltown, Equanil), rather than a psychotropic agent of the chlorpromazine (Thorazine) type because of the great potential toxicity of the latter agents in an individual who has some underlying serious disease that has brought him to his present state. I should certainly be very chary of using morphine, because of its depressant effect on the respiratory center, and it will not relieve the restlessness in a patient of this sort anyway.

W. Desmond Henry, Alan M. Mann. Diagnosis and Treatment of Delirium. Canad. M. J. 93:1156, Nov. 27, 1965.

DENGUE

"Here in the South we occasionally see a case of dengue, and have been able to offer nothing but symptomatic therapy. These people are pretty sick for a while, but they all seem to recover. Is there any specific therapy in the offing?"

Reply: I do not know what is brewing in the investigational laboratories that is of promise, but at the moment no specific drugs are available.

DEODORANTS

"Why have not dermatologists been inveighing against the use of zirconium-containing deodorants since they can cause granulomas, as I can testify from experience in a recent case?"

Reply: Why not, indeed? Reports of axillary granulomas due to zirconium-containing deodorants have been appearing in the literature since 1956.

G. Robert Baler (Boston). Granulomas from Topical Zirconium in Poison Ivy Dermatitis. Arch. Dermat. 91:145, 1965.

DERMATITIS HERPETIFORMIS

"A dermatologic associate of mine has been using the antileprosy drugs in his dermatitis herpetiformis cases and claims good results. I do not know anything about these agents and am wondering whether their use is justified."

Reply: Howard Linn, in Australia, reported on the use of Dapsone in 113 patients with dermatitis herpetiformis, pustular bacterid or eczematous dermatitis. Initial dosage was

100 mg. two or three times daily in adults, 25 mg. in children under 3, and 50 mg. in older children. Fairly good results were obtained in all categories, but there was considerable toxicity: cyanosis of lips, nail beds and eruption itself in 17 patients; vomiting in 7; headaches in 4; dermatitis medicamentosa in 3; acute hemolytic anemia in 2; arthralgia in 2; asthma in 1 and depression in 1. Adverse reactions required discontinuation of the therapy in 12 patients. The leprologists, who have their patients usually under close supervision, are using these drugs without often incurring excessive reactions, but I would expect them to cause considerable trouble in general dermatologic practice.

Howard W. Linn (Adelaide). Use of Dapsone in Dermatology. Australian J. Dermat. 6:203, 1962.

DERMATOMYOSITIS

"Is there any danger involved in using the corticosteroids in dermatomyositis?"

Reply: Be careful to avoid the fluorinated ones for they may only worsen the situation: fluprednisolone (Alphadrol), paramethasone (Haldrone), triamcinolone (Aristocort, etc.).

"I have a patient with dermatomyositis who is being treated rather unsatisfactorily with corticosteroids. Would there be any rationale in adding anabolic hormones to this therapy?"

Reply: Well, yes. To be sure, there is muscle fiber degeneration and inflammatory cell infiltration in dermatomyositis, but some muscle regeneration is also characteristic. The additional use of anabolic hormones to aid this regeneration, and possibly to counteract also the catabolic effect of long-term corticosteroid therapy, would appear to be sensible. In fact, W. R. Murdoch, in England, has reported the successful use of norethandrolone (Nilevar) and methandrostenolone (Dianabol) in 2 cases. Dosage of Dianabol was 30 mg. daily.

W. R. Murdoch. Anabolic Hormones in Dermatomyositis. Brit. M. J. 2:1929, Dec. 31, 1960.

DIABETES INSIPIDUS

"I have heard that in some cases of diabetes insipidus a good response is obtained from use of diuretic agents, but I do not understand this. Can you explain?"

Reply: In a great majority of instances this disease is due to a lack of the posterior pituitary hormone, vasopressin (Pitressin),

which enables the kidneys to form concentrated urine. And the treatment consists simply in supplying the missing hormone. But in a few instances there occurs a nephrogenic type of the disease, in which the hormone is formed abundantly but does not engender its usual response in the kidneys. It is in these latter cases that the thiazide diuretics have been found helpful. In 2 patients, seen by James Wenzl and associates at the Mayo Clinic, there was a decrease in urine of 25 and 35%, respectively, as a result of treatment with chlorothiazide (Diuril, etc.). I do not think that we have as yet achieved a satisfactory explanation of the phenomena involved here. In London, Havard and Wood expressed the tentative opinion that the antidiuretic effect of the thiazides in this situation is predominantly the result of sodium and water loss with consequent reduction in plasma volume and glomerular filtration rate; but in New York, Schotland's group failed to find a consistent change in the glomerular filtration rate in their cases.

John D. Crawford, Gordon C. Kennedy and Lisa E. Hill. Clinical Results of Treatment of Diabetes Insipidus with Drugs of Chlorothiazide Series. New England J. Med. 262:737, Apr. 14, 1960. Marilyn G. Schotland, Melvin M. Grumbach and José Strauss. Effects of Chlorothiazides in Nephrogenic Diabetes Insipidus. Pediatrics 31:741, 1963. C. W. H. Havard and P. H. N. Wood. Antidiabetic Properties of Hydrochlorothiazide in Diabetes Insipidus. Brit. M. J. 1:1306, 1960. James E. Wenzl, Gunnar B. Sticler, Donald A. Scholz and Raymond V. Randall. Nephrogenic Diabetes Insipidus: Report on Two Patients Treated with Chlorothiazide. Proc. Staff Meet. Mayo Clin. 36:543, Oct. 11, 1961.

DIABETES MELLITUS

"I have not been long in practice and am just beginning to assemble a sizeable group of diabetic patients. What can I hope for in these people; i.e., what is the prognosis in diabetes under modern drug therapy?"

Reply: Of course you must bear always in mind that in diabetes as in any other disease prognosis is an individual affair. However, it is certainly the consensus that adequate treatment—that is, treatment that is begun early and pursued faithfully and vigorously—will both prolong life and postpone complications. At the Joslin Clinic nearly 3000 "Life Expectancy" medals have been awarded to patients who have lived longer after the onset of diabetes than it was predicted they would live without it in life insurance tables. At this same famous clinic the "Quarter Century Victory" medal had been awarded in 1965, according to Howard Root, to 115 individuals, the granting conditions being: (a) proof of diabetes of 25 years' duration; (b) a healthy body; (c) no diabetic retinopathy; (d) absence of calcified arteries. Untreated diabetes in early life carries the greatest risk of rapid development of coma and death, but delay in diagnosis at any period of life encourages the premature development of vascular complications. Once the case has been diagnosed, there is good evidence that the length of the patient's life and the development of sequelae are dependent upon the quality of treatment and degree of control of the diabetic state. If one defines "good" control as a urine test at least once daily, a weighed diet for the first 6 weeks of training and thereafter at regular intervals and careful measurement of food at all other times, glycosuria in 24 hours not to exceed 5% of the total carbohydrate intake, no acetone bodies in the urine, and the majority of blood glucose levels no more than 130 mg./100 ml. before meals—in patients controlled to this extent, Root reports retinopathy in only 7% of 58 patients as compared with 43% in poorly controlled patients. Likewise with regard to nephropathy; this complication was present in only 7% of 86 patients who had had good control and in 30% of 380 patients whose control had been poor. So, other things being equal, prognosis pretty well paces the degree of care. The qualifying "other things," however, keep us from being entirely sure of ourselves because there are still many unsolved problems in diabetes. You will certainly do well to bear in mind that there is a greater incidence of coronary heart disease in the diabetic than in the nondiabetic individual, that gangrene and lower extremity infection are always a threat, that diabetes and infection exacerbate each other, that intercurrent tuberculosis in a diabetic constitutes a true medical emergency, that the course and outcome of pregnancy is affected more unfavorably by diabetes than is the diabetes by pregnancy and that there is an increase above the normal in both morbidity and mortality in the immediate newborn period of an infant born of a diabetic mother.

Howard F. Root. Prognosis in Diabetes. M. Clin. North America 49:1147, 1965. Alexander Marble. Relation of Control of Diabetes to Vascular Sequelae. M. Clin. North America 49:1137, 1965.

I have a patient who is becoming insulin resistant. I intend switching her to tolbutamide (Orinase) but do not know how long I should persist in the use of this oral drug in the face of failure to control the situation fully."

Reply: E. J. Segree (State University of New York, Syracuse) felt, as a result of experience in his case, that the oral antidiabetic should be continued for 1 or 2 weeks before being abandoned, since a therapeutic response may not occur during the first few days of treatment. Have you tried some of the other "tricks" in your patient? Taken advantage of the fact that crystalline insulin, given in a single dose subcutaneously, will have a more prolonged effect than when given in several separate smaller doses? Tried her on a pure pork insulin preparation, which may reduce the dosage by one-third? Made sure that the resistance is not due to an associated leukocytosis, eosinophilia or leukemia; or to increased production of adrenocortical or anterior pituitary hormones; or to diffuse liver disease with defective glycogen storage; or in association with hemochromatosis, hypothyroidism, hyperthyroidism, pituitary basophilism (Cushing's syndrome), specific infection such as with tuberculosis or syphilis or with rheumatoid arthritis?

Eugene J. Segrce. Diabetes Mellitus with Insulin Resistance: Report of Case Successfully Treated with Tolbutamide (Orinase). Metabolism 11:562, 1962.

"Very limited but favorable experience with the anabolic steroids in the treatment of diabetic retinopathy has caused me to wonder whether anyone has made extensive study of the general amelioration of the diabetic state under these compounds?"

Reply: There have been a few favorable reports, but they have not been supported by the findings of George Molnar's group at the Mayo Clinic. These investigators were able to demonstrate the induction of positive nitrogen balance in a small group of "brittle" patients with the daily administration of 6 mg. of stanozolol (Winstrol), but stabilization or amelioration of the diabetes, or any reduction in ketogenesis, did not occur. There was some reduction in levels of plasma cholesterol, total fatty acids, and phospholipids in 3 of 7 moderately hyperlipemic patients, but not in the other patients who were normolipemic initially. There was fasting blood sugar concentration reduction to some degree in 5 patients, but without change in other parameters of diabetic control. And there were no significant changes during therapy in serum protein fractions and in the concentrations of serum ketone bodies, free fatty acid, and blood urea as well as in retinopathy and in body weight.

George D. Molnar, John W. Rosevear, Clifford F. Gastineau and Karen E. Moxness. Effects of Anabolic Steroids on Diabetic Instability. Am. J. M. Sc. 249:280, 1965.

"Is there any reason to believe that the serum concentration achieved with the sulfonylureas in diabetes is related to the patient's body weight?"

Reply: Most diabetics responding satisfactorily to the sulfonylureas do so in the following dosage ranges providing there is concomitant carbohydrate restriction: tolbutamide (Orinase), 1.0–2.0 Gm./day; chlorpropamide (Diabinese), 100–250 mg./day; acetohexamide (Dymelor), 0.5–2.0 Gm./day. However, in studying the matter of serum concentration in urinary excretion of these drugs in 125 diabetics over periods of 8–18 months, Joanna Sheldon and associates (London, England) found 3 individuals in whom it was necessary to increase dosage in order to achieve therapeutic serum levels of the drugs, and 2 of these individuals were overweight.

Joanna Sheldon, John Anderson and Linda Stoner. Serum Concentration and Urinary Excretion of Oral Sulfonylurea Compounds, Relation to Diabetic Control. Diabetes 14:362, 1965.

"I have recently seen a patient in an emergency situation of hypoglycemic coma. After we pulled her out she revealed that she had been told by her physician 1 month previously that she had 'a trace of sugar' in the urine and that she should avoid sugar in her diet and take 125 mg. of chlorpropamide (Diabinese) three times daily. Whereupon she almost completely eliminated carbohydrate from her diet and took the drug as prescribed. Can we not do something to impress upon our fellow physicians that these are potentially dangerous drugs, these oral antidiabetic agents?"

Reply: Alfred Vogl, in reporting precisely this sort of case in New York, has very trenchantly made the point that the sulfonylurea compounds should be regarded not as antidiabetic but as hypoglycemic agents since, in sufficient dosage, they can lower the blood sugar concentration in normal persons. To designate them as "hypoglycemics" instead of "antidiabetics" might help to put practitioners on their guard.

Alfred Vogl. Chlorpropamide (Diabinese)-Induced Hypoglycemic Coma. Postgrad. Med. 36:400, 1964.

"I have heard that thrombocytopenia has been associated with chlorpropamide (Diabinese) therapy. Do you know of such an instance?"

Reply: At the Royal Melbourne Hospital, Morley and Hirsh have reported a case of thrombocytopenia that they thought may have resulted from a direct toxic effect of this drug on the patient's platelets, and this could have been the case because the individual had received high dosage: 3 Gm. daily for 1 week, 2 Gm. daily for another week and 1.5 Gm. daily for a third week, the lesions appearing 3 days after reduction to 1 Gm. daily. However, I think the possibility of a hypersensitivity reaction should not be ruled out because the in vitro tests, which were negative, were only performed 7 days after the appearance of purpura and then performed but one time.

A. Morley and J. Hirsh. Case of Thrombocytopenia Asso-ciated with Chlorpropamide (Diabinese) Therapy. M. J. Australia 2:988, Dec. 19, 1964.

"I have recently had a most interesting experience that I would like explained. The non-diabetic relative of a diabetic patient wanted to know whether she was possibly in a prediabetic state. So I performed a cortisone glucose tolerance test, using cortisone in dosage of 50 mg. orally 8½ and 2 hours before an oral glucose dose of 100 Gm. The result of this test showed her to be possibly prediabetic since there was a cortisone-induced glucose intolerance. She then requested therapy and I put her on a placebo, and thereafter she no longer responded as a prediabetic to the test. What was going on here?"

Reply: Now that is truly entertaining, suggesting as it does that the carbohydrate intolerance in the early stages of beginning diabetes may be influenced beneficently by psychologic factors. In Montreal, Douglas Wilansky and associates had some experiences comparable to yours, and they also found that phenformin (DBI) appears to retard development of the diabetic state in prediabetic individuals. So they reason that single or multiple short courses of phenformin may be capable of retarding the emergence and onset of clinical diabetes mellitus. This must and certainly will be put to extensive tests.

Douglas L. Wilansky, Inge Hahn and Reuben Schucher. Effect of Phenformin (DBI) on "Prediabetes." Metabolism 14:793, 1965.

"Cholestatic jaundice is reported as following the use of sulfonylurea drugs in the treatment of diabetes. Has it ever been associated with the use of phenformin (DBI)?"

Reply: No report of such an association has come to my attention.

"Animal studies have suggested that long-term tolbutamide (Orinase) may increase the functional capacity of the islet cells, but does this occur in man? In other words, if routine examination of an asymptomatic individual reveals an abnormal glucose tolerance test, am I likely to affect the test by instituting tolbutamide therapy?"

Reply: In the young asymptomatic diabetic, S. S. Fajans and J. W. Conn, at the University of Michigan, have reported improvement or normalization of oral glucose tolerance, often only after several months of therapy; less dramatic effects were obtained by Hugo Engelhardt and Thomas Vecchio, at Baylor University, in maturity-onset cases.

S. S. Fajans and J. W. Conn. The Use of Tolbutamide in the Treatment of Young People with Mild Diabetes Mellitus. A Progress Report. Diabetes 11: Supplement, 1962. Hugo T. Engelhardt and Thomas J. Vecchio. The Long-Term

Effect of Tolbutamide on Glucose Tolerance in Adult, Asymptomatic, Latent Diabetes. Metabolism 14:885, 1965.

"My young son, who has just joined me in practice, cannot quite understand why I am sometimes a bit hesitant regarding the use of the oral antidiabetic compounds. Would you kindly supply a statement of the accomplishments with insulin vis-a-vis the oral drugs?"

Reply: With the use of certain dietary alterations and insulin one is able to reduce the elevated blood sugar and cholesterol to normal, decrease serum inorganic phosphate and potassium, eliminate glycosuria and hence polyuria and polydipsia, promote normal storage of glycogen, promote the complete oxidation of fatty acids, stop the increased excretion of nitrogen resulting from protein destruction to augment the supply of glucose, and enable the patient to resume an active place in the competitive world. Even pregnancy will not offer a very great threat to the life of the well treated patient, provided she is not already over 30 years of age and has had diabetes since early childhood, and insulin will unquestionably increase her chances of becoming pregnant. But insulin is only an arresting medicament. Its use is only replacement therapy, and if we cease using it the patient will at once revert to his untreated state except in the mildest cases.

Insulin has apparently decreased the incidence of diabetic cataract and toxic amblyopia and has caused lipemia retinalis to become a rarity. But arteriosclerotic diabetic retinitis has become a more prominent complication, since its progress is not controlled by insulin. Diabetics properly treated with insulin certainly live much longer nowadays than formerly, but there is still no incontrovertible evidence that insulin protects fully against the sclerosing process that involves diabetic arteries earlier than others.

In summary, I think it may be said that, with certain exceptions so rare as to "prove the rule," any diabetic no matter what his age or status otherwise can expect the elimination of those of his symptoms that are directly attributable to faulty glucose utilization. His day-to-day living will be placed on a completely normal basis except for the attention to his diet, and his life will be very considerably prolonged and made much freer from incapacitating complications than would have been the case otherwise—provided he takes insulin under careful supervision of his physician.

Contrasting it with insulin therapy, the position of oral therapy is not nearly so strong. Admittedly, taking drugs by mouth is a much simpler thing than injecting oneself daily with a needle and syringe that must always be safeguarded against bacterial contamination, and measuring dosage in numbers of tablets is easier than measuring with great accuracy the amount of a liquid preparation drawn up into a syringe. But there are several serious drawbacks to this type of therapy. Not the least of these, though not so often called attention to as it deserves, is that the patient who is provided with a certain number of "pills" to take at his discretion is prone to abandon discretion after a short while, cease to test his urine as a guide to dosage, and forget altogether to maintain a safeguarding contact with his doctor. More obvious limitations are the facts that (a) childhood diabetes, and for the most part diabetes in very young adults ("growth-onset" cases), cannot be handled easily with the drugs; (b) patients with a more severe and labile form of the disease (unstable, "brittle," with sharply plunging and rising blood sugar levels on an unchanged dietary) are not often satisfactorily responsive; (c) severe acidosis, coma, increases in severity of the disease due to intercurrent infection, surgical or other stress, liver or renal disease—all of these things will often call for supplementary use of insulin and may require that insulin be used exclusively for the management of the case; (d) escape from "diabetic training" in the details of the permitted dietary and the injection technique is not really accomplished with the oral preparations because, in the first place, dietetics is the backbone of diabetes therapy no matter what type of drug is used, and, in the second place, the orally-treated patient may at any time have to resort to insulin therapy as a supplementary or emergency measure; (e) the oral drugs are more expensive than insulin.

The patient for whom the oral drugs provide the most satisfactory treatment is one whose diabetes is of a mild type that developed when he was middle-aged or older. Many of these patients are overweight and can be taken out of a diabetic class without the use of any drugs merely by reducing their weight and altering their eating habits. Something additional must be said in favor of the oral drugs, however, namely, that intercurrent pregnancy or surgery do not necessarily require resort to insulin if the patient has satisfied the requirements for oral therapy originally, and that individuals who respond poorly to insulin because they appear hyposensitive to it or are allergic to it, may sometimes be handled very well on the drugs. Furthermore, the possibility of dosing themselves orally can really be a boon to patients handicapped by poor vision, parkinsonism, hemiplegia or senility.

"I have just heard that the administration of a sulfonamide to a patient who is taking oral antidiabetic compounds may be dangerous. Is this true?"

Reply: The statement is probably too broad, since not all of the oral antidiabetics are sulfonylurea compounds; but tolbutamide (Orinase), chlorpropamide (Diabinese) and aceto-hexamide (Dymelor) are sulfonylureas and hence their hypoglycemic action may presumably be potentiated by the concomitant administration of a sulfonamide. L. K. Christensen and associates in Copenhagen found a severe hypoglycemic reaction provoked by the giving of sulfaphenazole (Sulfabid) to diabetics under treatment with tolbutamide; comparable experience is recorded by J. S. Soeldner and J. Steinke. Phenformin (DBI), not being a sulfonylurea, would not be involved in such an occurrence. Another drug that has been implicated in increasing the hypoglycemic effects of tolbutamide is phenylbutazone (Butazolidin), and one should bear this in mind when using the closely related compound, oxyphenbutazone (Tandearil).

L. K. Christensen, J. M. Hansen and M. Kristensen. Sulpha-phenazole-Induced Hypoglycaemic Attacks in Tolbuta-mide-Treated Diabetics. Lancet 2:1298, 1963. J. Stuart Soeldner and Jurgen Steinke. Hypoglycemia in Tolbuta-mide-Treated Diabetes. J.A.M.A. 193:398, Aug. 2, 1965.

"I have recently had an elderly diabetic patient on tolbutamide who had a much more prolonged period of hypoglycemia following a brief period of low caloric intake than seemed easily explainable. What might have accounted for this?"

Reply: Cherner's group (Jefferson Medical College) reported the case of a patient who had a severe hypoglycemic reaction following 3 days of poor food intake, whose serum reflected the presence of tolbutamide for 5 days after discontinuance of the medication and resumption of abundant carbohydrate administration. It appeared very much as though the aberration was an inability to metabolize or excrete tolbutamide rather than a depression of absorption or utilization. Probably a number of cases of this sort will become apparent as experience increases. One cannot be too cautious in the use of the sulfonylureas in elderly patients who are likely to be erratic and unpredictable in their dietary intake.

Rachmel Cherner, Carl W. Groppe, Jr., and Joseph J. Rupp. Prolonged Tolbutamide-Induced Hypoglycemia. J.A.M.A. 185:883, Sept. 14, 1963.

"Why is it that some patients who fulfill all the requirements for oral sufonylurea therapy never-theless come quickly out of control when transferred to the oral drug, though others who seem to resemble them in every way respond very consistently and well?"

Reply: The reasons for this can, of course, be very many and complex, but I have known of a number of such situations that were easily corrected by requiring that the patient be seen in the office much more often than when he was on insulin therapy. The trouble in these cases has been that the patient was one of the type whose relief when freed from the necessity of taking injections completely distorted his judgment and led to abandonment of all caution.

"It is the impression in our group that aceto-hexamide (Dymelor) is effective in about the same group of patients as responds to other sulfonylurea compounds, but that it seldom results in secondary failure. Is this the common experience?"

Reply: Lozano-Casteneda and associates, of the Joslin group in Boston, said they found two things that will possibly be advantages of this compound: one, that it is often effective in a single daily dose, and the other that secondary failure with it is unusual. My own feeling, however, and that of some of my associates, is that perhaps more time must pass and greater experience be gained before we can be certain about this latter point.

Oscar Lozano-Castaneda, Rafael A. Camerini-Dávalos, Leo P. Krall and Alexander Marble. Two Years' Experience with Acetohexamide (Dymelor). Metabolism 13:99, 1964.

"Have instances of blood dyscrasias or of liver damage been chalked up against tolbutamide (Orinase)?"

Reply: Yes, I have seen the report of an instance of pancytopenia associated with tolbutamide therapy, and another of cholestatic jaundice, liver decompensation and shock related to the use of the drug. But I should like to repeat here what I have said elsewhere on this head: "These things, hematologic and hepatic damage, are serious, but in these trying times it behooves us to be very chary of condemning any drug on the evidence of only one or a few adverse reports. There appears to be a growing tendency to accept one swallow as making a summer. Actually, these oral anti-diabetic compounds have been used in many thousands of cases, with excellent results and no serious reactions. Having long accepted calculated risks in other departments of medical practice, should we not be able to take these undesired results in our stride in view of the great good that has accrued to the vast majority of patients who have been treated with these drugs? I really feel so and think that in many instances a mere alteration in the package literature will take care of the situation rather than precipitously withdrawing the drug from the market."

Irving Chapman and Wan Ho Cheung (Elmhurst, N. Y.). Pancytopenia Associated with Tolbutamide Therapy. J.A.M.A. 186:595, Nov. 9, 1963. Thomas F. McMahon (Georgetown Univ.). Cholestatic Jaundice, Liver Decompensation and Shock Resulting from Tolbutamide: Report of Case. M. Ann. District of Columbia 32:509, 1963. Harry Beckman. 1964–1965 Year Book of Drug Therapy, p. 183.

"I have a patient on tolbutamide in whom there is appearing some evidence in the urine of slight disturbance of hepatic detoxication, but I cannot convince myself that this should be laid to the door of the drug. Is there any support for my position?"

Reply: Yes, I believe that there is. Dieter Müting (University of Homburg/Saar) studied a large number of patients from this standpoint and found that even in uncomplicated diabetes the detoxicating action of the liver can be disturbed, as manifested by a mild to moderate decrease in glucuronic acid and an increase in the free phenolic compounds in the urine. But he was unable to say that tolbutamide was primarily responsible for these disturbances, for slight relaxation in observance of diet, intercurrent infection and irregularity in taking the tablets, may in themselves considerably alter the oxidizing functions of the liver.

Dieter Müting. Hepatic Detoxication after Long-Term Treatment of Diabetes Mellitus with Sulfonylureas. Lancet 2:15, July 4, 1964.

"Among my associates there are some who feel that it is unnecessary to follow the carbohydrate metabolism very closely in individuals on sulfonylurea compounds, so long as ketosis is being prevented; but I do not feel entirely at ease in this attitude. Is there any recorded experience to bolster my disinclination to 'join up'?"

Reply: Yes, I believe that there is. For instance, Joseph Shipp and associates, at Harvard, reported the cases of three diabetics treated with sulfonylureas in whom it appeared that the drugs prevented the development of severe ketoacidosis but not of hyperglycemia. Severe hyperlipemia associated with lipemia retinalis and xanthomatosis appeared in these cases, but fortunately cleared with diet and insulin therapy. These were young patients, and perhaps it is questionable whether they should have been considered suitable candidates for sulfonylurea therapy in the first place, but I think the occurrences in these instances nevertheless justify the position that careful study of what is going on in the carbohydrate metabolism of the diabetic is mandatory whether he is on oral or needle therapy.

Joseph C. Shipp, Francis C. Wood, Jr., and Alexander Marble. Hyperlipemia Following Sulfonylurea Therapy in Young Diabetics. J.A.M.A. 188:468, May 4, 1964.

"In our group we seem to be returning to the suspicion that diabetics who have a 'secondary failure' to sulfonylurea therapy have certain distinguishing characteristics from the very inception of their disease. Has this point been recently clarified?"

Reply: No, I should say that it has not, but there does seem to be an increasing impression that this is the case. For example, of the 784 patients on long-term sulfonylurea treatment by Haden and associates (Royal Victoria Hospital, Belfast), 5.9% showed secondary failure and this group had a longer average history of diabetes before therapy. However, 7 of these patients, with an average age of 53, had a short history (1–3 months). Another item of interest in this study was that initial blood glucose levels of the secondary failure group were higher than those of the successful responders. More than half of the secondary failures in this study occurred within the first year of treatment, and several patients showed transient periods of secondary failure before the final failure ensued.

D. R. Hadden, D. A. D. Montgomery and J. A. Weaver. Secondary Failure to Sulfonylurea Treatment. Irish J. M. Sc. 469, 1963.

"I know that transient myopic alteration sometimes occurs in early diabetes, and I have seen the institution of insulin therapy associated with a hyperopic alteration. But now I have a patient in whom a small hyperopic correction became necessary almost immediately after starting him on tolbutamide (Orinase). Is such an occurrence on record?"

Reply: Yes, it is being seen occasionally, but I believe so far it has been only transient when use of the drug was persisted in. Of course, retinopathy is the more serious cause of visual disturbance in a diabetic.

Frederick M. Kapetansky (Ohio State University). Refractive Changes with Tolbutamide. Ohio M. J. 59:275, 1963.

"I have a relatively mild, maturity-onset diabetic woman under treatment with tolbutamide (Orinase), who at the age of 36 has become pregnant for the first time. Is the risk too great to justify trying to take her through her pregnancy on this drug?"

Reply: I am obliged to reply that the safety of such a course as routine practice has not been established. But of course patients have been so treated and brought safely through the period, when there has been the exercise of all possible precaution. Certainly if your patient has ever had ketosis or coma, or is not an altogether responsible and reliable person, I would not contemplate making the trial.

"In a diabetic patient who is under good insulin control but has a very high serum cholesterol level, would it be safe for me to try to reduce the latter through use of dextrothyroxin?"

Reply: Zinn and Schleissner's experience at the University of Southern California indicates that it might be risky. The blood sugar level was raised in their patients regardless of previous diabetic control, and in some instances the control was completely unbalanced and more insulin had to be given. Acidosis developed in 1 of the 8 patients and 8 of them showed extreme elevations of fasting blood sugar levels.

Willard J. Zinn and L. A. Schleissner. Effects of Dextrothyroxin in Diabetes. California Med. 101:240, 1964.

"I have a patient on oral antidiabetic compounds who experiences a severe Antabuse-type effect when she takes any sort of alcoholic drink. Has this matter been studied?"

Reply: Not studied, to my knowledge, but it has been reported in connection with use of the sulfonylureas.

R. Royer, G. Debry, M. Lamarche and P. Kissel (Nancy, France). Antidiabetic Sulfonamides and Antabuse Effect. Presse méd. 72:661, Mar. 7, 1964.

"A moderately severe diabetic patient of mine, who has been carefully controlled on insulin for many years, has begun to lose the usual warning symptoms of approaching hypoglycemia. He suddenly becomes belligerent, obstinate and resistant toward those who are familiar with his situation and are trying to treat the obvious hypoglycemia. His blood sugar level is not strikingly different from that which usually provides ample warning of approaching reaction, but he quickly flies into this confusion and unconsciousness. What is to be done?"

Reply: This is truly a serious state of affairs for which there is no specific preventive measure available. Some years ago, Balodimos and Root of the Joslin group in Boston, presented a study of 116 patients who had lost their ability to recognize an approaching reaction. The only recommendations they could provide were that, in addition to energetic

treatment of the hypoglycemic reaction by the usual methods, the best hope for prevention of recurrent episodes lies in careful readjustment of the diet, frequent testing of the urine and regular medical supervision. They often had their patients take as many as eight supplementary snacks during the waking hours, sometimes adding also some regular insulin to the basic dose before breakfast and again at bedtime. In some patients, division of the long-acting dose into two portions, taken one before breakfast and one before the evening meal, was helpful. In these people there must be constant emphasis on the necessity of regular hours in meals and exercise, the carrying of sugar or candy on the person, and the wearing of an identification and diagnostic card. One should not attempt to treat these patients with the oral antidiabetic compounds.

Marios C. Balodimos and Howard F. Root. Hypoglycemic Insulin Reactions without Warning Symptoms. J.A.M.A. 171:261, Sept. 19, 1959.

"Is there such a thing as a 'chronic hypoglycemia syndrome' in an insulin-treated diabetic? I think that I have seen such a case."

Reply: Yes, I believe that one may coin the term. The hypoglycemia developing from chronic overdosage of a long-acting insulin is often so gradual as to be almost symptomless, and the patient may have an unrecognized unphysiologic blood sugar level for weeks or months or even for years. Such individuals complain of headaches, backaches and leg aches associated with feelings of exhaustion and weakness with an incapacity for mental concentration, and their symptoms disappear when the insulin dosage is reduced. Sometimes, however, there is actual mental deterioration, and then recovery is much delayed. Chronically overtreated patients occasionally show paradoxical hyperglycemia, the explanation for which is far from clear; reduction in insulin dosage is the remedy.

"Please outline the use of drugs in the treatment of diabetic acidosis and coma."

Reply: Ketone bodies (acetoacetic and β-hydroxybutyric acids and acetone) are excessively formed in the liver when the insulin supply is insufficient. The kidneys secrete some of these bodies in the free form and as ammonium salts, some of the bicarbonates of the blood are split up to yield base for neutralizing purposes, and there is additional liberation of carbon dioxide. Ultimately, when these combined mechanisms fail to keep pace with the production of the acids, the fixed bases begin to be called upon and the body loses sodium. Since this latter step really amounts to a decrease in total salt concentration, there results a state of dehydration of the salt-depletion type because water is excreted to maintain isotonicity in the tissues. Chloride is often lost through vomiting, also. The patient is therefore acidotic (owing to reduction of the alkali reserve of the blood), hyperpneic (the liberated carbon dioxide must be eliminated) and dehydrated (because of the sodium chloride loss).

If the state of acidosis is allowed to persist, coma will supervene and there will be impairment of renal function, azotemia and oliguria. A notable rise in the plasma level and urinary excretion of phosphorus may also occur with resultant significant depletion of phosphorus stores, the reason probably being that phosphorylation of glucose is not taking place in the absence of insulin.

The very obvious aims of treatment of the acidotic state in diabetes are to put a stop to the defective metabolism of fat and utilization of carbohydrate, which are causing the ketosis, and to replace the fluid and salt that have been lost. In short, give insulin and physiologic saline solution. Frequently, glucose is administered also in the belief that it (a) promotes oxidation of glycogen; (b) reduces destruction of protein; (c) diminishes production of ketone bodies. Some observers feel, however, that glucose is contraindicated, at least in the beginning, because it delays restoration of the blood volume through promoting polyuria and perpetuates peripheral circulatory failure and extracellular dehydration. Some men compromise between the glucose-from-the-beginning and no-glucose-at-all viewpoints by administering physiologic saline alone at first, and then changing later to 5% glucose in saline in order to prevent disappearance of glycosuria before ketosis has been abolished. The latter occurrence is considered to be a real danger, since the carbohydrate store may be so low that the circulating sugar may represent the greater part of the carbohydrate reserve.

INSULIN AND GLUCOSE ADMINISTRATION. It is usual in some services to give insulin as follows, broadly speaking: 200 units intravenously to patients drowsy but easily rousable, 300 units to those rousable with difficulty, 400 units to those in coma. The intravenous saline drip is started at once and 500 ml. is given in the first 15 minutes; 500 ml. in the second 15–30 minutes; and perhaps a third 500 ml. at the same rate. Thereafter, 5% glucose in saline is used, usually at the rate of 500 ml. hourly, until after ketosis disappears and further vomiting is unlikely. The bladder is emptied by catheter at the very beginning and thereafter at 30 minute intervals, all specimens being tested for sugar and acetone bodies and at frequent intervals for urinary chloride (latterly many men are decrying catheteriza-

tion and substituting plasma ketone studies). Insulin continues to be injected into the drip tubing in 50 unit doses every 30 minutes until the urine or plasma is free of acetone bodies. The stomach is aspirated at regular intervals when vomiting is persistent.

Those who believe in initial heavy intravenous glucose administration give an average of 40–50 Gm. in the first hour to patients who are unconscious and not responsive to external stimuli, 20–30 Gm. in the second hour and 20–30 Gm. in the succeeding 2 hours. Initial insulin dosage is 100–200 units, with similar amounts every 2 hours until the blood sugar definitely falls. I think it should be remarked that the British, who probably deal with a larger proportion of serious coma emergencies than we do, practically all stoutly champion the liberal use of glucose.

A small dose–short interval method of giving insulin consists in giving 25 units subcutaneously at half-hour intervals until the patient is free from all signs of ketosis as judged by clinical and laboratory evidence, glucose and saline being used concomitantly.

SODIUM PHOSPHATE. Some observers feel that the loss of phosphorus during acidosis should be made up by administering sodium phosphate, 2.6 Gm. in 1000 ml. of water intravenously, during about 4 hours. One of the advantages of replenishing the phosphorus level is that in doing so the erythrocytes are caused to give up chloride ions to the plasma, thus helping to maintain the plasma sodium chloride level.

POTASSIUM CHLORIDE. Attention has been directed in relatively recent times toward the potassium deficiency that may occur in diabetic acidosis, especially when vigorously treated. Potassium migrates from cells to plasma when there is excessive excretion of sodium chloride and water, and this potassium is lost in the urine. Furthermore, insulin produces a striking decrease of serum potassium coincident with the decrease in blood sugar because the deposition of glycogen in the liver is accompanied by storage of potassium. Potassium deficiency causes flaccidity of striated muscles, paralysis of the diaphragm and intercostal muscles, fall in diastolic pressure, increase in venous pressure and electrocardiographic changes.

Potassium chloride is given intravenously, 1.5 Gm. as 2% solution, during one-half hour, or 1–2 Gm. orally for several doses. A method of administration introduced some years ago is to place 80 ml. of 10% potassium phosphate, diluted to 100 ml. with water, in the stomach, and as soon as the patient can take fluids without nausea, give him hourly feedings of 100 Gm. of fruit juice, broth or milk, to which 10–20 ml. of the potassium phosphate solution is added, continuing this regimen for 4–6 hours. However, there may be some danger in beginning potassium administration before adequate laboratory study has shown a potassium deficiency. In the beginning, before insulin, saline and glucose treatment has taken hold, there is likely to be hyperpotassemia, and to increase it might be disastrous.

SODIUM LACTATE OR BICARBONATE. If the function of the kidneys is so badly disturbed that hardly any ammonium can be formed, and fixed bases are therefore inordinately passed out in the urine, it may be advisable to administer alkalis because the sodium in the blood is likely to be held by the retained phosphates and sulfates. Those who use alkalis under these circumstances are usually guided by the carbon dioxide–combining power of the blood. If it has fallen below 20 volumes per 100 ml. they give not more than 2000 ml. of sixth-molar sodium lactate in 24 hours, or 1000 ml. of 2.5% sodium bicarbonate in 1 hour.

"How should one alter the therapy of an insulin-treated diabetic during an intercurrent infection?"

Reply: This is a real diabetic emergency because an infectious process considerably raises the insulin requirement. Speculative "explanations" are the following: (a) adrenocortical activation with release of steroids to reduce glucose tolerance and antagonize insulin's action; (b) increased destruction of insulin by proteolytic enzymes; (c) decreased hepatic formation and release of glycogen; (d) increased rate of cellular metabolism as the result of increased temperature.

Considerable advantage attends use of an intermediate or long-acting insulin (oral hypoglycemic agents will not suffice here) with the addition of quick-acting insulin at 4–6 hour intervals in these cases. If the Clinitest is orange, one should add 8–10 units; if it is tan, 4–5 units. When the emergency has passed and convalescence has begun, requirement for insulin may decline rather quickly and the supplementary doses must be diminished.

"Would you please outline the alterations in the care of a diabetic who is coming up for surgery?"

Reply: PREOPERATIVE CARE. If the patient is under good diabetic control and is coming up for an elective operation he should be given 6–10 ounces of orange juice and 10–12 units of insulin 2 hours before operation, 10 Gm. of glucose intravenously with another 5 units of insulin being added just before or during the operation if the carbon dioxide–combining power of the plasma is less than 40 volumes per 100 ml. If the patient is not under diabetic control, or if the operation is of an emergency nature or complicated by infection, the treatment had better be that of acidosis with threatened coma. The diabetic coming to operation for the relief of complicating hyperthyroidism should be treated as though his diabetes were complicated by infection, for hyperthyroidism, like infection, decreases the power of insulin. When the hyperthyroid state is relieved the diabetes is nearly always much ameliorated.

POSTOPERATIVE CARE. The total amount of insulin that the patient has been taking preoperatively in 24 hours should be given in the 24 hours succeeding operation, but divided into smaller portions and injected every 3–4 hours. During this period the amount of carbohydrate customarily allowed in the diet should be given in the form of intravenously administered glucose. In making dietary readjustment thereafter, one may find that the insulin requirement differs somewhat for a while from what it was preoperatively.

A simple basic adjustment that is made in some services is to divide the patient's usual dose of insulin in half, giving one-half before surgery and the other half when the operation is completed. The patient is given 1000 ml. of 5% dextrose in water in place of breakfast, and of course other intravenous fluids as developments dictate.

"How should one alter the therapy of a diabetic who becomes pregnant?"

Reply: Nausea and vomiting during the first trimester demand readjustment to prevent ketosis. Patients on an intermediate insulin mixture are usually given extra doses of quick-acting insulin before lunch and before the evening meal to prevent the excretion of glucose that is often excessive owing to the lowered renal threshold in pregnancy. Though unpredictable, the most marked fall in carbohydrate tolerance is likely to begin at the sixth to eighth month and return to the original level at or shortly before term.

Prolonged difficult labor, which is more frequent among diabetic than nondiabetic women because of the overweight of the child, centers attention upon the actual period of labor as the most trying from a diabetic standpoint. There is not only the possibility of a plunge into hypoglycemic shock upon the one hand or ketosis and coma upon the other, but perineal or cervical tears and postpartum sepsis are undoubtedly greater causes for concern in the diabetic than in the nondiabetic woman. Of course the antibiotics have considerably lightened the burden of these things in recent years. Many observers feel that delivery should take place about 3 weeks before term, the method to be individualized.

Diabetic women are seldom able to nurse their infants; nevertheless one must be on guard against a decrease in the blood sugar level, necessitating reduction in insulin dosage, when lactation begins.

"What is the best way to handle the situation when an insulin-treated diabetic has an acute gastrointestinal upset?"

Reply: If the patient cannot eat, or vomits what he does manage to get down, or is losing food and fluids through diarrhea, he is being deprived of carbohydrate and the consequent breakdown of body tissues may bring him closer to ketosis. Insulin should not be omitted, usually, but only cut down somewhat and the situation very carefully watched. The chief thing is to get food into and absorbed by the patient, covering with insulin of course. Individualization of treatment is absolutely necessary in these cases because in some instances the metabolic activities of the body may be so low that the administered insulin will, in effect, be hyperactive and the patient will go into hypoglycemic shock.

"What is the best way to handle the situation when an insulin-treated diabetic is forced to omit either insulin or food?"

Reply: If a classically treated diabetic cannot get his usual insulin, his best chance of minimizing acidosis is probably to continue eating his usual carbohydrate, but no fat and only a little protein. When the interrupted routine is resumed, extra insulin may be required to get back to the old status. If insulin supplies are running short, best procedure is to cut dosage in half and continue the usual diet but eliminate fat. If insulin is available but carbohydrate food is not, it is probably advisable for the severe diabetic to take one-third to one-half his usual insulin without food, taking the usual meal and the insulin as soon as food becomes available, or taking the usual food and only a half dose of insulin if the preceding dose had been taken within 6 hours.

"In treating diabetes how may one best take advantage of the insulin-sparing action of exercise?"

Reply: The mild diabetic is improved and the severe diabetic made worse by exercise. In general, the more exercise the less insulin will be needed. But for exercise to exert its maximum benefit, sufficient insulin must be available in the body at the time. Therefore the preferable sequence should be insulin, exercise and breakfast, not exercise, insulin and then breakfast.

"Would you kindly supply a comparison of the various insulins currently available?"

Reply: INSULIN INJECTION AND ZINC INSULIN CRYSTALS. These two insulins, often referred to simply as "amorphous" and "crystalline," are the fastest and the shortest-acting insulins, but this speed and brevity are not desirable assets in routine therapy because several injections may be necessary in the 24 hours in order to maintain something approximating normoglycemia. The two agents are therefore used very little nowadays except in combination with one of the intermediate insulins (see below) in order to sharpen its early effect, in emergencies when quick action is imperative and even intravenous administration may be desirable, and in certain "brittle" diabetics who do not do well on the intermediate preparations.

PROTAMINE ZINC INSULIN SUSPENSION. This preparation cannot be used for quick action in emergencies because it is a cloudy suspension suitable only for subcutaneous injection after thorough shaking. It is sometimes said of this insulin that it is like regular insulin with fivefold duration of action and fivefold loss of intensity at any one time. A single daily 60 unit protamine injection would be equivalent to 10 units of amorphous or crystalline insulin at 4 hour intervals or 20 units at 8 hour intervals, continuously. It is valuable to provide a sustained insulin effect through use of only a single injection daily in cases of only moderate severity in which high postprandial blood sugar rises are not expected and it does not much matter whether an insulin is at the peak of its activity at a certain time. In severe cases treated with this drug there is considerable likelihood of glycosuria appearing after meals even though the single daily dose is high enough to cause hypoglycemia during fasting. These patients often experience alternating glycosuria and insulin shock (hypoglycemia), the former by day and the latter at night or during exercise.

AMORPHOUS (OR CRYSTALLINE) AND PROTAMINE ZINC INSULIN, 2 : 1 MIXTURE. A formerly frequent practice (now largely superseded by use of lente insulin) was to employ a mixture of protamine and regular insulins, combined in fixed proportions in a syringe just before injecting, prior to taking the morning meal. Two parts of regular to 1 part of protamine insulin best fitted the needs of most patients most of the time. The 2 : 1 mixture was really a new insulin in the sense that it was an insulin-saturated protamine zinc complex releasing insulin more rapidly during the first than during the second 12 hours. There was enough rapid action to take care of the elevated insulin requirement provoked by the taking of food during the day, and enough slow or retarded action to provide for the diminished but continuing requirement for insulin in the fasting hours of the night. Glycosuria before breakfast indicated need for more of the late-acting protamine zinc insulin, and glycosuria before the evening meal, more of the early-acting regular insulin. Increments were usually 2–4 units. However, if the total requirement was more than 40 units of regular and 20 units of protamine insulin, many observers felt that only the quantity of regular insulin should be increased beyond this point, or the attempt to treat the patient with only a single daily injection should be abandoned and a supplementary injection of regular insulin be given before the evening meal. If a patient is being changed from either protamine zinc or amorphous (or crystalline) insulin alone to the mixture, it is advisable to start with a unit dosage of the mixture only two-thirds that previously taken and build up from there. If dosage is as high as 60 units it is probably best to give no insulin at all for 24 hours and then begin at two-thirds.

The protamine and quick-acting mixture must be made extemporaneously by the patient as follows: (a) inject a volume of air equal to the dose into the top of the vial of protamine zinc insulin and withdraw the syringe and needle empty; (b) inject air and withdraw the proper amount of quick-acting insulin from its vial; (c) invert the protamine zinc insulin vial several times and withdraw the dose of protamine into the syringe containing the quick-acting insulin; (d) holding the syringe with needle upright, draw an air bubble into it and invert and roll the bubble through to mix; (e) discharge the bubble and inject the mixture.

ISOPHANE INSULIN SUSPENSION (NPH INSULIN; NPH ILETIN). This preparation was designed to replace extemporaneous mixing of protamine zinc and quick-acting insulins, and had succeeded in doing so in a great many practices, though it is now largely replaced by lente insulin. Trial dosage in a previously untreated case is usually 10 units before breakfast, increasing 3–5 units daily until satisfactory control is reached. This agent can usually be substituted unit for unit in patients who have previously been on globin insulin (see below) or a 2 : 1 quick-acting and protamine mixture. If protamine zinc insulin has been used alone, it is considered advisable to reduce the initial isophane insulin dose 10–20% and build up from there.

The most conspicuous failures with iso-

phane insulin have been in patients, usually very young diabetics, with a greater requirement for rapidly acting than for slower-acting insulin. The addition of a smaller amount of quick-acting insulin to the single before-breakfast injection of isophane is quite feasible in such cases, but of course this marks a departure from the idea of no extemporaneous mixing, which underlay the introduction of isophane. It appears advisable to give mid-afternoon and perhaps bedtime feedings to such patients.

GLOBIN ZINC INSULIN INJECTION. Experience indicates that the effects achievable with globin insulin are not easily distinguishable from those with either the 2 : 1 quick-acting and protamine mixture or with isophane. We actually appear to have available nowadays four satisfactory insulins whose actions are intermediate between those of quick-acting and protamine insulin. Three of these, isophane, globin and lente, require no mixing for the single daily injection before breakfast. The other, 2 : 1 quick-acting and protamine, requires preparation before injecting.

A serious fault characterizing globin insulin is a tendency for its effect to diminish so rapidly in severe cases that an overnight rise in the sugar level occurs, heavy glycosuria appears before and after breakfast and doses large enough to reduce the level promptly are prone to cause afternoon insulin shock. However, it is usually possible to control this situation with small midafternoon feedings. In cases in which high insulin dosage is required, or in "brittle" individuals, best results are often obtained by giving 70% of the total globin insulin dose before breakfast and the rest at 3 P.M. The results were so satisfactory with globin insulin as a single-dose preparation under the circumstances of the blitz air raids in England during World War II that it remained the insulin of choice in many practices in that country until it began to be replaced by lente insulin.

INSULIN ZINC SUSPENSION (LENTE INSULIN, LENTE ILETIN). This preparation, being devoid of foreign protein (except that in the insulin itself), should ideally be used whenever possible to the exclusion of all others, except of course that it cannot be given intravenously. Actually the transfer of patients to it, and starting of new patients on it has become almost universal practice. Control is nearly always smoother and reactions fewer and milder in stable diabetics receiving this drug than with any previously used insulins. With few exceptions, lente can be substituted for isophane on a unit-for-unit basis; however, since some patients exhibit significantly better control with lente, it is wise to use a slightly lower dose at the outset. Ultra-Lente may be substituted very satisfactorily for protamine zinc insulin, or it can be mixed with lente to achieve an effect dependent upon the proportions in the mixture.

Mixtures of lente and quick-acting insulin can be employed, but conservative observers suggest that it is wise to confine the amount of the quick-acting insulin (preferably crystalline) to no more than 50% of the mixture to avoid disrupting the buffer mechanism that preserves the independent time-action potential of lente insulin. When crystalline insulin is drawn into the syringe containing lente no attempt should be made to mix the two types in the syringe before injecting.

"I have a patient who habitually has a headache after injection of epinephrine for quick control of a hypoglycemic reaction but does not experience this when glucagon is used. I give him roughly 30 μ/kg. body weight (2 mg. for his 160 pounds). What would be acceptable dosage for a child?"

Reply: Traisman and Newcomb used glucagon satisfactorily in dosage of 0.05–0.1 mg./kg. body weight in several children ranging in age from a newborn infant to a girl of 12.

H. S. Traisman and A. L. Newcomb. Illinois M. J. 117:81, 1960. Fred W. Whitehouse and Henry G. Bryan (Detroit). Glucagon for Treatment of Insulin Hypoglycemia: Its Use in Patient with Diabetes. Am. Pract. & Digest Treat. 10:1326, 1959.

"Some years ago I overheard, rather inattentively, of the treatment of diabetic retinopathy with estrogens. Now I have a case in which I would like to try this therapy; can you cite the evidence?"

Reply: In 1961, H. J. Roberts (West Palm Beach, Florida) reported the use of estrogens in 9 patients who were followed for periods up to 3 years, with improvement of the retinal lesions in 7. His criteria were demonstrable cessation of active retinal bleeding, with or without resorption of hemorrhages; no recurrence of bleeding in patients previously manifesting continual or repeated hemorrhage; sustained objective improvement in vision; and an exacerbation of visual impairment after withdrawal of estrogen or substitution of placebo therapy. The 2 patients who failed to respond had far advanced retinopathy with retinitis proliferans and glomerulosclerosis. Conjugated estrogens (Premarin) was used initially in 0.3 mg. dosage daily and later reduced to 0.3 mg. three times weekly in most cases.

H. J. Roberts. Treatment of Diabetic Retinopathy with Estrogens. J. Am. Geriatrics Soc. 9:655, 1961.

"Are the thiazide diuretics contraindicated in diabetes because of the well known ability to induce carbohydrate intolerance?"

Reply: I do not believe that they should be considered contraindicated, but it is nevertheless certain that ordinary diabetic vigilance should be much sharpened during the period of their use so that antidiabetic therapy can be adjusted if indicated. In studying the etiologic factors involved in thiazide hyperglycemia in the diabetic, Chazan and Boshell, in Birmingham, Alabama, felt that the following mechanisms might be in operation: (1) direct or indirect toxic effect on islet cells of the pancreas, (2) decreased sensitivity to insulin, (3) decreased secretion of insulin, (4) increased binding of insulin or (5) a secondary effect resulting from other biochemical alterations that often accompany thiazide treatment, such as hyperuricemia and hypokalemia.

Joseph A. Chazan and Buris R. Boshell. Etiologic Factors in Thiazide-Induced or Aggravated Diabetes Mellitus. Diabetes 14:132, 1965.

"Is insulin allergy, which fortunately now is a rare occurrence, likely to increase with the frequent intermittent use of insulin and oral hypoglycemic agents that is going on?"

Reply: Yes, I think that the switching between the classic agent and the newer oral compounds is almost certain to produce the result you foresee.

J. B. Aiken. Allergy to Insulin. Canad. M. A. J. 91:660, Sept. 19, 1964.

"It is generally believed that symptoms of allergy to insulin usually appear during the first month of therapy, but I have a patient in whom what appears to be a typical allergic manifestation has appeared only after 3 years of uninterrupted insulin injections. Is it likely that this is truly allergy, and if so, what do you recommend?"

Reply: It could certainly be an allergic reaction. Kenneth Kreines, University of Cincinnati, has reported a patient who had such a reaction after 4 years and another after 7. Antihistaminics have sometimes been used successfully in the usual way, or equal quantities of 1 : 1000 solution of diphenhydramine (Benadryl) injected with the insulin to prevent local reaction. The method of desensitization perhaps most frequently employed is to start with an intradermal injection of 1/1000 unit of whatever insulin is to be used and double the dose every 15–30 minutes, according to tolerance, to 1 unit. Thereafter the drug is injected subcutaneously in increasing amounts until the desired dose is reached. Some cases are also successfully handled by merely changing about among the different brands of insulin. In one of Kreines's cases the allergy was clearly specific for beef and pork insulins but not for sheep insulin or for pork insulin modified by dealanination. A few years ago, Henry Dolger reported the denaturation of insulin by boiling, stating that either of the two quick-acting insulins will lose only 10–20% of their activity during boiling for 15 minutes. He said that once the patient has been desensitized with such a denatured insulin, he may be treated with any of the other commercially available insulins without difficulty. In a typical case he boiled a vial of crystalline zinc insulin for 30 minutes and injected 10 units subcutaneously 4 hours after an allergic reaction had subsided; this was repeated in an hour and then every 2 hours until 60 units had been given and the patient was no longer acidotic; he was then kept on 20 units of denatured insulin twice daily for a month and thereafter transferred uneventfully to 40 units of globin insulin daily.

Kenneth Kreines. The Use of Various Insulins in Insulin Allergy. Arch. Int. Med. 116:167, 1965. H. Dolger. Management of Insulin Allergy and Insulin Resistance in Diabetes Mellitus. M. Clin. North America 36:783, 1952.

"I think we are all aware of the fact that it is often a very rewarding experience to reduce the weight of an obese diabetic patient, but this is certainly not an easy thing to do. What has been the experience of those who have sought to do this with the anorexigenic drugs under controlled conditions?"

Reply: In the study of S. K. Fineberg (Harlem Hospital, New York), which was a carefully controlled, triple-blind, crossover affair, the average trial period was 10 weeks and a significant weight loss occurred among 72% of the phenmetrazine (Preludin)-treated individuals and in only 12% of the untreated. The patients took one 25 mg. capsule three times daily 1 hour before meals, but were not informed of the purpose of the study and no dietary instructions were given. At the beginning of the study 16 patients were on insulin therapy and 7 on oral hypoglycemic agents; 12 of the insulin group noted a significant drop in insulin requirement and 6 of them were able to discontinue this medication. Of those taking oral hypoglycemics, 7 reduced their dosage sharply and 2 discontinued. Fineberg enthusiastically stated the belief that patients selected by the criteria for oral hypoglycemic medication would probably do much better on diet and anorexigenic medication instead. However, when Barbara Hazlett (University of Toronto) studied the matter under conditions more nearly comparable to those in private practice, she found that almost all patients who lost weight did so most effectively

in the first 2 months of treatment and that prolongation of therapy beyond 6 months was of little benefit. There were also side effects of the drug in one fourth of the patients, which caused discontinuance of its use in one eighth of them. It was possible to assess the effect of this anorexigenic therapy on diabetes on 33 of her patients who lost weight: insulin dosage could be reduced in 13 and discontinued in 3, but it had to be resumed in 2 as weight was regained. Five patients had repeated hypoglycemic episodes when they started phenmetrazine therapy, though warned to lower their insulin dose, and the reactions disturbed 2 patients sufficiently to influence them to refuse further therapy.

S. K. Fineberg. Obesity-Diabetes and Anorexigenics. J.A.M.A. 175:680, Feb. 25, 1961. Barbara E. Hazlett. Long-Term Anorexigenic Therapy in Obese Diabetic Patients. Canad. M. A. J. 85:677, Sept. 16, 1961.

"In a few instances in our hospital it has seemed that the administration of imipramine (Tofranil) to counteract depression in diabetics has reduced the glycosuria somewhat. Has anything of practical value come out of such an observation elsewhere?"

Reply: I do not think so. In 1960, Kaplan's group (University of Cincinnati) reported an observation of this sort in several mildly diabetic patients, but I have neither seen nor heard of any follow-up of this anywhere.

Stanley Kaplan, James W. Maas, John M. Pixley and W. Donald Ross. Use of Imipramine (Tofranil) in Diabetics: Effects on Glycosuria and Blood Sugar Levels. J.A.M.A. 174:511, Oct. 1, 1960.

"I have heard it rumored that tolbutamide (Orinase) has been used effectively in the treatment of skin diseases, but hesitate to try it. What is the record?"

Reply: I have seen only one report, that of Singh and associates at the Armed Forces Medical College, Poona, India, but it was upon the whole certainly favorable. The drug was given in dosage of 0.5–1.5 Gm. daily with meals in a wide variety of dermatoses. However, that was in 1961 and I hear no chatter about it nowadays. Two other bizarre uses of the drug that I have been aware of have come to nothing: in parkinsonism, and in thromboangiitis obliterans. So if you use it, I would suggest keeping your fingers crossed.

Inder Singh, M. L. Gaind and D. Jayram. Tolbutamide in Treatment of Skin Diseases. Brit. J. Dermat. 73:362, 1961.

"In a normal individual with a mildly elevated blood glucose during pregnancy would it be rational to administer tolbutamide (Orinase)?"

Reply: The data of Spellacy's group, at the University of Minnesota, show that tolbutamide is pancreatropic, i.e., that it stimulates the beta cells of the pancreas to release insulin during pregnancy. Therefore it would seem logical to use the drug in the situation you present. However, since pregnancy has been shown to be a strong stimulus to the pancreas, it appears to be even more logical to supplement the patient's deficient endogenous insulin production with enough injected insulin to maintain normal glucose values rather than to add an additional stimulus to the pancreas as would be done through giving tolbutamide. But the question really has not been answered in experience. Another objection that might be urged is that tolbutamide has been shown to be teratogenic in animals and possibly in humans also. However, insulin, too, has been shown to be teratogenic, and there is also an increased incidence of malformed infants born to women with diabetes in any case. So I do not feel that the alleged teratogenicity of the drug needs to be very seriously considered at the present time.

W. N. Spellacy, F. C. Goetz, B. Z. Greenberg and K. L. Schoeller. Tolbutamide Response in Normal Pregnancy. J. Clin. Endocrinol. 25:1251, 1965.

"Is chlorpropamide (Diabinese) capable of producing severe and prolonged hypoglycemia, as is tolbutamide (Orinase)?"

Reply: Yes. Hypoglycemia should always be considered when searching for the cause of a comatose episode in a diabetic who is using a sulfonylurea oral antidiabetic.

"How long should one wait before switching a diabetic patient from one drug to another?"

Reply: There is no ready-made answer to this question. You should be aware that glucose excretion fluctuates considerably in many patients from day to day and even from week to week, and that it therefore requires a considerable period of observation to determine just what is going on. In many instances if you will only wait long enough, which will sometimes be a matter of several weeks, you may find that rather than switching to another oral drug you will need only to alter the dosage in the one that you are presently using. Oral antidiabetic therapy must be absolutely individualized as much as insulin therapy. Are you satisfied with a urine that will yield less than 10 grams of glucose in 24 hours? Many men are.

"In our practice we do not see insulin allergy as often as statistics would lead us to expect, but a case is encountered occasionally nevertheless. To which of the insulins are these people most often hypersensitive?"

Reply: Perhaps closer inquiry would elicit information from some of your patients that would increase your incidence of allergic reactions to insulin? In some instances local allergic manifestations are rather slight— perhaps no more than a bit of pruritus and maybe slight induration at an injection site— and tend to disappear as the injection course is continued. The stoical type of individual would take this sort of thing in stride and perhaps not even report it. I cannot answer your question regarding the types of insulin most prone to cause allergic reactions, but I can cite the 5 interesting cases reported by Kenneth Kreines, in Cincinnati, as indicative of the spread. Two of these patients had generalized reaction: 1 a serum sickness type of reaction and the other generalized pruritus, the latter appearing to be dose-related. The other 3 patients had severe local cutaneous allergy only. In 1 patient the allergy was clearly specific for beef and pork insulins but not for sheep insulin or for pork insulin modified by dealanination. One patient was allergic to insulin from every available species including the human. In 2 patients allergy was temporary, disappearing in 1 after 1 month's treatment with dealaninated pork insulin and in the other after insulin was stopped for 3 days and then administered intravenously when ketoacidosis developed.

Kenneth Kreines. The Use of Various Insulins in Insulin Allergy. Arch. Int. Med. 116:167, 1965.

"What combination of chlorpropamide (Diabinese) and phenformin (DBI) has been most effective in the treatment of diabetes?"

Reply: I think that one can only answer this on the basis of individual experience because a large scale review of the matter has not been made, at least to my knowledge. In Cleveland, Joseph Goodman found the combination of 500 mg. chlorpropamide and 25 mg. phenformin twice daily a very efficacious one, but the various other combinations that were usually less satisfactory were not employed often enough to give the study statistical significance as a whole.

Joseph I. Goodman. Role of Phenformin (DBI) as an Adjuvant in Oral Antidiabetic Therapy. Metabolism 14:1153, 1965.

DIARRHEA

"Most of the nonspecific diarrheas that are encountered in a general practice are self terminating, but it is a comfort to be able to stop

them a bit sooner through the use of a drug. Most of my friends, like myself, switch about among the numerous preparations that are promoted for this purpose, but I am not quite at ease in doing so. Would you kindly compare the principal of these drugs from the standpoint of their potential toxicities?"

Reply: Of course old familiar *paregoric* is both effective and nontoxic, though admittedly the dose is a bit nasty to take. Addiction certainly need not be feared from this kind of use of the drug. *Lomotil* contains in addition to its antidiarrhea ingredient a small amount of atropine sulfate and should therefore be used with caution in elderly individuals in the glaucoma age or in those with prostatism or other type of urinary retention as well as in individuals with coronary disease, tachycardia from any cause, or pyloric obstruction. There appears to be the further possibility that Lomotil may be harmful in the presence of disturbed liver function; the fact that the principal ingredient of this preparation is related to some of the narcotics apparently need be no cause for concern from the standpoint of addiction. *Cantilyn* and *Cantilyn w/Neomycin* should be regarded as equivalent to Lomotil from the standpoint of contraindications to its use in situations where an anticholinergic agent would be undesirable. *Cremomycin*, containing both Sulfasuxidine and neomycin, of course has the toxic potentialities of both of these antibiotics. *Kaopectate* contains kaolin and pectin; I am not aware of any toxicity reported in connection with its use. The same thing may be said of *Quintess*, which contains pectin and attapulgite; but *Quintess-N* contains neomycin in addition, from which some toxicity may derive, though admittedly systemic toxicity from oral administration of this antibiotic is practically unknown. In using *Sorboquel* there may be some degree of cramping and bloating since this is a hydrophilic gel; the drug should probably be considered contraindicated in persons of advanced years and if there is any type of gastrointestinal stenosis; and one of the ingredients of this preparation is capable of atropine-like action. *Valmycin* contains pectin and kaolin and neomycin, ingredients of which I have already said enough. *Furoxone* is one of the nitrofuran derivatives that have caused a good many very serious reactions. However, nothing very alarming has been reported with Furoxone to my knowledge: some gastrointestinal disturbances, a few instances of rashes and very rarely partial deafness, dizziness, angioneurotic edema, fever and arthralgia.

"I see all sorts of fancy new, and expensive, antibacterial agents proposed for the prophylaxis and/or treatment of the familiar traveler's diar-

rhea. Are these drugs rationally employed since we really do not know the etiology of this malady?"

Reply: Do you really want an old timer's advice? A long time ago we used to use tannic acid derivative preparations quite effectively in this malady, and there are a few oldsters here and there who still do so. The familiar compounds at that time were acetyltannic acid and albumin tannate, and they are still commercially available as Tannigen and Tannalbin, respectively. Dosage of Tannigen is 3–10 grains (0.2–0.6 Gm.), four or more times daily, taken dry on the tongue followed by a swallow of water, or mixed with food, avoiding warm or alkaline liquids. Tannalbin dosage is 30 grains (2.0 Gm.) or more, in capsules or as a powder. Try one of these agents, since there is nothing to lose, for the attacks are self-terminating anyway.

"The usual criteria of efficacy of the anti-infective drugs in the diarrheal disorders of infancy, namely the effect on mortality, the duration of the diarrhea or the elimination of pathogens from the stools, are more or less unsatisfactory. Is there no way of measuring the effect on the volume of the stool?"

Reply: Kahn and associates (University of the Witwatersrand) developed a "diarrhea index" to correlate with stool volume and provided a formula for determination of this derived parameter. But the only trouble is that when I studied their report (which perhaps indeed I did not understand) it seemed to me that the intravenous administration of fluids would vitiate the whole calculation.

Eric Kahn, Harry Stein and Samuel Wayburne. Antidiarrheal Effect of Antibiotics. Lancet 2:703, Oct. 5, 1963.

"In the infantile diarrheas the organism, enteropathogenic *E. coli* (EPEC), appears frequently to be the causative agent and we can identify this organism in our hospital through fluorescent antibody techniques. But we have not had much success in treating the cases with either tetracyclines or chloramphenicol. What has been the experience elsewhere?"

Reply: In Houston, M. D. Yow obtained her best results when giving orally the nonabsorbable agents, polymyxin B, colistin (Coly-Mycin), neomycin, kanamycin (Kantrex) and furazolidone (Furoxone).

M. D. Yow. Antibiotic Management of Acute Infectious Gastroenteritis in Infancy. Pediat. Clin. North America 10:103, 1963.

"The attacks of diarrhea that are common in travelers, especially in tropical and subtropical areas, have not been shown to be amenable to any specific type of therapy in carefully performed studies, at least so far as I am aware. And yet one reads, or learns by word of mouth from one's associates, of any number of drugs that have been 'sure fire' in putting stop to individual cases or even to epidemics of the malady. Where does the truth lie in all of this?"

Reply: I do not think that any of these individual reports should be ridiculed. A doctor gives a drug, controls an epidemic, and can surely congratulate himself on having had an eminently satisfactory clinical experience. What does it matter that the fellow had no control cases and persuaded himself to overlook the fact that in many outbreaks of the "guppies" the stricken individuals frequently recover spontaneously within the time allotted to active treatment? "Curing" the patient is good doctoring, and spurious remedies are not always false ones.

"Iodochlorhydroxyquin (Vioform) is highly recommended in our part of the country for individuals who are going to travel into foreign countries. Is there really definite evidence that this agent is effective in the prophylaxis of traveler's diarrhea?"

Reply: Kean and Waters (Cornell University) performed a careful study in American students attending summer schools in Mexico City, and found the drug no more effective than placebo.

B. H. Kean and Somerset R. Waters. Diarrhea of Travelers: III. Drug Prophylaxis in Mexico. New England J. Med. 261:71, July 9, 1959.

DIPHTHERIA

"What is the drug of choice in diphtheria?"

Reply: I do not like precisely the phrasing of your question because it implies that specific drug therapy is the preferable approach in this disease. Which is of course not the case since antitoxin is *the* life-saving agent. For supplementary use, however, the penicillins, tetracyclines and erythromycin (Ilotycin, etc.) are useful in some cases. It should be distinctly understood that it is wrong to rush in and give these drugs before being certain of the diagnosis, because in doing so you may mask the symptoms sufficiently so that you will miss identification of the disease until it is too late.

DRUG ERUPTIONS

"I have recently had a near fatality in association with use of phenylbutazone (Butazolidin),

the lesion having been diagnosed by our dermatologist as toxic epidermal necrolysis. What other drugs may cause life-threatening drug eruptions and what are the principal dermatologic forms that these reactions assume?"

Reply: At the University of Illinois, Rostenberg and Fagelson have discussed the following as principal life-threatening drug eruptions: Stevens-Johnson syndrome, toxic epidermal necrolysis, systemic lupus erythematosus–like syndrome, and exfoliative dermatitis. They listed the following drugs in connection with these respective reactions: *Stevens-Johnson*: chlorpropamide (Diabinese), diphenylhydantoin (Dilantin), diphenylhydantoin and trimethadione (Tridione) together, amithiozone (Tibione), phenobarbital, sulfadimethoxine (Madribon), sulfamethoxypyridazine (Kynex), sulfadiazine, sulfamerazine and sulfamethazine (Sulfatriad), amithiozone, trimethadione and phenobarbital together. *Toxic epidermal necrolysis*: dapsone, diphenylhydantoin (Dilantin), nitrofurantoin (Furadantin), penicillin, phenolphthalein, phenylbutazone (Butazolidin), procaine penicillin, aqueous injection and oral mixed sulfonamide preparation, sulfadimethoxine (Madribon), sulfamethoxypyridazine (Kynex), sulfathiazole, methyl salicylate, tetracycline, diallylbarbituric acid with ethylmorphine hydrochloride (Diadol), neomycin, ipecac, opium, gold salts, antipyrine, acetazolamide (Diamox), barbiturates, antihistamines, oil of chenopodium. *Systemic lupus-erythematosus*: diphenylhydantoin and mephobarbital (Mebarol) and paramethadione (Paradione), hydralazine (Apresoline), griseofulvin (Grifulvin), procainamide (Pronestyl), sulfamethoxypyridazine (Kynex), tetracycline hydrochloride degraded, trimethadione (Tridione) and diphenylhydantoin (Dilantin). *Exfoliative dermatitis*: aminosalicylic acid, diphenylhydantoin (Dilantin), griseofulvin (Grifulvin), phenindione (Danilone, Hedulin, Indon), sulfamethoxypyridazine (Kynex).

Adolph Rostenberg, Jr. and Harvey J. Fagelson. Life-Threatening Drug Eruptions. J.A.M.A. 194:660, Nov. 8, 1965.

DRUGS IN THE DEVELOPING FETUS

"Can you acquaint me with authoritative opinion regarding the effect of drugs upon the developing fetus?"

Reply: I really do not believe that there can be "authoritative" opinion as yet on this subject for several reasons. In the first place, entirely satisfactory methods of studying the fetal effects of maternally administered drugs in experimental animals have not yet been devised. In the second place, we do not know with what assurance we can extrapolate the experimental findings into the problem as it is posed in human obstetrical practice. And finally, although we do have bits of information regarding the possible teratogenicity of some of the relatively new drugs, we do not have assurance that some of the old familiar agents may not all along have been exerting some degree of this type of action. Therefore the most authoritative pronouncement that can be made at the present time is that throughout the entire period of pregnancy administration of any drugs whatsoever should be held to the minimum consistently with nonneglect of such drug administration as is important for the obstetrical and general welfare of the patient. It is the period of organogenesis, from the beginning of the third week to the end of the tenth week of pregnancy, with which one is concerned, for it is during this time that deleterious effects upon the embryo may be exerted. To this tenth week of *known* pregnancy must be added the first 2 weeks of embryonic life in which the pregnant state is usually unsuspected, which gives us a period of 12 weeks in which drugs may exert an acute interference in the development of the fetus. But since we do not know that all action ceases when administration of the drug ceases, it is advisable to consider that the first 4 months of pregnancy is the danger period. The fact that the first 2 weeks during which the pregnancy may not be suspected is an unguarded period so far as refraining from drug use is concerned, is perhaps not a very serious matter, since, as Smithells says, there is a time lag of about a week between fertilization and implantation, maternal drugs are unlikely to affect the embryo before a close vascular relationship has been established between the two organisms, and a noxious factor affecting the embryo at this early and undifferentiated stage is more likely to cause embryonic death than survival with malformation.

The drugs to be avoided, other things being equal, during this first 4 month period are the following, if you understand that there is no reason to believe that this list is either valid or complete. Documentation is very poor in this entire area. The drugs listed here are those against which there is reasonable evidence of their deforming or lethal effect upon the fetus, but the actual fact is that until relatively recent times little attention has been paid to this matter and we are therefore ignorant of the possible association of some of our familiar drugs with interruptions in pregnancy or deformation of the fetus. Certainly the wisest policy at present is to refrain from using any drugs in at least the first trimester that are not considered to be of great importance in maintaining the state of health of the pregnant woman.

ANDROGENIC COMPOUNDS (testosterone and its derivatives) may possibly induce masculinization of the female fetus.

ANTIBIOTICS as a group may be used with impunity, but a few qualifying remarks need to be made. Considering the potential ototoxicity of streptomycin, it is surprising that only a few instances of damage to the hearing organ in the developing infant have been recorded; there seems to be doubtful indication for withholding this drug from a tuberculous mother in whom its use is required (but see a Reply in the section on Tuberculosis). A teratogenic effect of the tetracyclines has been suggested in the literature but not fully substantiated; but it may be that the prematurely born infant is retarded in skeletal growth when the mother has been given tetracyclines before delivery. It is apparently an established fact that yellowing and enamel defects in the teeth of the fetus of a tetracycline-treated woman occurs in a proportion of instances not yet established; the effect appears to be induced by ingestion of the drugs during midpregnancy and after.

ANTICOAGULANTS. There are strong indications, both experimental and clinical, that retarded development or even death of the fetus may result from bishydroxycoumarin (Dicumarol) during pregnancy. However, it appears that use of the drug for short periods just before delivery may be a safer procedure. The other orally administered agents should be held under suspicion also. Heparin is safe as it does not traverse the placental barrier.

ANTIDIABETIC DRUGS. Increased perinatal loss in mothers taking chlorpropamide (Diabinese) during their pregnancy has been reported, but the evidence is not convincing that these occurrences have been more than coincidental. A very small number of cases of malformed fetuses has been ascribed to tolbutamide (Orinase) treatment of the mothers, but again the cause-and-effect evidence is not entirely satisfactory. Phenformin (DBI) may questionably cause lactic acidosis.

ANTIMALARIALS. All the new synthetic antimalarials may apparently be administered safely to the pregnant woman in the dosage used in treating malaria, but it is a firmly entrenched clinical impression that quinine in such dosage is contraindicated in her and may cause serious visual and auditory disturbances in the infant. Satisfactory statistical study, however, has not substantiated this clinical impression regarding quinine, nor indeed overthrown it. The fact that malaria itself frequently causes abortion has made it difficult to prove that quinine importantly contributes to this. Thrombocytopenic effects in the infant have been attributed in rare instances to administration of quinine in antimalarial dosage to the mother during her pregnancy. When the newer synthetic antimalarials – such drugs as chloroquine (Aralen), hydroxychloroquine (Plaquenil) and amodiaquin (Camoquin) – are used in treatment of the collagen disorders, in dosage very much higher than is employed in malaria, there are evidences that congenital abnormalities may be induced occasionally. Pyrimethamine (Daraprim), another of these newer drugs, is favorably used in the treatment of toxoplasmosis in dosage much higher than employed in malaria; I have not seen evidence of deleterious action upon the fetus, though this might be anticipated since the drug is a folic acid antagonist like some of the antineoplastic agents.

ANTINEOPLASTIC COMPOUNDS. Other things being equal (and this is an important consideration in the patient with a malignant lesion), the alkylating agents (mostly nitrogen mustard type compounds), are contraindicated during the first trimester – such drugs as mechlorethamine (Mustargen), melphalan (Alkeran), chlorambucil (Leukeran), cyclophosphamide (Cytoxan), thiotepa (Thio-Tepa), triethylenemelamine (TEM), uracil mustard (Uracil Mustard), busulfan (Myleran). I think it important to note, however, regarding the last listed agent, busulfan, that I have seen the reports of 4 cases in which it was used throughout pregnancy without serious apparent damage to the fetus. The folic acid antagonists, aminopterin and amethopterin (Methotrexate), are considered to be capable of abortifacient action and hence contraindicated in at least the first trimester; aminopterin may also cause deformation of the fetal skull, it seems. I have seen no record of a study of the purine antagonist, mercaptopurine (Purinethol), in pregnancy, but would hold it suspect. The pyrimidine antagonist, fluorouracil (Fluorouracil) is a very toxic drug, difficult to handle, and I should think to be used with diffidence in pregnancy, although in fact its employment against gastrointestinal and breast cancer is predominantly in individuals beyond childbearing age. Dromostanolone propionate (Drolban) is a testosterone derivative sometimes used in breast cancer in women who are still premenopausal; masculinity of the fetus has not been reported, to my knowledge. I suppose one should consider it inadvisable to use the plant alkaloids, vinblastine (Velban) and vincristine (Oncovin), during the first trimester, but I have seen no record of teratogenic action attributable to them.

ANTITHYROID COMPOUNDS. All these agents – the thiouracils, iodides, perchlorates, radioactive iodine – cross the placental barrier and can cause fetal goiter since the fetal thyroid concentrates iodide at 14 weeks and synthesizes organic iodine compounds at 15–19 weeks. This goiter apparently reflects compensatory enlargement resulting from increase in thyroid-stimulating hormone when thyroxin production is inhibited. The infant may be hypothyroid at birth (this may be permanent if radioiodine has been used) or experience a period of transient hyperthyroidism. Authoritative opinion is that use of these drugs during pregnancy need not be interdicted if tight supervision is maintained.

ANTITUBERCULOSIS DRUGS. There is a higher incidence of malformation in the infants of women treated with these drugs during pregnancy (at least the three major ones: isoniazid, PAS and streptomycin), but it is not certain that the disease itself is not responsible.

BARBITURATES. These agents not only cross the placental barrier but, except for the very shortest-acting ones that are used as anesthetics, accumulate in the brain, liver and placenta. It is therefore important in the barbiturate-addicted patient (inquire into this; she is unlikely to volunteer the information that she has been taking one of these drugs for a long period of time) that the drug be gradually withdrawn during the pregnancy.

CORTICOSTEROIDS. Pregnancy does not contraindicate the use of these drugs. Some evidence has been produced of a causative relationship to cleft palate, but it is not convincing. The incidence of postnatal infantile hypoadrenalism has been too low to have significance.

DISULFIRAM (ANTABUSE). It is the consensus that if this drug is being used in the attempt to break the alcohol habit in a pregnant woman it is advisable to omit the alcohol test.

DISODIUM EDETATE (ENDRATE), an agent that will abstract calcium through a process of chelation, had best not be used, though I am not certain that calcium would be withdrawn by it from the fetus.

GANGLIONIC BLOCKING AGENTS: mecamylamine (Inversine), hexamethonium (Methium), pentolinium (Ansolysen), chlorisondamine (Ecolid), trimethaphan (Arfonad), trimethidinium (Ostensin). It is probably inadvisable to use these drugs in the pregnant hypertensive because there have been reports indicating that ileus and pneumonitis in the newborn may be increased by such therapy.

GLUTETHIMIDE (DORIDEN) is a drug of addiction with which there are associated quite severe withdrawal symptoms. I consider it unwise to prescribe this drug as a hypnotic for the pregnant woman, and if she is already taking it habitually when first seen, the withdrawal should be accomplished very gradually. Among the withdrawal symptoms in the adult are ileus and atony of the urinary bladder; I have not seen record of these things appearing in the neonate of a woman undergoing glutethimide withdrawal, but theoretically this could occur.

GOLD SALTS should probably be looked upon as contraindicated.

MAJOR TRANQUILIZERS. Most of these drugs are phenothiazines—chlorpromazine (Thorazine), promazine (Sparine), triflupromazine (Vesprin), mepazine (Pacatal), thioridazine (Mellaril), acetophenazine (Tindal), carphenazine (Proketazine), fluphenazine (Prolixin, Permitil), perphenazine (Trilafon), trifluoperazine (Stelazine), prochlorperazine (Compazine), thiopropazate (Dartal)—capable of such a diversity of reactions not only upon the central and autonomic nervous systems but of an allergic nature as well, that it seems only sensible to withhold them during pregnancy. I do not believe that the earlier suggestion that these drugs contribute significantly to neonatal hyperbilirubinemia has been satisfactorily substantiated, but it seems to me that caution is certainly the better part of valor here.

MECLIZINE (BONINE), CYCLIZINE (MAREZINE) AND CHLORCYCLIZINE (DI-PARALENE, PERAZIL) are three antihistaminic antiemetic agents that have been withdrawn from over-the-counter sale and a relabeling ordered by the Food and Drug Administration to warn against their use "without medical advice" by women who are or who may become pregnant. This action was said to have been taken because careful animal experimentation had shown that teratogenic effects can be demonstrated. That such findings cannot be automatically transferred to man, however, is implicit in two facts: first, that teratogenic effects may be present in one species of animal and not in another; and, second, even the lowest dosage producing teratogenic effects in animals has been 25–50 fold the therapeutic dose in man. Therefore, only studies in man can have validity, and the only three prospective studies of the matter that I have seen, in which adequate comparisons were possible, showed no teratogenic effects of these drugs. For example in the most recent of these studies, that of Yerushalmy and Milkovich, at the University of California, there were 330 gravidas for whom drugs of the meclizine/cyclizine group were prescribed during the first 12 weeks of pregnancy, 473 for whom other antinausea drugs were prescribed, and 3474 for whom no antinauseants were prescribed, although it is certainly possible that some of these latter may have procured such drugs over-the-counter. It was found that the abortion and perinatal mortality rates, and the number per 100 infants of nontrivial and of severe anomalies for the gravidas in the meclizine/cyclizine group, were nearly identical with those in the "other" antinausea drugs group. In the group

for whom no antinausea drugs were prescribed, the percentage of infants born with anomalies was the same as in the other two groups but the incidence of abortion was much higher. When the women in this latter group were subdivided into those who did and did not suffer nausea and vomiting early in pregnancy, it was found that gravidas who did not have nausea and vomiting had abortion rates three times as high as those who did. This latter finding was in confirmation of earlier suggestions in the literature.

So what is one to say? I suppose only that since the Food and Drug Administration has acted to prohibit over-the-counter sale of these agents, it is probably inadvisable to prescribe them during pregnancy. I would be inclined, then, to add to the list buclizine (Softran) and Bucladin (which contains buclizine and other ingredients).

OPIATES should be used in no more than a very few doses, if at all, during pregnancy for fear of addicting the mother and precipitating withdrawal symptoms in the addicted infant shortly after birth.

PHENELZINE (NARDIL). This drug, which is used to combat depressive illness, is capable of potentiating the action of so many other drugs that I believe it inadvisable to use it at any time during pregnancy.

PHENMETRAZINE (PRELUDIN). I do not believe we have substantial evidence of the teratogenicity of this drug. However, a few years ago there appeared a letter in the British Medical Journal suggesting that this may be the case: the patient took the drug during the first trimester of her first and third pregnancies, both of which produced infants with nearly identical malformations, while the second pregnancy, in which the drug was not taken, produced a normal child. To draw conclusions from this one report would of course be inadmissible; I have merely brought it to your attention.

PHENTOLAMINE (REGITINE). The death of both a mother and fetus when this drug was used to diagnose pheochromocytoma during pregnancy has been reported.

POTASSIUM SALTS. It is my personal belief, which I cannot support by citing specific cases, that the parenteral administration of potassium salts to the pregnant woman could seriously endanger the developing fetal myocardium.

PROGESTATIONAL COMPOUNDS. There have been several reports of masculinization of the female fetus in mothers treated with the newer synthetic compounds, sometimes proceeding as far as marked hypoplasia of the uterus and vagina as well as enlargement of the clitoris and labial fusion. Paradoxically, *estrogens* have also done this upon rare occasion, and it is not certain that all these instances were not merely coincidental.

RESERPINE. I have seen a report covering 77 reserpine-treated mothers of whom 16% of the infants were born with a snuffy nose and nasal discharge, retractions, cyanosis and anorexia, and 2 fatalities.

SALICYLATES in large amounts may cause neonatal bleeding.

SULFONAMIDES. These drugs are principally detoxified through reaction with glucuronic acid in the liver, a process that does not begin until several days after birth. Therefore an infant born of a mother who has recently received a drug of this group may have in its blood stream an amount of the agent with which it cannot cope. It is probably inadvisable to give sulfonamides in any form, but especially the long-acting members of the group, late in a pregnancy.

THIAZIDE DIURETICS. There has been some evidence that thrombocytopenia in newborn infants may be due to the administration of drugs of this group to women late in their pregnancies. In some of these instances there has been additional evidence of bone marrow depression, though none of these things were exhibited in the mothers.

VITAMIN D. There has been reported the case of an infant with severe hypercalcemia and cardiovascular lesions that resembled the findings in instances of experimental vitamin D intoxication. This may mean nothing, but admonition to the pregnant woman not to overstuff herself with vitamin D would not be amiss.

VITAMIN K. There has been some evidence that large doses of vitamin K given parenterally prior to delivery are responsible for hyperbilirubinemia and brain damage in the newborn. It is therefore advisable not only to refrain from such injections, giving the drug to the infant instead if there is a neonatal hemorrhagic disorder, but to caution the patient against taking vitamin tablets that contain vitamin K during her pregnancy.

It seems fitting, in closing this listing, to remind you that 2–3% of all infants have deformities recognizable at birth and that valid attribution of such deformities to drugs ingested during pregnancy cannot truly be made where only one or a few cases are involved. It is only when the type of abnormality occurring is identical in connection with a given drug that we are on reasonably safe ground.

James M. Sutherland, Irwin J. Light (Cincinnati). The Effect of Drugs upon the Developing Fetus. Pediat. Clin. North America 12:781, 1965. R. W. Smithells (Liverpool). The Problem of Teratogenicity. Practitioner, 194: 104, 1965. Alan K. Done (Salt Lake City, Utah). Developmental Pharmacology. Clin. Pharmacol. Therap. 5: 432, 1964. J. B. E. Baker. The Effects of Drugs on the Fetus. Pharm. Rev. 12:37, 1960. Erkki Varpela. The Effect Exerted by First-Line Tuberculosis Medicines on the Fetus.

Acta tuberc. et pneumol. scandinav. 45:53, 1964. Sidney Q. Cohlan. Fetal and Neonatal Hazards from Drugs Administered During Pregnancy. New York J. Med., Feb. 15, 1964, p. 493. Virginia Apgar. Drugs in Pregnancy. J.A.M.A. 190:840, Nov. 30, 1964. Herbert C. Flessa, Albert B. Kapstrom, Helen J. Glueck and John J. Will. Placental Transport of Heparin. Am. J. Obst. & Gynec. 93:570, 1965.
J. Yerushalmy and L. Milkovich. Evaluation of the Teratogenic Effect of Meclizine in Man. Am. J. Obst. & Gynec. 93:553, Oct. 15, 1965. R. W. Smithells and E. R. Chinn. Meclozine and Foetal Malformations: A Prospective Study. Brit. M. J. 1:217, 1964. G. W. Mellin and M. Katzenstein. Meclozine and Foetal Abnormalities. Lancet. 1:222, 1963.

DRUG REACTION INCIDENCE

"There is a great deal of talk nowadays about the serious drug reactions, but is not a good bit of this 'scare-head'? I do not believe we are seeing these things in our hospital."

Reply: Without wishing to be impertinent may I inquire whether you always recognize them when you see them? In a 350 bed teaching hospital which, because of its membership in the FDA Adverse-Drug-Reaction Reporting program, might be presumed to have a personnel peculiarly alert to matters of drug reactions as well as indications, MacDonald and Mackay have reported that nearly 2% of the deaths were directly associated with drug reactions. In a year in which there were 9557 inpatient and 35,018 outpatient admissions there were 98 reported reactions (about 1 to 100 admitted patients). Overdosage accounted for 25 of these, underdosage, 1; side effects occurred 26 times, secondary effects 4 times. More than 40% of the reactions were thought to have been allergic. Drugs producing the most reactions were penicillin, warfarin, chlorpromazine, phenobarbital, imipramine, secobarbital, digitalis and sulfisoxazole, in that order. The systems most often involved in reactions were the skin, hemopoietic, cardiovascular, central nervous system and urinary systems. Reactions were classified as serious in 27 instances, and death occurred in 7 of these cases.

Murdo G. MacDonald and Bruce R. Mackay. Adverse Drug Reactions: Experience of Mary Fletcher Hospital During 1962. J.A.M.A. 190:1071, Dec. 21, 1964.

"If a patient has an adverse drug reaction upon admission to hospital, is he likely to have a higher than ordinary incidence of additional drug reactions after hospitalization?"

Reply: Larry Seidl has said that of 714 patients admitted on a certain service at Johns Hopkins Hospital there was a 13.6% incidence of adverse reactions acquired within the hospital, but that in patients admitted specifically because of an adverse reaction the risk of second adverse reactions while in hospital was 30%. The overall incidence of reactions in this Hopkins study is much higher than in any other reports I have seen; the reasons for this escape me but, with regard to the answer that I am trying to supply to your question, I do not think that the absolute figures are of as great importance as the relationship between them.

Larry Seidl. Symposium: Adverse Drug Reactions; Meeting the Problem. J.A.M.A. 196:421, May 2, 1966.

DYSMENORRHEA

"I have been using oxyphenbutazone (Tandearil) for its anti-inflammatory effect in dysmenorrhea and have had a satisfactory response with it in about 8 out of 10 women, but I am wondering whether there is too much risk of toxic reactions to warrant continuing use of the drug month after month by those women who are relieved by it?"

Reply: Oxyphenbutazone is both an analogue and a metabolite of phenylbutazone (Butazolidine), and the incidence and severity of side actions to both drugs have been about the same except that oxyphenbutazone appears to cause less acute gastric irritation. With phenylbutazone itself side actions have occurred in about 40% of patients, causing discontinuance of the drug in about 15%. E. B. Mendel, in Texas, has had about the same experience as yourself regarding incidence of relief obtained with oxyphenbutazone, but I think it advisable to heed his list of contraindications: chronic edema, cardiac decompensation, history of peptic ulcer or drug allergy, hypertension or renal, cardiac or hepatic damage.

E. B. Mendel. Oxyphenbutazone (Tandearil) in Treatment of Dysmenorrhea. Texas J. Med. 61:44, 1965.

"I have not had much success in treating dysmenorrhea with progesterones, but the promotion for the new one, dydrogesterone (Duphaston) tempts me to try it. Has a definitive study been made?"

Reply: A double-blind trial was made by Fairweather, in England, on a small number of patients through 5 menstrual cycles. The drug was given in 5 mg. dosage two to three times daily from the fifth to the twenty-fifth day of the cycle. Nausea, vomiting and pain were all well relieved, and the only adverse effect noted was breakthrough bleeding which occurred in 3 patients during the first course of treatment, but without causing anxiety. It was not noticed that there was any carry-over effect of treatment in one cycle on the response in the next cycle. One is at a loss how to explain the effect of the drug in that, unlike the other progesterones, it does not inhibit ovulation, though a myometrial relaxing action has been shown in the experimental animal. The British findings have been confirmed here in the United States by Aydar and Coleman, in Georgia.

D. V. I. Fairweather. Duphaston in Dysmenorrhoea. J. Obst. & Gynaec. Brit. Common. 72:193, 1965. Cetin K. Aydar and Blanche D. Coleman. Treatment of Primary Dysmenorrhea: Double-Blind Study. J.A.M.A. 192:1003, June 14, 1965.

"I have heard that sequential estrogen-progestogen therapy is being used effectively in dysmenorrhea. Is this correct?"

Reply: At least its use has been favorably reported by Edwin Jungck and associates in Augusta, Georgia. They used a 0.1 mg. ethinyl estradiol tablet for 21 days beginning on day 5 of the menstrual cycle and using the Oracon preparation (which contains 25 mg. of dimethisterone in additon to the estrogen) during the last 5 days. A total of 195 patients used the sequential regimen for 844 cycles; 2 patients for as long as 24 cycles, 7 for 18 or more cycles and 15 for 12 or more cycles. Of the group, complete relief was obtained by 166 patients, partial relief by 8.

Edwin C. Jungck with collaborators. Sequential Estrogen-Progestogen Therapy in Gynecology. Am. J. Obst. & Gynec. 94:165, Jan. 15, 1966.

"Acting upon the long established impression that there is a correlation between certain areas of the nasal mucosa, the 'genital spots,' and cyclic changes of the endometrium, I recently used a long-acting oral nasal decongestant in a few patients with dysmenorrhea and obtained results that upon the whole were gratifying. Has this sort of thing been carefully studied?"

Reply: The only study I have seen reported in recent times was that of McCain and Olley (Emory University), who gave a sustained-release capsule containing 8 mg. chlorpheniramine maleate, 50 mg. phenylpropanolamine hydrochloride and 2.5 mg. isopropamide iodide (the total preparation known as Ornade) to 157 women with menstrual disturbances. Initially 1 capsule was taken every 12 hours, but often as frequently as every 6–8 hours. Considerable relief was experienced in a fair percentage of patients with menorrhagia, dysmenorrhea, endometriosis, and in the bleeding associated with leiomyoma of the uterus. But this was not a controlled study, and I think that really a double-blind and rather exhaustive one would be required to establish the worth of this therapy. It might not be wise to give a nasal decongestant systemically to pregnant patients.

John R. McCain and James F. Olley. Effect of Oral Nasal Decongestant on Menstrual Cycle. Am. J. Obst. & Gynec. 87:354, Oct. 1, 1963.

"I have been using isoxsuprine (Vasodilan) for the treatment of dysmenorrhea because the use of the drug for this purpose is actively promoted in our area. The results have been disappointing. Has it really any worth?"

Reply: Have your patients been taking the drug only at the onset of pain? When Alan Rubin (University of Pennsylvania) performed a double-blind study with the drug used in this way he was unable to establish real worth for it, but in an earlier study, Dennis Voulgaris (Wharton, Texas) reported that the drug satisfactorily relieved or prevented pelvic cramping in 44 of his 53 patients when taken for 1–3 days before the expected onset of menstruation. His initial dosage was usually a 10 mg. tablet four times daily, though it was sometimes necessary to increase the dose to 10 or 20 mg. four times daily. There was some drowsiness and gastric distress in 7 patients but not severe enough to necessitate reducing the dosage.

Alan Rubin. Isoxsuprine (Vasodilan) for Treatment of Dysmenorrhea: Double-Blind Study of 143 Subjects. Obst. & Gynec. 19:9, 1962. Dennis M. Voulgaris. Dysmenorrhea: Treatment with Isoxsuprine (Vasodilan). Obst. & Gynec. 15:220, 1960.

"How would you explain the relief that we sometimes obtain from the use of a belladonna alkaloid in the treatment of dysmenorrhea?"

Reply: In the experience of most physicians who use one of the belladonna alkaloids in the treatment of dysmenorrhea, the colicky pains are much more relieved than the headache, bearing-down in the lower abdomen, lassitude, etc., that characterize this disability. Usually the painfully menstruating uterus does not display any gross anatomic or histologic differences from one that does not menstruate painfully, but in the dysmenorrheic patient there are hypertonicity and dysrhythmia of uterine muscle plus apparent alterations in electrolyte metabolism and water retention. Atropine has a relaxing effect on the circular but not the longitudinal fibers of the excised human uterus, which probably explains the salutary action in some cases.

ECHO-COXSACKIE INFECTION

"Has any sort of specific drug therapy been developed for ECHO virus or Coxsackie virus infections?"

Reply: No.

ECLAMPSIA

"Despite contrary reports in the literature, we have the impression in our clinic that thiazides are of value in the prophylaxis of toxemia of pregnancy, particularly in women having their first baby; are there any definite contraindications to this measure?"

Reply: Actually, not all the findings in this matter have been adverse, for at the University of Mississippi, Norma Fallis and her group produced evidence which seemed to confirm the impression that you have gained in your own practice, and so too did Finnerty and Bepko at the District of Columbia General Hospital. Regarding contraindications, D. N. Menzies (University College Hospital Medical School, London) who studied the use of thiazides in treatment of early pre-eclampsia in 100 patients, agreed with the general viewpoint that diabetes mellitus is a definite contraindication to the use of these drugs but felt that all other pregnant women with hypertension, edema or excessive weight gain appear to be suitable for early and prolonged treatment with them. You must bear in mind, however, that the evaluation of oral carbohydrate tolerance in a pregnant patient on chlorothiazide is unreliable at present, as emphasized by Ladner's group at the Madigan General Hospital, Tacoma, Washington.

Norma E. Fallis, Warren C. Plauche, Lois M. Mosey and Herbert G. Langford. Thiazide Versus Placebo in Prophylaxis of Toxemia of Pregnancy in Primigravid Patients. Am. J. Obst. & Gynec. 88:502, Feb. 15, 1964. D. N. Menzies. Controlled Trial of Chlorothiazide (Diuril) in Treatment of Early Pre-eclampsia. Brit. M. J. 1:739, Mar. 21, 1964. Calvin N. Ladner, Jack W. Pearson, C. N. Herrick and H. E. Harrison. Effect of Chlorothiazide (Diuril) on Blood Glucose in Third Trimester of Pregnancy: Preliminary Report. Obst. & Gynec. 23:555, 1964. Frank A. Finnerty, Jr. and Frank J. Bepko, Jr. Lowering the Perinatal Mortality and the Prematurity Rate: The Value of Prophylactic Thiazides in Juveniles. J.A.M.A. 195:429, Feb. 7, 1966.

"In using a rauwolfia preparation for hypotensive effect in treating toxemias of pregnancy, I have found fewer side effects with syrosingopine (Singoserp) than with the other preparations of this group, but it has seemed to me that I have achieved a rapid and truly satisfactory hypotensive effect only in quite young patients; has this been general experience?"

Reply: At Baylor University, Jack Duffy's group recorded essentially such an experience; at least they found the drug most effective where there had been no evidence or history of renal damage, i.e., in the 18 primigravidas among their 49 patients. But be on guard; the rauwolfias may cause severe nasal congestion in the newborn infant.

Jack G. Duffy, David L. Bond and Stanley F. Rogers. New Hypotensive Agent for Toxemia of Pregnancy. Obst. & Gynec. 14:374, 1959.

"As obstetrician in a rather active group practice, I am being urged by one of my associates to try veratrum viride in eclampsia because he says that one of his friends in the South is doing so very effectively. What about this?"

Reply: I am very glad to have this question asked because it enables me to refer to a type of study that is the delight of the heart of any clinical investigator. At the University of Cincinnati, Richard Bryant and John Flemming have reported on the same basic treatment of this malady that they have followed consistently for 30 years, the elements of which are the use of a vasodilating or vasorelaxing drug, use of magnesium sulfate intramuscularly, and administration of at least 3000 ml. of fluid daily. And the vasodilating drug they have used is veratrum viride (Gartrone). It is given intravenously at a rate sufficient to reduce the blood pressure and stabilize it at about 75% of the systolic pressure at which the patient had a convulsion. Magnesium sulfate, in dosage of 5 ml. of 50% solution, is given every 6 hours during the first 24 and every 12 hours during the second 24. During the second day, an attempt is made to eliminate the intravenous administration of veratrum viride, but 0.3 ml. is given intramuscularly as often as necessary, usually at intervals of 1–4 hours. Without analyzing further their results, I can just say that they were pretty good and that perhaps your friend's friend has something good going for him down there.

Richard D. Bryant and John G. Flemming. Veratrum Viride in Treatment of Eclampsia: III. Obst. & Gynec. 19:372, 1962.

In our practice we have no doubt about the utility of magnesium sulfate as an anticonvulsant in severe pre-eclampsia, but it is our experience that the drug has an inhibiting action on uterine contractility. The latter point is contested by some of our associates. Has the matter been investigated?"

Reply: Yes, at Johns Hopkins Hospital, Kumar and associates found the spontaneous activity of excised myometrial strips from both nonpregnant and pregnant uteri was decreased when magnesium was added, and they furthermore observed uterine activity in vivo to be decreased in 10 of 12 patients,

this inhibitory effect not being limited to oxytocin-induced labor but occurring also in spontaneous onset of labor. The change was not significant in tonus or amplitude but occurred mainly in frequency of contractions, being apparent within 20 minutes after onset of magnesium administration and maximum after 40–50 minutes; full activity was resumed about 30 minutes after discontinuance of the drug.

D. Kumar, Pantelis A. Zourlas and Allan C. Barnes. In Vitro and In Vivo Effects of Magnesium Sulfate on Human Uterine Contractility. Am. J. Obst. & Gynec. 86:1036, 1963.

"My basic therapy in severe toxemia of pregnancy has consisted in a daily infusion of 2000 — 3000 ml. of 10% dextrose, a continuous intravenous drip of 1—2% magnesium sulfate, and the intravenous administration of 60–120 mg. of sodium phenobarbital every 6—8 hours. Would I likely gain anything by adding antihypertensive therapy, say through the use of hydralazine (Apresoline) to this regimen?"

Reply: At the Baltimore City Hospitals, Paul Molumphy and Raphael Garcia added 60–100 mg. of hydralazine to 1000 ml. of the 10% dextrose they used for infusion, regulating the rate of administration of the drip according to blood pressure response, reflex irritability, basic fluid requirements and urinary output. They found that this therapy had some advantages over other regimens but that it usually achieved only temporary control and rarely permitted long-term continuance of pregnancy. Ultimate control in their experience could be obtained only by terminating pregnancy. No serious complications developed in their series, although mild, transient hypotension occurred eight times in their 61 patients but always responded to withdrawal of hydralazine for short periods. Forty-eight patients maintained satisfactory urinary output or actually had diuresis; oliguria developed in 6 but progressed to satisfactory urinary output or diuresis as therapy continued. Of 64 infants delivered, 11 died; there were no maternal deaths, and no patient had convulsions.

Paul E. Molumphy and Raphael Garcia. Treatment of Severe Toxemia of Pregnancy with Intravenous Magnesium Sulfate and Apresoline. Obst. & Gynec. 14:193, 1959.

I was trained, in another part of the country than that in which I am practicing, in the belief that magnesium sulfate is an effective anticonvulsant agent in the toxemia of pregnancy. But the measure is unpopular here and so I do not use it. What can be at fault?"

Reply: I think it altogether likely that the measure was never tried in your present area with sufficient boldness. Magnesium sulfate is undeniably the most effective of all anticonvulsant drugs when used in sufficient amount. This matter of sufficiency is defined by Flowers' group (University of North Carolina) as an amount to give a plasma level of magnesium of 3–6 mg./100 ml. Since concentrations under 16 mg./100 ml. may be considered nontoxic, they feel that patients with normal renal function can safely be given 40–60 Gm. per 24 hours. Among their 71 patients with severe toxemia and eclampsia, no convulsions occurred after the initial injection of magnesium sulfate, and the drug did not have a hypotensive effect after the midbrain adjusted to the initial rapid intravenous injection. Renal excretion varied considerably but was fairly constant in individuals. In a typical case, a woman weighing 185 pounds was initially given 14 Gm. of the drug; in 6 hours the plasma magnesium level had risen from 0.75 to 4 mg./100 ml., and at 6 hour intervals 9 Gm. were given to maintain the plasma level at 6 mg./100 ml. During this 24 hour period 2 Gm. magnesium (equivalent to 20 Gm. magnesium sulfate) were excreted; therefore on the second day she received 5 Gm. every 6 hours. During this time she excreted 1.6 Gm. but the plasma magnesium level fell to 1.5 mg./100 ml. She therefore required 16 Gm. of magnesium sulfate on the third day to replace the 1.6 Gm. magnesium excreted and an additional 12 Gm. to raise the plasma magnesium level from 1.5 to 6 mg./100 ml. Of course to obtain this fine result the facilities for determining plasma and urine magnesium levels must be available. On this point, I quote the authors: "It would seem reasonable to expect hospitals to furnish these simple determinations on severe pre-eclamptic and eclamptic patients, particularly since the average obstetric service requests comparatively few laboratory procedures."

Charles E. Flowers, Jr., William E. Easterling, Jr., Franklin D. White, James M. Jung and J. Thomas Fox, Jr. Magnesium Sulfate in Toxemia of Pregnancy: New Dosage Schedule Based on Body Weight. Obst. & Gynec. 19:315, 1962.

"In a patient with toxemia of pregnancy, who requires an oxytocic drug, what is the best one to use?"

Reply: In a careful comparison, in Iowa, of oxytocin (Pitocin), methylergonovine maleate (Methergine) and a placebo in noneclamptic women, William Howard's group found that oxytocin produces fewer pressor responses than methylergonovine, though both produced more pressor changes than does a placebo. They therefore recommended that when, an oxytocic drug is required in a patient with toxemia of pregnancy, oxytocin be the one that is used.

William F. Howard, Philip R. McFadden and William C. Keettel. Oxytocic Drugs in Fourth Stage of Labor. J.A.M.A. 189:411, Aug. 10, 1964.

"I have just had a case in which a single dose of methylergometrine (Methergine) appeared to be suspiciously associated with a brief period of generalized eclamptic convulsions immediately postpartum. Has such an occurrence been documented?"

Reply: Several years ago, G. N. Casady and associates showed that, even in the normotensive woman, the blood pressure may be dangerously raised by the ergot preparations if a vasoconstrictor of the nature of a sympathomimetic amine is used before administration of the drug, but I have seen the report of only 1 case, that of Hassim and Lucas in South Africa, in which ergonovine (Ergotrate) was considered to be the provocative agent of eclamptic symptoms in a patient with previously normal blood pressure. In this case, 0.5 mg. of ergonovine was injected intramuscularly as the head crowned, the third stage was normal, blood loss moderate and placenta perfectly healthy. The blood pressure throughout labor had not exceeded 124/80 mm. Hg and urinalysis remained negative, but 12 minutes after the ergot injection it had risen to 170/115 and approximately 25 minutes later, despite reduction of the pressure under Pantopon, the patient developed a severe frontal headache, blood pressure rose to 170/110 mm. Hg and typical generalized eclamptic convulsions ensued. Sedative medication controlled the convulsions, and 5 hours after delivery the blood pressure had returned to normal.

A. M. Hassim and Cynthia Lucas. Ergometrine Maleate as a Causative Factor in Postpartum Eclampsia. South African Obst. & Gynec. 3:31, 5 June 1965. G. N. Casady, D. C. Moore and L. D. Bridenbaugh. J.A.M.A. 172:1011, 1960.

"I have been using bendroflumethiazide with potassium supplement (Naturetin W/K) in treating pre-eclamptic patients with good results upon the whole, but the preparation seems always to produce hyperuricemia. Should I be concerned about this?"

Reply: I do not think so, for the hyperuricemia that appears to characterize the action of the drugs of this class is of clinical importance very rarely.

Irving Siegel (Cook County Hosp.). Use of Bendroflumethiazide with Potassium Supplement in Toxemia of Pregnancy. Obst. & Gynec. 25:82, 1965.

ECZEMA

"Can eczema, or the history of same, predispose to sulfonamide reaction?"

Reply: G. Goerz and associates (Düsseldorf) on the basis of experience in several cases, have stated the opinion that this is so, but I wonder whether it would not be more accurate to say that eczema is merely an indicator of an allergic tendency and that, therefore, such a patient might be more likely to develop sulfonamide sensitivity.

G. Goerz, H. Ippen and H. G. Meiers. Sensitivity to Sulfonamides: Cross Reaction between Antibacterial and Diuretic Sulfonamides. Deutsche med. Wchnschr. 89: 1301, July 3, 1964.

EMPTYING STOMACH

"In a patient who has swallowed some potentially lethal agent and is seen shortly thereafter while still conscious and cooperative, shall I lavage or trust to the administration of an emetic?"

Reply: I think it is now the consensus that the use of an emetic drug is the more efficient way of emptying the stomach than the resort to lavage in the great majority of instances. Syrup of ipecac is always available in the hospital or in the patient's corner drug store. Usual dosage for infants and young children is ½–1 teaspoonful (2.5–5.0 ml.) followed by tepid water; 2–4 teaspoonfuls (10–20 ml.) may be given, and repetition of dosage may be made at intervals of a few minutes in older children and adults until effect is obtained. The only other emetic that is used to any considerable extent nowadays is apomorphine in dosage of 5 mg. (1/12 gr.) subcutaneously (no more than 1 mg. (1/60 gr.) for an infant); but use of this drug is always accompanied by some degree of central depression, and excessive dosage will cause collapse, loss of voluntary muscle tone and very irregular respiration. Nalorphine (Nalline) or levallorphan (Lorfan) are not always as effective antidotes for apomorphine as they are for morphine itself.

"Is the syrup of ipecac fully effective as an emetic when the offending agent swallowed has been an antiemetic?"

Reply: In the Poison Control Branch of USPHS, Mark Thoman and Henry Verhulst studied this matter and found that the answer is yes.

Mark E. Thoman and Henry L. Verhulst. Ipecac Syrup in Antiemetic Ingestion. J.A.M.A. 196:433, May 2, 1966.

"Copper sulfate has been in use as an emetic for a very long time; just how effective is it, really?"

Reply: The only study of this matter that has been reported in recent years, to my knowledge, was that of Franklin Mellencamp, who found that in 100 children who had ingested noncorrosive toxic materials, a 250 mg. dose of copper sulfate (dissolve the dry salt in a 1 oz. bottle, fill with tap water, and have the patient drink directly from the bottle) produced effective emesis in 86% of instances within 15 minutes. The second dose may be given within 10 minutes if vomiting has not occurred, but if this is not followed by effective vomiting within 5 minutes the patient should be lavaged immediately.

Franklin Mellencamp. Copper Sulfate as an Emetic. Journal-Lancet 85:261, 1965.

ENCEPHALITIS

"It seems to me that each year we are hearing of a new type of encephalitis. So far I have heard of Japanese B encephalitis, Australian X disease, Venezuelan encephalomyelitis, Russian tick-borne or spring-summer encephalitis and equine encephalomyelitis.

Some of these of course we do not have here in the United States, and in fact I have seen only one case of one of them, namely the mild western type of equine encephalomyelitis, but I am wondering whether there is any sort of specific therapy that might be used should one suddenly become involved in an outbreak of any of these maladies?"

Reply: No, these are all viral infections for which no specific therapy has been devised.

ENCEPHALOMYELITIS

"We have a case in hospital of encephalomyelitis that complicated rabies vaccination. The diagnosis was not made until quite late and nothing we have been able to do so far has been helpful. It seems most likely that we shall lose the patient, but what might have been done with drugs had the diagnosis been made earlier?"

Reply: Byron Waksman says that if corticosteroid, or corticotropin (ACTH), therapy is started within 2 days of the onset of the disease there may be dramatic improvement in as many as half of the patients with at least arrest of the progress of the disease in the others. But he warns also that there may be recurrence when this treatment is stopped.

Byron H. Waksman *in* Beeson & McDermott. Textbook of Medicine. Phila., W. B. Saunders Co., 1963, p. 56.

ENDOMETRIOSIS

"What is the effect of pseudopregnancy, as achieved through use of the contraceptive pill, upon surgical procedures that may subsequently be necessary in treating a case of endometriosis?"

Reply: It is the consensus, if indeed not the unanimous opinion, that this treatment not only makes the surgery itself easier but that, if it is reinstituted following the operation, there is high likelihood that it will curtail extension of the process and the formation of the adhesions that cause so much of the discomfort in advanced stages of this malady.

ENURESIS

"I have a very stubborn case of enuresis in a child of 10, in whom awakening devices and anticholinergic drugs have not been helpful. Has any new pharmacologic approach been developed?"

Reply: In recent years imipramine (Tofranil) has been used with considerable success in a number of practices. In Los Angeles, Alvin Poussaint and Keith Ditman reported a double-blind placebo-controlled study with crossover in which 47 enuretic children were treated for 8 weeks with imipramine in dosage of 25 or 50 mg. (the latter for children of 12 years or over). The drug was found markedly superior to placebo in decreasing the frequency of enuretic nights and the side effects were minimal. Seven of the children were completely dry at the end of the eighth week, and with manipulation of dosage thereafter between 25 and 75 mg., 11 children became completely dry and remained so after the drug was withdrawn following 2 months of complete dryness. The related drug, amitriptyline (Elavil), has also been favorably used.

Alvin F. Poussaint and Keith S. Ditman. A Controlled Study of Imipramine (Tofranil) in the Treatment of Childhood Enuresis. J. Pediat. 67:283, 1965. Alvin F. Poussaint, Keith S. Ditman and Richard Greenfield. Amitriptyline in Childhood Enuresis. Clin. Pharm. & Ther. 7:21, 1966.

EPIDEMIC PLEURODYNIA

"In our area we have just passed through a little bout of epidemic pleurodynia, which truly deserves its popular name of 'devil's grip.' We found neither antibiotics nor sulfonamides effective, but is there something in drug therapy that we did not know?"

Reply: No, this is one of the Coxsackie virus infections, and we have no specific therapy.

EPIDERMOLYSIS BULLOSA DYSTROPHICA

"I have a patient with epidermolysis bullosa dystrophica in whom all therapy has failed. Do you know of anything new that offers some hope for relief in this terrible disease?"

Reply: Fortunately, the malady is so rare that extensive study of it has not been possible. I do know, however, of the effective use of alpha tocopherol, described by H. D. Wilson (Ontario Hospital School, Orillia). He gave alpha tocopherol gelatin capsules, 400 units four times daily, and applied a tocopherol ointment to all affected areas twice daily. Improvement was progressive but slow, and dosage was finally raised to 1200 units four times daily. There was improvement, then deterioration when the medication was stopped, and improvement again when it was resumed. At the time of writing, the patient's physical condition was such that only one nursing hour daily was required, sedation was no longer necessary, and there had been considerable improvement in mental attitude.

H. D. Wilson. Treatment of Epidermolysis Bullosa Dystrophica by Alpha Tocopherol. Canad. M. A. J. 90:1315, June 6, 1964.

EPILEPSY

"I have an epileptic patient on diphenylhydantoin (Dilantin) and phenobarbital who has developed macrocytosis. Is it necessary to resort to folic acid therapy in this situation?"

Reply: Most authorities do not consider that it is necessary to do so, but of course megaloblastic anemia requires very serious attention. The latter is a quite rare occurrence, however, and seems most often to have been associated with the employment of diphenylhydantoin (Dilantin), primidone (Mysoline) and the barbiturates, singly or in combination. Penny (St. Vincent's Hospital, New York) has reviewed the reported cases and found that 20 responded to cyanocobalamine alone, 26 to folic acid alone and 8 to combinations of these factors; but in most patients who responded to cyanocobalamine there was a question whether the mere cessation of anticonvulsant therapy had produced the response.

John L. Penny. Megaloblastic Anemia During Anticonvulsant Drug Therapy: Case Report and Review of Literature. Arch. Int. Med. 111:744, 1963.

"I have a grand mal epileptic who requires a hydantoin drug together with phenobarbital for reasonable control, but I cannot keep her for any extended period on hydantoin without the development of severe megaloblastic anemia. What would you suggest?"

Reply: Have you tried the concomitant administration of folic acid? A dosage of 20 mg. daily would likely be sufficient to enable you to continue with the offending drug, or perhaps enable you to use one of the hydantoins if you switch about among them to find the least offensive.

G. I. Horsfield and J. N. Marshall Chalmers (Queen Elizabeth Hospital, Birmingham, England). Megaloblastic Anemia Associated with Anticonvulsant Therapy. Practitioner 191:316, 1963.

"I have a patient with grand mal epilepsy in whom it appears that diphenylhydantoin (Dilantin) has increased the incidence of seizures. Has such a thing been noted by others?"

Reply: There are numerous evidences that diphenylhydantoin may exert a toxic action on the central nervous system, but in none of the many reviews of the drug's action has an increase in epileptiform convulsions been recorded. However, at a VA hospital associated with Yale University, Lewis Levy and Gerald Fenichel observed 3 patients in whom it appeared that the drug did actually increase seizure incidence; indeed, in 1 of these cases the fact was substantiated by decreasing convulsive frequency when the drug was withdrawn and an increase when it was reintroduced after a 3 week period. It is also of interest that one instance of a myasthenia gravis–like syndrome has been observed in Switzerland in connection with the use of this drug.

Lewis L. Levy and Gerald M. Fenichel. Diphenylhydantoin Activated Seizures. Neurology 15, 716, 1965. F. Regli and P. Guggenheim. Myasthenisches Syndrom als seltene Komplikation unter Hydantoinbehandlung. Nervenarzt 36:315, 1965.

"I have an epileptic patient who has been on diphenylhydantoin (Dilantin) for several years and is now developing myasthenia gravis. Could this be ascribable to the drug?"

Reply: I should think it extremely unlikely, although Regli and Guggenheim, in Zurich, have reported an instance in which the association was suggested.

F. Regli and P. Guggenheim. Myasthenisches Syndrom als seltene Komplikation unter Hydantoinbehandlung. Nervenarzt 36:315, 1965.

"Is there any way to determine the likelihood of an individual to develop central nervous system toxicity when placed on diphenylhydantoin (Dilantin)?"

Reply: At Cornell University, Henn Kutt and associates studied 32 patients with this in mind and determined that clinical signs of toxicity developed when the following blood levels were approached: nystagmus, 20 μg./ml., with a range of 15–25 μg./ml.; ataxia, 30 μg./ml. and above; and mental changes, 40 μg./ml. and up. They did not, however, explain the fact that individuals on the same dosage of the drug, in terms of mg./kg., show considerable variations in blood levels – and from the practical bedside standpoint this can only mean that drug dosage must be most carefully titrated individually in each patient.

Henn Kutt, William Winters, Roy Kokenge and Fletcher Dowell. Diphenylhydantoin (Dilantin) Metabolism, Blood Levels and Toxicity. Arch. Neurol. 11:642, 1964.

"I have a 20-year-old mild grand mal epileptic who is not being controlled as well as I feel that he should be with the usual combination of diphenylhydantoin (Dilantin) and phenobarbital. What would you suggest?"

Reply: Have you looked into the actual serum diphenylhydantoin levels that you are achieving in the patient? In a study of 151 patients treated with this drug, Jakob Husby (University of Arhuus) found an average initial serum diphenylhydantoin level of 16.4 μg./ml. on a mean dosage of 4.6 mg./kg. body weight, but there was only a very rough correlation between the serum drug level and the dose ingested. He found that the ratio of serum level to dose decreases with increasing dosage, and that at all levels the ratio is smaller for younger patients.

Jakob Husby. Delayed Toxicity and Serum Concentrations of Phenytoin (Dilantin). Danish M. Bull. 10:236, 1963.

"One of my associates, who sees a good deal of epilepsy, uses chlordiazepoxide (Librium) almost routinely to supplement his more specific antiepileptic therapy, but I have tried this in a few instances and have not found that it reduced the frequency of seizures. What has been the experience of others?"

Reply: I do not think anyone feels that Librium is as effective as the hydantoins and phenobarbital in grand mal cases, but it is the consensus that the tranquilizing action of the drug is useful in damping the activity of hyperkinetic individuals and an aid in the control of behavior disturbances that are not uncommon in epileptic children. Regarding effect on frequency of seizures, I can only point out that Livingston's group, at Johns Hopkins, failed to control the frequency of seizures in any of their 26 patients who did not respond to the conventional antiepileptic drugs, though their dosage ranged from a daily average of 60–70 mg. to as high as 125 mg., the previous medication always being continued; whereas Watson's group, in Boston, found that seizure incidence was reduced – so there you have it.

J. Espinosa Iborra (Valencia, Spain). Chlordiazepoxide (Librium) in Epilepsy. Experiences with Epileptics with Grand Mal Seizures and Behavior Disturbances. Psychiat. et neurol. 145:235, 1963. S. Livingston, L. Pauli and J. B. Murphy. Ineffectiveness of Chlordiazepoxide Hydrochloride in Epilepsy. J.A.M.A. 177: 243, July 29, 1961. C. W. Watson, R. Bowker and C. Calish. Effect of Chlordiazepoxide on Epileptic Seizures. J.A.M.A. 188:212, Apr. 20, 1964.

"What is the status of diazepam (Valium) in the treatment of nonconvulsive forms of epilepsy?"

Reply: I shall cite below the two studies in which the drug was reported upon favorably, but since neither of these investigations was controlled, I am myself not yet convinced that the agent has the value that has been claimed for it.

H. Gastaut, J. Roger, R. Soulayrol, H. Lob and C.-A. Tassinari. Action of Diazepam (Valium) in Treatment of Nonconvulsive Forms of Generalized Epilepsy (Absences and States of Absence of Various Types.) Rev. neurol. 112:99, 1965. Roger K. Kalina. Diazepam (Valium): Its Role in a Prison Setting. Dis. Nerv. System 25:101, 1964.

"I have an epileptic in his 30's who has never been well controlled with diphenylhydantoin (Dilantin) and phenobarbital, and so last year I put him on mephenytoin (Mesantoin). In a few days on the new drug he developed symptoms that pointed toward the incidental development of Hodgkin's disease. Of course he was taken off the drug at once and returned to the former antiepileptic regime. Some months later, after the reaction had subsided, I tried Mesantoin again, with the same result. The man's epilepsy is very poorly controlled; what am I to do?"

Reply: This is a rare type of reaction, but it has been recorded with the other two hydantoin compounds as well, ethotoin (Peganone) and diphenylhydantoin (Dilantin). The likelihood is great that in your case you would not experience the same reaction with Peganone that you have with Mesantoin because you already know that you do not get it with Dilantin. In any case, if you do have the same trouble, you can always go back to Dilantin and settle for what control it will provide in combination with phenobarbital. None of the other antiepileptics are likely to give you as good control in grand mal cases as the hydantoins and phenobarbital.

A. P. Doyle and H. R. Hellstrom (VA Hospital, Pittsburgh). Mesantoin Lymphadenopathy Morphologically Simulating Hodgkin's Disease. Ann. Int. Med. 59:363, 1963.

"I have a patient with grand mal epilepsy who has repeatedly developed megaloblastic anemia under several different drug combinations. What do you suggest?"

Reply: At the University of Uppsala, Arne Hamfelt and associates have reported a case of precisely this sort. Since complete hematologic remission was induced by treatment with folic acid in each instance in their patient, the presumption might be made that this individual suffered from repeated attacks of folic acid deficiency induced by the anticonvulsant drugs. Experimental proof of such a thing is lacking, so far as I am aware.

Arne Hamfelt, Andreas Killander, Elis Malers and Carl-Henric de Verdier. Megaloblastic Anemia Associated with Anticonvulsant Drugs: Studies on Case with Four Relapses. Acta med. scandinav. 177:549, 1965.

"In the treatment of epilepsy nowadays it is frequently necessary to use several drugs in combination in order to obtain best effects. And the effects are in many instances very fine, but the drugs are all potentially quite toxic and it is not always easy to know which ingredient of a mixture is causing the most trouble, or when one introduces a new agent into the therapy of a particular case just what is to be expected of it in the way of reactions. Would you therefore kindly provide a comparison of all of the principal agents as to their toxic proclivities?"

Reply: PHENOBARBITAL causes incapacitating drowsiness and sluggishness in perhaps no more than 10% of patients who take it in full antiepileptic dosage. Sometimes amphetamine will counteract this effect satisfactorily. A very small proportion of patients, perhaps not even 1 in 100, develop an allergic scarlatiniform, morbilliform or other type of rash from phenobarbital, requiring discontinuance of the drug for a while. It must be permanently discontinued if the rash recurs on readministration, because there is then the possibility that exfoliative dermatitis may supervene. It is unusual for a patient to experience tremors, nystagmus or ataxia on usual dosage, but some individuals who take phenobarbital for a long time develop subjective symptoms difficult to substantiate in objective findings; this is perhaps referable to the effects on autonomic innervations.

If phenobarbital is to be withdrawn from a patient, whether an epileptic or not, it should be done very gradually to avoid throwing him into severe convulsive attacks.

DIPHENYLHYDANTOIN (DILANTIN) does not have the hypnotic properties of phenobarbital. Conduct and performance ratings are often improved by it. Sometimes, however, the patient becomes excessively excited and occasionally truly psychotic. Other reactions of more frequent occurrence than with phenobarbital are subjective tremulousness with a feeling of apprehension and tension, tremors, dizziness, ataxia, nausea and sometimes vomiting, burning sensation in the eyes, skin reactions, nosebleed, purpura and cardiovascular disturbances. Diffuse pulmonary fibrosis associated with the taking of the drug has been reported. Many individuals develop nystagmus and sometimes diplopia and blurring of vision. Hirsutism sometimes occurs, especially in adolescent girls. A peculiar hyperplastic reaction of the gums, superficially resembling that of scurvy, appears not infrequently. Major allergic occurrences are rare, although a fatal hypersensitivity with hepatitis, exfoliative dermatitis, eosinophilia and lymphadenopathy is recorded. Direct toxicity, in the sense of danger to life from the taking of a large overdose, seems to be slight, but a fatal case with hepatitis and exfoliative dermatitis has been reported.

MEPHENYTOIN (MESANTOIN), except for the hypertrophy of the gums and the diplopia, causes the same side effects as Dilantin, principally dizziness, muscular incoordination, ataxia, gastric discomfort, hyperirritability, restlessness, loss of weight and dermatitis. It may also cause drowsiness. Phenobarbital can be used to combat the restlessness and irritability, and amphetamine the drowsiness, but sometimes the severity of the reactions forces discontinuance of the Mesantoin. The drug is certainly not as toxic as Tridione but it is capable of causing agranulocytosis, aplastic anemia and skin rashes; lupus erythematosus disseminatus has also been reported in association with its use. It also distorts the electroencephalographic record in a way to obscure dysrhythmias or produce changes in records that might otherwise be normal. One case has been reported in which the inadvertent use of 0.3 Gm. as a beginning dose caused an intense cutaneous reaction followed by prostration and death. Toxic effects sometimes appear with dosage as low as 0.1 Gm., but usually they are not evident until dosage reaches 0.7 Gm. or more.

TRIMETHADIONE (TRIDIONE) is potentially toxic to skin, bone marrow and kidneys. Apparently it may stimulate as well as depress all bone marrow elements, though the latter is the more frequent reaction. The action on the kidneys causes nephrosis, apparently through provoking increased porosity of the glomeruli for proteins. The drug causes gastrointestinal distress, drowsiness and diplopia occasionally, photophobia frequently. Wells has drawn attention to the lack of correlation between the incidence of fatalities and the age or sex of the patient, the dosage of the drug used and the length of time during which it was administered.

PARAMETHADIONE (PARADIONE) toxicities are similar to those of Tridione but they occur less frequently.

PHENSUXIMIDE (MILONTIN) appears to be considerably less toxic than either of the other two principal petit mal drugs, but it sometimes causes gastrointestinal disturbances, drowsi-

ness, dreamlike states and muscular weakness. Skin reactions are unusual, and I believe that no serious hematologic complications have been reported.

PHENACEMIDE (PHENURONE) has such serious toxic proclivities that Yahr and Merritt say it should be tried only as a last resort in patients in whom severe and frequent psychomotor seizures cannot otherwise be controlled. The drug may produce not only gastrointestinal disturbances, skin eruptions, drowsiness, hepatitis and blood dyscrasias, but also personality disturbances with severe psychotic manifestations.

METHSUXIMIDE (CELONTIN) causes somnolence and unsteady gait not infrequently; other reported reactions are gastrointestinal disturbances, hepatitis, urinary evidences of kidney damage, skin rashes, fever, hiccup, severe diaphoresis, visual disturbances and psychic disturbances, the latter ranging from personality alterations to acute psychosis. A case of fatal aplastic anemia in association with use of the drug is on record.

ETHOTOIN (PEGANONE) appears to be less toxic than the other hydantoins. Parenchymatous organ damage has not been reported, to my knowledge, but there is record of lymphadenopathy mimicking malignant lymphoma as in the case of Dilantin. The following have been seen occasionally: dizziness, diplopia, drowsiness, headache, numbness, nystagmus, tension, depression, anorexia, nausea and vomiting, skin rashes, gastrointestinal disturbances.

PRIMIDONE (MYSOLINE) toxicity of a serious nature has not been reported often, though the account by Plaa and associates of several cases in which the symptoms appeared to be due to biotransformation of the drug into phenobarbital, was very interesting from the standpoint of presenting toxic potentialities not usually appreciated. Reported side effects of relatively infrequent occurrence include gastrointestinal disturbances, skin rashes, malaise, drowsiness, ataxia, vertigo, psychosis, anorexia, irritability, painful gums, dependent edema and edema of the eyelids.

ETHOSUXIMIDE (ZARONTIN) appears to be less toxic than Tridione and Paradione, with which it competes in the treatment of petit mal. The most frequent reactions are gastrointestinal disturbances, but one may also expect evidences of central nervous system involvements and also skin eruptions and psychic aberrations, the latter rarely. Hiccup in association with the drug has been reported, and there have been rare instances of attack upon the bone marrow.

C. E. Wells. Trimethadione; Its Dosage and Toxicity. Arch. Neurol. & Psychiat. 77:140, 1957. M. D. Yahr and H. H. Merritt. Current Status of the Drug Therapy of Epileptic

Seizures. J.A.M.A. 161:333, 1956. G. L. Plaa, J. M. Fujimoto and C. H. Hine. Intoxication from Primidone Due to its Biotransformation to Phenobarbital. J.A.M.A. 168: 1769, 1958.

"What are the most serious reactions to the anti-epileptic agents?"

Reply: The principal life-threatening reactions involve the bone marrow, liver and kidney, but skin reactions can be very severe, and if they are bullous the situation may not be relieved by switching about among the compounds.

"Rumor is rife in our circles here that some of the antiepileptic drugs are about to be forced off the market because they are capable of causing aplastic anemia. Is this true?"

Reply: Do you mean, is it true that they are going to be taken off the market or that they are capable of causing serious marrow depression? I shall answer the latter part of the question first, in any case. In 1962, M. M. Robins reviewed 48 cases of aplastic anemia secondary to anticonvulsant medication and found that most of them were associated with administration of mephenytoin (Mesantoin) and trimethadione (Tridione), but actually one could consider that the potential for marrow damage resides in all of these agents since for the most part they show a basic chemical structure. For example, Mann and Habenicht (Loma Linda University) have reported a fatal bone marrow aplasia associated with ethosuximide (Zarontin) employment. As for the first part of your question, I can only say that it would truly be tragic if we were to be deprived of the use of these tremendously valuable drugs. That they are being frivolously employed in some instances is undeniable (and this is true of all our drugs!), but it is sincerely to be hoped that the Food and Drug Administration will exhaust all possible warning measures before contemplating severe restriction in the use of the agents as a group.

Leslie B. Mann and Herald Allen Habenicht. Fatal Bone Marrow Aplasia Associated with Administration of Ethosuximide (Zarontin) for Petit Mal Epilepsy. Bull. Los Angeles Neurol. Soc. 27:173, 1962. M. M. Robins. Aplastic Anemia Secondary to Anticonvulsants. Am. J. Dis. Child. 104:614, 1962.

"One would think that when epileptic children are reasonably well controlled with the anti-epileptic drugs that the feeling of security this engenders would more than offset the sedative action of the drug (I am thinking principally of children controlled with phenobarbital almost exclusively), but this has not been the case in my experience. Has the matter been studied?"

Reply: Yes, Wapner's group in St. Louis did a controlled study, using several standard tests of intelligence and learning, and found no significant changes in these parameters, just as you have done.

Irwin Wapner, Don L. Thurston and Jean Holowach. Phenobarbital: Its Effect on Learning in Epileptic Children. J.A.M.A. 182:937, Dec. 1, 1962.

"I have under my care a 14-year-old boy who has twice been pulled out of status epilepticus only with greatest difficulty. Have the curare drugs ever been used to combat this situation?"

Reply: Yes, but then of course controlled respiration must be resorted to also. In the case reported by Nisbet (Liverpool), 15 mg. of d-tubocurarine was injected intravenously and controlled respiration instituted; when the effect of the drug began to wear off, in about 45 minutes, an additional 3 mg. was given and the controlled respiration continued for another 2 hours. After 3 hours, there were no more convulsions and respiration was assisted manually as it gradually returned to normal.

H. I. Armstrong Nisbet. Status Epilepticus Treated with d-Tubocurarine and Controlled Respiration. Brit. M. J. 1:95, Jan. 10, 1959.

"I have been using the new drug ethosuximide (Zarontin) effectively in the treatment of petit mal epilepsy, but now I have had one case of hypoplastic anemia that seemed definitely attributable to the drug, and I have become frightened. What has been the experience?"

Reply: In England, Heathfield and Jewesbury reported the treatment of 50 cases without undesirable side effects, but more recently in Ann Arbor, Weinstein and Allen were obliged to withdraw the drug in 9 of their 87 patients because of severe side effects: 7 because of gastrointestinal complaints; 1 because of leukopenia; and 1 because of hypoplastic anemia.

Kenneth W. G. Heathfield and Eric C. O. Jewesbury. Treatment of Petit Mal with Ethosuximide: Follow-up Report. Brit. M. J. 2:616, Sept. 5, 1964. Anita W. Weinstein and Richard J. Allen. Ethosuximide Treatment of Petit Mal Seizures. Am. J. Dis. Child. 111:63, 1966.

"I have heard that ethosuximide (Zarontin) is being very effectively used in treatment of petit mal cases, but I have not had very good success with it. How does the matter stand?"

Reply: In England, F. Lees and L. A. Liversedge found in a follow-up study of 121 patients that attacks were still being experienced by at least two-thirds and that only 5 not having therapy had lost their petit mal. But 2 other English investigators, Heathfield and Jewesbury, have been reporting the quite successful use of the drug for several years. So you see the matter does not "stand" anywhere just at present.

Kenneth W. G. Heathfield and Eric C. O. Jewesbury. Treatment of Petit Mal with Ethosuximide (Zarontin): Follow-Up Report. Brit. M. J. 2:616, Sept. 5, 1964. F. Lees and L. A. Liversedge. The Prognosis of "Petit Mal" and Minor Epilepsy. Lancet 2:797, 1962.

"I have a young patient with petit mal epilepsy that began at about the age of 3 years and is now, at the age of 9 years, perfectly controlled by trimethadione (Tridione). Since I understand that this type of epilepsy is very unlikely to carry over into adulthood, how should I treat this boy as adolescence approaches?"

Reply: I should add one of the drugs used to control grand mal seizures because as puberty approaches the petit mal individual is prone to develop grand mal. To have him under the influence of a grand mal drug at this time would appear a wise precaution, and after that you can determine the necessity for continued drug therapy of any sort by gradual withdrawals.

Samuel Livingston, Iluminada Torres, Lydia L. Pauli and Rowland V. Rider. Petit Mal Epilepsy. J.A.M.A. 194:227, Oct. 18, 1965.

"I've heard that trimethadione (Tridione) may cause myasthenia gravis. Is this true?"

Reply: I do not think that one can say so with assurance. A case has been reported, to be sure, of a child receiving trimethadione who developed myasthenia gravis and trimethadione toxicity simultaneously; but this is only 1 case and so far should be accepted as merely a reason for increasing one's watchfulness.

Hart DeC. Peterson. Association of Trimethadione Therapy and Myasthenia Gravis. New England J. Med. 274:506, Mar. 3, 1966.

"I have several epileptic patients in whom I have been forced to discontinue use of diphenylhydantoin (Dilantin) because of a severe degree of gingival hyperplasia. What is the incidence of this adverse reaction to the drug?"

Reply: It is apparently much higher than I had realized before your question provoked inquiry. Now I find that at a state hospital for epileptics, James Babcock has reported an incidence of 36% of this reaction in 369 patients ranging in age from 5 to 74 years. Edentulous patients were excluded from the study, but no attempt was made to group the patients according to other drugs they were receiving. In support of other observers, no significant differences were found in the prevalence of the reaction in relation to sex or race. The relationship to dosage appears to be a controversial matter.

James R. Babcock. Incidence of Gingival Hyperplasia Associated with Dilantin Therapy in a Hospital Population. J. Am. Dent. A. 71:1447, 1965.

ERYSIPELAS

"Is penicillin still fully effective in erysipelas?"

Reply: Yes.

ERYSIPELOID

"What agent is most effective in the therapy of erysipeloid?"

Reply: Penicillin usually clears up the process in a few days.

ERYTHROBLASTIC APLASIA

"I have a patient in whom there is reason to suspect that erythroblastic aplasia was associated with the use of an antituberculosis drug. Is there such an instance on record?"

Reply: There have been a few documented cases of pure erythroblastic aplasia resulting from drug therapy. One of these was in a tuberculous patient who was treated with both isoniazid and PAS; complete aplasia of red cell precursors and lack of peripheral blood reticulocytes occurred on two separate occasions while the patient was taking the drugs, and recovery occurred each time the drugs were stopped. But unfortunately the patient moved out of the physician's practice before he could determine with certainty which of the two drugs caused the trouble.

Stephen B. Goodman and Matthew H. Block. Case of Red Cell Aplasia Occurring as a Result of Antituberculous Therapy. Blood 24:616, 1964.

ESTROGEN DOSAGE EQUIVALENCE

"In various publications dealing with the use of estrogens in therapy, one frequently sees dosage stated as a certain amount of one preparation 'or its equivalent.' What are some of the estrogen 'equivalents'?"

Reply: I believe that the following may be accepted as equivalents to 0.5 mg. diethylstilbestrol (Stilbestrol): 0.625 mg. estrone sulfate, 0.625 mg. conjugated equine estrogen (Premarin, etc.), 0.025 mg. ethinyl estradiol (Eticylol, etc.).

EXANTHEMATA OF VIRAL CAUSATION

"What of that group of viral diseases that is characterized by cutaneous lesions; is there

nothing approaching specific therapy in any of them?"

Reply: The answer is unfortunately obliged to be no, although secondary infections are of course often effectively combated by the specific antibiotic determined through laboratory studies.

EXTRAPYRAMIDAL SYNDROME

"I have a young patient with a progressive extrapyramidal syndrome of choreo-athetoid type in whom both diagnosis (there was originally a faulty diagnosis of congenital cerebral palsy) and therapy have been puzzling. Have you anything to suggest?"

Reply: In the matter of drugs, I can only cite the report of Mucklow and Metz, in London, in which there were described the cases of 3 children affected in this way who responded extremely well to trihexyphenidyl (Artane) as used in the treatment of Parkinsonism.

E. S. Mucklow and H. T. Metz. Remarkable Response to Benzhexol Hydrochloride (Artane) in Children with an Unusual Progressive Striatal Syndrome. Develop. Med. Child Neurol. 6:598, 1964.

FACTOR X (STUART-PROWER) DEFICIENCY

"I have a young woman patient with factor X (Stuart-Prower) deficiency whose bleeding tendency has twice corrected spontaneously during pregnancies, only to return a few months after delivery. I am tempted to try norethynodrel (Enovid) to create an artificial pregnancy just as one does when using the agent as a contraceptive. Is there any precedent for this?"

Reply: Yes, Seymour Haber (Kansas City General Hospital) did precisely that in a 31-year-old woman and maintained her in an asymptomatic state during the therapy. Bleeding recurred 2 months after discontinuance of the drug, but this stopped when administration was resumed.

Seymour Haber. Norethynodrel in Treatment of Factor X Deficiency. Arch. Int. Med. 114:89, 1964.

FAMILIAL HYPOPHOSPHATEMIA

"Are any drugs helpful in the treatment of familial hypophosphatemia? Of course I understand that vitamin D must be given."

Reply: The vitamin D, as you probably know, must be given in very high dosage; even 100,000 units daily seldom suffices. No other drugs are specifically helpful.

FAMILIAL MEDITERRANEAN FEVER

"I am treating a case of familial Mediterranean fever with a low-fat diet and cannot say that much is being accomplished. Are there any drugs that might be helpful?"

Reply: None of which I am aware, but in the related etiocholanolone fever (which the laboratory people can distinguish for you from the Mediterranean fever), attacks can apparently be terminated by administration of corticosteroids.

FANCONI SYNDROME

"Are any of the diverse and really multitudinous symptoms of the Fanconi syndrome favorably affected by drug therapy?"

Reply: Yes, the use of vitamin D and calcium salts is definitely remedial in the rickets and osteomalacia, the former more likely to be seen in children and the latter in adults. Alkalinization, too, is helpful; Shohl's solution is recommended in dosage of 30 ml. three times daily to restore the electrolyte balance: 140 Gm. of citric acid and 98 Gm. of hydrated crystalline sodium citrate in 1000 ml. of water.

FEVER OF UNKNOWN ORIGIN

"If a patient enters the office with a history of fever for the past week or so and I am unable to obtain any localizing signs of infectious disease upon routine physical examination, am I justified in initiating an antibiotic regimen on the assumption that infection is responsible for the fever nevertheless?"

Reply: I should say that in numerous instances you would be correct in your assumption of an underlying infection but wrong in your therapy because that infection is likely to be subacute bacterial endocarditis, and to coast along for a week or two with merely routine antibiotic therapy in this malady may be disastrous. In a patient of the sort that you have in mind you simply have to institute the most thoroughgoing diagnostic investigation before beginning therapy of any kind. He may have another sort of infection, to be sure, namely tuberculosis, and your relatively superficial office examination would have been unlikely to disclose a disseminated form of this disease. Then there are the difficultly detectable lymphomas, or asymptomatic regional enteritis, or atypical rheumatoid arthritis, or fever due to drugs. And there are a number of other possibilities. No, I should say that this man needs to be hospitalized and be given the benefit of exhaustive study before entertaining the thought of treatment.

Louis Weinstein (Boston). The Use and Abuse of Anti-microbial Agents. Med. Sci. 14, 35, 1963.

FOOD POISONING

"Following a small outbreak of salmonella food poisoning in an institution for retarded children the organism continues to be excreted in the feces of sample cases. Would this have been the case had we treated the affected children vigorously with antibiotics during the acute course of the malady?"

Reply: We do not understand the mechanism whereby the intestine clears itself of salmonella organisms nor does it seem possible to hasten the process through the action of drugs. In England, J. M. S. Dixon treated 67 children infected in an outbreak of food poisoning due to *Salmonella typhimurium* with antibiotics to which the strain was sensitive in vitro. Not only did antibiotic treatment fail to shorten the period of symptomless excretion of the organisms, but it appeared possible that it prolonged it, possibly by interference with the normal clearance mechanism.

J. M. S. Dixon. Effect of Antibiotic Treatment on Duration of Excretion of Salmonella Typhimurium by Children. Brit. M. J. 2:1343, 1965.

FOOT-AND-MOUTH DISEASE

"I now have in hand my first case of foot-and-mouth disease, and am finding that none of the antibiotics or chemotherapeutic agents are being helpful. What has been the general experience?"

Reply: Precisely what yours has been.

FRIEDREICH'S ATAXIA

"Is there any drug therapy that is helpful in Friedreich's ataxia?"

Reply: No, but the physiotherapists and orthopedic people can often be very helpful in these cases if their ministrations are begun very early.

FROSTBITE

"Each year in our clinic we see a number of cases of severe frostbite of the hands and feet, and have learned that rapid thawing in a water bath at a temperature 104–107.5 F. (40–42 C.) appears to be more beneficial than slow thawing at room temperature. We have not used sympathectomy as a therapeutic measure, being convinced that the acute vasoconstriction that occurs when the cooling takes place is replaced by vasomotor dilatation and hyperemia as soon as thawing occurs. By the same reasoning, we do not use intra-arterial vasodilator agents. But do you think that anticoagulants and fibrinolysin, or low molecular weight plasma expanders, would be helpful?"

Reply: Heparin would of course be the logical anticoagulant since its action is much more rapid than that of the orally administered coumarins, but the few reported results have been equivocal. It would seem to me logical that to prevent blood sludging with plasma expanders, or the use of fibrinolysin to reverse the thrombotic process would be logical, but these measures still await full clinical evaluation.

Gilbert Hermann, David C. Schechter, J. Cuthbert Owens, Thomas E. Starzl (Denver, Colorado). The Problem of Frostbite in Civilian Medical Practice. Surg. Clin. North America, April, 1963. Israel Penn and S. I. Schwartz. Evaluation of Low Molecular Weight Dextran in the Treatment of Frost Bite. J. Trauma 4:784, 1964. N. LeRoy Lapp and John L. Juergens. Frostbite. Mayo Clin. Proc. 40:932, 1965.

FUNGUS INFECTION, SUPERFICIAL

"I find my patients—and myself!—growing impatient with the use of griseofulvin (Grifulvin, Fulvicin) in the treatment of superficial fungal infections. Can an agent that acts so slowly, if at all, really be an effective one?"

Reply: Yes. This drug is fungistatic and not fungicidal in its action, and the former is a much slower process than the latter. Just give it time, that commodity which is never in short supply.

"I have been frightened by the rumor that griseofulvin (Fulvicin, etc.) may cause exfoliative dermatitis, since I have been prescribing the drug rather freely. What is the actual fact?"

Reply: I have seen only one case report of exfoliative dermatitis in association with use of this drug, that of Leonard Reaves, in Florida. Most of the griseofulvin reactions have been transient and reversible and usually not of a serious nature: urticaria, angioneurotic edema, skin rash and transient albuminuria, gastrointestinal disturbances, arthralgia. And there have also been a few reversible central nervous system involvements: headache, vertigo and diminished hearing are all that have come to my attention. However, here in Milwaukee we have had reported by Alexander Berman and Richard Franklin what appeared to have been a case of inadvertent precipitation of acute intermittent porphyria by griseofulvin therapy for a superficial fungus infection.

Leonard E. Reaves. Exfoliative Dermatitis Occurring in Patient Treated with Griseofulvin (Fulvicin, etc.). J. Am. Geriatrics Soc. 12:889, 1964. Alexander Berman and Richard L. Franklin. Precipitation of Acute Intermittent Porphyria by Griseofulvin Therapy. J.A.M.A. 192:1005, June 14, 1965.

"Is it true that a patient who is taking phenobarbital has difficulty in obtaining a full effect from griseofulvin (Fulvicin, etc.)?"

Reply: In England, Busfield and associates observed appreciably lower blood levels of the drug in such persons, but more work needs to be done to establish this as having clinical significance.

D. Busfield, K. J. Child, R. M. Atkinson and E. G. Tomich. Effect of Phenobarbitone on Blood Levels of Griseofulvin in Man. Lancet 2:1042, Nov. 16, 1963.

GAMMA GLOBULIN

"I suppose one could hardly consider gamma globulin a drug, yet since it is often used in prophylaxis and sometimes in therapy of acute infectious diseases I am wondering whether you would care to provide a listing of the entities in which its use is really justified?"

Reply: The agent is effectively prophylactic in the following entities: infectious hepatitis (Holland's group at the National Institutes of Health failed with it in post-transfusion hepatitis), measles, pertussis, vaccinia. *Infectious hepatitis*: recommended dosage is 0.01–0.02 ml./pound (some observers would have dosage as high as 0.05–0.06 ml./pound used), to be given as soon as possible after exposure. *Measles*: the attenuating dose, to be given during the first 6 days after exposure and much preferred by many men to the fully preventive dose because the attenuated attack practically always confers permanent immunity, is 0.02 ml./pound for children under 2 years and 0.04 ml./pound for others. The fully preventive dose is 0.1 ml./pound for children under 2 years. *Pertussis (whooping cough)*: preventive dosage is 2.5 ml. for infants as soon as possible after exposure and repeated once after 5 days. *Vaccinia*: there is a specially prepared Vaccinia Immune Globulin available through the Red Cross to be used according to special directions for the prevention of disseminated vaccinia in persons exposed to recently vaccinated individuals and who are themselves unvaccinated. *Agammaglobulinemia*, congenital or acquired, subjects the patient to recurrent infections against which he may be protected by initial dosage of 0.6 ml./pound with maintenance dosage of 0.3 ml./pound intramuscularly at monthly intervals for children and 2 week intervals for adults. It is the consensus that the prophylactic efficacy of gamma globulin has been convincingly demonstrated in no other entities than those listed above, and this includes its use in dosage of about 20 ml. in attempted prevention of rubella during the first trimester of pregnancy.

There is one therapeutic use of gamma globulin that seems to be justified by experience, namely, in the treatment of eczema vaccinatum. For this purpose the Vaccinia Immune Globulin, above referred to, is employed.

Paul V. Holland, Richard M. Rubinson, Andrew G. Morrow and Paul J. Schmidt. Gamma Globulin in Post-transfusion Hepatitis. J.A.M.A. 196:471, May 9, 1966.

GAS GANGRENE

"What is the drug of choice in gas gangrene?"

Reply: The penicillins in high dosage, but some men like to use a broad-spectrum antibiotic in addition, to hedge against intercurrent infection with other organisms. Of course the surgeon or the gynecologist are often the most important figures in the treatment of one of these cases.

GASTROENTERITIS

"I have a patient in whom a sprue-like syndrome has developed immediately after recovery from a bout of acute gastroenteritis, in which no antibiotic or chemotherapeutic agents had been used. Is there a likely relationship of the one malady with the other?"

Reply: In East Pakistan, John Lindenbaum studied the matter of malabsorption during and after recovery from acute intestinal infection in 95 patients who spent a few days in a hospital ward for the treatment of acute diarrheal illness. Using xylose, folic acid and vitamin B_{12} absorption as indicators, he found that both during infection and during the first week after clinical recovery there was a considerable but usually transient impairment of absorption from the small intestine. In a few instances this malabsorption continued for weeks or months after the acute infection, but it was not certain that these instances of prolonged disturbance were not due to an underlying bowel disorder which preceded the intestinal infection.

John Lindenbaum. Malabsorption During and After Recovery from Acute Intestinal Infection. Brit. M. J. 2:326, 1965.

"It has been my experience, and is generally conceded, that the result of antibacterial therapy in childhood gastroenteritis has been something

short of brilliant. In the adult, we often attribute these cases to a dietary indiscretion or an emotional upset, and prescribe a tranquilizing agent with some success. Would it not be rational to try a tranquilizer in the youngster?"

Reply: I certainly think so, but do not know of anyone who has reported a study of such a trial.

GENITAL ABNORMALITIES

"Would you please make a brief statement of the indications for and uses of the sex hormones in hypogonadism, eunuchoidism, cryptorchism and Fröhlich's syndrome?"

Reply: The desired clinical effects with chorionic gonadotropin (or with testosterone) in *hypogonadism*, whether or not associated with eunuchoidism, are of course a reversal of the characteristic signs and symptoms; namely, infantile genitalia and secondary sexual characteristics, female distribution of fat, pale and sallow complexion, poor muscular development, diminished libido and possibly both overgrowth of the long bones and psychiatric manifestations.

If *eunuchoidism* is due primarily to failure of the luteinizing hormone of the anterior pituitary to stimulate the testicular androgen production, then the patient is said to have the hypogonadotropic type of the malady and he may be benefited by chorionic gonadotropin. But if the aberration is of the hypogonadotropic type in which there is primary failure of the testis itself, due to intrinsic defect or to atrophy and fibrosis of the interstitial cells as the result of a toxic attack upon them by roentgen rays or the mumps virus, then only testosterone will succeed. Most cases of eunuchoidism are actually of the latter type.

In *cryptorchism* there is failure of one or both of the testes to descend into the scrotum at birth or shortly thereafter, and the hoped-for result of therapy is correction of the associated evidences of endocrine dysfunction as well as promotion of descent of the testes. Usually there is some obstruction causing the failure, I believe, and treatment is necessarily surgical, but in cases associated with evidences of endocrine dysfunction the use of chorionic gonadotropin or testosterone is sometimes successful. Chorionic gonadotropin is used first and then, if it fails, testosterone. It is the gonadotropin that most often succeeds (or would descent have occurred in all these patients had they been left untreated until puberty?).

Fröhlich's syndrome seems to be satisfactorily treated only when it is associated with cryptorchism.

Neither chorionic gonadotropin nor testosterone influences the anterior pituitary production of follicle-stimulating hormone that engenders spermatogenesis in the seminiferous tubules of the testes, but supermatogenesis is nevertheless occasionally promoted in a eunuchoid individual by use of these hormones.

In one of the types of eunuchoidism the therapy consists in injection of 1000 units of chorionic gonadotropin (Antuitrin-S) twice daily for two courses of 3 months with a 6 month rest period between. Usual dosage in cryptorchism is 500–1000 units two or three times weekly, to be discontinued if progressive descent has not occurred during 8 weeks or if signs of precocious maturity have appeared.

In treating most cases of eunuchoidism, testosterone propionate is injected intramuscularly in 25 mg. dosage (range 10–50 mg.) three times weekly. Methyltestosterone tablets are given orally in three to five times the dosage of the injected preparation. Tablets for buccal absorption are given in 30–40 mg. dosage daily. These dosages are also sometimes stated as follows: buccal, 1 mg./kg. daily, increased or decreased according to indication; oral, twice as much; intramuscular, 1 mg./5 kg. of body weight twice weekly, increased or decreased according to indications. Crystalline testosterone is used intramuscularly in the same dosage as the propionate, and both compounds may be implanted subcutaneously in the back using the specially devised trocar. Three 75–100 mg. pellets are usually placed at two sites at 6–8 month intervals in eunuchoidism.

"In implanting testosterone for the treatment of testosterone deficiency in the male, what is the preferred preparation?"

Reply: From the vantage point of his extensive experience in London, Tiberius Reiter has said that pure testosterone only should be used in the form of fused testosterone crystals, in adequate dosage (at least 4000 mg. every 6–7 months). There is a 2–3 weeks latent period after introduction before the effects are apparent. Reiter accompanies each testosterone implantation with implantation of one 20 mg. pellet of estradiol (Dimenformon, etc.); the two active hormonal ingredients are incorporated in 3–4 ml. of 2% lignocaine (lidocaine) with 1 : 80,000 epinephrine (Adrenaline).

Tiberius Reiter. Testosterone Implantation: The Method of Choice for Treatment of Testosterone Deficiency. J. Am. Geriatrics Soc. 13:1003, 1965.

GIARDIASIS

"What is the preferred agent in the treatment of giardiasis?"

Reply: Quinacrine (Atabrine) is the standard drug. Usual adult dosage is 100 mg. three times daily for 5–7 days; keep the dosage down to 100–200 mg. daily in children under 10 years of age. Amodiaquin (Camoquin) has also been used successfully in India in a single dose of 3 tablets of 0.2 Gm. for adults, 2 tablets for patients aged 5–15 years, 1/3 tablet three times daily for 2 days for infants and young children.

N. R. Konar, A. N. Sen Gupta, S. P. Bhattacharjee and Gita Chandra. Camoquin in Treatment of Giardiasis. J. Indian M. A. 23:52, 1953.

GLANDERS

"What is the best drug to use in a case of glanders?"

Reply: Actually there has been very little written on the specific therapy of this disease since Howe and Miller reported, in 1947, that their results with sulfadiazine in 6 cases warranted further adequate trial of the agent. Nowadays, in addition to a sulfonamide, it is considered advisable to use streptomycin or tetracycline or chloramphenicol (Chloromycetin). It is said to be advisable to excise the local nodule where possible, though in an outbreak of 7 cases on the Continent reported a number of years ago 5 terminated fatally in spite of the fact that the original focus was eliminated in each case.

C. Howe and W. R. Miller. Glanders. Ann. Int. Med. 26:93, 1947.

GLYCOGEN STORAGE DISEASE

"In hepatic glycogen storage disease every effort is made to improve nutrition and of course correct the hypoglycemia and acidosis. Will any drugs help in mobilizing the glycogen stores?"

Reply: Thyroxine, glucagon, corticotropin (ACTH) and the androgens are all resorted to, but it is difficult to determine how effective any of these agents really are because these children tend to improve as they grow older, and there really is not a sufficient backlog of cases against which to determine the true efficacy of remedial drug measures.

GOITER

"What has been the result of thyroid medication of nontoxic diffuse goiter?"

Reply: In Sydney, Australia, I. B. Hales and associates treated 81 patients and obtained complete disappearance of goiter in 49% of them and a decrease in size in an additional 40%. It did not seem that either the duration of the goiter or the initial thyroidal iodine uptake influenced the response. The drugs used were thyroid substance or levothyroxin (Synthroid). At the Roswell Park Memorial Institute, Buffalo, J. Badillo's group had comparable results with sodium liothyronine (Cytomel), and so too did Norman Schneeberg's group at Philadelphia General Hospital.

I. B. Hales, J. Myhill, T. S. Reeve and F. F. Rundle. Nontoxic Diffuse Goiter: Factors Influencing Effect of Thyroid Medication. Brit. M. J. 1:977, Apr. 7, 1962. J. Badillo, K. Shimaoka, E. M. Lessmann, F. C. Marchetta and Joseph E. Sokal. Treatment of Nontoxic Goiter with Sodium Liothyronine (Cytomel). J.A.M.A. 184:29, Apr. 6, 1963. Norman G. Schneeberg, Theodore J. Stahl, Godofredo Maldia and Hyman Menduke. Regression of Goiter by Whole Thyroid or Triiodothyronine (Cytomel). Metabolism 11:1054, 1962.

"Should my patient with a multinodular goiter be treated medically or surgically?"

Reply: We all know that deaths from cancer of the thyroid are extremely rare while nodular goiter is common. The known incidence of thyroid cancer, according to U.S. Public Health statistics, is only 25 cases per year per million with 8 deaths per million. Extrapolating to a population of 180 million, that would be 4700 cases and 1440 cancer deaths. One cannot jump to the conclusion, however, that some of these 1440 patients might have been saved by surgery because we do not know how many *did* have surgery. At the Massachusetts General Hospital, Claude Welch has made earnest attempt at statistical calculation of the number of deaths that could theoretically be saved by prophylactic thyroidectomy and has concluded that the number of deaths from prophylactic surgery is about the same as those from cancer without surgery. Which is what one is obliged to call a stalemate, and this brings us to the point of trying to determine what clinical features may be used to select the patient who should have surgery. Welch has listed these features to be the following in his judgment: (1) a large gland; (2) surgical signs that suggest malignancy, such as extreme hardness, fixation of the trachea, hoarseness, painful mass, or a positive needle biopsy; (3) palpable lymph nodes, particularly the Delphian; (4) a multinodular gland with one dominant particularly hard nodule; (5) a gland that increases in size or becomes harder on thyroid therapy; (6) a gland that has a cold nodule on scintiscans (scanning); (7) a gland associated with distant metastases proved to be of thyroid origin.

It seems that at the Massachusetts General Hospital about 25% of patients with multinodular goiter are advised to have operation at the time of initial study and that an additional 10% develop signs or symptoms under observation that indicate the desirability of surgery.

Claude E. Welch. Therapy for Multinodular Goiter. J.A.M.A. 195:339, Jan. 31, 1966.

GOUT

"An associate of mine recently injected 2 ml. of 2% procaine into the appropriate interspinous spaces in an acute attack of gout and said that almost immediately the patient was able to move his swollen and seemingly immobile extremity freely and without pain. Colchicine was given in addition to complete the relief, but what do you think of this?"

Reply: In Hawaii, Reichert and Burden reported the treatment of 10 patients with such an injection, with instant relief in all instances. But I believe that most men would settle for the slower relief that can be obtained with colchicine alone. One does incur risks with intraspinous injections, you know.

Frederick Leet Reichert and J. Alfred Burden. Method for Instant Relief of Pain in Cases of Gout. Hawaii M. J. 22:116, 1962.

"Do the corticosteroids have any usefulness in the treatment of acute gout?"

Reply: I do not recall a large-scale study of this matter, but a few years ago John Staige Davis and Samuel Hashim, at St. Luke's Hospital, New York, reported that they were usually able to abort an acute attack of gout with a single dose of 1 mg. colchicine and 0.75 mg. dexamethasone (Gammacorten).

John Staige Davis and Samuel Hashim. Treatment of Osteoarthritis and Other Collagen Diseases with Dexamethasone (Gammacorten). Rheumatism 19:74, 1963.

"I have heard that in England the new drug, indomethacin (Indocin), is being used effectively in the treatment of acute gout. Do you know anything of this?"

Reply: At Westminster Hospital, in London, F. Dudley Hart has reported the use of the drug. In the 26 patients given indomethacin, it was said that response was good in 61.5%, fair in 19.2% and nil in 19.2%; response to phenylbutazone (Butazolidin) good in 12.5% of 16 patients, fair in 56.25% and nil in 31.25%; response to colchicine in 16 patients was good in 12.5%, fair in 12.5% and nil in 75%. This certainly makes the new drug look very good, but I have my tongue in cheek regarding this report because I do not believe that colchicine would provide such poor relief if given properly, i.e., in adequate dosage and early enough.

P. L. Boardman and F. Dudley Hart. Indomethacin (Indocin) in Treatment of Acute Gout. Practitioner 194:560, 1965.

"I would like so much to use aspirin as a uricosuric agent in my gout patients instead of probenecid (Benemid) or sulfinpyrazone (Anturan), but none of them has been able to stay with it very long. Do most men succeed with this therapy?"

Reply: None that I know. Despite the statements of the men – there are very few – who champion aspirin as a uricosuric agent, I do not believe that any patient who says that he is taking 1 Gm. of the drug five times daily, week in and week out, is actually *doing* it.

"I have a patient with gout, being treated with sulfinpyrazone (Anturan), in whom I have discovered quite incidentally a decrease in the platelet count definitely ascribable to action of the drug. Has this any significance?"

Reply: J. F. Mustard's group, in Canada, found that, in male subjects with primary gout, platelet survival is shortened and platelet turnover correspondingly increased, and they felt that the increased tendency to vascular disease in subjects with gout might possibly result from this increased platelet turnover. H. A. Smythe and associates, of the same Canadian group, have found in a deliberate study of the matter, as you did accidentally, that sulfinpyrazone has a considerable influence on platelet economy in addition to its uricosuric action. I think that this is all very interesting, but its practical significance appears still somewhat doubtful.

H. A. Smythe, M. A. Ogryzlo, E. A. Murphy and J. F. Mustard. Effect of Sulfinpyrazone (Anturan) on Platelet Economy and Blood Coagulation in Man. Canad. M. A. J. 92:818, Apr. 10, 1965. J. F. Mustard, E. A. Murphy, M. A. Ogryzlo and H. A. Smythe. Blood Coagulation and Platelet Economy in Subjects with Primary Gout. Canad. M. A. J. 89:1207, 1963.

"I am aware that normal renal function, as determined by phenolsulfonphthalein (P.S.P.) excretion, cannot be accurately assessed in a patient who is being treated with probenecid (Benemid). Is this true also of the newer drug, sulfinpyrazone (Anturan)?"

Reply: Yes, Newcombe and Cohen (Massachusetts Memorial Hospital) have found this to be the case.

David S. Newcombe and Alan S. Cohen. Uricosuric Agents and Phenolsulfonphthalein Excretion. Arch. Int. Med. 112:738, 1963.

"Does the newer uricosuric agent, sulfinpyrazone (Anturan), increase the plasma level of concomitantly administered penicillin as does probenecid (Benemid)?"

Reply: No, Howard Duncan (Royal North Shore Hospital, Sydney) has reported that it does not.

Howard Duncan. Effect of Sulfinpyrazone (Anturan) on Plasma Levels of Penicillin. M. J. Australia 1:588, Apr. 18, 1964.

"I have a patient with gout who also has renal disease and is relatively insusceptible to the action of both probenecid (Benemid) and sulfin-pyrazone (Anturan). Is there any other drug that might be useful?"

Reply: Yes, at the Mount Sinai Hospital in New York, Ts'ai Fan Yü and Alexander B. Gutman have shown allopurinol (Zyloprim) capable of suppressing uric acid production without undue hazard of toxicity, doing so even in the presence of renal damage sufficient to render uricosuric drugs virtually impotent. The dosage usually employed was 200–300 mg./day orally in two or three divided doses, but some of their patients received as much as 400 or 600 mg./day. Colchicine prophylaxis was maintained concurrently in most of the cases. This drug does not act like the uricosuric agents, i.e., to promote elimination of urates, but rather it inhibits the action of xanthine oxidase, an enzyme that catalyzes conversion of hypoxanthine to xanthine and xanthine to uric acid. Therefore when using it one does not increase the risk of uric acid urolithiasis, as may be the case with the uricosuric agents.

Ts'ai Fan Yü and Alexander B. Gutman. Effect of Allopurinol (Zyloprim) (4-Hydroxypyrazolo-(3,4-d) Pyrimidine) on Serum and Urinary Uric Acid in Primary and Secondary Gout. Am. J. Med. 37:885, 1964.

"One of my associates has been making a study of the new drug, allopurinol (Zyloprim) in the treatment of gout, and reports himself very satisfied with it. Has this been the general experience?"

Reply: I believe the most satisfactory report has been made by Wayne Rundles and his group at Duke University. They made most exhaustive studies in 46 patients with well-documented, acute intermittent or chronic, or both intermittent and chronic manifestations of gout. About one third of the patients had mild or moderately severe disease and the remainder were selected because of having severe disease characterized by early onset, poor control with standard agents, an eventual production of large tophi, joint destruction, neuropathy, etc. Their evidence made it appear that this is going to be an important addition to the armamentarium for gout, particularly useful in patients with severe disease, extensive tophaceous deposits, nephropathy and in those tending to form urate stones. Patients with mild or moderately severe gout required 200–300 mg. daily for optimal control, and those with severe disease, 400–800 mg./day. Colchicine was used when necessary to prevent acute attacks, and probenecid (Benemid) and allopurinol were used together to increase renal clearance and the excretion of uric acid without evidence of major drug incompatibility. When the drug was used alone, episodes of acute gouty arthritis continued to occur for several weeks but then gradually became less frequent, milder and more responsive to symptomatic therapy. Disability was reduced, and in most patients tophi gradually became smaller or disappeared. And with the reduction in uric acid excretion, stones ceased to be formed.

R. Wayne Rundles, Earl N. Metz and H. R. Silverman. Allopurinol in the Treatment of Gout. Ann. Int. Med. 64,229, 1966.

"In what sort of dosage must probenecid (Benemid) be used for its uricosuric effect in chronic gout?"

Reply: A. B. Gutman and T. F. Yü, in New York, who are close students of this subject, have found 0.5 Gm. effective in 10% of their patients, 1.0 Gm. in 50%, 1.5–2.0 Gm. in 25% and 2.5–3.0 Gm. in 15%. The smaller doses are usually given only once daily, the larger doses divided between two or three administrations. Because there is the possibility of urate gravel or stone formation in the urinary passages, it is conservative practice to neutralize the urine through oral administration of about 2.5 Gm. (½ teaspoonful) of sodium bicarbonate twice daily during the first 2–3 weeks and require that enough fluid be taken to produce 2000 ml. of urine daily. It is not known how probenecid therapy causes acute gouty attacks when its use is begun, but concomitant prophylactic use of colchicine will prevent this. Probenecid therapy need not be discontinued during an acute attack though it will not contribute toward its amelioration.

There are records of the continuous ingestion of probenecid for as long as eight years without major toxic reactions. In Boger and Strickland's review of 2502 patients treated with the drug there were gastrointestinal symptoms, usually mild and not requiring cessation of therapy, in 3.1% of instances, fever and rash in 1.35%, precipitation of acute gout in 1.2%, and a spate of diverse and mild reactions in a small number of instances; renal colic or passage of urate stones had an incidence of 0.68% and a reducing substance appeared in the urine in 0.55% of instances. However, one cannot be entirely nonchalant with regard to this drug, for

Reynolds and associates observed fatal massive hepatic necrosis as a manifestation of hypersensitivity to it.

A. B. Gutman and T. F. Yü. Prevention and Treatment of Chronic Gouty Arthritis. J.A.M.A. 157:1096, 1955. Protracted Uricosuric Therapy in Tophaceous Gout. Lancet 2:1258, 1957. Renal Regulation of Uric Acid Excretion in Normal and Gouty Man: Modification by Uricosuric Agents. Bull. New York Acad. Med. 34:287, 1958. W. P. Boger and S. C. Strickland. Probenecid (Benemid); Its Uses and Side Effects in 2502 Patients. Arch. Int. Med. 95:83, 1955. E. S. Reynolds, R. C. Schlant, H. C. Gonick and G. J. Dammin. Fatal Massive Necrosis of the Liver as a Manifestation of Hypersensitivity to Probenecid. New England J. Med. 256:592, 1957.

"When probenecid (Benemid) is being used for its uricosuric action in gout may the patient use aspirin now and then in treatment of a headache?"

Reply: Salicylates should not be administered in full uricosuric dosage while probenecid is being used because they nullify the effect in some manner not understood; this interdiction does not apply to the usual small analgesic doses of aspirin as used in the treatment of a headache.

"I have a patient with a highly allergic background and personal history in whom gout has now been diagnosed. Will it be dangerous to use probenecid (Benemid) in this individual?"

Reply: I do not think that you can be accused of taking undue risk in doing so because the number of reported reactions of an allergic type, usually in the form of mild skin rashes, has been extremely small in comparison with the very wide use to which this drug has been put. In fact, I have seen only three reports of such reactions.

Norbert A. Hillecke (California). Acute Anaphylactoid Reaction to Probenecid. J.A.M.A. 193:740, Aug. 30, 1965.

"I have a patient with gout whose formerly recurrent attacks are well prevented by prophylactic use of colchicine except that now and then there is a 'breakthrough.' Is there any way in which I might anticipate and thus hope to prevent these very undesirable occurrences?"

Reply: Probably the best way is to prohibit excesses in eating and drinking and advise avoidance as much as possible of unusual stresses of other natures. In the experience of perhaps the most knowledgeable pair of investigators of gout in this country, Yü and Gutman (Mount Sinai Hospital, New York), the stepping up somewhat of colchicine dosage in anticipation of unusual events, or if an attack seemed to be starting, was found often to be profitable. In reporting on a series of 205 patients in whom they attempted the prevention of attacks over a mean period of 5 years, 76 of the patients being more or less incapacitated because of four or more disabling attacks annually, they describe their initial colchicine dosage as 1 or 1.2 mg. daily, often reducing to 0.5 mg. daily, and in a very few instances succeeding with 0.5 mg. on alternate days only. Extra doses, usually to a total of 2 or 3 mg. for a day or two, were used for the special situations previously referred to. They found that in any patterns of employing colchicine and uricosuric agents, it was only the colchicine that was responsible for preventing the attacks.

Ts'ai Fan Yü and Alexander B. Gutman. Efficacy of Colchicine Prophylaxis in Gout: Prevention of Recurrent Gouty Arthritis over Mean Period of Five Years in 208 Gouty Subjects. Ann. Int. Med. 55:179, 1961.

"I have several patients with gout who have been on prophylactic colchicine dosage for 2 years. Need I fear the sudden appearance of cumulative toxic effects?"

Reply: No.

"I have a patient with gout who is severely intolerant to colchicine. What may I use to bring the situation under control during one of his acute attacks?"

Reply: Wallace and Nissen gave griseofulvin (Fulvicin, etc.) to 20 patients in total dosage of 6–9 Gm., according to body size, giving 2 Gm. every 4 hours until the total dose was taken. Fifteen of the patients responded with a 50% or greater clearing of objective inflammatory changes within 24–48 hours. There were no more side effects than mild to moderate nausea.

Stanley L. Wallace and Anthony W. Nissen. Griseofulvin in Acute Gout. New England J. Med. 266:1099, May 24, 1962.

"What is to be expected if an irascible patient takes an excessive amount of colchicine in the attempt to relieve his attack of gout?"

Reply: The principal toxic reaction to colchicine is a rather severe abdominal colic and profuse watery diarrhea; this occurs in nearly all individuals receiving full dosage for treatment of an acute attack of gout. In the prophylactic employment these symptoms do not appear.

In relatively rare instances colchicine in full therapeutic dosage causes loss of body hair, which is usually confined to the scalp region.

Excessive dosage exaggerates the toxic action on the bowel and damages the kidneys and myocardium. There are bloody, watery stools, hematuria and oliguria, and death from shock and dehydration. Several hours elapse between the taking of a large excessive dose and the appearance of symptoms, suggesting the formation of a toxic product in the interim.

"How is colchicine used prophylactically in gout?"

Reply: Some experienced gouty patients recognize prodromal symptoms of an attack and abort it by taking three or four hourly doses of colchicine. Others use the drug prophylactically in 0.5 mg. dosage three times daily for 2 or 3 days each week. I have seen the record of a patient who had been maintained free of gouty symptoms, previously frequent and severe, by taking 0.5 mg. of colchicine twice daily for 5 years.

"How is colchicine best used to effect relief in an acute bout of gout?"

Reply: It is perhaps the most usual practice to give a 0.5 mg. (1/120 grain) tablet every hour until diarrhea begins, which will usually occur at the seventh to tenth dose, but Hoffmann tries to avoid the diarrhea by giving 1 tablet every hour for four doses, then 1 tablet every 3 hours. In an attack that is not already several days old when treatment is started, either of these methods of dosing should bring relief in 24–48 hours. As soon as relief is obtained, which happens very sharply, further administration is stopped, and the gastrointestinal symptoms are attended to through giving a dose of paregoric every 3 hours until the distressing diarrhea ceases. Sometimes it is necessary to start the opiate therapy before relief from pain is achieved, but this is unusual unless treatment was begun late in the attack.

Intravenous administration has been described on the basis of limited experience; dosage has usually been 1 mg., repeated at 3–6 hour intervals for 3–12 doses, depending upon the response; or 2 mg. may be given at 8 hour intervals. Carmichael recorded 4 cases in which no gastrointestinal disturbances had been experienced, and others have had like results.

It is frequent practice to give 0.65–1.0 Gm. doses of acetylsalicylic acid (aspirin) to promote uric acid excretion while giving colchicine in the acute attack. The drugs do not potentiate each other's actions; neither do they interfere with each other.

L. P. Carmichael. Treatment of Acute Gout with Injection of Colchicine. J.A.M.A., 170:1410, 1959. W. S. Hoffmann. Some Unsolved Problems of Gout. M. Clin. North America 43:595, 1959.

"Do you advocate the parenteral administration of colchicine in an acute attack of gout rather than to wait for the slower action of the orally administered drug?"

Reply: No, I do not. Unless there are very pressing reasons for doing so I would not give the drug parenterally, because of the increased risk of severe toxicity incurred. The well recognized side effects of colchicine when given orally are nausea, vomiting, abdominal pain and diarrhea and some anorexia and malaise. But that is all unless ordinary dosage has been greatly exceeded; but when giving the drug parenterally there is the danger of inducing in addition fever, alopecia, hepatotoxicity and severe damage to the nervous and hematopoietic systems.

Albert A. Carr (National Institutes of Health). Colchicine Toxicity. Arch. Int. Med. 115:29, 1965.

GRAM-NEGATIVE INFECTIONS

"I am becoming much disturbed by all the present talk of gram-negative or coliform infections and am not sure that I know precisely just what these organisms are or when one may expect to encounter such infections and what antibiotics to use. Can you enlighten me?"

Reply: Your confusion is not surprising, for this subject has come to the fore-front of attention only relatively recently, since these organisms tended to be looked upon prior to the antibiotic era as not being very pathogenic. The term "coliform organisms" is loosely used to include various gram-negative bacilli that are normal inhabitants of fecal flora, such as *Escherichia coli, Klebsiella-Aerobacter, Proteus* species and *Pseudomonas aeruginosa;* and the *Herellea* species, which occur frequently in the genitourinary tract, are also included. All these organisms are often naturally resistant to the widely used antibiotics or have become more resistant to them with the passage of time. And they are the cause of an increasing number of deaths. The subject has been well reviewed by Francis Sweeney and Joseph Rodgers, of Jefferson Medical College, and I shall follow their report in attempting to provide a brief answer to your questions. Infections occur most frequently in hospital but they are seen in the community also, and they affect the very young and elderly more often than individuals in other age groups. The degenerative and chronic debilitating diseases such as diabetes mellitus, leukemia, lymphomas, neoplasms, agranulocytosis, chronic pulmonary disease, various types of vasculitis and collagen disorders predispose. Most of the gram-negative infections are encountered in the urinary tract, but they may be associated with acute pulmonary infections in elderly and debilitated individuals and in patients treated with corticosteroids, antimetabolites or antimicrobial drugs. They may in fact cause infections in almost any part of the body but are only occasionally involved in respiratory tract infections. They cause meningitis in the newborn frequently but rarely in other age groups. Bacterial endocarditis is rarely caused by a gram-negative organism, but severe burns are frequently so contaminated, particularly with *Pseudomonas*. The antibiotics presently available for treatment of gram-negative infections are streptomycin, the tetracyclines, chloramphenicol (Chloromycetin), kanamycin (Kantrex), ampicillin (Penbritin, Polycillin), cephalothin (Keflin), polymyxin B (Aerosporin) and colistin (Coly-Mycin). Some of the infections can also be successfully attacked with penicillin G in quite massive dosage. If a gram-negative infection is suspected it is advisable to begin treatment with kanamycin intravenously or intramuscularly if renal function is adequate, and then modify the therapy according to the result of bacteriologic studies. But if the patient has entered the hospital with the infection, i.e., if it is "community acquired," therapy may be begun with chloramphenicol or a tetracycline, the latter being preferred because of the hematologic complications associated with chloramphenicol. *Escherichia coli* is frequently sensitive to the tetracyclines and chloramphenicol and almost always sensitive to kanamycin, polymyxin B and colistin, but only 25–50% of these infections are sensitive to streptomycin. In addition to the initial chloramphenicol or tetracycline it may be necessary to employ a second agent if the organism is *Klebsiella-Aerobacter, Proteus* or *Pseudomonas. Klebsiella-Aerobacter* organisms are resistant to streptomycin, the tetracyclines and ampicillin and some of the strains also to chloramphenicol; a few are sensitive to cephalothin and most to kanamycin, polymyxin and colistin. *Proteus* is nearly always sensitive to kanamycin and cephalothin and to chloramphenicol about three quarters of the time, and it is frequently sensitive to ampicillin. However, *Proteus* strains other than *mirabilis* are practically susceptible only to kanamycin. Most strains of *Pseudomonas* are sensitive to polymyxin B or colistin but resistant to other antibiotics except for a few strains that are sensitive to streptomycin or one of the tetracyclines. Extremely high dosage of penicillin G may eradicate *Proteus* bacteremias and the majority of strains of *Escherichia coli, Klebsiella-Aerobacter* and *Proteus mirabilis*. The other strains of *Proteus* and all of the *Pseudomonas* species do not respond to such therapy.

Francis J. Sweeney, Jr. and Joseph F. Rodgers. Therapy of Infections Caused by Gram-Negative Bacilli. M. Clin. North America 49:1391, 1965.

"In our hospital the gram-negative bacilli are fortunately encountered principally in infections of the urinary tract, but occasionally we do see them as systemic invaders. What is one to do in the emergency situation when the patient is admitted in what appears clinically to be a state of gram-negative bacteremic shock?"

Reply: At Jefferson Medical College, Francis Sweeney, Jr., and Joseph Rodgers have recently dealt with this subject. They say it is their policy to begin treatment with kanamycin (Kantrex), 0.5 Gm./8 hours, or cephalothin (Keflin), 2 Gm./4 hours until the etiologic organism and antibiotic sensitivities are available. Change the antibiotic therapy then according to the sensitivity pattern: tetracycline dosage should be 500 mg./6 hours; no chloramphenicol unless no other suitable antibiotic is available; streptomycin probably has no place in this therapy; polymyxin, 2 mg./kg., should be used for any suspected case of bacteremia due to *Pseudomonas* species; certain *Proteus* species are sensitive to ampicillin, 2 Gm./4 hours, or penicillin G, 20,000,000 units/day. It is essential that all antibiotics be given intravenously until the blood pressure is stabilized and be continued for a minimum of 10 days. Concomitant renal or hepatic insufficiency will necessitate reduction of dosage of some of the more toxic antibiotics. Since the initial effects of antibiotic therapy may be intensification of the shock syndrome through rapid liberation of large amounts of endotoxin, corticosteroids should be administered along with the appropriate antibiotics as soon as the diagnosis is established: 500 mg. of hydrocortisone intravenously/4–6 hours, or other corticosteroids in equivalent dosage. Continue the corticosteroids until the blood pressure has remained within normal limits for 24–48 hours without use of vasopressors. The use of vasopressor drugs in this malady is controversial, but these investigators recommend that metaraminol (Aramine) be given in dosage sufficient to keep the systolic blood pressure at 20–30 mm. above the preshock level, which can usually be achieved with 100 mg. of the drug/1000 ml. of 5% glucose in water. Restoration of blood volume, correction of electrolyte or water imbalance, adequate oxygenation, treatment of associated underlying diseases, drainage of abscesses, and relief of obstructions in the genitourinary or biliary systems should all be accomplished.

Francis J. Sweeney, Jr. and Joseph F. Rodgers. Therapy of Infections Caused by Gram-Negative Bacilli. M. Clin. North America 49:1391, 1965.

"I have been wondering whether we have abandoned the use of penicillin inadvisedly in gram-negative infections merely because early studies showed that these organisms were not suppressed by in vitro levels that were feasible to use when penicillin was in short supply. Has this matter been reconsidered at any time?"

Reply: An important subject, and it has been reconsidered. At Tufts University, Louis Weinstein's group, approaching the matter from precisely your standpoint, studied the role of penicillin G in the management of serious gram-negative infections from both the microbiologic and the clinical standpoint. Laboratory studies, using the tube-dilution method, indicated that the bulk of strains of gram-negative organisms such as *Escherichia coli, Aerobacter aerogenes, Alcaligenes faecalis*, salmonella, shigella and indole-negative *Proteus (mirabilis)* were inhibited by concentrations of penicillin G ranging from 2.5 to 625 units/ml. in most cases. Pseudomonas and indole-producing proteus, on the other hand, were suppressed only by quantities of 5000–10,000 units/ml. Seventeen patients with a variety of infections due to several species of gram-negative bacilli were treated with "massive" doses of penicillin G (20,000,000–60,000,000 units/day). Though the presence of serious underlying noninfectious disorders in some of these patients led to relapse or death, unrelated to infection, many cures were achieved even though some of the cases were complicated by bacteremia. Studies of serum concentrations of penicillin G revealed peak levels as high as 737 units/ml., which were well in excess of those required to inhibit growth of the causative organisms in vitro. The only untoward effects resulting from such therapy were related to cerebral irritation and consisted of generalized seizures, but these appeared only in patients with renal failure or with underlying central nervous system disease; and in some instances these reactions did not recur after reduction in dosage. This study, although certainly not a definitive one, invites further investigation of the subject and may mean that a resort to massive penicillin G dosage in some gram-negative infections that are not responding to other antibiotics may at times be a life-saving measure.

Louis Weinstein, Phillip I. Lerner and William H. Chew. Clinical and Bacteriologic Studies of the Effect of "Massive" Doses of Penicillin G on Infections Caused by Gram-Negative Bacilli. New England J. Med. 271:525, Sept. 10, 1964.

GROWTH

"Methandrostenolone (Dianabol) has been promoted for several years as a strongly anabolic agent with slight androgenic side effects. Is it perfectly safe to use this preparation for its anabolic effects on linear growth and weight gain in prepubertal children of short stature?"

Reply: In a small series of children, Whitelaw and associates, in San Jose, California,

found doses of this drug as low as 1 mg. to be androgenic, and they therefore concluded that the agent should not be given to children or to adult female patients. I think it very doubtful that noticeable differences would appear between the newer anabolic steroids, to which group this drug belongs, if careful double-blind comparative studies could be made of them on an exhaustive basis. However, note should perhaps be made of the fact that in evaluating another one of them, stanozolol (Winstrol) in debilitated children, bedridden and crippled by a variety of birth injuries and congenital deformities, C. H. Carter, in Florida, felt that the improvement effected in general condition far outweighed in clinical importance the acceleration of sexual development.

M. James Whitelaw, Thomas N. Foster and William H. Graham. Methandrostenolone (Dianabol): A Controlled Study of its Anabolic and Androgenic Effect in Children. J. Pediat. 68:294, 1966. C. H. Carter. The Anabolic Steroid, Stanozolol: Its Evaluation in Debilitated Children. Clin. Pediat. 4:671, 1965.

GUILLAIN-BARRÉ SYNDROME

"Is there anything of promise at all in the therapy of Guillain-Barré syndrome? I have a most distressing case presently in my practice."

Reply: I can only cite the experience of K. N. V. Palmer, in Aberdeen, who reported that in a single case in which there had been no improvement with steroid therapy in high dosage there was a dramatic and sustained return of muscular power associated with the return to normal in strength-duration curves and a fall in cerebrospinal fluid protein when the patient was placed on 6-mercaptopurine (Purinethol). Spontaneous remission could not be ruled out in this case but it was nevertheless felt that the result obtained with the drug was actually ascribable to its action.

K. N. V. Palmer. Polyradiculoneuropathy (Guillain-Barré Syndrome) Treated with 6-Mercaptopurine. Lancet 1:733, Apr. 3, 1965.

HARTNUP'S DISEASE

"I have heard that a case of the rare malady, Hartnup disease, has appeared in one of the hospitals of our city. Is there any effective drug therapy?"

Reply: I believe that nicotinamide is used just as in the treatment of pellagra.

HEMOCHROMATOSIS

"In addition to frequent phlebotomies and the treatment of the diabetes if present, is there any drug therapy that might be helpful in hemo-chromatosis?"

Reply: Vitamin B complex is often found useful.

HEMOPHILIA

"I have a hemophilic patient whose bouts of hematuria are not as easily controllable with fresh frozen plasma as are the hemarthroses. Aside from the use of Factor VIII concentrate, which has not been as successfully used here in the United States as in Scandinavia, what else might I use with some hope of success in stopping this bleeding?"

Reply: At the University of Illinois, Charles Abildgaard and associates effected cessation of hematuria in 3 hemophilic patients following treatment with corticosteroids. The patient was kept at bed rest and given hydrocortisone intravenously (100 mg./day) for 2 days, followed by prednisone, 25 mg. orally/6 hours for five doses. Gross hematuria cleared within the first 24 hours, and there was no further bleeding except for a few clots in one specimen on the second day.

Charles F. Abildgaard, Joseph V. Simone and Irving Schulman. Steroid Treatment of Hemophilic Hematuria. J. Pediat. 66:117, 1965.

"I have a hemophilic patient in whom I am tempted to try the new agent, aminocaproic acid (Amicar). What is the record?"

Reply: There have been a few favorable uncontrolled studies, but the only controlled one that has come to my attention was unfavorable. At the Children's Hospital Medical Center, in Boston, Herbert Strauss and associates placed 7 patients with severe classic hemophilia on a schedule of aminocaproic acid and placebo, alternated each month so that each patient served as his own control, the duration of the study varying from 8 to 13 months and lasting for 12 months in half the patients and for 8 months in only 1. The dose was 100 mg./kg. body weight given four times daily during waking hours. Upon completion of the study, monthly observations and impressions of the parents and the patients and investigators regarding the amount and frequency of hemorrhage and general feeling of well-being were tabulated, together with the objective evidence of severe bleeding requiring replacement therapy. By both subjective and objective criteria, no difference between the two treatment groups was observed.

Herbert S. Strauss, Sherwin V. Kevy and Louis K. Diamond. Ineffectiveness of Prophylactic Epsilon Aminocaproic Acid in Severe Hemophilia. New England J. Med. 273: 301, Aug. 5, 1965.

HEMOPHILIC MALINGERING

"I have a 'bleeder' patient whom I strongly suspect to be taking an anticoagulant drug surreptitiously. How can I establish this?"

Reply: These are of course difficult cases because the differential diagnosis necessarily includes all the known bleeding states. However, there are tests by which the presence of both coumarin and indandione anticoagulants can be demonstrated in the blood. In addition, Bowie and associates, at the Mayo Clinic, have pointed out that the prothrombin time of Quick is invariably prolonged to a striking degree if bleeding is attributable to an oral anticoagulant. The prothrombin time test consists of adding tissue thromboplastin and ionic calcium to oxalated plasma and timing the formation of the clot. The malingering situation in which an anticoagulant drug is employed is probably quite rare, although it is very likely that the 20 cases reported to date do not truly reflect the incidence.

E. J. Walter Bowie, Margaret Todd, John H. Thompson, Jr., Charles A. Owen, Jr. and Irving S. Wright. Anticoagulant Malingerers (the "Dicumarol-Eaters"). Am. J. Med. 39:855, 1965. Robert A. O'Reilly and Paul M. Aggeler. Surreptitious Ingestion of Coumarin Anticoagulant Drugs. Ann. Int. Med. 64:1034, 1966.

HEMORRHAGE

"Considerable use is made in our hospital of a complex preparation known as Adrenosem Salicylate in the attempt to control bleeding not only postpartum and postoperative but also in cases of purpura, epistaxis, hematuria, retinal hemorrhage, etc. Does this drug really have established hemostatic action?"

Reply: There have been some enthusiastic reports but only one double-blind one has come to my attention. In it Adrenosem, the conjugated estrogenic substance (Premarin) and the oxalic and malonic acid preparation (Koagamin) were compared and none found more effective than a placebo in controlling hemorrhage during tonsillectomy. I do not find any sound evidence that Adrenosem really has hemostatic action in any type of bleeding, but one must say for the preparation that it does seem to be harmless.

S. Thajeb, M. Kurkcuoglu and A. E. McElfresh. The Value of Systemic Hemostatic Drugs. Arch. Otolaryng. 70:72, 1959.

"Is there any drug that might be helpful in a patient whose blood appears to be in a hypercoagulable state though he continues to bleed?"

Reply: What about the degree of fibrinolysis? In Stockholm, Irene von Francken and associates recorded the cases of 3 bleeding patients who in addition to shortened coagulation time and shortened plasma recalcification time were found to have increased fibrinolysis. They regarded the shortened coagulation and plasma recalcification times as expressions of hypercoagulability and felt that the bleeding was due to the increased fibrinolytic activity secondary to hypercoagulability. They therefore administered heparin, and in 2 patients the hypercoagulable state was normalized and bleeding ceased. In the third patient bleeding seemed to decrease after an initial dose of 50 mg. of heparin, but hematemesis occurred 6 hours after a second dose, and she died 1 hour later. Who can say whether the surmise was correct in these cases? The bleeding did stop in 2 of the 3, however.

Irene von Francken, Lennart Johansson, Per Olsson and Eric Zetterqvist. Heparin Treatment of Bleeding: Clinical Observations. Lancet 1:70, Jan. 12, 1963.

"One of my associates is fond of using conjugated estrogenic substance (Premarin) postoperatively to control hemorrhage, but I cannot find it at all helpful. What is the evidence?"

Reply: In the immediately preceding Reply I have cited a comparison of this drug with others in which it was shown that none of them had value. I have seen some enthusiastic reports on the use of Premarin but the only one that was well controlled actually failed to show that the drug had any value in controlling blood loss during or following prostatic surgery.

W. H. Cooner and H. M. Burros. Clinical Evaluation of the Effect of Premarin on Bleeding During and Following Prostatic Surgery. J. Urol. 83:64, 1960.

"In our area considerable use is made of a medicated chewing troche, known as Orabiotic, to prevent secondary hemorrhage in the post-tonsillectomy period. Has this preparation ever been shown to be really effective?"

Reply: At the Children's Hospital in Evanston, John Elsen dispensed this preparation randomly in a double-blind study in which 80 children were given the medication and 51 an identical-seeming placebo. Secondary post-tonsillectomy hemorrhage occurred in 1 (1.2%) of the children using the active preparation and in 6 (11.8%) of those using the control preparation. Elsen said that by both subjective and objective evaluations the results were considered good or excellent in 90% of the children who used the active preparation and in only about 50% of those who used the other one. The Orabiotic troche contains 3.5 mg. of neomycin and 0.25 mg. of gramicidin and in addition 2 mg. of propylaminobenzoate for analgesic effect. If infection is the most important cause of secondary post-tonsillectomy hemorrhage, then I suppose it may be considered that this troche acts through control of the infection.

John Elsen. Post-Tonsillectomy Effects of a Medicated Chewing Troche. Arch. Otolaryng. 82:78, 1965.

HEMOSIDEROSIS

"I have a case of idiopathic pulmonary hemosiderosis in my practice and do not know what to do. Can you advise?"

Reply: In their report of a single case, seen in Budapest, Steiner and Nabrady recounted the amazingly effective use of azathioprine (Imuran), giving the drug initially in dosage of 2.5 mg./kg./day, and later in half dosage for 6 months. Spleenectomy, another antineoplastic agent, 6-mercaptopurine (Purinethol), and corticosteroids have been used with moderate success in some instances.

B. Steiner and J. Nabrady. Immunoallergic Lung Purpura Treated with Azathioprine. Lancet 1:140, Jan. 16, 1965.

"I have a case on my hands of transfusional hemosiderosis in consequence of chronic blood replacement for a refractory anemia. Is there any drug that will be helpful in getting rid of some of this iron?"

Reply: Desferrioxamine (Desferal) appears to be the most satisfactory agent currently available for this purpose, though not all observers have found it very useful except in treatment of acute iron intoxication. At Mount Sinai Hospital, in New York, Norman Gevirtz's group used it effectively, however, in 2 patients with hemochromatosis. The agent has to be given intravenously because it is unabsorbable from the gastrointestinal tract.

Norman R. Gevirtz, Dina Tendler, Gertrude Lurinsky and Louis R. Wasserman. Clinical Studies of Storage Iron with Desferrioxamine (Desferal). New England J. Med. 273:95, July 8, 1965.

HEPATITIS

"I have heard of the use of antileukemic drugs in the treatment of chronic hepatitis, but would like to know what the chances are of success before beginning the use of such potentially toxic agents."

Reply: At the Royal Melbourne Hospital, in Victoria, Australia, Ian Mackay and associates used a long-term maintenance therapy for 3–12 months with 6-mercaptopurine (Purinethol) and azathioprine (Imuran) for 12 short and 7 long courses in 15 patients with chronic liver disease (both active chronic and lupoid hepatitis). Of this number, 7 did not respond favorably. Effective dosage was 50–100 mg. of 6-mercaptopurine and 100–200 mg. of azothioprine daily. At times, the side effects required stopping treatment for 2–3 weeks: anorexia, nausea and vomiting, diarrhea, hyperbilirubinemia, leukopenia.

Ian R. Mackay, Sara Weiden and Berta Ungar. Treatment of Active Chronic Hepatitis and Lupoid Hepatitis with 6-Mercaptopurine (Purinethol) and Azothioprine (Imuran). Lancet 1:899, Apr. 25, 1964.

"Has the value of corticosteroid therapy in viral hepatitis really been established?"

Reply: The early reports were upon the whole favorable, but when de Ritis and associates (University of Naples) performed a thorough study of the matter they found no statistically significant differences in their biochemical determinations, and the disease was not shortened or its severity lessened.

F. de Ritis, G. Giusti, L. Mallucci and M. Piazza. Negative Results of Prednisone Therapy in Viral Hepatitis. Lancet 1:533, Mar. 7, 1964.

"I hear it said that viral hepatitis is likely to be more severe among heroin addicts than among nonaddicted individuals for the reasons that the former eat very little, inject the organism intravenously with the drug, and share the needle with other individuals and thus assure rapid serial transfer. Has the matter actually been put to the test?"

Reply: Yes. At Lincoln Hospital, New York, Myron Schoenfeld and associates compared 68 consecutive addicts with viral hepatitis with 60 hepatitis patients who were not addicts, and found the disease no more severe, indeed perhaps milder in the addicts than in the nonaddicts. They felt that the mildness of the disease in the addicts might be partly ascribed to the immunity conferred on them by repeated exposure to the virus through frequent use of the needle; they thought also that there might be a difference both in virus type and in the size of the inoculum between orally acquired and needle-acquired cases.

Myron R. Schoenfeld, Norman Shacknow, Keyhan Farian and Charles R. Messeloff. Severity of Hepatitis Among Heroin Addicts. J. New Drugs 4:79, 1964.

"I have not had success in the several patients with coma in acute hepatitis through use of corticosteroids; what has been the result of using these drugs in a significant series of patients?"

Reply: Katz and associates (University of Chile) treated 23 patients, 19 of whom were in deep coma when treatment was begun and 4 of whom became comatose a few hours later. They used cortisone, 500 mg. intramuscularly every 8 hours, prednisolone (Delta-Cortef, etc.), 100 mg. intramuscularly every 8 hours, or dexamethasone (Decadron, etc.), 16 mg. intramuscularly or intravenously every 6 hours. They also gave intravenous glucose, broad-spectrum antibiotics and, in women, testosterone propionate; the electrolyte balance was also maintained. When consciousness returned, glucose and antibiotics were discontinued and steroids were reduced and terminated in most patients within 3 weeks. In the 9 patients who recovered, consciousness returned in 12 hours to 7 days after start of the treatment; 13 of the 14 patients who died did so without showing any response to therapy. It appeared that advantageous factors were relative youth, early appearance of coma, short duration of jaundice before coma and symptoms of severe liver failure for no more than 4 days before coma began. The only laboratory tests that seemed to be of prognostic significance were an early rise of the prothrombin complex and labile factor concentrations.

Ricardo Katz, Marta Velasco, Jaime Klinger and Hernan Alessandri. Corticosteroids in Treatment of Acute Hepatitis in Coma. Gastroenterology 42:258, 1962.

"In our clinic we have just made the diagnosis of cholangiolitic hepatitis, sometimes known also as primary biliary cirrhosis, in a woman of 42 years of age in whom the affliction has apparently been present for several years. I am aware that the disease will ultimately be fatal, but would very much like to know whether it would be advisable to start the patient on corticosteroids?"

Reply: In reviewing their experience in 21 cases of this malady, William Longmire and associates in Los Angeles said that corticosteroids had been of little value in treatment. Discussing their report, Francis Moore, of Boston, went further and said that the use of these drugs is not only disappointing but also dangerous because of the very high incidence of severe Cushing's syndrome in these people.

At the University of Chicago, Goldgraber and Kirsner were unable to find evidence of an alteration in the basic disease process through the use of this therapy. Some clinical alteration was effective, however: 3 of the patients experienced increase in appetite and sense of well-being, but 1 died despite decreases in temperature and pulse to normal; itching disappeared in 2; bilirubin decreased remarkably in 1, slightly in another and did not change in the 2 in whom there was a low value before therapy; serum albumin decreased in

1 and increased in 1; serum globulin decreased in 3; serum alkaline phosphatase decreased in 2 and increased in 1 before slowly declining; total cholesterol rose significantly in 3 of the 4 patients; thymol turbidity and cephalin-cholesterol flocculation were unaffected.

William P. Longmire, Jr., William L. Joseph, Philip M. Levin and Sherman M. Mellinkoff. Diagnosis and Treatment of Cholangiolitic Hepatitis (Primary Biliary Cirrhosis). Ann. Surg. 162:356, 1965. Francis D. Moore. Ibid. (Discussion). Moshe B. Goldgraber and Joseph B. Kirsner. Use of Adrenal Steroids in Subacute and Chronic Cholangiolitic Hepatitis: Clinicopathologic Correlation. Arch. Int. Med. 103:354, 1959.

HERPES SIMPLEX

"Herpes simplex involving the eye has been successfully treated with IDU, but what of the ordinary herpes simplex (cold sore) around the mouth and nose?"

Reply: In England, Hall-Smith and associates treated 11 patients with this malady through use of a 0.1% topical solution and 2 patients with a 0.5% ointment. There was relief from symptoms and marked resolution of the eruption within 24–72 hours in 12 of the patients, and no recurrences during a short follow-up. And in Los Angeles, Corbett and associates had good results in a much larger series. However, I have seen 1 patient who was made distinctly worse by topical application of the commercially available ointment.

S. P. Hall-Smith, M. J. Corrigan and M. J. Gilkes. Treatment of Herpes Simplex with 5-Iodo-2'-Deoxyuridine. Brit. M. J. 2:1515, Dec. 8, 1962. Max B. Corbett, Chester M. Sidell and Murray Zimmermann. Idoxuridine in the Treatment of Cutaneous Herpes Simplex. J.A.M.A. 196: 441, May 2, 1966.

HIATUS HERNIA

"A 'visiting fireman' in our area recently advocated the full peptic ulcer therapy in treatment of hiatus hernia. Of course since many people are not disturbed by their hernia, and indeed don't even know they have it until it is revealed in the course of a routine examination, it would be absurd in my opinion to put such individuals on such a regimen. And even when the individual has symptoms of some degree, I am wondering whether the advice is entirely sound?"

Reply: Well, I would go along with it insofar as frequent feedings and the use of antacids is concerned. But I should certainly avoid the use of anticholinergic drugs such as propantheline (Pro-Banthine), adiphenine (Trasentine), diphemanil (Prantal) and the many other members of this group, because they are likely to promote regurgitation and retention of material in the esophagus through delaying the emptying of both it and the stomach.

HICCUP

"What drugs offer the best hope of controlling an attack of severe hiccup?"

Reply: I think one may say that chlorpromazine (Thorazine) has proved to be the most effective agent. In Friedgood and Ripstein's series of 50 cases the medical and surgical conditions provoking the hiccup included chest or abdominal surgery, prostatectomy, nephrectomy, acute coronary thrombosis, congestive heart failure and uremia. Symptoms had persisted from days to weeks and had not responded to heavy sedation, carbon dioxide inhalation or other therapy, including phrenic nerve crush in five instances. In this series, 41 of the 50 patients were relieved almost immediately by chlorpromazine without recurrence of symptoms; 4 did not respond (the causal factors had not been concomitantly treated), and in 5 the drug only reduced the intensity and frequency of the hiccups but did not abolish them.

Just how carbon dioxide can be helpful in hiccup I do not know unless it be that through the improvement it effects in cerebral circulation it makes the necessary metabolic adjustment at some site of abnormal motor discharge. That it can be and often is helpful is fully established; simply breathing and rebreathing into a paper bag is a well known home remedy, and the full treatment with gas mask and apparatus is not infrequently used in recalcitrant cases in hospital.

In cases of seriously persistent hiccup, quinidine seems sometimes to be effective when other measures have failed. If hiccup is due to spasmodic contractions of the diaphragm and other muscles of respiration, as appears to be the case, the action of quinidine might be explained as a direct depression of these muscles with possibly also a blocking of nerve impulses at myoneural junctions. The latter action would be comparable to the vagus block that the drug sometimes effects in the heart.

C. E. Friedgood and C. V. Ripstein. Chlorpromazine (Thorazine) in Treatment of Intractable Hiccup. J.A.M.A. 157: 309, 1955.

HIRSCHSPRUNG'S DISEASE

"What drug, if any, has been consistently most helpful in the treatment of Hirschsprung's disease?"

Reply: It is presently considered that congenital megacolon (Hirschsprung's disease) is an expression of autonomic nervous system dysfunction with relative decrease in parasympathetic stimulation of the colon, hence the colonic relaxation and dilatation and the rationale of employing cholinergic drugs. Among these, bethanechol (Urecholine) appears to be especially effective because of its pronounced activity in the gut, its prolonged action due to absence of cholinesterase destruction and the fact that the only annoying side action as the drug is used here is the promotion of micturition. Under 5–10 mg. dosage orally, or subcutaneously if necessary, abdominal distention often disappears, daily spontaneous stools occur without laxatives or enemas, and the barium enema shows a decrease in size of the sigmoid and the descending colon.

HYDROCEPHALUS

"I have a 2-year-old child in my practice whose head is beginning to enlarge abnormally, and of course the parents are becoming frantic. Is there any nonsurgical therapy worth trying?"

Reply: At the Massachusetts General Hospital, Peter Huttenlocher obtained a therapeutically useful effect with orally administrated acetazolamide (Diamox) when abnormal head enlargement was occurring at a rate of 1.5 cm. per month. Of the 15 children treated, aged 5 weeks to 16 years, there was cessation of the abnormal head growth in 8, in 3 of whom there was aqueductal stenosis and in the other 5 communicating hydrocephalus. The drug was also effective in a young adult in whom decompensation of hydrocephalus had led to papilledema and to symptoms of intracranial hypertension. Dosage was 30–50 mg./kg./day, increased to 100 mg. if necessary and administered in two to four divided doses. There have been a few other favorable reports of this sort, but also some that were unfavorable. It would appear that the therapy is worth a trial in any case in which the increase in head size or the signs of increased intracranial pressure have been active during the immediately preceding weeks provided there is absence of brain tumor, subdural hematoma or other surgically correctable lesions, since about 50% of untreated patients die in infancy or childhood and there are numerous instances of mental or neurologic deficits among the survivors. Acetazolamide has been shown experimentally both to lower intraocular and cerebrospinal fluid pressure and to decrease the rate of production of the cerebrospinal fluid. The fact that in 3 of Huttenlocher's cases withdrawal of the drug resulted in resumption of head enlargement makes it appear that the success achieved was not due to spontaneous arrest of the process.

Peter R. Huttenlocher. Treatment of Hydrocephalus with Acetazolamide. J. Pediat. 66:1023, 1965.

HYPERPARATHYROIDISM

"Is there any drug therapy that is helpful in hyperparathyroidism?"

Reply: The treatment is surgical, and postoperatively it is that of tetany in many instances.

HYPERTENSION

"Upon what does the successful drug therapy of moderately severe hypertension depend?"

Reply: I suppose you want an answer in two words. Well, I shall try to provide it in twenty: be alert to the necessity for alterations in drugs and dosage according to the vicissitudes of the individual case.

"When undertaking the treatment of a severely hypertensive individual with the hope of preventing the occurrence of cerebrovascular episodes, how much time must pass before one can feel that this has possibly been accomplished?"

Reply: At the widely known Hypertension Clinic in Dunedin, New Zealand, this matter was carefully studied in 457 patients by R. M. Douglas, who derived the opinion that the most dangerous time for the occurrence of such episodes appears to be during the first 4 months after initiation of hypotensive therapy, this being the time of most erratic blood pressure control in most patients. In his study some of the episodes occurred when blood pressure was high, but others were definitely precipitated by falls in blood pressure, though many of the latter were minor. There can be no doubt, I believe, that the patient who is in greatest danger is the one who takes his treatment into his own hands with an "on-again, off-again" performance regarding his use of drugs.

R. M. Douglas. Hypertensive Cerebrovascular Disease Considered in Relation to Treatment with Hypotensive Drugs. M. J. Australia 2:525, Oct. 3, 1964.

"When I begin antihypertensive therapy in a patient, will the state of his retinal vessels provide any inkling of the likelihood of a cerebrovascular episode?"

Reply: In his thorough study of this matter

in Dunedin, New Zealand, R. M. Douglas found the incidence of cerebrovascular symptoms in patients with severe grades of hypertensive retinopathy higher than in patients with mildly affected retinal vessels.

R. M. Douglas. Hypertensive Cerebrovascular Disease Considered in Relation to Treatment with Hypotensive Drugs. M. J. Australia 2:525: Oct 3, 1964.

"In private practice my greatest interest in hypertension is in treating the individual with mild or only moderately advanced disease, because in him the chance for accomplishment is greatest. The challenge here is to know just how to combine the drugs for best effects. Studies of hospitalized groups of patients are not very helpful because of the pressure-lowering effect of hospitalization itself. I like to use a thiazide derivative and combine it with other agents when necessary. Has there been published a recent study on a significant number of patients in which a thiazide was combined with another mildly acting antihypertensive and with one that was more potent, under conditions comparable to those of office and home practice?"

Reply: The study that would most nearly meet your requirement is perhaps that reported by William M. Smith's group from the double-blind controlled evaluation of several antihypertensive regimens involving chlorothiazide conducted in 305 patients in 7 Public Health Service Hospitals for a period of 3–18 months of continuous treatment. The blood pressure–lowering effect of the drugs was measured by comparing the average of home blood pressure recordings during the final month of therapy with the average of home blood pressures determined during a 1 month pretreatment control period. All patients were ambulatory throughout this study. Each of the treatment regimens (chlorothiazide alone, chlorothiazide and rauwolfia, chlorothiazide and hydralazine) was significantly more effective than placebo. The combination of chlorothiazide (Diuril), 500 mg., and rauwolfia serpentina (crude root), 100 mg. twice daily, was the most effective regimen, resulting in a lowering of the mean pressure by 20 mm. Hg to less than 140/90 mm. Hg in 68% of cases. This was statistically more effective than the same amount of the thiazide alone or in combination with hydralazine (Apresoline), 200 mg. daily. Side effects were not serious and led to discontinuance of treatment in only 6 of the 305 patients. This same group of observers have made a comparison of mebutamate (Capla) with a combination of mebutamate and chlorothiazide and with a chlorothiazide-rauwolfia preparation such as used in the preceding study. With the exception of white women, who comprised a small proportion of

their group of 151 patients who completed at least 3 months of therapy, they did not find mebutamate lowering blood pressure significantly, though the rauwolfia-chlorothiazide combination again yielded excellent results. However, there is another study, that of William Parsons, Madison, Wisconsin, in which mebutamate was found to have moderate antihypertensive activity in some, but not all, individuals in a private office practice. Obviously, more experience of this newer agent is needed under the variable conditions of practice.

William M. Smith, Anthony N. Damato, Nicholas J. Galluzzi, Claude F. Garfield, Ernest G. Hanowell, William H. Stimson, Richard H. Thurm, John J. Walsh and Louis Bromer. The Evaluation of Antihypertensive Therapy: Cooperative Clinical Trial Method. Ann. Int. Med. 61:829, 1964. William B. Parsons, Jr. Treatment of Hypertension with Mebutamate Alone and in Combination with Hydrochlorothiazide. J. New Drugs 4:188, 1964. William M. Smith, Anthony N. Damato, Claude F. Garfield, Ernest G. Hanowell, Richard H. Thurm, William B. Furgerson, Jr., Charles E. Koch, Jr., Stanley D. Korfmacher and Louis Bromer. Evaluation of Antihypertensive Therapy. J.A.M.A. 193:727, Aug. 30, 1965.

"Like everyone else, I have hypertensive patients who are completely asymptomatic. Again like everyone else, I usually consider it advisable not to attempt lowering of the pressure through the use of specific antihypertensive drugs; but occasionally it seems to me that an individual patient would profit by and should have treatment with such an agent. What drug shall I use?"

Reply: Giving thought to this subject, Agnew's group (Auckland, New Zealand) concluded that none of the drug combinations that they had tried was really suitable because their blood pressure–lowering activity was accompanied by undesirable side actions, and of course this is truly the case. The ideal drug for the hypertensive patient without symptoms should certainly be free from deleterious side actions, for there is no point in making the man sick just for the satisfaction of a lowered blood pressure reading. At least this is my feeling.

T. M. Agnew, R. O. H. Irvine and J. D. K. North. Methyldopa (Aldomet) and Hydrochlorothiazide (Hydro-Diuril, Etc.) Compared with Reserpine and Hydrochlorothiazide in Hypertension. Brit. M. J. 2:781, Sept. 28, 1963.

"A simple question: just what is accomplished by the use of antihypertensive drugs other than making the patient more comfortable?"

Reply: Such experienced observers as Irvine Page and Harriet Dustan (Cleveland Clinic) have concluded that if blood pressure can be adequately lowered and maintained long enough, the controlling mechanism may be reset; i.e., that persistent and adequate treatment with antihypertensive drugs will finally permit the omission of these drugs without recurrence of hypertension in a considerable proportion of patients. Will, then, meticulous use of the drugs also prolong life? I do not believe that Page and Dustan have made this claim, but in New Zealand, the very able group around Smirk have shown that mortality is indeed very favorably affected. In the United States, Perera found the opposite to be true, but his conditions were nothing like those in the studies of Page and Dustan and Smirk. For example, he had in his series only patients with long-standing hypertension, with signs of myocardial damage generally associated with cardiac hypertrophy and sometimes with possible early nephrosclerosis. Furthermore, there were not in his series the features which were distinctive of the Page and Dustan regimen: round-the-clock study of pressure, or insistence on a low (below 100) supine reading. Nevertheless, Perera's observations cannot be disregarded. And finally, let us fill the cup of skepticism to the full; I quote from William Goldring and Herbert Chasis, of New York University School of Medicine: "After about 15 years of data collecting, we believe that the alleged usefulness of antihypertensive drugs rests on conclusions drawn from notoriously uncertain statistical compilations compounded by equally uncertain estimates of morbidity and mortality in the natural history of a disease of highly unpredictable course."

I thank you, Sir, for your question, and you have been answered!

Irvine H. Page and Harriet P. Dustan. Persistence of Normal Blood Pressure After Discontinuing Treatment in Hypertensive Patients. Circulation 25:433, 1962. J. V. Hodge, E. G. McQueen and Horace Smirk (Univ. of Otago). Results of Hypotensive Therapy in Arterial Hypertension. Ibid. 1:1, Jan. 7, 1961. George A. Perera (Columbia University). Antihypertensive Drugs Versus Symptomatic Treatment in Primary Hypertension: Effect on Survival. J.A.M.A. 173:11, May 7, 1960. William Goldring and Herbert Chasis, in F. J. Ingelfinger, A. S. Relman and M. Finland, eds. Controversy in Internal Medicine. Phila., W. B. Saunders Co., 1966, p. 83.

"How is it that the thiazide derivatives, that are merely diuretic agents, will reduce blood pressure in my hypertensive patients who have no symptoms or signs of congestive heart failure and no edema?"

Reply: This fascinating question is not yet answered to the satisfaction of all of us. Despite such studies as that of Wilson and Freis (Georgetown University), which suggest the importance of the decrease in plasma volume in producing the hypertensive effect, the inescapable fact remains that other potent diuretics are not as hypotensive as these drugs. Dustan and associates (Cleveland Clinic) have expressed the unique opinion that the thiazides enhance responsiveness to the other antihypertensive drugs by causing oligemia, which intensifies vasomotor tone; since this increases the fraction of the hypertension that is sustained by the vasomotor system, there is established a degree of neurogenic hypertension of the sort susceptible to relief by the other antihypertensive agents. With regard to a possible action antagonistic to the sympathomimetic amines, Aleksandrow's group found that a short course of thiazide therapy reduced the pressor effect of norepinephrine in 20 patients with mild hypertension, this occurring without constant lowering of plasma volume and with very little changes of the basal blood pressure levels. Actually, in animal experimentation, Preziosi and associates have shown that chlorothiazide decreases the vasopressor responses to epinephrine and norepinephrine and exerts a depressant action on peripheral vascular smooth muscle. A simple answer to your question, therefore, cannot be supplied, by me at least.

Ilse M. Wilson and Edward D. Freis. Relationship Between Plasma and Extracellular Fluid Volume Depletion and Antihypertensive Effect of Chlorothiazide (Diuril). Circulation 20:1028, 1959. H. P. Dustan, G. R. Cumming, A. C. Corcoran, and I. H. Page. A Mechanism of Chlorothiazide-Enhanced Effectiveness of Antihypertensive Ganglioplegic Drugs. Circulation 19:360, 1959. D. Aleksandrow, W. Wysznacka, and J. Gajewski. Influence of Chlorothiazide Upon Arterial Responsiveness to Norepinephrine in Hypertensive Subjects. New England J. Med. 261:1052, 1959. P. Preziosi, A. Bianchi, B. Loscalzo and A. F. de Schaepdryver. On the Pharmacology of Chlorothiazide with Special Regard to its Diuretic and Antihypertensive Effects. Arch. Internat. Pharmacodyn. 118:467, 1959.

"We are told to pay careful attention to the electrolyte balance of patients on thiazide derivatives, but this cannot always be easily done in private practice. What are the conditions most likely to upset this balance?"

Reply: Hypokalemia, the cause of most concern, may result from excessive perspiration in hot weather, in any situation in which there is associated vomiting, where there is postoperative loss of electrolytes, during digitalis or corticosteroid or corticotropin administration, in the cirrhotic patient and in the one who is elderly and debilitated, and in the patient with severe renal disease in whom there is pre-existing potassium depletion; diarrhea may also cause potassium depletion as paracentesis will do also.

"When I give chlorothiazide (Diuril) to my pregnant patient will there be action on the fetus also?"

Reply: There should be, since James Garnet (Pennsylvania Hospital, Philadelphia) showed that in 15 cases maternal and fetal plasma levels of the drug were comparable, though in 2 cases the drug could not be found in either maternal or fetal blood and in 2 others it was found only in the maternal plasma.

James D. Garnet. Placental Transfer of Chlorothiazide (Diuril). Obst. & Gynec. 21:123, 1963.

"Since the thiazide-induced hyperuricemia can be reversed by the concomitant use of a uricosuric agent, would it not be rational therapy to use a drug from each of the categories in combination in routine therapy?"

Reply: Maybe so, but I am too old-fashioned to feel quite at ease in suggesting that the use of an antidotal agent be employed each time we give an active drug. I simply don't like the thing, though admittedly Beisel and Forsham (University of California) have shown it to be feasible. With their hydrochlorothiazide (Hydro-Diuril), 50 mg. every 8 hours, or their chlorthalidone (Hygroton), 100 mg. daily, they combined probenecid (Benemid), 250 mg. every 8 hours; likewise, with 100 mg. of chlorthalidone daily they combined 50 mg. of sulfinpyrazone (Anturan) every 8 hours.

William R. Beisel and Peter H. Forsham. Reversal of Thiazide-Induced Transient Hyperuricemia by Uricosuric Agents. New England J. Med. 267:1225, Dec. 13, 1962.

"In treating hypertension it seems to me that I fail with thiazide diuretic combinations (with or without reserpine) in about half my patients. Should I do better than this?"

Reply: That seems to be par or perhaps just a bit above. A recent report of representative experience was that of Bryant and associates at Bellevue Hospital, who found it necessary in a group of 100 ambulatory outpatients with moderate to severe essential hypertension to augment such combinations as you have mentioned with a postganglionic sympathetic blocking agent in 42 instances.

J. Marion Bryant, Lucian Fletcher, Jr., Natalio Schvartz, Harrison Fertig and Richard B. F. Quan. The Role of Postganglionic Sympathetic Blockade in Antihypertensive Therapy. J.A.M.A. 193:1021, Sept. 20, 1965.

"One of my associates has been using chlorthalidone (Hygroton) instead of the thiazide diuretics under the impression that it is less toxic, but now he has a case of acute hemorrhagic pancreatitis on his hands. Has this been seen before?"

Reply: Yes it has, and in fact it would seem to be a wise precaution to consider this drug to be about equivalent to the thiazide derivative diuretics in its toxic potentialities, although it does differ somewhat from them chemically.

Martin F. Jones and John R. Caldwell (Henry Ford Hospital). Acute Hemorrhagic Pancreatitis Associated with Administration of Chlorthalidone: Report of a Case. New England J. Med. 267:1029, Nov. 15, 1962.

"I have a hypertensive patient on hydrochlorothiazide (Hydro-Diuril, etc.) in whom I would not like to resort to a blocking agent for more blood pressure-lowering effect than I am getting with the thiazide drug; would I gain anything by adding the new drug, ethacrynic acid?"

Reply: At the University of Michigan, Conway and Leonetti studied this matter and found ethacrynic acid to have antihypertensive properties similar to those of hydrochlorothiazide and that its addition to hydrochlorothiazide augmented the hypotensive effect of the latter. The more severely hypertensive patients in their series had a fall in mean blood pressure on combination therapy from 210/122 to 168/112 mm. Hg and a reduction in body weight of 12 pounds. The patients felt well and continued working, but there was an average rise in BUN of 18.6 mg./100 ml.

James Conway and Gastone Leonetti. Hypotensive Effect of Ethacrinic Acid. Circulation 31:661, 1965.

"In a recent patient who had been on reserpine for some time for treatment for hypertension, I was unable to withdraw the drug as recommended by the manufacturers before elective surgery. Nothing unfortunate occurred. What is the recorded experience?"

Reply: It is of course the fear of significant hypotension and bradycardia during surgery in the patient taking the drug that has provoked the manufacturer's warning. Wayne Munson and John Jenicek observed considerable lability of neurocirculatory balance in about half of a small group of patients who continued on reserpine therapy up to 5 days or less before surgery, and they concluded that rauwolfia derivatives should therefore probably be withdrawn 10–14 days before elective operations. They therefore withdrew 16 patients from reserpine therapy 8 days or more before operation, and found that despite this withdrawal 7 of them exhibited neurocirculatory instability during the induction of general anesthesia. Since this incidence of undesirable effects did not differ significantly from that in their original series, they returned to the policy of continuing reserpine therapy in the period before elective surgery. They also made no alterations in preanesthetic medication or in the choice of a general anesthetic agent, but it is to be noted that, unless contraindicated, they used scopolamine for belladonna effect; this is probably important as a preventive measure against hypotension and bradycardia.

Wayne M. Munson and John A. Jenicek. Effect of Anesthetic Agents on Patients Receiving Reserpine Therapy. Anesthesiology 23:741, 1962.

"What can be accomplished with the rauwolfia preparations in hypertension and what are the dosages of the several preparations and the side actions?"

Reply: In mild and uncomplicated hypertension a modest fall in blood pressure can be accomplished in perhaps a third, certainly no more than a half, of the cases. Rauwolfia is of little value when used alone in protracted employment in cases of more severe hypertension, but use of the preparations in conjunction with more potent hypotensive agents often enables the latter to achieve their blood pressure reduction and symptom alleviation with much reduced dosage.

Usual dosages of the Rauwolfia preparations employed in treating hypertension are as follows: alseroxylon (Rauwiloid), 2–4 mg. daily; deserpidine (Harmonyl), 0.25 mg. three or four times daily, possibly less as effect is established; rauwolfia (Raudixin, Rauserpa, Rauval), 200–400 mg. daily in divided doses; rescinnamine (Moderil), 0.5 mg. daily, possibly less after several weeks; reserpine (Reserpoid, Serpasil, etc.), orally, 0.25–1.0 mg. daily in two or three divided doses (sometimes lower dosage after a while), intramuscularly, 5–10 mg.; syrosingopine (Singoserp), 1 mg. daily for 2 weeks, then increasing very slowly up to 3 mg. if necessary.

In the lower dosage range that may sometimes be employed when the rauwolfia drugs are used in combination with other antihypertensives they are not very toxic. But numerous annoying side actions occur not uncommonly (nasal stuffiness, sometimes accompanied by dryness of the mouth; increased gastrointestinal activity and diarrhea; weight gain; rise in free and total hydrochloric acid and increase in volume in gastric secretion that does not respond to anticholinergic or antihistaminic drugs; and rarely peptic ulceration, epistaxis and skin eruptions). When full dosage must be used the disturbances are of considerable magnitude, with severe mental depression leading the list. These depressions do not always resolve quickly upon withdrawal of the drug, and this can be a catastrophic thing.

On the basis of some disturbing experiences several observers have considered that reserpine promotes fluid retention, which might contribute to heart failure in susceptible subjects. Orthostatic hypotension occasionally occurs following parenteral administration. The drugs have caused so few allergic reactions that doubt of their allergenicity has been expressed. Observers several years ago found that administration of reserpine alleviated the symptoms of thyrotoxicosis without changing the blood protein-bound iodine level and warned that the increasing use of the drug for other purposes might cause some cases of hyperthyroidism to go undetected. Attention has been drawn to the danger of severe reactions when combining reserpine and electroconvulsive therapy and the establishment of a reversible parkinsonism-like state has been reported. The changes in kidney function, output of urine and sodium excretion are not indicative of specific action of the drug on the kidneys. Reduce dosage radically if there has been a recent stroke.

"The conventional recommendation for parenteral administration of reserpine in hypertensive crises is that it be given in dosage of 2.5 – 10 mg.; but if a patient has recently had a stroke, is this still safe dosage?"

Reply: Whether it may properly be considered "safe" or not I do not know, but Stanley Leonberg, Jr., and associates (Pennsylvania Hospital, Philadelphia) have shown that such patients do not need large amounts since they will often respond to doses as small as one fiftieth or one hundredth of those commonly used. They reason that a cerebrovascular accident may increase an already elevated blood pressure by peripheral vasoconstriction and release of norepinephrine from arterial walls; the sudden introduction of reserpine would then rapidly deplete the remaining peripheral norepinephrine stores to deplete vasomotor tone and cause an abrupt fall in blood pressure. Another speculation was that serotonin release by clotted blood within the brain would cause local vasoconstriction and sensitize the hypothalamus and reticular formation; then sudden introduction of reserpine would produce a response greater than would otherwise occur.

Stanley C. Leonberg, Jr., Joseph B. Green and Frank A. Elliott. Response of Stroke Patients to Very Small Doses of Parenteral Reserpine. Ann. Int. Med. 60:866, May, 1964.

"One hears the 'rauwolfia derivatives' glibly referred to but never with a listing. What are the principal members of this group and what are the reactions to them?"

Reply: Reserpine (Reserpoid, Serpasil, etc.), an ester alkaloid obtained from rauwolfia root. Rauwolfia (Raudixin, Rauserpa, etc.), the powdered whole root of the rauwolfia plant. Alseroxylon (Rauwiloid), an alkaloidal fraction from rauwolfia root. Deserpidine (Harmonyl), an alkaloid from rauwolfia root. Rescinnamine (Moderil), an alkaloid of the alseroxylon fraction of rauwolfia root. Syrosingopine (Singoserp), a preparation made from reserpine by hydrolysis and re-esterification.

The more serious reactions are excessive drowsiness, fatigue and a sense of weakness, sometimes with aching of the extremities, insomnia and nightmares, excitement and irrational behavior or an incapacitating degree of agitated depression. Sometimes, but unpredictably, the concomitant use of a central nervous system stimulant will satisfactorily counteract the depression, but the patient frequently reaches the depths of despair, and there have been a number of suicides.

On the basis of some disturbing experiences several observers have considered that reserpine promotes fluid retention, which might contribute to heart failure in susceptible subjects. Orthostatic hypotension occasionally occurs following parenteral administration. The drugs have caused so few allergic reactions that doubt of their allergenicity has been expressed. Observers several years ago found that administration of reserpine alleviated the symptoms of thyrotoxicosis without changing the blood protein-bound iodine level and warned that the increasing use of the drug for other purposes might cause some cases of hyperthyroidism to go undetected. Attention has been drawn to the danger of severe reactions when combining reserpine and electroconvulsive therapy, and the establishment of a reversible parkinsonism-like state has been reported. The changes in kidney function, output of urine and sodium excretion are not indicative of a specific action of the drug on the kidneys.

"Two of my patients on guanethidine (Ismelin) medication for hypertension have mentioned that they have experienced difficulty in ejaculation upon occasion, and therefore wondered whether the drug might not be effectively promoted as a male contraceptive?"

Reply: As a matter of fact, Kiessling and Huhnstock (Heidelberg) investigated this matter of ejaculation disturbance, which they said had been reported in as many as 63% of men who were studied with this in mind, and concluded that the thing might be regarded as due to a selective, reversible arrest of secretions of the prostate gland and seminal vesicles in spermatogenesis, the ejaculation mechanism not being directly involved. They questioned whether testicular damage had occurred in their patients. So far as use of the drug as a male contraceptive is concerned, I should think that the only men who could be interested would be those, if there are such, who employ intercourse only as a form of exercise.

W. Kiessling and K. Huhnstock. Aspermia After Peroral Guanethidine (Ismelin) Medication. Klin. Wchnschr. 41:948, Oct. 1, 1963.

"I have a patient in whom symptoms resembling those of systemic lupus erythematosus have persisted for somewhat more than a year after cessation of the administration of hydralazine (Apresoline) that appeared to be the inducing agent. Has there been other experience of this sort?"

Reply: There is a group of occurrences with this drug, none having a very high incidence, that comprise the "hydralazine syndrome," which is not always completely reversible soon after cessation of the drug's use. In fact, Eugene Hildreth and associates (University of Pennsylvania) noted the persistence of some aspects of this syndrome in at least 4 of their 11 patients several years after the drug had been withdrawn. A rheumatoid arthritis–like condition, as well as lupus erythematosus, hepatosplenomegaly, and accelerated sedimentation rate have probably been the principal manifestations of this persisting deleterious action of the drug.

Eugene A. Hildreth, Carlos E. Biro and Thomas A. McCreary. Persistence of "Hydralazine Syndrome": Follow-up Study of 11 Cases. J.A.M.A. 173:657, June 11, 1960.

"Since methyldopa (Aldomet) has seemed in my practice to control blood pressure in the hypertensive patient about as do the other autonomic blocking agents, i.e., with a predominant effect on standing pressure, I have not been able clearly to determine what advantage there is in using it. Am I overlooking something?"

Reply: Have you not found that in the early treatment of severe cases with this drug you can sometimes effect a quick pressure adjustment without incurring the prolonged hypotension that may characterize guanethidine's (Ismelin) action? Some men have had this experience with fair regularity, but admittedly the drug may occasionally be ineffective when used alone as an agent for long-term control in cases of severe hypertension. In some practices it is used with an oral diuretic in cases of mild or moderate severity, and with guanethidine, with or without the diuretic, in more severe cases.

James Conway, Andrew J. Zweifler and Stevo Julius (Univ. of Michigan). Place of Methyldopa (Aldomet) in Treatment of Severe Hypertension. J.A.M.A. 186:266, Oct. 19, 1963. J. W. Leonard, Ray W. Gifford, Jr., and D. C. Humphrey. Treatment of Hypertension with Methyldopa Alone or Combined with Diuretics and/or Guanethidine. Am. Heart J. 69:610, 1965.

"Without reference to their respective incidences, my associates and I have recorded the following occurrences in connection with the use of methyldopa (Aldomet) in our hypertensives: orthostatic hypotension, excessive sedation, mouth dryness, fever, bradycardia, gastrointestinal disturbances, slight liver function disturbances, arthralgia, edema, leukopenia, dizziness and giddiness, reversible psychic depression. What else have we missed? This is a good drug, but we would like to know the whole story."

Reply: That is about the list, except for recent intimations of hemolytic anemia associated with the drug's use. Impotence has been reported in rare instances; have you seen this? And occasionally a breakdown of the drug or of its metabolites will provide a very dark urine, about which of course the patient complains.

"I have a hypertensive patient under treatment with guanethidine (Ismelin), whose gain in weight appears to be due to fluid retention. Is this a correct assumption?"

Reply: There have been reports of fluid retention associated with the use of practically all of the more potent antihypertensive agents. True explanation of this is lacking, but the speculations are that the retention results from impairment of renal function consequent on postural hypotension, venous pooling in the extremities or reduction in cardiac output.

"It is common experience with all of us that we frequently get better results in treating hypertension through the use of several of the hypotensive agents in low dosage combinations than through the use of any one of them in full dosage. Since the combined drugs often act differently and at different sites, might this mean that the pathologic anatomy in the disease resides at different sites?"

Reply: Could be, but that is all I can say.

"Can you suggest anything to control an otherwise intractable headache in a hypertensive?"

Reply: At the Cleveland Clinic, H. Saint-Pierre's group used sodium thiocyanate effectively in 11 of 15 patients of this sort, only 1 of whom required a second intravenous injection; relief was less in 3 others and 1 (an

early case) was not helped at all. The effect was manifest in a few hours after the injection and lasted 5 days or more. *Dosage:* 1.396 Gm. of sodium thiocyanate to make 20 ml. of solution. This injection is unlikely to be associated with any reactions, but the drug is potentially very toxic and therefore one should be constantly on guard and discontinue these injections if any sort of untoward symptoms appear other than perhaps mild lassitude and weakness. Nausea, vomiting and striking weakness are often significant of beginning severe toxicity, in which there may also be a component of serious mental disturbance.

H. Saint-Pierre, A. C. Corcoran, R. D. Taylor and H. P. Dustan. Relief of Hypertensive Headache by Intravenous Injection of Thiocyanate. J.A.M.A. 152:493, 1953.

"I have recently had a patient who was on a combination of pargyline (Eutonyl) and hydrochlorothiazide (Hydro-Diuril) and was given meperidine (Demerol) and scopolamine as premedication for necessary surgery. He quickly went into coma, from which he recovered only after many hours and rather frantic resuscitory measures on our part. What was involved here and what might have hastened the recovery?"

Reply: What happened was that Eutonyl, a monoamine oxidase inhibitor, had potentiated the depressant action of Demerol. The drugs of this group, i.e., the monoamine oxidase inhibitors—Marplan, Nardil, Niamid, Eutonyl, Parnate—have been known to have this effect upon not only nonopiate analgesics such as Demerol but upon the narcotic analgesics, barbiturates, sympathomimetic agents, antihistamines and the ganglionic blocking agents. As to what sort of measure might have been helpful in hastening recovery, Vigran (Los Angeles) suggests the use of acidifying agents, such as intravenous sodium biphosphate, lysine or arginine hydrochloride, to aid in removal of Demerol from the body. I doubt, however, whether this would be very helpful because less than 10% of the drug is usually excreted unchanged, most of it being rather quickly destroyed in the liver. Did your patient have disturbed liver function?

I. Myron Vigran. Dangerous Potentiation of Meperidine (Demerol) Hydrochloride by Pargyline (Eutonyl) Hydrochloride. J.A.M.A. 187:953, Mar. 21, 1964.

"Occasionally in a patient with hypertension I have prescribed a 5 mg. oral dose of pilocarpine to antidote the overaction of a ganglionic blocking agent such as pentolinium (Ansolysen) with good effect, but I am always apprehensive lest the patient take an overdose of the pilocarpine and compound the situation through the toxic effects of this drug. What would be the signs and symptoms of excessive pilocarpine action?"

Reply: They would essentially be those of the overaction of the group of acetylcholine congeners, with sweating, lacrimation, salivation, vomiting, urinary urgency and incipient pulmonary edema predominating; confusion, tremor and mild convulsions might occur before death through cardiac failure and/or pulmonary edema.

"I think that we have all seen instances in which straining at stool has directly provoked a cerebrovascular accident. Has the incidence of this sort of thing been higher in individuals who are taking the antihypertensive drugs?"

Reply: I do not believe that a study of the matter has ever been reported, but some of these drugs, notably the ganglionic blocking agents, are quite likely to cause stubborn constipation. Laxative drugs could of course successfully combat this effect and obviate the complication you fear.

"Sometimes it has seemed to me that when starting the treatment of a new hypertensive patient merely with a placebo to determine the extent of his reactivity to the therapy situation alone, the individual with very high pressure responds better to this approach than one with a more moderate pressure. Has this sort of thing ever been looked into?"

Reply: Only indirectly, I should say. Grenfell and associates (University of Mississippi) observed, in the course of their controlled double-blind comparative study of a number of antihypertensive drugs, that oral placebo caused a significant drop in pressure in individuals with pressures exceeding 200/120 mm. Hg but not in those with pressures between 150/100 and 200/120 mm. Hg. I do not know what significance this has, if any, but feel sure that it is not universal placebo experience. Very interesting it is, however.

Raymond F. Grenfell, Arthur H. Briggs and William C. Holland. Antihypertensive Drugs Evaluated in Controlled Double-Blind Study. South. M. J. 56:1410, 1963.

"I have heard it rumored that antithyroid drugs have been effectively used in maligant hypertension when the true antihypertensive agents have failed, but I hesitate to try this. Is this really effective therapy?"

Reply: I know of only one man who is in the literature with the antithyroid agents in this situation and no one personally who is using them. George Perera (Columbia University) feels he has evidence that such an antithyroid drug as methimazole (Tapazole) may interfere with the progression of the accelerated form of hypertension. He has speculated that the drug interferes with autonomic nervous system responses, that there occurs a check to necrotizing arteriolitis at a local tissue level, or that antithyroid drugs affect sodium balance. I wish that someone would study the matter independently.

George A. Perera. Methimazole (Tapazole) in "Malignant" Hypertension: Report of Patient's Progress after Two Years. Am. J. M. Sc. 247:175, 1964.

"One of my associates is using mebutamate (Capla) with results that please him in cases of mild hypertension. Has a controlled study of this drug been made in this situation?"

Reply: Yes, at Oak Forest Hospital, in Illinois, Eugene Chesrow and associates treated 36 patients with mild essential hypertension with mebutamate, phenobarbital and a placebo in a comparative study conducted under double-blind conditions. Statistically significant reductions in blood pressure were obtained with mebutamate, but not with the other preparations, and it appears that symptoms associated with this mild hypertension (chiefly headache, dizziness and shortness of breath) also responded better to mebutamate. Usual dosage of the drug was 300 mg. four times daily.

Eugene J. Chesrow, Max Bernstein, Donald Weiss and Gilbert H. Marquardt. Comparison of Mebutamate, Phenobarbital, and Placebo in the Treatment of Mild Essential Hypertension. Am. J. M. Sc. 251:166, 1966.

"What is the best drug to use in attempting to control the acute crisis of severely elevated pressure in a hypertensive?"

Reply: This is a very serious situation because such a crisis may quickly damage the brain, retina, heart and kidneys, and if you drop the pressure too rapidly through use of a very potent agent you are in danger of inducing renal failure or causing respiratory arrest if there is papilledema with encephalopathy. I cannot nominate a "best" drug because any one of those to be discussed may be "best" or "worst" in a given individual.

HEXAMETHONIUM (BISTRIUM, ETC.). In using this drug intravenously to control a hypertensive crisis, the attempt is usually made to lower the mean blood pressure 20–30 mm. Hg or even more in the absence of excessive side actions, through slow injection of 50–100 mg. during 10–20 minutes while watching the blood pressure. In my opinion the drug should be considered contraindicated in the presence of a damaged myocardium, and in a patient with diabetes mellitus, in whom it may precipitate severe hypoglycemic reactions, and it may also direly affect the individual who has recently hemorrhaged severely because it will very likely prevent compensatory vasoconstrictor responses. There have been several reports of pulmonary lesions associated with hexamethonium therapy for hypertension. The drug has no toxic action on parenchymatous organs, the central nervous system or the hematopoietic system.

VERATRUM PREPARATIONS. These drugs are given by intravenous injection or effusion or by spaced intramuscular injections. When veratrum is given parenterally the blood pressure response has two phases: (1) a sharp and often fluctuating decrease in arterial pressure, pulse rate and peripheral blood flow; (2) a steady state of reduced arterial pressure and pulse rate with return of renal, hepatic and muscle blood flow to control volumes. In the second phase, cardiac output is the same as in the pretreatment period. It appears, therefore, that a decrease in resistance occurs in all peripheral areas without the compensating tachycardia and palpitation that characterize the action of such peripheral vasodilators as the ganglionic blocking agents. With the normal cardiac output and unreduced supply of blood to the vital organs, circulatory equilibrium is maintained despite the lowered arterial pressure.

Initial parenteral dosage of protoveratrine A and B (Veralba) in crises is usually 0.3–0.5 ml. (0.06–0.1 mg.), increasing by small increments after several hours if necessary. Whatever response is to be had from a single intravenous dose is usually present in less than 30 minutes and lasts from 1½ to 3 hours. Sometimes the preparation is given in dilute solution of 2 mg. in 200 ml. of 5% glucose, infusing in the beginning at the rate of 3–6 ml. per 10 minutes, later at only half this rate.

The unfortunate and limiting feature of veratrum's employment is that toxic effects, which seem to be an integral part of the reflex pattern of the drug's action, occur with almost prohibitive frequency. Symptoms are nausea and vomiting; substernal tightness; excessive salivation; paresthesias about the mouth, jaws, hands and feet; excessive hypotension and bradycardia; and collapse. Blurring of vision is a rare occurrence. Transient oliguria sometimes reflects a period of antidiuresis of obscure nature. It is best not to use the drug in cases complicated by renal failure because lowering of blood pressure may make the failure worse. Previously damaged kidneys do not seem to be harmed, but it should be considered that Adams-Stokes disease and carotid sinus irritability are contraindications. Veratrum is not a myocardial depressant and does not lower cardiac output, hence congestive failure in individuals with hypertension may actually be improved if the drug causes pressure to fall. Atropine sulfate, 1 mg. (1/60 grain)

intramuscularly or intravenously, is effective against bradycardia and to some extent against the vomiting; ephedrine sulfate, 50 mg. (5/6 grain) intramuscularly, acts against the hypotension.

RAUWOLFIA PREPARATIONS. The shortcoming of these drugs is that their full hypotensive effect is usually not achieved under 2 hours and is quite variable. Serpasil intramuscular dosage is 5–10 mg. The numerous annoying side actions occur not uncommonly but some of them, by reason of their very nature, need not be anticipated in this emergency use of the drug; they are discussed in an earlier Reply in this Hypertension section.

SODIUM NITROPRUSSIDE. This drug has been very little used, but upon the occasion of receiving an honorary degree at one of the European Universities in mid-1965, Irvine Page said that he still knows of no drug that more effectively lowers blood pressure than sodium nitroprusside. Some years ago it was said that at the Mayo Clinic the drug is stored in stoppered bottles of 60 mg. in 25 ml. of 0.9% sodium chloride, adding this to a liter of 5% glucose for infusion. Such an infusion, administered at 10–30 drops/minute, must be done under close supervision at all times because the induced blood pressure drop is precipitous and small variations in rate of flow may cause wide pressure fluctuation. Apprehension, restlessness, perspiration and retching indicate excessive speed of delivery.

TRIMETHAPHAN CAMPHORSULFONATE (ARFONAD), a ganglion-blocking agent, is popular just now because it both acts and is disposed of very quickly. Most men dissolve it, 1 mg./ml., in 5% glucose and inject at the rate of about 4 ml./minute; be very careful after 50 mg. have been introduced.

PENTOLINIUM (ANSOLYSEN). Some men use this drug in crisis, but it is very hard to handle because it may suddenly cause excessive hypotension. However, this matter of induced hypotension is the tricky aspect of the whole approach to the hypertensive crisis, because you may suddenly compound the felony by having an anuric patient on your hands. Inject pentolinium slowly intravenously in a solution of 10 mg./20 ml. under constant monitoring of the blood pressure.

SUCROSE. Sometimes sucrose injections adequately substitute for venesection to deplete the circulation in hypertensive encephalopathy. Blood pressure is little affected, but spinal fluid pressure usually falls promptly, and during the 8–12 hours before it returns to the previous level there may have been considerable subsidence of headache, vomiting, vertigo and twitching. Dosage is 300–500 ml. of 50% solution, diuresis beginning in 2 hours and usually lasting for 6 hours. Sucrose appears in the spinal fluid in very low concentration, even when there are hemorrhages in the central nervous system. The use of sucrose is much restricted by the fact that it causes characteristic lesions of the renal convoluted tubules in both experimental animals and man, and also because there is always some risk attached to intravenous injection of large quantities of any fluid in a cardiovascular disturbance.

"I have used sodium nitroprusside recently with good effect in a hypertensive emergency. Would it be feasible to continue the use of this agent for a prolonged period?"

Reply: I am unaware of any evidence that the drug would lose its efficacy when used for a prolonged period, but I would draw your attention to the experience of David Nourok and associates (University of California at Los Angeles), whose patient, though having her blood pressure effectively lowered through continuous intravenous infusion of the drug for 21 days, also developed hypothyroidism and retention of thiocyanate.

David S. Nourok, Richard J. Glassock, David H. Solomon and Morton H. Maxwell. Hypothyroidism Following Prolonged Sodium Nitroprusside Therapy. Am. J. M. Sc. 248:129, 1964.

HYPOMETABOLISM WITHOUT THYROIDAL DEFICIENCY

"What is the evidence that use of thyroid preparations is efficacious in the treatment of patients with hypometabolism without thyroidal deficiency?"

Reply: It does not seem to me that there is any good evidence. At Washington University, Marvin Levin made a double-blind control study of therapy in 18 patients with this alleged malady, employing liothyronine (Cytomel), levothyroxine (Synthroid) and a placebo. All of the patients said they felt less weak, less fatigued and less nervous after 1 month regardless of the agent they had been given, and the placebo as well as the active drugs was sometimes associated with an elevated B.M.R. In the study of Charles Reynolds and E. Perry McCullagh, at the Cleveland Clinic, there was observed a striking absence of response of both symptoms and B.M.R. to high dosage of both liothyronine (Cytomel) and desiccated thyroid. I think that most observers agree with Levin that the term "metabolic insufficiency" is vague and misleading and could well be dropped since the patients tagged with this diagnosis probably do not have a discrete biochemical lesion but an underlying psycho-logic disorder that does not directly involve the thyroid.

Charles W. Reynolds and E. Perry McCullagh. Desiccated Thyroid and l-Triiodothyronine Administration in Hypometabolism Without Thyroidal Deficiency. Cleveland Clin. Quart. 28:70, 1961. Marvin E. Levin. "Metabolic Insufficiency": Double-Blind Study Using Triiodothyronine, Thyroxin and Placebo; Psychometric Evaluation of Hypometabolic Patient. J. Clin. Endocrinol. 20:106, 1960.

HYPOPARATHYROIDISM

"One of my associates has had a patient with post-thyroidectomy hypoparathyroidism on probenecid (Benemid) with very good effect for about 2 years. What could be the explanation of the drug's action in such a case?"

Reply: The renal tubular reabsorption of phosphorus is lessened by probenecid, which will result in a decreasing of hyperphosphatemia and an increasing of phosphaturia. This interesting drug effects several other changes as a result of its action in the kidneys: lessening of tubular reabsorption of excessive urates, which justifies its use in gout; increasing the plasma titer of penicillin and para-aminosalicylic acid, which is not of as great importance nowadays as formerly; and lessening the urinary excretion of phenolsulfonphthalein and Diodrast.

Barkley Beidleman (Pensacola, Florida). Treatment of Chronic Hypoparathyroidism with Probenecid (Benemid). Metabolism 7:690, 1958.

HYPOPITUITARISM

"In a case of hypopituitarism that has been in our practice for some time we failed to effect much relief through use of corticotropin (ACTH) in the beginning but are now quite satisfied with the result obtained through use of corticosteroids, though we find we can use these drugs only in rather low dosage since the patient seems very prone to develop symptoms of overaction. Would it be safe to give her estrogens in the attempt to provoke a menstrual cycle?"

Reply: The answer is yes, and actually testosterone may provide a puny sort of libido in the male.

HYPOTHYROIDISM

"For many years I have been using desiccated thyroid with satisfaction in my hypothyroid patients, but recently I have heard that a spot check by Government officials has found some of these thyroid preparations to be substandard

despite fulfilling U.S.P. specifications. Should I abandon the desiccated thyroid substance for one of the newer preparations?"

Reply: Unfortunately, the Pharmacopoeia fails to specify the species source of the thyroid, and this can make a difference between preparations since the metabolic activity of pig thyroid is much greater than that of cattle or sheep. But you are completely safeguarded if you use exclusively the thyroid tablets of a single manufacturer because you can count on invariably achieving the result in subsequent cases that you obtained the first time these tablets were used, which might not always be the case if you switch to the tablet of another manufacturer whose source may be different or in whose processing methods there may be slight differences. In order to insure that your patient obtains full value from the prescribed tablet it might be an advisable precaution to have him chew it instead of swallowing it whole because some of the tablets tend to become less absorbable with age; but this might be an objectionable thing for some patients. Abandoning your practice of using desiccated thyroid substance in favor of one of the newer compounds might make it difficult for you to follow the course of the patient's progress until you become acquainted with certain differences in the effects of these agents if you use the protein-bound iodine (PBI) of serum rather than a B.M.R. determination to guide you. At Yale University, Paul Lavietes and Franklin Epstein treated patients with hypothyroidism with U.S.P. desiccated thyroid, thyroglobulin (Proloid), sodium levothyroxine (Synthroid Sodium) and sodium liothyronine (Cytomel), using all of the drugs in dosage that was roughly equivalent in effectiveness. They found that in patients treated with U.S.P. thyroid substance the PBI was low to midnormal, in those treated with thyroglobulin it was subnormal, in those treated with levothyroxine it was high normal to supernormal and in those treated with liothyronine it was almost nil. The same effects can be obtained with levothyroxine as with thyroid substance, but experience with the drug is still relatively limited in comparison with the considerable experience with thyroid substance, and it seems to me to have no apparent advantages over the natural product for continuous maintenance use in chronic hypothyroid states provided one uses always a familiar thyroid preparation. As for liothyronine, you must remember that it has a short duration of action in comparison with thyroid substance and levothyroxine, and that its omission may cause distressing withdrawal symptoms. Of course if a myxedematous patient needs the rapid and powerful action it can provide in order to be saved from death, then its use would certainly be indicated.

Paul H. Lavietes and Franklin H. Epstein. Thyroid Therapy of Myxedema: Comparison of Various Agents with Note on Composition of Thyroid Secretion in Man. Ann. Int. Med. 60:79, 1964.

"In a patient who has both hypothyroidism and adrenal insufficiency, which should be corrected first?"

Reply: Use the corticosteroids first because in the presence of adrenal insufficiency the thyroid preparations may engender an increased tissue demand for the adrenocortical hormones and thus precipitate an acute adrenal crisis.

"I have a myxedematous patient who is responding to thyroid therapy unusually in that there are periods in which the usually effective dosage does not seem fully protective. What could cause such variations in response to the drug?"

Reply: The two most usual reasons for such a situation are that the patient is not ingesting the drug with necessary regularity or that she is shopping about for less expensive thyroid tablets and at times using some that are substandard. Of course intercurrent episodes of diarrhea might conceivably lessen absorption of the hormone, and it might be worthwhile drawing your attention to the case reported by Aldo Pinchera and associates at the Massachusetts General Hospital, in whose cretinous patient with milk allergy it was found that a soy bean formula strikingly decreased the absorption of thyroxine. Could it be that your patient goes on "debauches" of Chinese food with large amounts of soy sauce?

Aldo Pinchera, Margaret H. MacGillivray, John D. Crawford and Allan G. Freeman. Thyroid Refractoriness in an Athyreotic Cretin Fed Soybean Formula. New England J. Med. 273:83, July 8, 1965.

"I have a patient with hypothyroidism who has responded well to desiccated thyroid in all particulars except the severe constipation. Is it possible that a switch to one of the newer thyroid compounds would be more effective in the control of this symptom?"

Reply: The matter has never been studied in a significant number of cases, to my knowledge, but I can cite the experience of Bengt Skanse (University of Lund) in 7 women with hypothyroidism. In these patients the constipation continued resistant even when he raised thyroid dosage sufficiently that the signs and symptoms of overdosage appeared. Then he returned the thyroid dosage to about its original level and added liothyronine (Cytomel) or placebo tablets in a double-blind study for 4 weeks at a time. It was said that frequency of bowel movements increased significantly in 5 of the 7 patients, without significant change in the B.M.R. readings. There were signs of thyroid overaction only in the 2 patients in whom there was no effect on the constipation. The patients who responded to the combination of thyroid substance and liothyronine were said to have remained free from constipation for follow-up periods of 6 months to 4 years.

Bengt Skanse. Supplemental Triiodothyronine in Treatment of Constipation of Hypothyroidism Resistant to Desiccated Thyroid. Acta med. scandinav. 173:251, 1963.

"What would be the usual differences in cost to the myxedematous patient of desiccated thyroid substance and the new synthetic preparations?"

Reply: At Johns Hopkins Hospital, Prout has made the following estimate of annual cost to the patient taking desiccated thyroid substance in dosage of 128 mg. and the other preparations in comparable amounts: thyroid U.S.P., $1.82; trade named thyroid, $5.50; Synthroid, $10.85 (reduced to $4.20/1000 when bought in lots of 5000); Cytomel, $47.52.

T. E. Prout. Desiccated Thyroid, Thyroxin and Triiodothyronine. Bull. Johns Hopkins Hosp. 117:195, 1965.

IDIOPATHIC HYPERCALCEMIA

"In the treatment of idiopathic hypercalcemia through reduction of the vitamin D intake as much as possible by dietary measures and use of corticosteroids, and the use of a low calcium diet, are there any drugs that are of positive value?"

Reply: None that I know of.

IDIOPATHIC HYPOGLYCEMIA

"I have an infant with idiopathic hypoglycemia that I have gotten past the acute stage through use of intravenous glucose, but what sort of long-haul drug therapy shall I make preparation for?"

Reply: If you will give feedings four or five times daily of a diet that is high in protein and low in carbohydrate, and supplement this with 2 mg./kg. of prednisone (Meticorten, etc.) in divided doses daily, you should be able to prevent acute episodes. If not, however, 1 mg. of glucagon intramuscularly, or even 0.1–0.3 ml. of epinephrine (Adrenalin) 1 : 1000 solution subcutaneously, may be necessary. Fortu-

nately, these cases seem to be self-terminating after a few years.

IMPETIGO

"In the average and ordinary case of impetigo is it advisable to treat fully with penicillin systemically as one would for a streptococcic pharyngitis?"

Reply: It is doubtful if rheumatic fever is ever traceable to an impetiginous infection, and the reported incidence of nephritis associated with this lesion varies widely from 7 to 68%. However, in studying a large series of children with impetigo, Milton Markowitz's group, in Baltimore, found evidence of streptococcic infection on a basis of combined bacteriologic and serologic studies in 48%. I should give a full 10 days' penicillin treatment, or equivalent in a long-acting preparation.

Milton Markowitz, H. David Bruton, Ann G. Kuttner and Leighton E. Cluff. Bacteriologic Findings, Streptococcic Immune Response and Renal Complications in Children with Impetigo. Pediatrics 35:393, 1965.

INBORN ERRORS OF METABOLISM

"For which of the maladies that are reflections of inborn errors of metabolism do we have drug therapy that is to some degree effective?"

Reply: Alcaptonuria, familial hypophosphatemia, etiocholanolone fever, Fanconi syndrome, glycogen storage disease, gout, Hartnup's disease, hemochromatosis, porphyria, renal tubular acidosis, Wilson's disease. The others, in which drug therapy has nothing to offer: acatalasia, alpha-beta-lipoproteinemia, aminoaciduria, argininosuccinic aciduria, beta-aminoisobutyricaciduria, cystinosis, disorders of melanin pigmentation, fructosuria, galactosemia, Gaucher's disease, hypophosphaturia, maple syrup urine disease, Niemann-Pick disease, McArdle's syndrome, oxalosis, pentosuria, phenylketonuria, renal glycosuria, renal tubular acidosis, Tay-Sack's disease.

INDOLENT ULCER

"I have a patient with an indolent skin ulcer that has failed to respond to antibiotics or any other sort of routine treatment. Could you suggest any new drug therapy?"

Reply: A somewhat unorthodox treatment that I bring to your attention is the use of isoniazid (Rimifon, INH, etc.) by John Martyn and H. Hoyle Campbell, at St. Michael's Hospital, Toronto, in a small series of nontuberculous patients with various lesions exhibiting delayed healing. They used the drug in dosage of 3 mg./kg. orally and in some instances a 2% ointment topically, and felt that the production of healthy granulation tissue was considerably stimulated.

John W. Martyn and H. Hoyle Campbell. Isoniazid (Rimifon, INH, etc.) and Wound Healing. Canad. M. A. J. 88:229, Feb. 2, 1963.

"In our clinic we have been treating varicose leg ulcers with corticosteroids in combination with antibiotics with good effect, but recently ulcers in 2 patients turned necrotic under such treatment. How might this be explained?"

Reply: Could it be that you changed your corticosteroid? In Gothenburg, Sweden, Björnberg and Hellgren obtained precisely this effect when they switched from hydrocortisone to fluocinolone acetonide (Synalar) in their ointment. Four patients had their ulcers treated with an ointment containing fluocinolone acetonide, 0.025%; neomycin sulfate, 0.5%; propylene glycol, 5.0%; hydrogenated lanolin, 10%; and paraffin to make 100%. The ointment was applied once daily in a thick layer on the ulcer and covered with a gauze bandage; in 2 patients the entire ulcer was treated, in 2 others only a part of it, the other part being treated with neomycin-bacitracin powder (0.5 Gm., 25,000 international units/100 Gm.) and chloramphenicol ointment (1%), respectively. Adverse effects of a necrotic nature occurred in all of the 4 patients, but in the 2 who had partial treatment with the neomycin-bacitracin powder and the Chloromycetin ointment there were no adverse reactions in the portions of the ulcers so treated. The investigators felt that the fluocinolone reaction reflected pronounced local vasoconstriction.

Alf Björnberg and Lars Hellgren. Necrosis in Leg Ulcers. Arch. Dermat. 92:52, 1965.

"The Medicare hoard is advancing upon us with its chronic skin ulcers. Is there anything new?"

Reply: At Northwestern University, Malcolm Spencer has had good success with a new enzymatic debriding agent (Biozyme) that contains 10,000 Armour units of proteolytic activity with 3.5 mg. neomycin palmitate/gram. He said the therapy did not prove to be a panacea but that it had greatly reduced the time and effort involved in patient care in his experience, comparable results being achieved with both open and closed applications of the ointment. And the use of gold leaf, though not new, has had an auspicious revival under Marion Wolf's group in Columbia, Missouri. After cleansing and debridement, the ulcers are wetted with 95% alcohol, covered with 4–8 layers of goldleaf, and protective dressings are applied; the procedure is repeated every 48 hours. Adverse reactions have not been observed, but deterrents to the therapy are hemoglobin below 12 grams/100 ml., excessive friction, undermining of ulcer edges, ringing of the lesion with scar tissue, and copious purulent discharge.

Marion Wolf, Paul C. Wheeler and Lester E. Wolcott. Goldleaf Treatment of Ischemic Skin Ulcers. J.A.M.A. 196: 693, May 23, 1966. Malcolm C. Spencer. Enzymatic Treatment of Chronic Skin Ulcers. J.A.M.A. 193:272, July 26, 1965.

INFECTIOUS DISEASE ERADICATION

"What are the prospects for the eradication of infectious disease?"

Reply: In a few instances in history diseases have disappeared, but never because of organized health efforts. At the moment, fine control of some diseases in some places has been achieved, and for a few diseases in many places, but John Gordon (Massachusetts Institute of Technology), in a splendid review of the subject, has pointed out that there is practical value in recognizing eradication for what it is—a hope, a laudable ambition, a goal to which to aspire, but which, for even the first infectious disease of man, lies a long way ahead. He says that an area may be described, for example, as "clear of malaria"—a statement which describes the situation exactly, since it gives no promise of what is going to happen in the future and does not imply that the existing state is either lasting or irreversible. In short, such a statement recognizes that, should world conditions change sufficiently, the existing trends in communicable disease could reverse sharply. In the less developed countries, which still today include more than two thirds of the world, the acute infections remain the principal cause of death. And the world global population crisis casts a dour shadow over the picture.

John E. Gordon and Theodore H. Ingalls. Preventive Medicine and Epidemiology. Am. J. M. Sc. 250:346, 1965.

INFECTIOUS MONONUCLEOSIS

"It has been rumored that chloroquine (Aralen) is a cure for infectious mononucleosis. Is this true?"

Reply: Unfortunately it is not. Hope ran high when Loren Gothberg (Spokane, Washington) reported a dramatic result in 1 case, but then Schumacher's group (U.S. Naval Hospital, Portsmouth, Va.) failed completely with the drug in 5 cases.

Loren Gothberg. Severe Infectious Mononucleosis Treated with Chloroquine (Aralen) Phosphate. J.A.M.A. 173:53, May 7, 1960. Harold R. Schumacher, William A. Jacobson and Carl R. Bemiller. Treatment of Infectious Mononucleosis. Ann. Int. Med. 58:217, 1963.

INFERTILITY

"One of my associates has been urging that we begin using the contraceptive pill in treatment of infertility. What has been the record?"

Reply: The first report of an increase in the fertility potential after withdrawal of progestogens taken for contraception was made by John Rock and associates, in 1956. Since that time the position of these pioneer investigators has been both supported and contradicted by other studies, but I think that the affirmative findings are winning out. A recent report from the Infertility Center at the Royal Victoria Hospital in Montreal was certainly favorable in the main. Arrata and Arronet, of this group, gave norethynodrel with mestranol (Enovid) to infertile women in the attempt to achieve a successful rebound phenomenon in cases of idiopathic infertility with normal ovulatory function and in subovulatory and anovulatory patients. They used the drug also to treat patients with proved luteal-phase inadequacy. For the rebound phenomenon, therapy was started on day 5 of the cycle and was continued for 20 days, the 36 patients treated receiving Enovid for an average of 4.6 cycles/patient. The 20 patients with proved luteal-phase inadequacy were given the drug just after the basal body temperature rise for at least 10 days and the therapy was resumed in the subsequent four or five cycles if a pregnancy test was negative or if bleeding ensued on withdrawal of the drug. Of the total 56 patients, 24 conceived after treatment; 7 improved in ovulatory or menstrual status, and 25 showed no improvement. Most failures were in anovulatory patients with histories of primary infertility.

John Rock, Gregory Pincus and Celso Ramon Garcia. Effects of Certain 19-Nor-Steroids on the Normal Human Menstrual Cycle. Science 124:891, 1956. W. S. M. Arrata and George H. Arronet. Norethynodrel with Mestranol (Enovid) in Infertility. Fertil. & Steril. 16:430, 1965.

"How often are infertile, hypothyroid women made to conceive through the use of thyroid substance?"

Reply: Some years ago, F. S. Hassler (Wilmington, Delaware) evaluated the effect of liothyronine (Cytomel) in 38 hypothyroid women who had not conceived after trying for 1–10 years. The optimum Cytomel dosage was considered to be the maximum that the patient could tolerate without side effects; in most instances this ranged from 25–50 mg. daily. In 24 of the women there were definite objective improvements, 14 conceiving and the other 10 becoming normal in menses and ovulation. There were no undesirable effects from the therapy, once the dosage had been adjusted, but one should use the drug cautiously if there is complicating cardiovascular disease and not at all if there is an uncorrected adrenal insufficiency.

F. S. Hassler. Liothyronine (Cytomel) Therapy in Female Infertility. Fertil. & Steril. 9:555, 1958.

INSOMNIA

"In our hospital considerable emphasis is placed upon the distinction between the long, intermediate and short acting barbiturates as hypnotics. For practical purposes, are we really justified in this?"

Reply: The comparative effectiveness of hypnotic agents is a very difficult thing to determine. The fact that the patient is or is not asleep is in itself not always easy to establish, and one has also to contend with the individual variations in people, the complex motives by which they are activated, and the degree of their perversity and crotchetiness. And how one wrong nurse, who entertains a low opinion of the study, can vitiate the findings! However, there are a couple of recent small scale investigations, those of Parsons in Glasgow, and Hinton, in London, in which no evidence appeared justifying the classification of barbiturates according to the duration of their hypnotic action.

T. W. Parsons (Western Infirmary, Glasgow). Clinical Comparison of Barbiturates as Hypnotics. Brit. M. J. 2:1035, Oct. 26, 1963. J. M. Hinton (Middlesex Hospital, London). Comparison of Effects of Six Barbiturates and a Placebo on Insomnia and Motility in Psychiatric Patients. Brit. J. Pharmacol. 20:319, 1963.

"The modern school denies the efficacy of alcohol as a drug, but I have several times found it useful under certain circumstances as a sleep-producer. Does it not really have some other valuable therapeutic attributes?"

Reply: Alcohol as a *hypnotic* has its limitations but is nevertheless very useful in one particular class of patient. In elderly individuals who are troubled by inability to sleep and rebel at the nastiness of chloral hydrate, and in whom one is fearful of the barbiturates both because of the possibility of some diminution in liver function and the likelihood of obtaining an excitatory rather than a quieting effect, the use of a whiskey toddy or a glass of heavy wine sipped while propped up in bed all ready for sleep may be a very successful measure provided neither of the two following reservations apply: (1) that the individual is not enough of a steady drinker so that moderate indulgence at bedtime will not constitute a "treat" of a relaxing nature; (2) that the individual is not hypersensitive to alcohol to such extent that the heart rate is annoyingly increased by imbibing it. I believe this bedtime "toping" to be the only valuable hypnotic use of the drug.

Alcohol as an *analgesic* agent merits mention. It is the pain reliever par excellence in dysmenorrhea, as many patients know without being so instructed by the physician, but it is probably true that alcoholic addiction has started in some women through use of whiskey or gin, or nowadays vodka, for this purpose. In more serious situations alcohol may be given intravenously for its analgesic effect in 5–10% solution in 5% glucose, but the inebriation this causes is often very objectionable to the patient. Intrathecal alcohol injections may give long-lasting relief from pain, but this is a radical procedure since the spinal cord may be injured. The risk is sometimes justified, however, in instances of intractable pain in association with cancer. The intrathecal alcohol injection may interfere with locomotion and cause some neuritic pain. It does not relieve claudication. Injection of alcohol or alcohol-containing vehicles into the region of the medial globus pallidus, as well as the thalamus, in treatment of such basal ganglion disorders as parkinsonism, is called chemopallidectomy.

Alcohol is definitely useful as a *vasodilator* in desperate situations. Taken as "hard liquor" without much dilution in peripheral vascular diseases, it often causes greater peripheral vasodilation than any other drug. In clinical investigation a larger increase in blood flow has been found in the fingers than in the toes, but practical experience has nevertheless shown alcohol to be the most effective analgesic agent in Buerger's disease. The unfortunate inebriating and habituating effects of alcohol are the only serious deterrents to its use in this distressing malady. In another situation, peripheral arterial embolism, in which pain is sometimes so severe that even the opiates will not control it, alcohol not infrequently affords considerable relief. The impression that alcohol is effective in relieving the acute attack of angina pectoris has failed to find support in careful studies; in many instances indeed the increased sense of wellbeing is without associated objective improvement, which could conceivably provoke the

patient into physical activity beyond his capacity. Actually, it is probably too much to expect that alcohol would be of analgesic value in the acute anginal attack because it takes longer for the drug's effects to be exerted upon the circulation than such an attack usually lasts. Moderate drinking on the chronic basis may have a most salutary effect, however, if the beverage used is not the bloating beer and if the drinker allows himself to be relaxed and not "busied up" by his imbibing.

Alcohol strikingly relaxes the *cerebral palsy* patient of the athetotic type, but of course we cannot well propose the use of the drug upon a chronic basis by such individuals; still it is undeniable that here, as in Buerger's disease, we have a potent symptomatic remedy in the agent. Alcohol has also been successfully used to relax individuals, particularly children, with *status asthmaticus*; aspirin, given together with a hot whiskey toddy, is a potent mixture that will occasionally conquer even severe paroxysms of asthma – but unfortunately an occasional asthmatic patient is allergic to aspirin, and most allergists show signs of distress themselves at the mere mention of this drug.

Alcohol has been effectively used intravenously in combination with a barbiturate to increase communicativeness and speech productivity in *narcosynthesis*; in fact this merely comprises the employment professionally of the layman's age-old method of "pumping" an unwary friend.

An interesting use of alcohol is as a vapor to be inhaled in the treatment of *pulmonary edema*, the desired effect being nonsystemic but based on the antifoaming action exerted locally in the air passages.

The only situation known to me in which experience has been alleged to indicate some therapeutic value attaching to actual intoxication with alcohol is in cases of *milk sickness*, the snake-root or rayless goldenrod poisoning that was a Midwestern scourge in pioneer days and is still diagnosed a few times each year.

And of course the carminative or gas-dispelling properties of alcohol are generally well known.

"I have a patient who had been taking several tablets of ethchlorvynol (Placidyl) daily when I hospitalized him for study of a malady not directly related to his alleged insomnia. Two days later he suddenly had a grand mal convulsion and another the next day and then began to have hallucinations, which have continued unabated now for more than a week. Could this sort of thing have been due exclusively to withdrawal of his drug?"

Reply: Did your patient have a history of psychiatric disturbances of any sort? I ask this because, in the reports that I have seen of this sort of thing attributable to ethchlorvynol, the patients have all been individuals with pathologic or inadequate personalities. But the drug has been shown to be one of addiction, and therefore it is not unlikely that it could cause such withdrawal symptoms even in a psychiatrically normal individual; others among the newer hypnotics have done so.

Monica D. Blumenthal and Melvin J. Reinhart. Psychosis and Convulsions Following Withdrawal from Ethchlorvynol (Placidyl). J.A.M.A. 190:154, Oct. 12, 1964.

"A patient in our hospital is able to avoid nightly 'doping' only if he can successfully fight off the entire nursing staff. Is all this use of hypnotics necessary?"

Reply: Certainly not. Of course it keeps the floor quieter than it might otherwise be and definitely eases the burden upon the night staff of calls to cantankerous and hypochondriacal patients, but as a therapeutic measure it is indefensible nevertheless.

"Would you care to say something about the use of hypnotics in insomnia?"

Reply: I have said a good deal upon this subject in my time, but here it is in essence. I think it very doubtful that any of the newer hypnotic agents are superior to the barbiturates, and I also feel that one need not be greatly concerned about the host of barbiturates currently available since a very few of them will accomplish all that is required. For example, secobarbital (Seconal) is a rapidly acting member of the group in average adult dosage of 100–200 mg., although it has seemed to many observers that its action is not sufficiently prolonged for the patient whose difficulty is in remaining asleep. However, it certainly will not make him logy the next day. Amobarbital (Amytal) does not act so rapidly but the effect is possibly more prolonged (I say *possibly* because there has been recent questioning of the alleged differences in the duration of action of all of the barbiturates, average adult dosage is 100–300 mg. Pentobarbital (Nembutal) seems to me to differ very little in rapidity and duration of action from amobarbital, but it is preferred in many practices for its presumed longer action; average dosage is 100 mg. Phenobarbital (Luminal) is slower acting than the others, but the effect is undoubtedly more prolonged; average dosage is 100–200 mg.; it is particularly well employed in the nervous jittery individual by distributing the hypnotic dose into three or four portions given at intervals throughout the day.

Chloral hydrate is a very excellent drug despite its objectionable taste and the fact that it is sometimes irritating to the stomach; actually the taste may be pretty well disguised for all but the most squeamish of people and the gastric irritation does not occur nearly so often as the proponents of the newer drugs would have us believe. Try it in the following mixture: chloral hydrate 30 Gm., fluidextract glycyrrhiza, 60 ml., and syrup of orange to make 120 ml.; give a teaspoonful of this well diluted 1 hour before retiring. Admittedly such a prescription as I have suggested is out of fashion nowadays, but the drug is available in tablet or capsule form as Beta-Chlor, Periclor, Felsules and Somnos; in fluid form as Noctec and Somnos; and in a rectal suppository as Rectules. The patient on ordinary dosage of 2 grams at bedtime may perspire a little, as a reflection of moderate vasomotor center depression, and should therefore remain under at least light bedclothing if in a cool or breezy room. But heart disease does not contraindicate chloral hydrate in moderate dosage, and very little hangover accompanies use of the drug.

Bromisovalum (Bromural) and carbromal (Adalin) are neither simple inorganic bromide salts nor barbiturates, though derived from urea and having some bromine attached. Either of them in a dose of 300 mg. three or four times daily, or 600 mg. to 1.2 gram an hour before bedtime, is useful in the type of insomnia in which sedatives rather than stronger hypnotics are indicated. Bromoderma is a very rare occurrence and habit-formation comparable to that with the barbiturates has not been reported. Recently there have been a few reports, however, of confusional states and coma, even a few deaths. A few rashes and one instance of jaundice associated with use of these drugs have come to my attention, but I think that they may still be considered a very safe group in relationship to the barbiturates and the newer hypnotics.

As "newer" hypnotics I list the following: Ethchlorvynol (Placidyl), 500 mg. at bedtime or 200 mg. three times daily; ethinamate (Valmid), 500 mg. about 20 minutes before bedtime, but higher dosage may be required or an additional dose may be given during the night; glutethimide (Doriden), 500 mg. at bedtime or 250 mg. three times daily; methyprylon (Noludar), 300 mg. at bedtime or 50–100 mg. three or four times daily; methaqualone (Quaalude), 150 mg. at bedtime. These drugs have not proved to be as devoid of the drawbacks of the barbiturates as had been hoped. In the case of ethchlorvynol, for example, nausea and vomiting, dermatitis, excitement and hangover have been reported, and in the case of methyprylon there have been occasional occurrences of nausea and vomiting, vertigo, pruritus and dermatitis and hangover. With glutethimide the incidence of gastric irritation, nausea and vomiting is slight, but there is sometimes anorexia and occasionally hangover, dizziness and light-headedness on the next day, and dermatitis has been seen. Addiction is also occurring with this drug, and there have sometimes been severe withdrawal symptoms: pupillary dilatation, paralytic ileus and atony of the urinary bladder, late hyperthermia, hypotension, delirium and convulsions, high incidence of pulmonary complications, and occasionally sudden unexpected apnea.

INTERSTITIAL FIBROSIS

"I have a patient with idiopathic interstitial fibrosis of the lungs in whom I have been able to accomplish nothing with the corticosteroids. Are these drugs ever helpful here?"

Reply: In Sweden, Malmberg's group obtained improvement of ventilatory capacity and gas exchange only in cases without radiological honeycomb lesions.

Rolf Malmberg, Erick Berglund and Lars Andér. Idiopathic Interstitial Fibrosis of the Lungs II. Reversibility of Respiratory Disturbances During Steroid Administration. Acta med. scandinav. 178:59, 1965.

JAUNDICE

"In our group we have been using steroid therapy on a somewhat tentative basis in jaundice, but it begins to appear that something of diagnostic value may be emerging from the experience. Has a suggestion of this sort been reported by any of the research groups?"

Reply: At the Royal Free Hospital, London, Roger Williams and Barbara Billing studied the effect of steroids on bilirubin metabolism in jaundice patients and felt the results might be of help in distinguishing hepatitis with long-continued jaundice from extrahepatic obstruction. In the obstruction cases the fall in serum bilirubin was rarely as great as in the hepatitis cases and, furthermore, it occurred in the first few days of treatment and then the level remained constant, which was quite different from the type of response in infective hepatitis. One is obliged to remark with regard to these observations, however, that their usefulness is limited by the fact that some cases of hepatitis do not respond to corticosteroid therapy.

Roger Williams and Barbara H. Billing. Action of Steroid Therapy in Jaundice. Lancet 2:392, Aug. 19, 1961.

"I understand that anion-exchange resins which form unabsorbable complexes with bile acid in the intestine have been used to some effect in combating the pruritus of obstructive jaundice. Can you cite any of the data?"

Reply: In the studies of Datta and Sherlock (Royal Free Hospital, London), and Van Itallie's group (New York), the resin, cholestyramine, was used. Eight of the British patients received 10 Gm. daily and 2 received 6.6 Gm. In 8 patients, pruritus was completely relieved in 4–11 days; 1 patient who was not relieved took the drug for too short a period, and the other was thought probably to have had total biliary obstruction. There was no constant effect on the depth of jaundice. Somewhat higher dosage, 15 Gm. per day in divided doses, was used in the American cases; all 5 of these patients were dramatically relieved from itching within 1–3 weeks, relief being sustained for as long as treatment was continued.

D. V. Datta and Sheila Sherlock. Treatment of Pruritus of Obstructive Jaundice with Cholestyramine. Brit. M. J. 1:216, Jan 26, 1963. Theodore B. Van Itallie, Sami A. Hashim, Richard S. Crampton and David M. Tennent. Treatment of Pruritus and Hypercholesteremia of Primary Biliary Cirrhosis with Cholestyramine. New England J. Med. 265:469, Sept. 7, 1961.

"Is there any new speculation regarding the pruritus of jaundice that has led to reasonably effective therapy?"

Reply: At Johns Hopkins Hospital, Juan Alva and Frank Iber obtained effective relief of itching of obstructive jaundice by methandrostenolone (Dianabol) in dosage of 5 mg. every 8 hours for from 4 to 42 days. If it is postulated that bile salts reach the area of itch fibers by active transport, possibly in the sweat glands, then it might be speculated that methandrostenolone relieves pruritus by interfering with accumulation of bile salts in the skin, at least according to these observers. In any event, their success with this therapy is worth noting even though it might rest upon no more than an empirical basis.

Juan Alva and Frank L. Iber. Relief of Pruritus of Jaundice with Methandrostenolone (Dianabol) and Speculations on the Nature of Pruritus in Liver Disease. Am. J. M. Sc. 250:60, 1965.

"In a patient with jaundice that can be shown not to be due to primary hepatic or hematologic disorders, what drugs should be thought of in the causative role?"

Reply: The phenothiazine-derivative compounds that are used in treatment of the psychoses; the indandione type of anticoagulants (such drugs as Hedulin, Danilone, Eridione); isoniazid (Nydrazid, Rimifon, etc.); PAS; the long-acting sulfonamides (such agents as sulfamethoxazole [Gantanol], sulfadimethoxine [Madribon], sulfamethoxypyridazine [Kynex, Midicel], and the acetyl form of the latter [Kynex Acetyl]); methyltestosterone (Metandren, Neo-Hombreol [M], Oreton-M); the monoamine oxidase inhibitors; chlorpropamide (Diabinese); methyldopa (Aldomet); nitrofurantoin (Furadantin); propylthiouracil; methimazole (Tapazole); imipramine (Tofranil); probenecid (Benemid); erythromycin estolate (Ilosone); novobiocin (Cathomycin, etc.); oxacillin (Prostaphlin); tetracyclines (in high dosage); thioridazine (Mellaril); thiazide diuretics; 6-mercaptopurine (Purinethol); norethandrolone (Nilevar); phenylbutazone (Butazolidin); tolbutamide (Orinase); urethane; tranylcypromine (Parnate); polythiazide (Renese); isocarboxazid (Marplan); pyrazinamide; gold salts. In most instances these will be rare reactions of hypersensitivity but occasionally there will be true toxic reactions.

"Where I am practicing it is almost prohibitively difficult to obtain an exchange transfusion for an infant with neonatal jaundice. Has any other reasonably successful therapy been devised?"

Reply: The most promising thing that has come to my attention is the use of charcoal, that has been introduced by John Canby at the Martin Army Hospital, Fort Benning, Georgia. Taking advantage of the fact that any unconjugated bilirubin which may reach the intestinal lumen is rapidly reabsorbed into the blood stream, he undertook to block this circulation by the use of charcoal to absorb bilirubin. All newborns exhibiting an unusual degree of jaundice from whatever cause were admitted to the study and given activated charcoal (Darco 60) suspended in water as a 10% solution. Administration was by gavage in 5 ml. increments, each containing approximately 0.5 Gm. of charcoal, every 2 hours, the program being continued until age 120 hours with normal full term infants and up to age 168 hours with the smallest premature infants, or until the abnormal serum bilirubin levels had fallen to more acceptable levels. During the control period there were 3009 live births and 53 exchange transfusions were performed on 27 infants. During the experimental (charcoal) period there were 1562 live births and only 12 exchange transfusions on 9 infants. This was of course only a preliminary study, but the results are very interesting.

John P. Canby. Charcoal Therapy of Neonatal Jaundice. Clin. Pediat. 4:178, 1965.

KELOIDS

"Has any effective drug therapy been developed for keloids?"

Reply: Henry Maguire, Jr., at the University of Pennsylvania, reported a very satisfactory response to the injection of large amounts of intralesional corticosteroid suspension into multiple large keloids in a single patient. At 4–6 week intervals during a period of about 2 years a total of 2–6 ml. of 1% triamcinolone acetonide (Kenalog) aqueous suspension was injected. The firm keloids accepted little of the drug in the beginning, but as treatment progressed they softened and became easy to infiltrate. The injections were only slightly painful.

Henry C. Maguire. Treatment of Keloids with Triamcinolone Acetonide Injected Intralesionally. J.A.M.A. 192:325, April 26, 1965.

KIDNEY DISORDERS

"I am employing peritoneal dialysis in a patient in whom it is also necessary to give oral antibiotic therapy for treatment of systemic infection. Am I going to drain away enough of the antibiotic in the dialysate to warrant increasing the dosage of the systemically administered drug?"

Reply: This matter was studied at the Walter Reed Hospital by Leroy Shear's group, who found that significant amounts of tetracycline and methicillin (Dimocillin-RT, Staphcillin) were not extracted in the peritoneal dialysate. However, they also concluded that patients with peritonitis should receive intraperitoneal as well as systemic antibiotic unless very high blood levels are being maintained through systemic administration. In Seattle, Bulger and associates, studying the intraperitoneal administration of broad-spectrum antibiotics, found intraperitoneal cephalothin (Keflin) and ampicillin (Polycillin) potentially superior to tetracycline and chloramphenicol (Chloromycetin) because tetracycline may be toxic, since the kidney is the major route of excretion of this drug, and chloramphenicol will achieve a low serum concentration.

Leroy Shear, James H. Shinaberger and Kevin G. Barry. Peritoneal Transport of Antibiotics in Man. New England J. Med. 272:666, Apr. 1, 1965. Roger J. Bulger, John F. Bennett and S. T. Boen. Intraperitoneal Administration of Broad-Spectrum Antibiotics in Patients with Renal Failure. J.A.M.A. 194:1198, Dec. 13, 1965.

"In a patient having a penicillin G–resistant staphylococcus infection, the commonly used anti-

biotics are methicillin (Dimocillin, Staphcillin) and oxacillin (Prostaphlin, Resistopen). But suppose the patient then develops renal failure requiring hemodialysis; which drug becomes the preferred one and why?"

Reply: Theoretically, the only molecules that pass through the membrane of the artificial kidney are those that are not bound to serum protein. Therefore methicillin, which is bound only to the extent of 15–20%, would be preferred to oxacillin, which is 85–90% bound. However, Bulger's group (Seattle) actually found that oxacillin disappeared from the blood more rapidly than methicillin. See what risks we take when venturing into gratuitous assumptions in the realm of drug therapy!

Roger J. Bulger, Dale D. Lindholm, John S. Murray and William M. M. Kirby. Effect of Uremia on Methicillin (Dimocillin, Staphcillin) and Oxacillin (Prostaphlin, Resistopen) Blood Levels: Excretion and Inactivation in Renal Failure and Hemodialysis. J.A.M.A. 187:319, Feb. 1, 1964.

"In our hospital we are increasingly resorting to peritoneal dialysis in cases of severe renal disease and are adding the broad-spectrum antibiotic, tetracycline, to each exchange of dialysis solution as a prophylactic measure against peritonitis. What is the fate of this antibiotic when so introduced?"

Reply: At the VA Hospital in Milwaukee, Harold Rose and associates found that in severely azotemic patients receiving peritoneal instillation of tetracycline at the rate of 25 mg./L./hour, a peak serum level in the therapeutic range was reached between 16 and 24 hours. The possibility of a systemic or toxic effect of the tetracycline when added to peritoneal dialysis solutions caused them to discontinue such additions at their hospital. An additional reason for taking this step was that the majority of the hospital-acquired infections in their institution are caused by tetracycline-resistant strains of *Staphylococcus aureus* or the enteric gram-negative bacilli, which are also the species most likely to be introduced into the peritoneal cavity during dialysis.

Harold D. Rose, Donald A. Roth and Marie L. Koch. Serum Tetracycline Levels During Peritoneal Dialysis. Am. J. M. Sc. 250:66, 1965.

"I have a patient with nephrosis who has not responded to the corticosteroids. Can you suggest anything?"

Reply: At the Kaiser Foundation Hospital, Oakland, Martin Shearn gave 14 courses of mercaptopurine (Purinethol) to 10 patients with nephrotic syndrome of diverse causes but all resistant to corticosteroids, as is your patient. Clinical remission, consisting in marked decrease in proteinuria, loss of edema and rise in serum albumin to normal levels, occurred in half the patients. It is likely that the toxicity of the drug will greatly limit its usefulness in nephrosis since in virtually all of these patients there was a high incidence of bone marrow suppression. Dosage used was high: 3 mg./kg. daily for 3 weeks, and if at this time there had been neither a therapeutic effect nor a toxic reaction the dose was increased.

Martin A. Shearn. Mercaptopurine in the Treatment of Steroid-Resistant Nephrotic Syndrome. New England J. Med. 273:943, Oct. 28, 1965.

"I have a child with the idiopathic nephrotic syndrome whom I have placed on corticosteroid therapy with good immediate effects. What is the long-time prognosis?"

Reply: At the Mayo Clinic, Robert Brown and associates concluded from their experience in 135 such children that corticosteroid therapy appreciably lengthens life or improves prognosis or both, but they felt that one could not be statistically assured that this is the case since, for humane reasons, they had no untreated controls in their series. The 5 year survival rate was 76.4%, which is similar to the figures published by other observers. Complete remission appeared to occur in 55.8% of the patients who had survived 5 or more years, while continued therapy for control of their symptoms was still required by 25%.

Robert B. Brown, Edmund C. Burke and Gunnar B. Stickler. Studies in Nephrotic Syndrome. I. Survival of 135 Children with Nephrotic Syndrome Treated with Adrenal Steroids. Mayo Clin. Proc. 40:384, 1965.

"Now I shall pose a difficult question: how is one to treat uremic patients found to be seriously infected with gram-negative organisms that are sensitive only to antibiotics that are reputedly provocative of renal damage?"

Reply: It seems to me that Atuk and associates (University of Virginia) met this problem quite triumphantly by simply using these agents *in reduced dosage*. They had a series of 12 uremic patients in the condition you describe. Oliguric patients among them received a loading dose of 1 Gm. kanamycin or 100–150 mg. polymyxin B, or colistin (in divided doses) intramuscularly, followed by injections of half the loading dose at intervals of 2–4 days. Individuals recovering from the oliguric phase of acute tubular necrosis, and uremic patients whose glomerular filtration rate was estimated to be greater than 10 ml./minute, received the same loading dose and subsequent doses of half the loading dose at intervals of 1–2 days. All but 1 patient survived both infection and therapy. The patient who died had inexorable renal failure despite cure of infection.

Nuzhet O. Atuk, Alfon Mosca and Calvin Kunin. Use of Potentially Nephrotoxic Antibiotics in Treatment of Gram-Negative Infections in Uremic Patients. Ann. Int. Med. 60:28, 1964.

"I have used a cation-exchange resin in a few patients with chronic renal disease and hyper-kalemia with no more untoward clinical reactions than occasional nausea and vomiting and consti-pation. I am wondering, however, whether I might not be endangering the patient through the opera-tion of something that does not usually meet the eye in this situation?"

Reply: The cation-exchange resins do not regularly disturb the normal absorption of phosphates, chlorides and sulfates, and the evidence of serious interference with mag-nesium, iron, manganese, copper, cobalt or amino acid absorption is not clear cut. How-ever, one must carefully guard against devel-opment of the low-sodium syndrome, severe acidosis and deficiencies in other cations. Really, the use of an agent of this sort is never safe unless you can follow the serum electro-lyte pattern closely at all times, which is often impracticable.

"Why is it that results with corticosteroids are so much better in the nephrotic syndrome in chil-dren than in adults?"

Reply: I do not know the answer.

Harry Sonnenschein, Arnold A. Minsky and Benjamin Kramer (Brooklyn). Treatment of Uncomplicated Nephro-tic Syndrome in Children with Triamcinolone (Aristocort): Six-Year Study. Clin. Pediat. 3:263, 1964. H. Gotze, W. T. E. McCaughey and R. A. Womersley (Queen's University, Belfast). Steroids in Treatment of Nephrotic Syndrome in Adults. Brit. M. J. 1:351, Feb. 8, 1964.

"It seems to me that mannitol has acquired a certain aura in the treatment of acute renal failure leading one to expect rather fabulous results from its use. But I have not had astounding success with it; what may I be doing incorrectly, or not doing?"

Reply: Really this drug does not work at all in any mysterious ways its wonders to perform. It is merely an osmotic diuretic precisely like urea. As a nonreabsorbable constituent of the glomerular filtrate, it requires water to satisfy osmotic relationships, and its diuretic action

rests solely upon the prevention of reabsorp-tion of this water. In nephrotic edema, it is the consensus that best results would be achieved through using concomitantly a mercurial tubular blocking diuretic. Have you done this?

"What is the safest, practical measure in the emergency management of hyperpotassemia in the uremic syndrome?"

Reply: The hyperpotassemia in uremia is often accompanied by acidosis, hyponatremia, hypocalcemia, alterations in body water and changes in cellular metabolism. If these asso-ciated electrolyte abnormalities are corrected there is often an accompanying improvement in the ECG manifestations of the potassium imbalance. Kuno Schwarz's group (Cornell University), and others, have found that cor-rection of the bicarbonate deficit with sodium bicarbonate lowers plasma potassium directly, apparently through intracellular transfer of potassium ions, since urinary potassium excre-tion is negligible. Serial pH determinations also give some evidence of some effect on the hydrogen ions by repletion of buffer alkali; correction of extracellular alkali deficit re-stores intracellular bicarbonate as well. It appears that the reduction in plasma potas-sium reflects a shift of potassium as well as bicarbonate into the cell with the correction of intracellular acidosis because potassium is the major intracellular cation. Correction of the acidosis is accompanied not only by lowering of the plasma potassium but also reversal of the ECG signs. Another useful measure, introduced by Samuel Bellet and Fred Wasserman (Philadelphia), is the intra-venous injection of 100 ml. of molar sodium lactate followed by an infusion at 30–60 drops/minute. Use of this agent requires great care, however, if there are cardiac arrhythmias present.

Kuno C. Schwarz, Burton D. Cohen, Glenn D. Lubash and Albert L. Rubin. Severe Acidosis and Hyperpotassemia Treated with Sodium Bicarbonate Infusion. Circulation 19:215, 1959. Samuel Bellet and Fred Wasserman. Indi-cations and Contraindications for Use of Molar Sodium Lactate. Circulation 15:591, 1957.

"Pyelonephritis, underlying other disorders, is often the progressive and unrelenting cause of death. What is one to do?"

Reply

"Oh, dear me, and my Dear too,
     what will me and my Dear do?"
Thus my grandmother long years ago when I was a very small boy. Of course we youngsters were frantic to know the answer—what *will* me and my Dear do? But it was never forth-coming. Indeed, I think it had been lost in the

dim backward of time and that my grandmother knew it no more nearly than we did. And thus it is also with pyelonephritis, it seems to me; knowing neither the "dear me" nor the "my Dear too," how can we know what to "do"? I have seen everything fail and so have you. We must gain real understanding of the etiology of pyelonephritis, and then the effective therapy will fall in place.

The clearest delineation of the factors involved that I have seen is that of William McCabe and George Jackson, at the University of Illinois. They found hypertension, renal insufficiency, structural abnormalities and mild obstructive uropathy not influencing the frequency of eradication of the infecting organism but each appearing to predispose to reinfection. Patients with these abnormalities acquired new infections at a rate 20–40 times that of the general population. Susceptibility to reinfection can also result partly from impaired capacity of the bladder to clear bacteria. Sulfonamides were the least effective drug they used, but no significant differences were found among the others: tetracycline, chloramphenicol (Chloromycetin), nitrofurantoin (Furadantin), colistin (Coly-Mycin), kanamycin (Kantrex) and nalidixic acid. Combinations of these agents were not more effective than the single drugs, bearing out the antagonisms between components of the combinations that were demonstrable in vivo; and there was poor correlation between in vitro serum antibiotic activity and eradication of bacteriuria.

William R. McCabe and George Gee Jackson. Treatment of Pyelonephritis: Bacterial, Drug and Host Factors in Success or Failure Among 252 Patients. New England J. Med. 272:1037, May 20, 1965.

"Why is it that we can often prevent the occurrence of acute rheumatic fever if we treat an acute streptococcic infection vigorously with penicillin but seem never able to prevent acute glomerulonephritis in the same way?"

Reply: I wish I knew.

"What drugs may it be dangerous to use in acute renal failure?"

Reply: Use of the following drugs is not interdicted, but if you do employ them you should greatly reduce their dosage: digitalis glycosides, barbiturates, diuretics, narcotics, salicylates, tetracycline (Achromycin, etc.), oxytetracycline (Terramycin), streptomycin, vancomycin (Vancocin); sulfonamides and nitrofurantoin (Furandantin) should not be used, and kanamycin (Kantrex), polymyxin B (Aerosporin) and colistin (Coly-Mycin) not unless there are no effective alternatives; even penicillin dosage should probably be somewhat reduced; use of the anticoagulants could be extremely hazardous.

Norman G. Levinsky. Management of Emergencies: Acute Renal Failure. New England J. Med. 274:1016, May 5, 1966. Dale D. Lindholm and John S. Murray. Persistence of Vancomycin in the Blood During Renal Failure and Its Treatment by Hemodialysis. New England J. Med. 274:1047, May 12, 1966.

LABOR

"In recent years in our hospital we have reduced the degree of fetal depression resulting from drugs administered during labor by reducing the dose of meperidine (Demerol) used for analgesia and amnesia and substituting a phenothiazine for the omitted portion of the dose, the latter drug not only synergizing the meperidine apparently but being also antiemetic and tranquilizing. We have been using these drugs in combination intramuscularly, but now we are wondering whether we would gain anything by giving them intravenously?"

Reply: In San Francisco, Kliger and Nelson found that a 50 mg. dose of meperidine plus 20 mg. of propriomazine (Largon), a phenothiazine agent, given intravenously every 2 hours for a total of two or three doses, provided excellent relief from pain in most patients. If they added 0.4 mg. of scopolamine to the mixture in one of the doses, 80% of the individuals were rendered amnesic. It was found that 100 mg. of meperidine was as useful as the combination of 50 mg. of meperidine with 20 mg. of propiomazine, but if the 100 mg. dose was repeated the rate of infant depression rose considerably.

Benjamin Kliger and H. Bristol Nelson. Analgesia and Fetal Depression with Intravenous Meperidine and Propiomazine. Am. J. Obst. & Gynec. 92:850, 1965.

"I have used relaxin (Releasin, Cervilaxin) in a few instances and always unsuccessfully. What is the real status of this drug in obstetrics?"

Reply: Relaxin, a water-soluble polypeptide obtained from the ovaries of pregnant sows, has been found in the blood stream of pregnant women, increasing in concentration to term and then rapidly decreasing. It has been alleged that the relaxation of pelvic joints that occurs in normal human pregnancy is relaxin-induced, and also that relaxin inhibits contractility of the myometrium; but I do not think that these things have been proved. Admittedly, Sands and Ko reported favorably on the use of the drug in term labor under certain circumstances; but on the other hand, Embrey and Garrett (Oxford University), in a tocographic study of the effect on contractility of human pregnant uterus, found no significant immediate or delayed effect in 9 of their 10 patients. In the tenth patient there was only a transient inhibition of uterine contractility following a large dose of the hormone. However, the contribution of Maclure and Ferguson (Miami, Florida) should be mentioned: in 9 of their 11 patients in whom gestation lasted 28–40 weeks before fetal death occurred they felt that relaxin had effected definite cervical softening before the induction of labor with Pitocin.

R. X. Sands and J. H. Ko. (St. Luke's Hospital, New York). Term Labor—Its Facilitation by Relaxin (Releasin, Cervilaxin): Preliminary Report. Canad. M. A. J. 80:886, June 1, 1959. Mostyn P. Embrey and William J. Garrett. Effect of Relaxin (Releasin) on Contractility of Human Pregnant Uterus: Tocographic Study. J. Obst. & Gynaec. Brit. Emp. 66:594, 1959. J. G. Maclure and J. H. Ferguson. Use of Relaxin in Management of Retained Dead Fetus. Am. J. Obst. & Gynec. 79:801, 1960.

"In a limited experience I have sometimes thought that the addition of an antihistaminic compound to analgesic agents has shortened labor, but have hesitated to adopt the measure routinely. What has been the experience?"

Reply: Rotter and associates have postulated the release of histamine during the stretching and tearing of the cervix, with a resultant stimulating action on uterine muscle and possibly cervical spasm; the use of an antihistaminic agent was thus rationalized to accelerate cervical dilatation. They found such a measure shortening labor by as much as 30% and decreasing the amount of additional sedatives required. Scott's group confirmed these findings and also reported the potentiation of other analgesics, but at the Radcliffe Infirmary, Oxford, England, Kenneth Cooper conducted a double-blind trial of the method in 200 patients, giving 100 mg. of dimenhydrinate (Dramamine) or an identical placebo with the first injection of a potent analgesic. At the time of injection a vaginal or rectal examination was made and the cervical dilatation recorded. He failed to substantiate the earlier claims, and therefore it seems that we really do not know where the truth lies in the matter.

Kenneth Cooper. Failure of Dimenhydrinate (Dramamine) to Shorten Labor. Am. J. Obst. & Gynec. 86:1041, Aug. 15, 1963. C. W. Rotter, J. L. Whitaker, J. Yored. Use of Intravenous Dramamine to Shorten the Time of Labor and Potentiate Analgesia. Am. J. Obst. & Gynec. 75:1101, 1959. R. S. Scott, K. H. Wallace, D. N. Dadley, B. H. Watson. Use of Dimenhydrinate in Labor. Am. J. Obst. & Gynec. 83:25, 1962.

"In my area there are a good many Puerto Rican women who often react very apprehensively to labor and thus require inordinate dosage of depressants in order to maintain the delivery room only reasonably quiet. Has anyone made a good study of this situation?"

Reply: Yes, at the Harlem Hospital, New York, Eisenstein's group used propiomazine (Largon) in combination with meperidine (Demerol) in 182 patients and found that while the progress of labor did not appear to be altered there was a rapid onset of desirable depression and relaxation and great reduction in noise in patients of this type. *Dosage:* propiomazine, 40 mg., meperidine, 50 mg.; in about 20% of instances the drugs were given intravenously, intramuscularly in the others. The patients were in labor when medicated, and as many as four doses, as required, were given at intervals of 2–4 hours.

Morris I. Eisenstein, Emanuel J. Rubin, Murray Arnold and A. Charles Posner. Propiomazine Hydrochloride (Largon) in Obstetrics. Am. J. Obst. & Gynec. 88:606, 1964.

"Sparteine sulfate (Tocosamine) is being proclaimed by some enthusiasts as an oxytocic that can be administered intramuscularly, does not require constant supervision, may shorten the duration of labor, has no known side effects and has a wide margin of safety. Is all of this true?"

Reply: The European clinical literature on this drug is voluminous and characterized more notably by an absence of accounts of severe toxicity than by its definite establishment of the usefulness of the compound. Here in the United States, Plentl and Gray at Columbia University undertook a large scale study of the drug as a prophylactic postpartum oxytocic and found that for its effect on the incidence of uterine atony it has no advantage over oxytocin; but for induction or stimulation of labor they found it unique, with lack of side effects, relative safety and ease of administration. However, the drug is *not* harmless; at the University of Iowa, Van Voorhis' group found a hypertonic state of the uterus and fetal bradycardia definitely more common than in the controls, and Harry Boysen, at the University of Illinois, has brought us up sharply with report of a rupture of the uterus under its influence. It certainly seems the part of wisdom to be just as careful in using sparteine sulfate as one would be in using oxytocin.

Albert A. Plentl, Emanuel A. Friedman and Mary Jane Gray. Sparteine Sulfate: Clinical Evaluation of Its Use in Management of Labor. Am. J. Obst. & Gynec. 82:1332, 1961. Harry Boysen. Sparteine Sulfate and Rupture of Uterus: Report of a Case. Obst. & Gynec. 21:403, 1963. Lee W. Van Voorhis, Leo J. Dunn and Darrol Heggen. Effect of Spartine Sulfate on Amniotomy Induction. Am. J. Obst. & Gynec. 94:230, 1966. Burritt W. Newton, Ralph C. Benson and Colin C. McCorriston. Sparteine Sulfate: A Potent, Capricious Oxytocic. Am. J. Obst. & Gynec. 94:234, 1966.

"Because anesthesia is a hazard to the fetus

and the mother during delivery, I have tried numerous methods of medication in order to avoid it. In recent times I have been using the meperidine (Demerol) and scopolamine combination with fair success so far as analgesia is concerned but with a disturbing amount of vomiting. How might I improve this situation?"

Reply: Chlorpromazine (Thorazine) has been found quite helpful in many practices. At the University of Kansas, Rogers' group found that the incidence of vomiting was reduced from 12–20% to 2% by adding chlorpromazine to the meperidine-scopolamine mixture. Their patients prepared for spontaneous labor were given 25 mg. chlorpromazine by deep intramuscular injection and after 30–45 minutes 100 mg. meperidine and 3 mg. scopolamine intravenously. If the patient was in active labor and apprehensive, she was given the meperidine and scopolamine shortly after receiving the chlorpromazine. Thereafter, when she became restless she was given small doses of meperidine, regardless of the amount previously given or the estimated proximity of delivery. If sedation was required beyond 5–6 hours after initial chlorpromazine injection, a second one of 12.5–25 mg. was given. If a patient was to have induction, she was given 25 mg. chlorpromazine intramuscularly, and then in 30–45 minutes intravenous oxytocin (Pitocin) was started with 150 mg. meperidine and 0.6 mg. scopolamine introduced into the tubing of the infusion set.

C. D. Rogers, C. P. Wickard and M. R. McCaskill. Labor and Delivery without Terminal Anesthesia: Report on Use of Chlorpromazine (Thorazine). Obst. & Gynec. 17:92, 1961.

"The obstetrician in our group tells me that he recently had the rather rare experience of dealing with a constriction ring dystocia and that when epinephrine failed him he got himself out of the difficulty through use of magnesium sulfate. And he is now enjoying considerable satisfaction from the fact that all of this puzzles me. Why would he resort to drugs of such different types and how would they act in this situation?"

Reply: In explanation of the constriction ring episode it is necessary to say that there are three natural uterine rings—the external os, the histologic internal os at the upper end of the cervix, and the anatomic internal os. The constriction ring, bearing no relationship to these natural rings, may occur at any time during labor and at any level of the upper or lower segments of the uterus. The normal rings rise (retract) during labor, but this constriction ring contracts down around some depression of the fetal body or below it. It is a spasmodic uterine contraction presumably comparable to the tetanic contractions occurring in other types of muscle following exces-

sive use. In its failure to relax it may cause the mother to traumatize herself in attempting to assist delivery, or it may injure the fetus through birth trauma or intrauterine asphyxia. Sometimes deep surgical anesthesia with ether is necessary to relax this ring sufficiently to permit forceps delivery, or even resort to cesarean section; more often, however, the systemic administration of either epinephrine or magnesium sulfate suffices, and even the inhalation of amyl nitrate will sometimes turn the trick. The matter of epinephrine's action was carefully studied by Kaiser and Harris in 140 patients, 121 of whom were in the twenty-sixth to fortieth weeks of pregnancy but not in labor, and 19 of whom were in labor. Uterine activity was recorded with the tocodynamometer, an instrument that picks up reflections of the contractions directly on the abdomen. The findings showed that epinephrine is strikingly inhibitory to uterine activity when used in very low concentration and that sudden withdrawal of these minute amounts is followed by increased uterine activity. The inhibition was the same in patients in labor as in those not in labor except that the greater uterine activity of the former group made it more striking. The explanation of magnesium sulfate's ability to relax the constriction ring is simply that it is a depressant of all types of muscle including that of the uterus; usual dosage is 20 ml. of 20% solution intravenously. Epinephrine is by far the preferable drug because its effect is only fleeting while that of magnesium sulfate is likely to last about half an hour.

I. H. Kaiser and J. S. Harris. Effect of Adrenalin on the Pregnant Human Uterus. Am. J. Obst. & Gynec. 59:775, 1950.

"Does the synthetic oxytocin, the product known as Syntocinon, have any advantage over the naturally occurring hormone (Pitocin)?"

Reply: It has replaced Pitocin in a good many practices because it costs just about the same and appears to be less prone to cause allergic reactions or an elevation in blood pressure.

"Oxytocin (Pitocin) stimulates the smooth muscle of the uterus and to some extent the blood vessels; does it have an effect of this sort on any other smooth muscle?"

Reply: No.

"Several years ago I saw a report indicating that the addition of hyaluronidase to ergonovine (Ergotrate) when the latter is injected intramuscularly enhances the effect. Has the matter been further investigated?"

Reply: Yes, Embrey and Garrett, in England,

looked into the matter and concluded that it is doubtfully advisable to use this combination routinely.

M. P. Embrey and W. J. Garrett. Ergometrine with Hyaluronidase: Speed of Action. Brit. M. J. 2:138, 1958.

"If the uterus appears to be excessively stimulated under the influence of oxytocin (Pitocin), ergonovine (Ergotrate) or methylergonovine (Methergine), what is the best antidotal measure?"

Reply: This uterus can be relaxed by intravenous administration of 10 ml. of 20% magnesium sulfate solution.

"It seems to me that the ergot preparations are used very loosely in obstetrical practice in our area. What are the 'principles' of this therapy?"

Reply: The action of these drugs, ergonovine (Ergotrate) and methylergonovine (Methergine), is more prolonged than that of oxytocin (Pitocin) and therefore they are not used interchangeably with it in the first two stages of labor. During the third stage, separation and expulsion of the placenta are complete within 6 minutes after delivery in nearly all anesthetized patients if the baby has delivered slowly, whether an oxytocic has been used or not. Without an oxytocic, however, more blood is lost when the placenta is expelled and considerably more afterward. Many obstetricians remove the placenta manually if it has not spontaneously come away in 20 minutes, earlier if there is excessive bleeding. Practically all remove it manually if it does not come away in an hour. Packing of the uterus to control excessive postpartum hemorrhage is nowadays only a very last-resort measure, not only because it is rarely effective and the risk of infection is great even though antibiotics are used, but also because of the relative ease with which bleeding can be prevented or controlled by the use of oxytocic drugs.

The champions of the early, and preferably intravenous, administration of ergot in the third stage say it reduces, though it does not completely eliminate, the occasions for manual removal of the placenta; they also point to the fact that through controlling hemorrhage it reduces the number of transfusions necessary when the third stage is abnormal. An abnormal third stage is considered by such observers to exist when the stage lasts more than 1 hour without hemorrhage, if more than 1 pint of blood is lost, or if there is a gush or trickle of blood from the vulva with more than three uterine contractions. In the series of 1000 patients given ergonovine early and 1000 controls not so treated reported by Martin and Dumoulin, the incidence of significant postpartum hemorrhage was lowered from 13.1% to 1.2%.

Many obstetricians give 0.2 mg. of either drug intramuscularly, or preferably intravenously, at once after the birth of the anterior shoulder in order to have strong contractions to close the sinuses as soon as the placenta is expelled. Others, fearing the too drastic ergot action so soon, wait until the placenta is expelled before giving the drug. Others give oxytocin (Pitocin) as soon as the placenta is expelled and one of the ergot drugs 20 minutes later, claiming that the muscle fibers of the cervix are caused to retract better into the body of the uterus when oxytocin is given at once after birth of the placenta than when ergot is given at this time. Their point is that oxytocin more effectively promotes the physiologic processes of both contraction and retraction, with earlier obliteration of the bleeding areas. Since the oxytocin action lasts about 20 minutes, they give the ergot intramuscularly at the end of that time.

Randall has pointed out that elimination of heavy inhalation anesthesia is an important aid in overcoming uterine atony. The intravenous injection of a calcium salt immediately after intravenous injection of the ergot preparation is alleged to enhance the oxytocic action, but it seems to me that in view of the risks associated with parenteral calcium administration this mineral should not be injected in the obstetric situation unless there is a compelling necessity to do so.

J. D. Martin and J. G. Dumoulin. Use of Intravenous Ergometrine to Prevent Postpartum Hemorrhage. Brit. M. J. 1:643, 1953. J. H. Randall. Bleeding During and After Third Stage of Labor. Jour.-Lancet 75:237, 1955.

"Please discuss the uses of oxytocin (Pitocin) in labor."

Reply: Since the term, oxytocic, is derived from two Greek roots meaning, when put together, swift birth, it is to be expected that a drug called oxytocin would shorten labor. And this is precisely what it does, both in cases of delayed initiation of labor and in instances of its prolongation. So we may speak of using oxytocin to induce labor or to promote effective contractions when labor is already in progress. Apparently also its employment will in most cases reduce the necessity of rotating an occiput posterior or occiput transverse presentation manually or with forceps. According to Greenhill, this action of the drug is especially helpful when conduction anesthesia is used because there is a high incidence of these positions associated with this form of anesthesia. When toxemia necessitates the interruption of pregnancy the drug may also be helpful, and it is sometimes used effectively to promote expulsion of the dead fetus in cases of missed abortion. Oxytocin is also effective in preventing excessive blood loss in cases of abruptio placentae and marginal placenta previa and in postpartum bleeding due to uterine atony, often precluding the use of such drastic measures to save the patient's life as hysterectomy and ligation of the uterine arteries.

In order to understand the action in postpartum hemorrhage it is necessary to know that there are three layers of muscular tissue in the wall of the uterus, laced together by many intervening muscle strands, and that the many blood vessels serving the uterus are enmeshed in the complex network resulting from the crossing and recrossing of the fibers. Uterine bleeding is normally controlled by the contraction and retraction of the interlacing muscle bundles and fibers, which constrict the vessels and sinuses almost as effectively as ligation. Thus bleeding is stopped when the placenta is delivered. But more than this must happen if the hemorrhage is to be assuaged more than momentarily, for muscle not only contracts — it relaxes, too. It is necessary also for the muscle fibers to shorten themselves, in the process called retraction, in order for hemostasis to become permanent. If the musculature is atonic and uterine retraction slow, there is postpartum hemorrhage. Oxytocin promotes retraction.

The intravenous technique described by Fields's group in reporting the use of the method in 3754 cases is practically that routinely employed throughout the world (some men preceding the Pitocin rather routinely with a sedative injection of 100 mg. meperidine [Demerol] and 0.4 mg. of scopolamine). A solution of commercially available oxytocin (Pitocin) is prepared by adding 10 units to 1000 ml. of 5% glucose solution and initiating the infusion at a rate of 6–8 drops/minute; this is then slowly increased, after the 30 seconds to 10 minutes required to establish the contractions, to the rate necessary to maintain the state desired. The usual rate is between 15 and 25 drops/minute. During the administration of the drug, fetal heart tones and the frequency of the uterine contractions must be carefully checked by a physician in constant attendance; oxytocin infusion is not a procedure to be presided over by any nurse alone, no matter how well trained she may be. It is the practice in some obstetric services to allow the infusion to continue until well after the termination of the third stage, particularly if there are bleeding problems associated with the labor.

In treating postpartum uterine atony with oxytocin infusion, the dilution found effective during labor is often inadequate and must be strengthened by using 20 instead of 10 units of Pitocin to make the 1000 ml. of 5% glucose

solution, and the dripping rate must sometimes be cautiously increased to 60 drops/minute. Sometimes even this solution is not completely effective in certain cases, particularly following severe abruptio placentae or other instances of severe atony, and it is felt necessary to increase the amount of oxytocin per 1000 ml. of solution to 40 units. Loudon reported the necessity to use higher dosage also in the management of missed abortion.

If blood is being transfused the drug may be added to this fluid instead of to a glucose solution.

J. P. Greenhill. Editorial Comment: Pitocin in Labor. 1955–56 Year Book of Obstetrics and Gynecology. Chicago, Year Book Publishers. p. 150. H. Fields, J. W. Greene, Jr., and R. R. Franklin. Intravenous Pitocin in Induction and Stimulation of Labor. Obst. & Gynec. 13:353, 1959. J. D. O. Loudon. The Use of High Concentration Oxytocin Intravenous Drips in the Management of Missed Abortion. J. Obst. & Gynec. 66:277, 1959.

"In suitable cases I have been electively inducing labor with amniotomy. Will I increase the risk to the patient by adding oxytocin (Pitocin) drip?"

Reply: I think that most obstetricians who have employed such a combination of methods agree with the report of George Schaefer (New York Hospital, Cornell Medical Center) a few years ago, who stated that the hazards of artificial rupture of the membranes alone and oxytocin induction alone are not cumulative when these procedures are performed together. Indeed, Schaefer felt that in many instances complications are avoided by using both procedures. However, all of this is predicated upon the correct choice of a candidate for induction. I shall list here Schaefer's criteria of suitability for elective induction, though I am aware that not all obstetricians would agree with him on all heads: (1) The patient is a multipara who has had at least one but less than five vaginal deliveries. (2) The cervix is not less than 3 cm. dilated and at least 60% effaced. (3) The cervix is centrally located in the axis of the vagina and is not posterior or difficult to reach. (4) The presenting part is a vertex at station −1 or lower. (5) The infant's weight is estimated between 6 and 8½ lb. (6) The pelvis is ample and there is no evidence of cephalopelvic disproportion. (7) There is no history of previous difficult labor or delivery. (8) The patient is within 10 days of the expected date of confinement as determined by her menstrual history. (9) The patient is psychologically prepared and knows what to expect.

George Schaefer. Elective Induction of Labor with Oxytocin and Amniotomy. Obst. & Gynec. 15:465, 1960.

"One of my young associates has been telling me that when I combine the use of a vasoconstrictor with an oxytocic drug in labor I am increasing the risk to the patient. Is this true?"

Reply: Several years ago, Casady and associates, in Seattle, studied the matter; the records of their 741 women indicated that the combined effect of a vasoconstrictor and an oxytocic drug, given 3–6 hours apart, led to severe hypertension in 4.6% of the cases. Prophylactic administration of a vasoconstrictor when regional block anesthesia is used was also found undesirable.

Gilbert N. Casady, Daniel C. Moore and L. Donald Bridenbaugh. Postpartum Hypertension After Use of Vasoconstrictor and Oxytocic Drugs: Etiology, Incidence, Complications and Treatment. J.A.M.A. 172:1011, Mar. 5, 1960.

"In our hospital methylergonovine (Methergine) has largely replaced ergonovine (Ergotrate) in the third stage of labor. Is this newer drug really superior to the older, which is often less expensive?"

Reply: The findings of neither Walter Groeber and Edward Bishop, in Philadelphia, nor Russell deAlvarez at the University of Washington, provided statistically significant evidence of such a superiority, and I think that many obstetricians have made such an evaluation in their own practice.

Walter R. Groeber and Edward H. Bishop. Methergine (Methylergonovine) and Ergonovine (Ergotrate) in Third Stage of Labor. Obst. & Gynec. 15:85, 1960. Russell R. deAlvarez. Synthetic Ergonovine (Methergine) and Ergonovine (Ergotrate): Comparative Evaluation of Effect on Postpartum Uterus. Obst. & Gynec. 15:80, 1960.

"In secondary arrest of dilatation in the active phase of the first stage of labor, what are the limiting criteria of a therapeutic trial of oxytocin (Pitocin) stimulation?"

Reply: In Friedman and Sachtleben's study of this matter, at Columbia University, they found that, in the absence of disproportion, the relative increase in the dilatation rate after successful oxytocin therapy, as compared with the prearrest rate, is of critical prognostic importance. Nearly all of their patients delivered normally if they responded after secondary arrest with a rate of dilatation over 1–1.5 cm./hour greater than the prearrest rate.

Emanuel A. Friedman and Marlene R. Sachtleben. Dysfunctional Labor: V. Therapeutic Trial of Oxytocin in Secondary Arrest. Obst. & Gynec. 21:13, 1963.

"How do the oxytocic drugs compare in the fourth stage of labor?"

Reply: In Iowa City, William Howard and associates assessed the effects of oxytocin

(Pitocin), methylergonovine maleate (Methergine) and a placebo upon the fourth stage of labor in 1459 parturient women in a controlled double-blind study. Although patients in the placebo group had a higher incidence of hemorrhage and more often required additional treatment in the form of an oxytocic agent, 88% of this group had no difficulty and atony developed in 5% of those who did receive treatment. It appeared that routine use of oxytocic drugs was of benefit to only 7% of patients postpartum. However, from the standpoint of efficacy, oxytocin and methylergonovine differed little in the management of the fourth stage; oxytocin produced fewer pressor responses than methylergonovine, though both produced more than did the placebo. But it should be noted that one third of the control group exhibited some pressor response and that in one third of these the blood pressure rise was striking; therefore it may not be admissible to attribute a marked rise in pressure following delivery to an oxytocic drug.

William F. Howard, Philip R. McFadden and William C. Keettel. Oxytocic Drugs in Fourth Stage of Labor. J.A.M.A. 189:411, Aug. 10, 1964.

"What are the cardiovascular effects of rapid intravenous injection of oxytocin (Pitocin) during cesarean section?"

Reply: At the University of Florida, Thorkild Andersen and associates found the effects to be very consistent; all of their 22 patients showed transient profound decreases in systolic and diastolic blood pressures and all but 3 a striking increase in heart rate. In all 16 patients in whom cardiac output was determined, oxytocin caused a marked increase in output and a profound decrease in the calculated total peripheral resistance. The electrocardiographic changes observed were nonspecific. Blood pressure in patients under spinal or epidural analgesia appeared to fall less than in those receiving other types of anesthesia, but the differences were not statistically significant.

Thorkild W. Andersen, C. B. DePadua, V. Stenger and H. Prystowsky. Cardiovascular Effects of Rapid Intravenous Injection of Synthetic Oxytocin During Elective Cesarean Section. Clin. Pharmacol. & Therap. 6:345, 1965.

"One of my associates has used oxytocin (Pitocin) in a breech presentation and says that he will do it again when opportunity presents. What do you think of this?"

Reply: I can cite the experience of Karl Neimand and Alexander Rosenthal, at the Long Island Jewish Hospital, who reported on a series of 328 patients with breech presentation in approximately one half of whom oxytocin stimulation of labor was used. There was no maternal mortality and the corrected perinatal mortality was low in patients who received the drug. This was also true for perinatal morbidity and indicated to these observers that oxytocin stimulation of labor is a safe procedure in the patient with breech presentation. The measure was also used in 23 patients with multiple gestations where at least 1 baby presented and was delivered as a breech presentation; there was no perinatal mortality in this group. However, this is only one report, and I am sure you are aware that there is almost universal disapproval of the use of oxytocin in the management of labor in breech presentation.

Karl M. Neimand and Alexander H. Rosenthal. Oxytocin in Breech Presentation. Am. J. Obst. & Gynec. 93:230, 1965.

"With some apprehension I have used hyaluronidase (Wydase) in a few instances in attempting to reduce the requirement for episiotomy. Success has been pretty good, but I would like to know what the experience of others has been, particularly whether there have been complications."

Reply: At Columbia-Presbyterian Medical Center, in New York, James O'Leary and Selcuk Erez made a study of this matter in 50 nulliparas or primiparas at term vaginal delivery, with a similar untreated control group; patients with breech and premature births were excluded. They injected 5–10 ml. of hyaluronidase before delivery into the perineal body, hymen and any previous episiotomy scars. An intact perineum was three times more frequent in the hyaluronidase-treated group than in the controls, and lacerations were less common; there was also a decreased incidence and size of the episiotomies. Post partum and at 6 weeks there was the same amount of perineal support in both groups of patients. It was also said that less medication was required in the study group, probably because of the fewer episiotomies. No intrapartum or postpartum complications that could be related to the use of the enzyme were noted.

James A. O'Leary and Selcuk Erez. Hyaluronidase as Adjuvant to Episiotomy. Obst. & Gynec. 26:66, 1965.

"One of my obstetrical associates is using ethchlorvynol (Placidyl) as a sedative in labor. He gives the patient two 500 mg. capsules of the drug to be taken at home at the onset of labor, and then at the hospital after routine preparation 2 more capsules are taken. Meperidine (Demerol), promethazine (Phenergan) or phenobarbital are injected also as indicated. He finds that less analgesic and adjunctive medication is required in patients so treated than in those not using the ethchlorvynol, finding the procedure especially useful in multiparas with rapid labor in whom it is difficult to effect adequate analgesia. Is this entirely safe medication?"

Reply: This drug, together with the other members of its group of newer nonbarbiturate sedatives—ethinamate (Valmid), methyprylon (Noludar) and glutethimide (Doriden)—appears much less likely to produce deep depression in dosage that is satisfactorily sedative than are the barbiturates. However, overdosage with any one of them will certainly produce very deep sedation, and I should therefore think it advisable not to provide the patient with more than 2 of the capsules to take on her own at home. In fact, Harold Boros and Maurice Priver, in Los Angeles, found that 2 of the 500 mg. tablets taken at home induced excessive sedation in a few of their patients, notably in those weighing less than 130 pounds. So it would appear a wise precaution to cut the home dosage in half for smaller women.

Harold H. Boros and Maurice S. Priver. Ethchlorvynol as a Sedative in Labor. Am. J. Obst. & Gynec. 89:1016, Aug. 15, 1964.

"In former times we used Pituitrin injections to stimulate labor, which I always felt to be dangerous practice; then came the intravenous drip of Pitocin, which is a practicable measure; to be followed by intranasal applications and even by a transbuccal method of administration. What advantage could the last of these methods have?"

Reply: It appears that the chief advantage claimed for this method is that the oxytocin effect can be quickly terminated by removal of the tablet from the mouth. It has not gained a large following, though a 200 mg. buccal tablet is available. In their recent report, Douglas and Dillon, at Cornell University, said they place such a tablet in a parabuccal space and an additional one every 20 minutes as needed to produce active progressive labor and delivery, removing tablets if the intensity of contractions becomes too great or the patient can no longer maintain protection of her airway.

R. Gordon Douglas and Thomas F. Dillon. Use of Transbuccal Oxytocin for Induction and Stimulation of Labor. South. M. J. 58:914, 1965. J. M. Ritchie and J. M. Brudenell. Routine Use of Buccal Oxytocin After Amniotomy for Induction of Labor. Brit. M. J. 1:581, Mar. 5, 1966.

"One of my associates has high praise for the intranasal route of administering oxytocin (Pitocin) in the induction of labor, but I have hesitated to try it. What is the consensus?"

Reply: I do not know that a consensus has been reached as yet, but there are certainly detractors as well as champions of the method. At Emory University, Clement's group reviewed the records of their patients who had received the drug intranasally during labor. They found that the measure had been successful in 91.5% of 47 primigravidas and 79.4% of 184 multiparas. There had been no latent period longer than 4 hours. When the induction had been for medical reasons it was successful in 85.6% of 14 primigravidas and 94.4% of 36 multiparas. At Mount Sinai Hospital, New York, Jacques Cohen and associates determined the response of the gravid uterus at term to intranasal oxytocin by intra-amniotic fluid pressure recordings and found that each of their 15 patients showed uterine response within 3–10 minutes after administration of the drug. This finding was interpreted to mean that 1 oxytocin spray in each nostril was approximately as effective as intravenous administration of standard dosage for 15 minutes. Their conclusion was that the intranasal spray is a safe method of administering relatively small quantities of oxytocin but that intravenous administration is more precise and more readily controlled and is the method of choice under ordinary conditions. Then in Indianapolis, Stander's group obtained continuous recordings of amniotic fluid pressure under the influence of intranasal oxytocin and found the measure most often successful in patients requiring only minimal enhancement of uterine contractility; included were those at term with ruptured membranes in whom labor had not begun and those in whom labor failed to progress normally because of infrequent or low-intensity contractions. Their conclusion was also that the intranasal spray can be efficacious, but, because of the variability of response, they still prefer intravenous infusion when oxytocin is indicated. In Australia, Bradfield also emphasized the lack of precision in the drug's action and observed significant uterine hyperactivity and hypoxic fetal heart rate changes. Finally, at the Medical College of Georgia, Eduardo Talledo and associates evaluated the response of the uterus at term, as measured by intra-amniotic pressure changes, to intranasal administration of oxytocin, the response of pain being compared to one produced by known concentrations of oxytocin given intravenously in an effort to estimate the amount of drug absorbed through the nasal mucosa. The purpose was not to initiate labor, but to create measurable responses and to assay the applicability of the intranasal administration of the drug in clinical obstetrics. The study was very carefully performed and the conclusion reached was that the unpredictability of absorption and uterine response makes the intranasal route of administration relatively unsafe, and these investigators were unwilling to recommend it for routine management of the pregnant patient.

Alan Bradfield. Reservations on the Safety of Oxytocin Nasal Spray. Aust. New Zeal. J. Obstet. Gynaec. 5:138, 1965. Eduardo Talledo, Suzanne F. Adams and Frederick P. Zuspan. Response of Pregnant Human Uterus to Oxytocin Given Intranasally. J.A.M.A. 189:348, Aug. 3, 1964. J. Edwin Clement, Walton C. Harwell and John R. McCain. Use of Intranasal Oxytocin for Induction and/or Stimulation of Labor. Am. J. Obst. & Gynec. 83:778, Mar. 15, 1962. Jacques Cohen, John Danezis and Michael S. Burnhill. Response of Gravid Uterus at Term to Intranasal Oxytocin as Determined by Intra-amniotic Fluid Pressure Recordings. Am. J. Obst. & Gynec. 83:774, 1962. Richard W. Stander, Joseph F. Thompson and Charles P. Gibbs. Evaluation of Intranasal Oxytocin by Amniotic Fluid Pressure Recordings. Am. J. Obst. & Gynec. 85: 193, 1963.

LACTATION

"I am confused by the methods and the hormonal preparations used both to support and to discourage lactation. Can you give me a bit of help?"

Reply: I shall cite three studies. First, those of Jones and Tanner (Baroness Erlanger Hospital, Chattanooga, Tenn.), and Jules Napier and associates (University of Oregon), and without going into the details of what was done, here is the impression I gained from this work. I hope it is correct and not too simple. If you want to aid your patient in *not* nursing her baby, give her a pure estrogen preparation. If you want to *support and aid her* in nursing, give a simple testosterone preparation. If you anticipate that she may change her mind and wish to nurse after having decided not to do so originally, give her a preparation that contains both hormones. Herewith the preparations employed in the two studies cited—Delestrogen: estradiol valerate, 10 mg./ml.; thus merely a simple estrogen preparation. Deladumone: testosterone enanthate, 90 mg., estradiol valerate, 4 mg./ml.; thus an androgen-estrogen preparation. Deladumone 2X: both the ingredients of the above in twice the strength. Delatestryl: testosterone enanthate, 200 mg./ml.; thus merely a simple androgen preparation. And now for the third study: At the National Maternity Hospital, in Dublin, Dermot MacDonald and Kieran O'Driscoll carried out a double-blind study with an estrogen and a placebo in 500 women and were unable to observe that one was more effective than the other in preventing uncomfortable breast engorgement. You have asked for a "bit" of help; I wonder if my answer qualifies?

Harry E. Jones and Jack E. Tanner. Suppression of Lactation: Use of Single Androgen-Estrogen Injection. Obst. & Gynec. 19:51, 1962. Jules Napier, Ralph C. Benson and Carl E. Hopkins. Effect of Delahormones on Lactation in the Nursing Mother: New Approach. West. J. Surg. 69:377, 1961. Dermot MacDonald and Kieran O'Driscoll. Suppression of Lactation: A Double-Blind Trial. Lancet 2:623, Sept. 25, 1965.

"In attempting the suppression of lactation and

breast engorgement in nonnursing mothers, I have injected the testosterone enanthate-estradiol valerate preparation, Deladumone, immediately after the third stage of labor, but the results have not been very striking. Could you suggest anything?"

Reply: I wonder if your dosage has been adequate? At the Mary Imogene Bassett Hospital, Cooperstown, New York, Douglas Barns found that when 3 or 4 ml. of this preparation was injected, fair to good relief was obtained in about 90% of instances. Or you might even try giving the injection immediately after the first stage of labor, as was done by Presto and Caypinar, at St. John's Episcopal Hospital, Brooklyn. It was said by the latter observers that complete prevention of lactation and its sequelae was achieved in 91.5% of their patients and that the subsequent course of labor was in no way altered.

Douglas H. Barnes. Suppression of Postpartum Lactation and Prevention of Breast Engorgement in Nonnursing Mothers. Am. J. Obst. & Gynec. 81:339, 1961. Benjamin Lo Presto and Erol Y. Caypinar. Prevention of Postpartum Lactation by Administration of Deladumone During Labor. J.A.M.A. 169:250, Jan. 17, 1959.

LANDRY'S PARALYSIS

"Is there any specific or near-specific drug therapy in Landry's paralysis (acute idiopathic polyneuritis)?"

Reply: No.

LEAD ENCEPHALOPATHY

"What is the position of oral penicillamine (Cuprimine) vis-à-vis a parenteral lead chelator such as calcium disodium edetate (EDTA) in the treatment of lead poisoning?"

Reply: Several years ago, C. E. C. Harris, at St. Mary's Hospital, Montreal, concluded that the slight inferiority of penicillamine to versenate was outweighed by its greater ease of administration, lower cost and lower toxicity. More recently, at the Western Infirmary, Glasgow, A. Goldberg's group also found penicillamine to be the superior of the two drugs. A 300 mg./day dose was felt to be sufficient to effect significant lead excretion provided the patient is not exposed to further lead intoxication.

Cecil E. C. Harris. Comparison of Intravenous Calcium Disodium Versenate and Oral Penicillamine in Promoting Elimination of Lead. Canad. M. A. J. 79:664, Oct. 15, 1958. A. Goldberg, Jacqueline A. Smith and Ann C. Lochhead. Treatment of Lead Poisoning with Oral Penicillamine (Cuprimine). Proc. Staff Meet. Mayo Clin. 38: 203, May 22, 1963.

"Lead poisoning still has not only a high case fatality rate but leaves the survivor with some damage to the central nervous system in a surprising proportion of cases. Most of us in our industrial area occasionally see a case of lead encephalopathy which we treat with EDTA without being entirely pleased with our results. Might the use of hemodialysis together with the chelating agent be helpful?"

Reply: In Cincinnati, Smith and associates put this to the test in an attempt to accelerate the removal of lead from the soft tissues of 4 children with lead encephalopathy, and found the combined therapy ineffective at least under the conditions of their study. Hemodialysis itself is not without some risks and is certainly a laborious procedure.

Hugo Dunlap Smith, Lionel R. King and E. Gordon Margolin. Treatment of Lead Encephalopathy. Am. J. Dis. Child. 109:322, 1965.

LEISHMANIASIS

"A case of American mucocutaneous leishmaniasis, with much facial disfigurement, has troubled me greatly because it has not responded to treatments with antimony, the usual antibiotics, 'stimulating' roentgen therapy and even local application of chromic acid. What should I do now?"

Reply: At the University of Munich, Schirren and Neuner treated such a case that had been imported from Venezuela with triweekly infusions of amphotericin B with 0.25 mg./kg. slowly increased to 1 mg./kg. They dissolved the drug in 500 ml. of 5% dextrose solution and added 25 mg. Solu-Decortin; and an antipyretic was given with each infusion, which was administered in a darkened room during 4 hours. During the treatment, nitrogen retention rose from 25 to 40% and the hemoglobin level sank sufficiently to justify two blood transfusions. But the patient was discharged in fairly good condition after 2 months.

C. G. Schirren and Y. Neuner. Influence of Amphotericin B Infusions on American Mucocutaneous Leishmaniasis. Hautarzt 14:473, 1963.

LEPROSY

"Just how much can be accomplished in the 'specific' therapy of leprosy nowadays?"

Reply: The sulfones are established in a position of undoubted supremacy to chaulmoogra oil and other agents that were used earlier; such compounds as diamino-diphenylsulfone (Avlosulfon), sulfoxone (Diasone) and glucosulfone (Promin). Clinical improvement of skin and mucous membrane lesions is definite and universal; involution to the point of complete disappearance may occur, but there are usually some residuals. Healing of the inflammatory mucosal lesions and the nasal and laryngeal ulcerations brings relief from nasal obstruction, epistaxis, dyspnea and hoarseness, and there is also relief from the discomfort, odor and unpleasantness of secondarily infected lesions. Formation of new leprous lesions is prevented and surgical and orthopedic corrections of deformities are facilitated. Unfortunately, however, disappearance of lepra bacilli from the lesions lags far behind clinical improvement, which is of course a serious deficiency in the drugs. Macular lesions may become negative after $1\frac{1}{2}$–3 years, but nodular and diffuse lesions sometimes require 3–5 or more years of treatment. I believe it is the consensus of leprologists that opportunity for contact of leprous and nonleprous individuals should be curtailed until the organisms can be recovered only with considerable difficulty. Unfortunately, the disease tends to relapse when sulfone administration stops, but the incidence of this may apparently be held to no more than 5% by continuing the use of one-third usual dosage after apparent arrest of the disease.

LEPTOSPIROSIS

"A case of leptospirosis has appeared in my practice in a patient who has just returned by jet plane from abroad. Is there an effective antibiotic therapy for this disease?"

Reply: No, unfortunately there is not. In his study comparing symptomatic treatment with penicillin therapy, Kocen (British Military Hospital, Taiping, Malaya) thought that most of the acute symptoms were more rapidly reduced with the antibiotic, but the final incidence of hemorrhagic manifestations, jaundice, renal involvement or stiff neck was 80% in each of the treated groups. This is really an intolerable situation in a malady that is very debilitating and of fairly high incidence in numerous parts of the world.

R. S. Kocen. Leptospirosis: Comparison of Symptomatic and Penicillin Therapy. Brit. M. J. 1:1181, Apr. 28, 1962.

LETTERER-SIWE DISEASE

"We have just diagnosed a case of Letterer-Siwe disease in our hospital and feel very helpless and hopeless. What can we do?"

Reply: As your question implies, you are aware that these cases are usually quickly fatal. However, in The Netherlands, Grosfeld and Spaas observed a girl with the typical

cutaneous changes of Letterer-Siwe disease who showed distinct improvement on histologic examination after oral treatment with dexamethasone (Decadron), and the child had continued in good condition for some time when they made their report. And in California, Howard Bierman reported the 17 year survival, in apparently good health, of a pair of identical twins who had been treated with multiple antibiotics.

J. C. M. Grosfeld and J. Spaas. Letterer-Siwe Disease: Favorable Results After Treatment with Dexamethasone. Dermatologica 128:387, 1964. Howard R. Bierman. Apparent Cure of Letterer-Siwe Disease. J.A.M.A. 196:368, Apr. 25, 1966.

LÖFFLER'S SYNDROME

"I have a patient with Löffler's syndrome who has responded quite dramatically to corticosteroid therapy. He moves about the country a good bit and it is difficult to control his therapy. How long should I continue the treatment?"

Reply: In reporting on 2 cases of this disease, seen at the Mayo Clinic, Dines and Donoghue expressed the opinion that corticosteroid treatment should be continued at the lowest dosage that will prevent a recurrence of symptoms and infiltration of the lungs, which often amounts to continuous treatment for a year. Relapse is also common if the dosage is tapered off too quickly. If there is a positive tuberculin reaction the therapy should be supplemented by the use of isoniazid, especially if prolonged corticosteroid therapy is being contemplated.

David E. Dines and F. Edmund Donoghue. Loeffler's Syndrome. J.A.M.A. 192:254, April 19, 1965.

LUPUS ERYTHEMATOSUS, DISCOID

"I have tried all the local treatments known to me for discoid lupus erythematosus, with no permanent effects. Is there something that I may not have tried?"

Reply: Perhaps you haven't heard of Wesley Wilson's study down in Tampa, Florida? He injected hydroxychloroquine (Plaquenil) intralesionally into 46 patients, using a solution of 40 mg./ml. in dosage of 0.1–0.5 ml./sq. cm., allegedly without discomfort. Treatment was repeated every 2 or 3 weeks. He said that sometimes one or two injections resulted in clearing, but that most patients required 8–12 injections for maximum improvement. Following one third of the patients for about 2 years, only 2 were found to manifest new lesions. I do not doubt that this happened as Dr. Wilson said, but his results were also so good in larva migrans and warts that the study well deserves repeating in independent hands.

Wesley W. Wilson. Clinical Evaluation of Intralesional Administration of Hydroxychloroquine Sulfate (Plaquenil) in Several Diseases. South. M. J. 56:794, 1963.

"Having failed to convince myself of the true efficacy of any of the many drugs that I have tried in a rather large experience with chronic discoid lupus erythematosus, I find myself quite discouraged. *Is there anything approaching specific therapy in this malady?*"

Reply: Many claims have certainly been made for many drugs, but it is easy to accept the conclusion reached by Kraak's group, in Amsterdam, as the result of an exhaustive review of the literature, that the information given in most of the reports is insufficient for evaluation of the therapies employed. Even in their own careful study of the effect of hydroxychloroquine (Plaquenil) they felt obliged to stress the point that the drug had no effect whatever in some cases though in others it appeared to be more effective than placebo. In a group of patients treated by them for a whole year with placebo, the natural history of the disease could be studied. The findings were that most of the exacerbations and relapses occurred in spring and early summer and that spontaneous improvement and even cure are not rare, especially in the last 5 months of the year. If one throws this finding across the reported results with drugs of diverse types, one's skepticism increases.

J. H. Kraak, W. G. van Ketel, J. R. Prakken and W. R. van Zwet. The Value of Hydroxychloroquine (Plaquenil) for the Treatment of Chronic Discoid Lupus Erythematosus: A Double-Blind Trial. Dermatologica 130:293, 1965.

LUPUS ERYTHEMATOSUS, SYSTEMIC

"I have a patient with undoubted systemic lupus erythematosus that seems to be pursuing a mild course so far; i.e., there are only minimal complaints such as dermatitis and a nondisabling arthropathy without objective joint signs. *Should I institute corticosteroid therapy?*"

Reply: A categorical answer to such a question regarding an individual case would of course be too hazardous to be admissible, so I shall only say that at the University of California, Jack Posnick decided, as a result of his study, that the corticosteroids are of little or no benefit in patients with mild systemic lupus erythematosus and that limiting therapy to rest and salicylates seems warranted in such cases. The increased survival time in patients with moderate disease appears to support the use of corticosteroids there, and when involvement is severe, intensive corticosteroid therapy is indicated.

Jack Posnick. Systemic Lupus Erythematosus: Effect of Corticotropin and Adrenocorticoid Therapy on Survival Rate. California Med. 98:308, 1963.

"I have heard that the antineoplastic agents are being effectively used in the treatment of systemic lupus erythematosus. *Is this correct?*"

Reply: I do not know about the antineoplastic agents as a group, but I have seen the report of Cheng Siang, Seah and associates, in Singapore, who had a very good response to cyclophosphamide (Cytoxan) in 3 of 9 patients and a moderately good response in 3 others. The only serious complications they had with the drug occurred in the 3 who did not respond to it: severe alopecia, severe leukopenia and aggravation of mucosal ulcerations in 1 of the patients. These investigators felt that patients presenting with serious complications should be given the benefit of corticosteroid therapy first and that cyclophosphamide should then be introduced later, when it will be found usually to lower the corticosteroid requirement.

Cheng Siang, Seah, K. H. Wong, Andrew G. K. Chew, F. J. Jayaratnam. Cyclophosphamide in the Treatment of Systemic Lupus Erythematosus. Brit. M. J. 1:333, Feb. 5, 1966.

"I have a patient with lupus erythematosus that I am inclined to ascribe to the taking of procainamide (Pronestyl) because she developed lupus-like symptoms (not recognized as such at the time) after a prolonged period on this drug for the correction of atrial fibrillation; and then when the drug was withdrawn the symptoms receded, only to reappear with reinstitution of the procainamide therapy. I know that a number of drugs have been established in association with the development of lupus, but *has procainamide been included in the list heretofore?*"

Reply: Yes, I have seen reports of several such instances and we have recently had a case in our own hospital in which such an association was strongly suspected.

Jerrold M. Kaplan, Herbert L. Wachtel, Stephen W. Czarnecki and John J. Sampson. Lupus-like Illness Precipitated by Procainamide Hydrochloride. J.A.M.A. 192:444, May 10, 1965. Robert Paine. Procainamide Hydrochloride and Lupus Erythematosus. J.A.M.A. 194:23, Oct. 4, 1965.

"I have an epileptic patient under treatment with diphenylhydantoin (Dilantin) and phenobarbital who has now developed systemic lupus erythematosus. *Is there reason to believe that the malady may be drug-induced?*"

Reply: Possible association of drugs with

the onset of SLE has involved agents in the anticonvulsant, antituberculosis, antihypertensive, cardiac depressant and sulfonamide groups, so far as they have come to my attention. Regarding specifically the anticonvulsants, the study of Kenneth Wilske's group at the University of Washington may be cited. In their group of 120 institutionalized patients, half on chronic anticonvulsant therapy, 5 individuals developed multiple abnormalities commonly associated with SLE, and all 5 were in the drug-treated group. However, the wider experience regarding all of the drugs in the categories that I have mentioned points to an incidence of drug association so low that one is obliged to believe that the individuals who are affected are only those in whom an underlying genetic diathesis is triggered by some sort of stimulus supplied by the drug that they are taking.

Kenneth R. Wilske, Ivan E. Shalit, Robert F. Willkens and John L. Decker. Findings Suggestive of Systemic Lupus Erythematosus in Subjects on Chronic Anticonvulsant Therapy. Arthritis & Rheum. 8:260, 1965.

LYMPHEDEMA

"I have a patient with primary lymphedema in whom I am accomplishing very little with diuretics. What has been the experience of others?"

Reply: The reports on the effectiveness of this therapy have certainly been conflicting. The best results that have come to my attention were those reported by W. R. Cattell and associates, in London, who performed a double-blind crossover trial of chlorothiazide (Diuril) in 1 Gm. daily dosage for 5 days a week in 25 patients. They felt that considerable improvement had been achieved in a third of the cases when analyzing the effects in terms of the subjective assessment by the patient, change in body weight, and change in limb circumference and volume. It was not felt that their experience provided any basis for prediction of which patients would respond to the therapy. A 3 month trial was suggested in all cases.

W. R. Cattell, G. W. Taylor and D. Artken. Diuretic Therapy of Primary Lymphedema. Lancet 2:312, Aug. 14, 1965.

MACROGLOBULINEMIA

"I have a patient with the rare disease, macroglobulinemia; what do I do?"

Reply: At the University of Wisconsin, Dallas Clatanoff and Ovid Meyer successfully used chlorambucil (Leukeran) in their 2 cases. Hemoglobin rose, total serum protein and macroglobulin decreased and albumin concentration increased. Dosage was started at 12 mg. daily and continued for 2 weeks, then reduced to 4 mg. daily for the next month; at one time in 1 of the patients there was a reversal and dosage had to be resumed at 8 mg. daily and discontinued for 4 weeks 1 month later because of leukopenia. Maintenance dosage of 2 mg. daily seemed satisfactory later.

At the Mayo Clinic, Edwin Bayrd and associates have continued chlorambucil treatment for 1½–5 years in daily doses of 2–8 mg. Three patients had a relapse when treatment was discontinued – 1 in 3 months, 1 in 12 months and 1 after 36 months. Two of these 3 patients died, but all of the other 9 patients who continued treatment were still alive at the time of the report. Bouroncle's group has also used the drug successfully in 3 cases at Ohio State University.

Dallas V. Clatanoff and Ovid O. Meyer. Response to Chlorambucil (Leukeran) in Macroglobulinemia. J.A.M.A. 183:40, Jan. 5, 1963. Edwin D. Bayrd, Albert B. Hagedorn and Warren F. McGuckin. Macroglobulinemia. J.A.M.A. 193:724, Aug. 30, 1965. B. A. Bouroncle, P. Datta and W. J. Frajola. Waldenström's Macroglobulinemia: Report of 3 Cases Treated with Cyclophosphamide. J.A.M.A. 189:729, 1964.

MALARIA

"We have not yet had a soldier return from Vietnam to our area with P. falciparum malaria, but we expect to have this happen at any time. How shall we treat him?"

Reply: He should be given quinine sulfate, 0.65 gm. (2 tablets of 5 gr. each), every 8 hours for 7–10 days. Keep him in bed during this time because of the tendency of some patients to develop postural hypotension while under the drug; and watch the urine output and discontinue the drug temporarily if oliguria develops. If the patient cannot retain the quinine or is in coma, the drug may be given intravenously. But you should be aware that this is a hazardous procedure, to be resorted to only under the conditions stated. Use quinine dihydrochloride, 600 mg. in 600 ml. of normal saline, and give it *very slowly* by intravenous drip with constant monitoring of the blood pressure and the pulse to detect hypotension or arrhythmia. This dose may be repeated at 8 hour intervals as required, returning to oral medication (by stomach tube if necessary) as soon as possible. If the patient responds to the therapy but later undergoes a recrudescence of the disease, repeat the quinine course and if necessary continue it for 3 weeks or even more if he can tolerate it. If the patient is responding well clinically but nevertheless has asexual parasites in the blood stream, you should give him 50 mg. daily of pyrimethamine (Daraprim) for 3 days, together with 0.5 Gm.

of sulfadiazine every 6 hours for 5 days. And see that he remains well hydrated throughout the therapy.

Dept. of Health, Education & Welfare, Communicable Disease Center, Malaria Special Report. 66–1, Jan. 17, 1966.

"Many of us practicing in the north Temperate Zone are asked with increasing frequency to recommend malaria prophylaxis for patients whose business takes them for longer or shorter periods into areas where malaria is endemic, principally nowadays into Africa. My practice is to prescribe 2 of the 250 mg. chloroquine diphosphate (Aralen) tablets to be taken on the same day each week, one-fourth this dosage for infants under 4 years of age, one-half for other children. And I like for the patient, with his family if they have accompanied him to the tropics, to see me upon his return so that I can admonish him to continue the Aralen regimen for 4–6 weeks when back at home again. I like to combine this also with 15 mg. of primaquine once daily for 14 days, because very occasionally one can see a 'relapse' of vivax malaria in an individual who has not continued the Aralen for as long as 2 years after leaving the endemic area. Now, however, since this regimen is somewhat cumbersome and numerous individuals simply will not follow through with it, I am wondering whether the new drug we have heard so much about, that is supposed to protect for 9–12 months through the taking of a single dose, is about to become available for our prescribing?"

Reply: The reference is, of course, to the drug developed by Thompson and his associates at Parke, Davis & Co., and known provisionally as Camolar. The answer is that this drug is still under investigation, both in voluntary malaria patients in this country and in endemic areas in Africa and elsewhere, but has not yet been freed for prescription use.

G. Robert Coatney, Peter G. Contacos and Joseph S. Lunn. Further Observations on Antimalarial Activity of CI 501 (Camolar) Against the Chesson Strain of Vivax Malaria. Am. J. Trop. Med. & Hyg. 13:383, 1964. Peter G. Contacos, G. Robert Coatney, Joseph S. Lunn and John W. Kilpatrick (Nat'l. Inst. of Health). Antimalarial Activity of CI 501 (Camolar) Against Falciparum Malaria. Am. J. Trop. Med. & Hyg. 13:386, 1964.

"A young patient in my practice, recently returned from a brief sojourn in tropical America, has presented with vivax malaria and a considerable therapeutic problem because she fought tigerishly against oral medication, supported by her overprotective neurotic mother. Had I succeeded in getting a rectal suppository of chloroquine (Aralen) into this little vixen, with the mother lured out of the room of course, might I have expected to achieve a satisfactory blood level of the drug?"

Reply: Yes, but Bruce-Chwatt and Gibson, in Nigeria, found that the drug was only one-third as effective when given in suppository form as when given orally. It took a week to clear their 6 children of parasites when they were given intrarectal doses of 300 mg. of the hydrochloride salt daily for 5 days. The drug acts very rapidly when given intramuscularly.

L. J. Bruce-Chwatt and F. D. Gibson. Chloroquine (Aralen) per Rectum for Malaria in Children. Brit. M. J. 1:894, Apr. 4, 1959.

"We hear much nowadays about the resistance of Vietnam falciparum malaria to chloroquine (Aralen). Has vivax malaria also become resistant to the drug?"

Reply: No, the vivax organism is still practically completely susceptible to chloroquine. The accepted oral therapy is 1.0 Gm. of chloroquine diphosphate (Aralen) immediately and 0.5 Gm. 6 hours later, and the latter dose then repeated once daily for 2 succeeding days.

MALIGNANCY: LYMPHOMAS AND LEUKEMIAS

"I have a young patient with acute leukemia who is in relapse after conventional therapy with corticosteroids, methotrexate, 6-mercaptopurine. Associates advised me to use cyclophosphamide (Cytoxan), and I did so but without effect. What has been the recorded experience?"

Reply: In the experience of Fernbach and associates, there was complete hematologic and clinical remission in 8 of 44 children. Remissions occurred with each of several dosage schedules, lasted 100–453 days with a mean of 206 days, and were not related to concomitant or antecedent corticosteroid therapy. There were partial remissions in an additional 5 patients.

Donald J. Fernbach, Wataru W. Sutow, William G. Thurman and Theresa J. Vietti. Clinical Evaluation of Cyclophosphamide (Cytoxan): New Agent for Treatment of Children with Acute Leukemia. J.A.M.A. 182:30, Oct. 6, 1962.

"What are the principal pitfalls that may be encountered in the drug therapy of leukemia in childhood?"

Reply: Donald Pinkel, in Memphis, has listed the following chiefly important things: discontinuance of antimetabolites too early (6-mercaptopurine [Purinethol] and methotrexate may require 3–8 weeks of administration before providing maximal benefit); failure to adjust dosage to individual tolerance (not only is there great variation in the sensitivity of patients to the toxic effect of the drugs, but malnutrition, infection, prior treatment with ionizing radiation or cytotoxic agents, impaired renal function and marrow infiltration with tumor may provoke severe reactions to moderate doses); misinterpreting leukopenia occurring during the treatment of acute leukemia (such leukopenia does not always indicate drug toxicity, for during induction it may indicate a favorable response or progressive disease and during remission it may indicate relapse; when leukopenia occurs a bone marrow examination is necessary to clarify its significance); continuous use of prednisone (this may cause severe disabilities, generalized osteoporosis with pathologic fractures, disabling muscular atrophy, hypertension); failing to protect the child from exposure to infectious disease; failure to regard fever during leukemia as a symptom of infection; failure to treat neutropenia during leukemia complicated by infection (infusion of fresh white blood cells, collected from 1 or 2 liters of fresh human blood by differential centrifugation, often appears to be beneficial).

Donald Pinkel. Pitfalls Concerning Tumors and Leukemia. Pediat. Clin. North America 12:299, 1965.

"What is the preferred chemotherapeutic agent in chronic granulocytic leukemia?"

Reply: Busulfan (Myleran) appears still to hold this position.

"Since the results of therapy with any one drug are so disappointing in adult acute myelogenous leukemia, I am tempted to begin therapy at once with a combination of several drugs in my next case. Is there any precedent for this?"

Reply: Yes, at the Boston City Hospital, Thompson and associates have used a four-drug combination in 38 such patients and reported preliminary results suggesting an improvement over previous therapy. The drugs used included vincristine, 1.2 mg. intravenously per week, amethopterin, 2.5 mg. given by mouth daily, 6-mercaptopurine, 100 mg. by mouth daily, and prednisone, 60 mg. by mouth daily. Drug toxicity was said to have been mild and controllable in this experience and there were no deaths directly related to use of the drugs.

Ian Thompson, Thomas C. Hall and William C. Moloney. Combination Therapy of Adult Acute Myelogenous Leukemia. New England J. Med. 273:1302, Dec. 9, 1965.

"I have used busulfan (Myleran) for the first time in a patient with chronic myelocytic leukemia and have easily brought the leukocyte count down to 10,000/cu. mm. Shall I continue the therapy or stop it for a while; if the latter, when shall I resume; and what may I expect to be the ultimate results?"

Reply: In the 30 patient series of Haut and associates in Wintrobe's group at the University of Utah, most patients were given 4–6 mg. busulfan orally each morning until the count fell to 10,000/cu. mm. or under, and then there was a respite from therapy until the count rose to 50,000/cu. mm. or more. Additional courses of this sort were then given as long as there was acceptable response. The first course was responded to well by all but 1 patient, defining response as subjective improvement, decline in number of leukocytes, decrease of anemia and subsidence of physical signs of the disease. Response to subsequent courses tended to appear later and the remissions to be shorter; i.e., after the first course there was a remission of 6 months or more in 85% of the patients, but after the fifth course this occurred in only 19%. If the anemia was not relieved and a large spleen not reduced 50% in size after a course of the drug, the prognosis was poor and the acute phase imminent. In 15 patients complete resistance to the drug occurred on development of the acute, myeloblastic phase of the disease. The group as a whole had a median survival period of 42 months in contrast to the median survival of 31 months in Minot's untreated control series.

A. Haut, W. S. Abbott, M. M. Wintrobe and G. E. Cartwright. Busulfan in Treatment of Chronic Myelocytic Leukemia: Effect of Long-Term Intermittent Therapy. Blood 17:1, 1961.

"In treatment of the lymphomas has it been definitely determined whether vinblastine (Velban) or cyclophosphamide (Cytoxan) is the better drug?"

Reply: Certainly not definitively as yet but the study of Stutzman's group at the Roswell Park Memorial Institute yielded interesting findings. These observers compared the two drugs in a random fashion in 69 patients with various types of lymphoma in a total of 96 courses of therapy. They did not use "loading" doses and adjusted dosage at weekly visits according to effect and toxicity. It was found that vinblastine, to which 28 of 33 patients responded, was strikingly superior to cyclophosphamide in Hodgkin's disease. But in reticulum cell sarcoma and lymphosarcoma, cyclophosphamide was superior, with a response appearing in 12 of 20 patients. These investigators recommended vinblastine as the initial agent in Hodgkin's disease unless a prompt response is necessary.

Leon Stutzman, Ediz Z. Ezdinli and Margaret A. Stutzman. Vinblastine Sulfate vs. Cyclophosphamide in the Therapy for Lymphoma. J.A.M.A. 195:173, Jan. 17, 1966.

"I have a patient with Hodgkin's disease in whom fever persists despite a satisfactory response to cytotoxic agents and employment of the usual antipyretic measures. Can you suggest anything?"

Reply: At Duke Hospital, Harold Silberman and associates used the new drug, indomethacin (Indocin) effectively in 9 such cases. Optimal control of fever was achieved by dosage of 25–50 mg. at 6 hour intervals.

Harold R. Silberman, Thomas G. McGinn and William B. Kremer. Control of Fever in Hodgkin's Disease by Indomethacin. J.A.M.A. 194:597, Nov. 8, 1965.

"In using chlorambucil (Leukeran) in the treatment of lymphomas and chronic lymphocytic leukemia, will intermittent therapy suffice or is it advisable to employ long-term or maintenance therapy?"

Reply: In their study of this therapy in 126 patients with pathologically confirmed diagnoses of Hodgkin's disease, chronic lymphocytic leukemia, lymphosarcoma and reticulum cell sarcoma at the Roswell Park Memorial Institute, Buffalo, E. Z. Ezdinli and L. Stutzman used the drug mainly on an outpatient basis and intermittent therapy, for they felt that it would be necessary to show prolonged survival or an increase in the total months of disease control throughout the patient's course in order to argue successfully that the trouble and expense of long-term or maintenance therapy is worthwhile. And such differences have not been shown. The median survival in this series was 5.3 years for the Hodgkin's disease group, 5.2 years for chronic lymphocytic leukemia, and 4.1 years for the lymphosarcoma group (including the small number of reticulum cell sarcoma cases). The usual mode of therapy consisted of daily oral doses of chlorambucil, 6–12 mg., during a period of 4–8 weeks, therapy being continued until a therapeutic result was obtained or until evidence of hematologic toxicity appeared. Average duration of remission following initial therapy in 26 responsive patients with Hodgkin's disease was 5.7 months, in 26 responsive patients with chronic lymphocytic leukemia it was 13.2 months, and in 11 responsive patients with lymphosarcoma it was 16.5 months. The response of 41 patients who were retreated in 79 courses of therapy were quite similar to the initial responses, with no apparent differences among the diagnostic groups.

Ediz Z. Ezdinli and Leon Stutzman. Chlorambucil Therapy for Lymphomas and Chronic Lymphocytic Leukemia. J.A.M.A. 191.444, Feb. 8, 1965.

"What is currently the preferred chemotherapeutic agent in chronic lymphocytic leukemia?"

Reply: I believe that in most circles it is considered that chlorambucil (Leukeran) still holds that position.

"Vinblastine (Velban) and vincristine (Oncovin) have had some efficacy in acute leukemia in children; are they useful in chronic granulocytic leukemia in adults?"

Reply: At the National Institutes of Health, Paul Carbone and associates did not find them to be so. In fact, these investigators found no evidence of action on the chromosomes, which is surprising since most antineoplastic drugs affect nucleic acids or their synthesis.

Paul P. Carbone, J. H. Tjio, Jacqueline Whang, Jerome B. Block, William B. Kremer and Emil Frei, III. Effect of Treatment in Patients with Chronic Myelogenous Leukemia: Hematologic and Cryogenic Studies. Ann. Int. Med. 59:622, 1963.

"I have heard that long periods of partial or complete remission in chronic lymphocytic leukemia and lymphosarcoma can be obtained through high corticosteroid dosage on 1 or each of 2 successive days each week. Is this true?"

Reply: It has been reported to be so by a group of observers at Washington University and the University of Miami, but this is certainly something new. Their patients had to fulfill one or more of certain criteria: evidence of refractoriness to an alkylating agent or radiotherapy, hemoglobin below 9 Gm./100 ml., platelet count below 100,000/cu. mm. or a near-total replacement of the bone marrow by lymphocytes, with difficulty in aspiration. Dosage was 60–145 mg. prednisone (Meticorten, etc.) or equivalent dosage of methylprednisolone (Depo-Medrol, etc.), dexamethasone (Decadron, etc.), triamcinolone (Aristocort, etc.) or betamethasone (Celestone) for 1–5 weeks. When improvement appeared to have reached a plateau, the drug was tapered to discontinuance, with maintenance dosage of 100–150 mg. prednisone, or its equivalent, beginning 7 days after the last dose on 1 or each of 2 successive days each week.

Richard A. Burningham, Alberto Restrepo, Reginald P. Pugh, Elmer B. Brown, Stuart F. Schlossman, Philip D. Khuri, Howard E. Lessner and William J. Harrington. Weekly High-Dosage Glucocorticosteroid Treatment of Lymphocytic Leukemias and Lymphomas. New England J. Med. 270:1160, May 28, 1964.

"In our trials of vinblastine (Velban) and vincristine (Oncovin) we have always found that Hodgkin's disease was the most responsive lesion. Does cross-resistance develop between these two drugs or between these drugs and the alkylating agents?"

Reply: In the study of Carbone and associates (National Cancer Institute) such cross-resistances were not observed.

Paul P. Carbone, Vincent Bono, Emil Frei, III, and Clyde O. Brindley. Clinical Studies with Vincristine. Blood 21:640, 1963.

"Some of my associates say that available chemotherapeutic agents can add nothing to the results achievable with radiation therapy in early Hodgkin's disease. Is this fair?"

Reply: I think one is obliged to say that since 20–40% of all cases of Hodgkin's are diagnosed in stage I or early stage II, when most susceptible to possible radical cure with adequate radiation, this modality *is* to be used in these cases to the exclusion of chemotherapy. However, some of the drugs are being used effectively upon an experimental basis by investigators in this field and we should certainly be receptive to any news that comes out of the research centers.

"Is it still the consensus that use of the corticosteroids is contraindicated in chronic lymphocytic leukemia?"

Reply: I would not say precisely that, but rather that use of other chemotherapeutic agents and irradiation are the preferred measures except perhaps for patients with complicating hemolytic anemia and/or thrombocytopenia, and those with refractory disease and bone marrow failure.

Richard K. Shaw, Dane R. Boggs, Harold R. Silberman and Emil Frei, III (National Institutes of Health). Study of Prednisone Therapy in Chronic Lymphocytic Leukemia. Blood 17:182, 1961.

"I have heard that the plasma uric acid level may be used as a guide to the corticosteroid treatment of acute leukemia. Is this true?"

Reply: No, it is not. But Edward Shanbrom (City of Hope Medical Center, Duarte, California) has shown that the uric acid excretion in the urine may have some predictive value when corticosteroids are being given in acute leukemia. He felt that patients excreting 4–10 Gm./24 hours in the first 2–3 days of therapy can be expected to go into complete hematologic remission. Of his 22 patients with acute lymphocytic leukemia, 7 showed a marked rise in uric acid excretion and obtained complete remissions; but regardless of dosage, patients with granulocytic and monocytic leukemia rarely exhibited a urine uric acid output greater than 2 Gm./24 hours, and none of these patients experienced hematologic remission.

Edward Shanbrom. Prognostic Value of Uric Acid Excretion in Steroid Therapy of Acute Leukemia. Am. J. M. Sc. 243:13, 1962.

"I have heard that massive corticosteroid therapy is more effective than conventional dosage in the treatment of acute leukemia. Is this true?"

Reply: At the City of Hope Medical Center, Duarte, California, Shanbrom and Miller did not find it so. In their series, remissions occurred with both conventional 50 mg. doses of prednisolone (Hydeltra, etc.) and massive 500 mg. doses. Hematologic improvement appeared more rapidly with the higher dosage, but many more patients were made worse by this dosage than by conventional dosage.

Edward Shanbrom and Sherwood Miller. Critical Evaluation of Massive Steroid Therapy of Acute Leukemia. New England J. Med. 266:1354, June 28, 1962.

"I have a pregnant woman with chronic granulocytic leukemia whom I have had on busulfan (Myleran) therapy; dare I continue use of this drug without fear of damage to the conceptus?"

Reply: I have seen 4 recorded cases in which use of busulfan during pregnancy was not conducive to congenital defects in the infant.

Lavere G. White (Fort Lauderdale, Florida). Busulfan (Myleran) in Pregnancy. J.A.M.A. 179:973, March 24, 1962.

"Our quite variable results with the chemotherapeutic agents and corticosteroids in acute leukemia have left us without means for predicting the outcome of such therapy in individual cases. Are there any helpful guideposts?"

Reply: To a limited extent, yes. At the National Institutes of Health, Freireich's group studied 178 consecutive patients with acute leukemia, all of whom were treated with mercaptopurine (Purinethol), amethopterin (Methotrexate) or corticosteroids. They found that in acute lymphatic leukemia the frequency of response to therapy was best in young children and progressively lower as age advanced. The difference in response did not vary with age in acute myelocytic leukemia, but there was a significantly longer median duration of complete remission in patients with myelocytic leukemia than in adults with lymphatic leukemia. Another observation was a trend toward shorter survival the higher the white count at diagnosis. The distribution of presenting symptoms was not found to be of prognostic value.

Emil J. Freireich, Edmund A. Gehan, David Sulman, Dane R. Boggs and Emil Frei, III. Effect of Chemotherapy on

Acute Leukemia in the Human. J. Chron. Dis. 14:593, 1961.

"When meningeal leukemia develops in a patient who is in bone marrow remission on drugs other than the anti–folic acid compounds, is it necessary to alter the dosage schedule of these drugs when adding intrathecal aminopterin to combat the meningeal involvement?"

Reply: According to Morse's group (National Institutes of Health) this is not necessary provided citrovorum factor protection is given with intrathecal aminopterin. They administered intramuscular citrovorum factor in dosage 10 times that of aminopterin: one eighth of the dose every 6 hours through 48 hours, the first dose 10–15 minutes after the intrathecal injection of aminopterin.

Edward E. Morse, David P. Rall, Emil Frei, III, and Emil J. Freireich. Intrathecal Aminopterin Therapy of Meningeal Leukemia. Arch. Int. Med. 111:620, 1963.

"It has been customary in our hospital in treating chronic granulocytic leukemia to withhold busulfan (Myleran) therapy until the patient is no longer responding to radiotherapy, but recent experience in a single case has led us to wonder whether this attitude is strictly correct?"

Reply: It is my impression that increasing numbers of the profession are hesitantly using the drug in initial therapy; at the Royal Victoria Hospital, Belfast, Bridges' group reported the achievement of complete clinical and hematologic remissions in 14 of 16 patients who had received no treatment for the malady before busulfan was started. Their initial dosage was 4–6 mg. daily, with maintenance dosage adjusted to keep the white blood cell count in the range of 10,000–20,000/cu. mm., but preferably below 12,000. In a multi-university study here in the United States, reported by Huguley's group, in which busulfan and mercaptopurine (Purinethol) were compared, it was found that busulfan provided a good or excellent response in 89% of instances whereas mercaptopurine did so in only 33% of instances. Busulfan was slower in action but its effect was more prolonged, and the granulocyte count tended to fluctuate more under mercaptopurine than under busulfan. These observers felt that if busulfan control becomes difficult because of the unique platelet-depressing action of the drug, mercaptopurine will probably offer control with greater safety.

J. M. Bridgoo, Dorothy M. Hayes and M G. Nelson. Busulfan in Treatment of Chronic Granulocytic Leukemia. Brit. J. Cancer 15:468, 1961. Charles M. Huguley, Jr., James Grizzle, R. Wayne Rundles, Warren N. Bell, Charles C. Corley, Jr., W. B. Frommeyer, Jr., B. G. Greenberg, William

Hammack, John C. Herion, G. Watson James, III, William E. Larsen, Virgil Loeb, Louis A. Leone, Jeffress G. Palmer and Sloan J. Wilson. Comparison of 6-Mercaptopurine and Busulfan in Chronic Granulocytic Leukemia. Blood 21:89, 1963.

"In the treatment of chronic lymphocytic leukemia or lymphosarcoma, when are the corticosteroids to be preferred to the specific chemotherapeutic agents?"

Reply: In Kyle, McParland and Dameshek's (Boston) study of 44 patients treated chiefly with large doses of prednisone or prednisolone there were the following reasons for starting corticosteroid therapy: disease far advanced and unresponsive to conventional therapy; depression of the bone marrow contraindicating further irradiation or chemotherapy; complications such as autoimmune thrombocytopenic purpura, vascular purpura or autoimmune hemolytic anemia.

Robert A. Kyle, Clifton E. McParland and William Dameshek. Large Doses of Prednisone and Prednisolone in Treatment of Malignant Lymphoproliferative Disorders. Ann. Int. Med. 57:717, 1962.

"What is the 'composite cyclic therapy' of leukemia of which one hears?"

Reply: In 1955 Wolf Zuelzer, at Wayne State University, adopted the treatment which has come to be known as you have designated. In his 1964 report he says that of a group of 175 children with a diagnosis of acute stem cell (lymphoblastic) leukemia who were treated by his method and lived at least 1 month after diagnosis, 50% lived 17.2 months, 25% 27.5 months and 10% 45 months. Six patients were alive in uninterrupted remission at the close of the study, 4–9 years after diagnosis. Patients with initially low white blood cell counts had twice the mean survival of those with higher counts; of the 44 patients who lived 2 years or more only 1 had an initial white count of more than 20,000.

Method: Initial treatment is with prednisone (Meticorten, etc.) orally 2 or 3 mg./kg./day for a month, then reducing by half on alternate days and discontinuing within a week (critically ill patients receive hydrocortisone [Cortef, etc.] intravenously). Concurrently, all patients able to tolerate oral medication receive 6-mercaptopurine (Purinethol) in a single daily dose of 2.5 mg./kg. irrespective of the white blood count; this is maintained for 3 months, and then methotrexate is substituted in daily oral dosage of 1.25–5 mg. depending on the patient's size. Drug dosage is adjusted or temporarily discontinued when the usual signs of toxicity appear. After 3 months of methotrexate therapy, 6-mercaptopurine is resumed, and thereafter the antimetabolites are alternated at regular intervals, this regimen being maintained indefinitely or until relapse. With relapse, corticosteroid therapy is resumed in full dosage for 1 month and the antimetabolite currently in use is replaced by its alternate.

Wolf W. Zuelzer. Implications of Long-Term Survival in Acute Stem Cell Leukemia of Childhood Treated with Composite Cyclic Therapy. Blood 24:477, 1964.

"I have heard that intrathecal methotrexate has value in central nervous system leukemia but would want to know whether the results attained with it are superior to mere lumbar puncture itself?"

Reply: At the Children's Hospital at Los Angeles, Carol Hyman's group reported that lumbar puncture without injection of methotrexate was followed by symptomatic improvement in 19 of 36 children, but that improvement in abnormal cerebrospinal fluid findings was less frequent, and the pressure and white cell count remained abnormal. With intrathecal methotrexate they induced complete symptomatic relief in 43 of 67 episodes and partial relief in an additional 14. The course of therapy comprised 0.2 mg. methotrexate/kg. intrathecally every other day for four doses. Symptoms improved within 48 hours after injection in 40 episodes and the response lasted a median of about 2½ months. One patient had favorable responses to repeated courses for 7 recurrent episodes.

Carol B. Hyman, James M. Bogle, Charles A. Brubaker, Kenneth Williams and Denman Hammond. Blood 25:13, 1965.

"Can one expect as good results with methotrexate in the acute leukemia of adults as in children?"

Reply: This has not been the case, but at Emory University, Charles Huguley and associates have described a method of therapy that appears to be a considerable advance in our approach to this malady in the adult. In 24 patients who were unresponsive to, or who had become refractory to, mercaptopurine (Purinethol) they gave 5 day courses of methotrexate in divided daily dosage of 1.25–3.75 mg. every 6 hours for 20 doses (5 days), stopping treatment if toxicity developed. Toxicity was indeed often severe but recovery was rapid. Definite improvement was seen in 46% of these patients and complete remission in 32%; patients living long enough to receive three courses of therapy had a complete remission rate of 47%. Duration of remissions averaged 98.5 days.

Charles M. Huguley, Jr., William R. Vogler, James W. Lea, Charles C. Corley, Jr., and Michael E. Lowrey. Acute Leukemia Treated with Divided Doses of Methotrexate. Arch. Int. Med. 115:23, 1965.

"What advantage, if any, is there in using the newer drugs, chlorambucil (Leukeran) and cyclophosphamide (Cytoxan) over nitrogen mustard preparations in treating lymphocytic leukemia?"

Reply: Both of these new drugs cause much less gastrointestinal disturbance than do mechlorethamine (Mustargen) and triethylenemelamine (TEM), which of course makes them easier to use. The patient should be warned, however, that cyclophosphamide is very likely to cause temporary but complete baldness.

David T. Kaung, R. M. Whittington and M. E. Patno. Chemotherapy of Chronic Lymphocytic Leukemia. Arch. Int. Med. 114:521, 1964.

"Is there any drug that could be used with the chemotherapeutic agents in the leukemias and lymphomas to increase the safety with which these drugs may be used?"

Reply: In New York, Irwin Krakoff and Richard Meyer have shown that at least the hyperuricemia and uric acid nephropathy that sometimes complicate the use of antineoplastic agents may be lessened by the use of allopurinol (Zyloprim). They used the drug in dosage of 100–200 mg. orally three or four times daily. They warned, however, that if allopurinol is used in a patient who is on 6-mercaptopurine (Purinethol) the dose of the latter should be reduced to 25% of its conventional dose to avoid serious bone marrow depression.

Irwin H. Krakoff and Richard L. Meyer. Prevention of Hyperuricemia in Leukemia and Lymphoma: Use of Allopurinol (Zyloprim), a Xanthine Oxidase Inhibitor. J.A.M.A. 193:89, July 5, 1965.

"I am discouraged by my inability to correct the anemia occurring in chronic lymphatic leukemia. Can you suggest anything?"

Reply: At the University of Minnesota, B. J. Kennedy used the androgenic hormones, fluoxymesterone (Halotestin, etc.), 20–50 mg. orally per day, and testosterone enanthate (Delatestryl) 400–1800 mg. per week intramuscularly in divided doses; 2 months was regarded as a minimum period of effective therapy. With the hormones he gave corticosteroids because of the observation that combined therapy appears to potentiate the stimulation of erythropoiesis. There were 9 patients with chronic lymphatic leukemia and 3 with subacute lymphatic leukemia; hemolysis was excluded as a major cause of the anemia, and corticosteroids had not been effective in its treatment. There was a striking increase in erythropoietic activity and a resultant increase in hemoglobin in 7 of the patients.

B. J. Kennedy. Androgenic Hormone Therapy in Lymphatic Leukemia. J.A.M.A. 190:1130, Dec. 28, 1964.

"I have a patient with an isolated lesion of mycosis fungoides. Might one hope for good results from the topical treatment of such a lesion with mechlorethamine (Mustargen)?"

Reply: The palliative effect of mechlorethamine administered systemically in mycosis fungoides has been well documented in a few instances, but little topical use of the agent has been recorded. At the Walter Reed Army Hospital, William Vineyard and Donald Mitchell applied a 0.25 mg./ml. solution, and after 1 week the area was essentially normal except for a mild, nonspecific dermatitic reaction. Subsequently the lesion was treated with a 0.5 mg./ml. solution for 3 consecutive days, with again a reaction that gradually subsided. There was no adverse systemic effect, and 10 weeks after therapy only an asymptomatic, macular, nonindurated erythematous flush remained. At the University of Szeged, Sipos found it beneficial to combine x-ray therapy with the topical nitrogen mustard.

William R. Vineyard and Donald E. Mitchell. Local Therapy of Mycosis Fungoides with Cytotoxic Agents: Case Report. Arch. Dermat. 84:928, 1961. K. Sipos. Painting Treatment of Nitrogen Mustard in Mycosis Fungoides. Dermatologica 130:3, 1965.

MALIGNANCY: MISCELLANEOUS TOPICS

"Has research in cancer chemotherapy progressed to the point at which there is now a specific agent for a specific cancer?"

Reply: No, I do not think one can say that this is truly the case. But the agents are certainly beginning to be sorted out sufficiently that it is possible to compile a list of drugs of choice in typical lesions, bearing in mind always that chemotherapy is indicated only if radiotherapy or surgery is not indicated and that palliation is the most that can be hoped for in practically all instances. Based on a large experience at the Columbia-Presbyterian Medical Center and the Francis Delafield Hospital in New York City, George Hyman has offered the following tentative list of chemotherapeutic agents of choice in neoplasms of the following types. Lung carcinoma: nitrogen mustard, Cytoxan; breast carcinoma: 5-fluorouracil, thio-TEPA; ovary carcinoma: thio-TEPA, chlorambucil, triethylene melamine; colon and stomach carcinoma: 5-fluorouracil;

bladder carcinoma: 5-fluorouracil; pancreas carcinoma: 5-fluorouracil; hepatoma: 5-fluorouracil; endometrium carcinoma: progesterone, Cytoxan; choriocarcinoma (female): methotrexate; choriocarcinoma (male): methotrexate, chlorambucil, actinomycin D; Wilms' tumor: actinomycin D plus radiotherapy; retinoblastoma: triethylene melamine plus radiotherapy; neuroblastoma: thio-TEPA, actinomycin D, Niticomin; osteogenic sarcoma: actinomycin D plus methotrexate plus chlorambucil; chondrosarcoma: actinomycin D plus methotrexate plus chlorambucil; embryonal rhabdomyosarcoma: actinomycin D plus methotrexate plus chlorambucil.

Among the lymphomas, which are sensitive to radiotherapy, Hodgkin's disease seems to respond best to nitrogen mustard, Cytoxan or Velban; giant follicular lymphosarcoma to nitrogen mustard, Leukeran or Cytoxan or the corticosteroids; small lymphocytic lymphosarcoma to nitrogen mustard or Leukeran; large lymphoblastic lymphosarcoma to Cytoxan; reticulum cell sarcoma to Cytoxan.

George A. Hyman. Management of Metastatic Cancer of the Lung by Newer Chemotherapeutic Agents. Am. J. M. Sc. 250:374, 1965.

"The profound depression of the bone marrow associated with the use of chemotherapeutic agents or radiation in the treatment of neoplastic disease is the major limitation of this therapy in most instances. Is bone marrow transfusion worth the effort?"

Reply: In most studies of the matter, such as that of Dunnigan and Brown (Glasgow Royal Infirmary), there has not developed clear evidence of the effectiveness of this measure; and this is very disappointing since rodents, dogs and primates can be protected against otherwise lethal doses of radiation by such transfusions. It appears that there is an immunologic problem in man that is still unsolved.

M. G. Dunnigan and Alexander Brown. Autologous Bone Marrow and Large Doses of Cytotoxic Drugs in Treatment of Malignant Disease: Report of a Controlled Trial. Lancet 2:477, Sept. 7, 1963.

"One of the chief drawbacks in the use of vincristine (Oncovin) in the treatment of neoplastic disease is the likelihood of producing neuromuscular complications. Are there any agents available that will reverse these manifestations?"

Reply: None have come to my attention.

"One often yields to the temptation to use broad-spectrum antibiotics in patients with malignancies who have fever without demonstrable infection. I wonder whether this is a harmful thing to do?"

Reply: At the National Institutes of Health, Boggs's group found it so. A total of 44 febrile episodes in 42 patients were studied and no differences in duration or severity of fever were demonstrated between patients given tetracycline and those given a placebo. But more infections developed in the tetracycline group and they were more severe than in the placebo group.

Dane R. Boggs, Emil Frei, III, and Charles H. Zierdt. Fever in Malignant Neoplastic Disease: Controlled Study of Tetracycline Therapy. Ann. Int. Med. 53:754, 1960.

"I have recently had considerable success in the control of malignant effusions through the use of quinacrine (Atabrine). How would you explain the action of this and other antimalarial compounds in nonmalarious maladies?"

Reply: The discovery was made some years ago that quinacrine has a cytotoxic action on tumor cells in tissue culture, but it is not possible to explain all of the nonspecific uses of the synthetic antimalarials—in rheumatoid arthritis, lupus erythematosus, Sjögren's syndrome, polymorphous light eruptions, pemphigus, cardiac arrhythmias—on the basis of this type of action. The use in rheumatoid arthritis came about quite accidentally when Page noted the striking amelioration of joint symptoms in 2 patients who had been treated with an antimalarial for chronic discoid lupus erythematosus. In explanation of the action in the latter malady, McChesney and associates proposed the hypothesis that it is simply a screening out of harmful wave lengths, thereby preventing the photonic activation of the process. The ameliorating action in polymorphous light eruptions has suggested to some dermatologists that perhaps in many instances these eruptions are actually subclinical or latent manifestations of lupus erythematosus; perhaps Sjögren's syndrome may also be a form of systemic lupus erythematosus. In the arrhythmias the action is simply a cardiac depressant one comparable to that of quinidine and procainamide. In the peritoneal cavity quinacrine provokes a marked fibrotic reaction and in the thoracic cavity it causes obliterative pleuritis.

F. Page. Treatment of Lupus Erythematosus with Mepacrine. Lancet 2:755, 1951. E. W. McChesney, F. C. Nachod and M. L. Tainter. Rationale for the Treatment of Lupus Erythematosus with Antimalarials. J. Invest. Dermat. 29:97, 1957.

"How is one to know whether a patient with cancer is a proper candidate for chemotherapy?"

Reply: I do not know that opinion has yet sufficiently crystalized to supply an entirely satisfactory answer to your question.

However, John Laszlo, at Duke University, has stated certain criteria for selection of patients that I think would probably not be vigorously opposed by most investigators in this field. First, any patient with a drug-sensitive malignancy who is not a candidate for cure by surgery or x-ray should be offered chemotherapy regardless of the degree of involvement or severity of illness, because one sometimes witnesses gratifyingly dramatic responses in patients apparently terminally ill with leukemia, lymphoma, myeloma, choriocarcinoma, breast or prostatic cancer, with restoration to good health for prolonged periods of time. On the other hand, there are patients terminally ill with characteristically unresponsive widespread malignancies whom it would be unreasonable to burden with the additional morbidity of chemotherapy before death; patients in this group would likely have such unresponsive tumors as adenocarcinoma of lung, cervix and pancreas, hypernephroma, malignant melanoma and sarcomas. Then there is a large intermediate group of patients in whom drug responses do occur, but uncommonly; individuals with such lesions as cancer of the bowel or liver and squamous carcinoma of the head, neck and lung. In cases of the latter sort the decision regarding chemotherapy must rest principally upon factors other than efficacy of the drug, such as availability of the patient for frequent medical follow-up, economic factors, and the wishes of the patient and family.

John Laszlo. Cancer Chemotherapy for Practicing Physicians. J. Chron. Dis. 18:681, 1965.

"What is the present position of vinblastine (Velban) in the treatment of cancer?"

Reply: The Eastern Cooperative Group in Solid Tumor Chemotherapy and the Acute Leukemia Cooperative Group reported in late 1965 on therapeutic trials of this drug in a group of 13 research hospitals in the Eastern States, the total number of patients studied having been 195. Their data confirmed and extended previous observations that vinblastine produces a significant degree of antitumor activity in Hodgkin's disease. Almost 20% of the patients with this malady had complete tumor regression and 82% had partial or complete regression. The median duration of regression was 13 weeks and all of the patients who achieved complete regression, and 20 of 24 who achieved partial regression, had complete abatement of symptoms referable to their Hodgkin's disease during remission. Vinblastine also produced objective tumor regression in 23% of patients with lymphosarcoma: this is less evidence of activity than is reported with the alkylating agents and with vincristine (Oncovin). There were three partial regressions in 33 patients with carcinoma of the lung and in 3 of 16 patients with carcinoma of the breast. One of 7 patients with carcinoma of the ovary responded, and 1 of 14 patients with malignant melanoma had a partial regression. None of 15 patients with adenocarcinoma of the colon and rectum responded.

Reports from investigators other than the present group have shown some responsiveness to vinblastine in carcinoma of the cervix, uterus, ovary, stomach, kidney, and for a variety of other malignancies including rhabdomyosarcoma, melanoma, seminoma and teratoma. The initial dosage in the study discussed was 0.1 mg./kg. and if no toxicity occurred the dose was increased at weekly intervals by 0.1 mg./kg. increments to a maximum of 0.3 mg./kg. The major toxic manifestation was leukopenia and an effort was made to adjust the dose to maintain the white cell count at 2000–4000/cu. mm. Adjustments in dosage were occasionally made because of platelet depression, gastrointestinal or neurological symptoms. Treatment was planned for a minimum of 42 days in patients with lymphoma and for 56 days in patients with carcinoma. If there was objective tumor regression the study was continued until relapse or prohibitive toxicity occurred.

Emil Frei, III (reporting for a cooperative group). Neoplastic Disease: Treatment with Vinblastine. Arch. Int. Med. 116:846, 1965.

"One hears the antineoplastic agents spoken of as antimetabolites, alkylating agents, etc. What are the compounds in these respective groups?"

Reply: The antimetabolites, being analogues of purines, pyrimidines and folic acid, displace the structurally similar compounds and interfere with nucleic acid synthesis by inhibiting enzyme binding, substituting a fraudulent for a genuine substance, or by interfering competitively with a normal substrate. The three principal members of this group are 6-mercaptopurine (Purinethol, 6-MP), methotrexate (MTX) and 5-fluorouracil (5-FU, FU).

The alkylating agents are compounds with two or more end groups (alkyl groups) that are either unsaturated or cyclic or that can be converted to such forms. They are extremely reactive compounds because these end groups may attach to other molecules through a sulfur, an oxygen or a nitrogen atom; and the antineoplastic effect achieved with them is believed to reflect a denaturing or inactivating action on desoxyribonucleic acid (DNA) of such nature that the biologic properties of the nucleic acid are altered. The members of the group are: melphalan (Alkeran), cyclophosphamide (Cytoxan), chlorambucil (Leukeran), busulfan (Myleran), mechlorethamine or nitrogen mustard (Mustargen), uracil mustard, triethylenemelamine (TEM), and triethylenethiophosphoramide (Thio-TEPA).

The plant alkaloids, vinblastine (Velban) and vincristine (Oncovin), derived from the periwinkle plant, are likely to be ultimately classified as antimetabolites because they appear to act by interfering with glutamic acid metabolism and inhibiting formation of nucleotides containing adenine and guanine.

If we can make a group of just one substance we can then speak of the antibiotics, which are presently represented only by dactinomycin or actinomycin D (Cosmegen), which seems to alter the physical properties of DNA so that abnormal complexes are formed.

Then we do really have a class of hormonal antineoplastics, for the estrogens, progestogens, androgens and corticosteroids all have specialized activities in certain of the malignant states.

And finally there are the radioactive isotopes (sodium phosphate-P^{32} and gold-Au^{198}) and the really unclassifiable agent, urethan (ethyl carbamate), with its questionable value in multiple myeloma.

"I have a cancer patient who has had several courses of 5-fluorouracil and is now becoming myxedematous. Could this be attributable to the drug?"

Reply: At the University of Wisconsin, Stephen Blomgren and Fred Ansfield studied this matter in 13 patients, 10 of whom had had at least 21 courses of fluorouracil. They concluded that long-term therapy of this sort does not significantly impair thyroid function.

Stephen E. Blomgren and Fred J. Ansfield. Thyroid Status Following Prolonged Therapy with Fluoropyrimidines. J.A.M.A. 193:51, July 5, 1965.

"The chemotherapy of malignant disease is getting out of the research hospitals into private practice nowadays, but I am not certain that we are all fully aware of the contraindications to the use of these drugs. What, for example, are the specific contraindications to the use of the fluorouracils?"

Reply: Moertel and associates, at the Mayo Clinic, in an evaluation of 5-fluorouracil (5-FU) and 5-fluorouracildeoxyriboside (5-FUDR) in patients with advanced malignant disease of the adenocarcinoma type known or presumed to have originated in the gastrointestinal tract, stated the following contraindications to this therapy: moribund state;

senility or severe emotional disturbance; recent major surgery; recent abdominal exploration and biopsy; recent "flu syndrome"; recent therapy with other chemotherapeutic agents; severe malnutrition, anorexia or frequent vomiting; leukopenia or thrombocytopenia; and previous total pelvic irradiation of significant degree.

Charles G. Moertel, Richard J. Reitemeier and Richard G. Hahn. Fluorinated Pyrimidine Therapy of Advanced Gastrointestinal Cancer. Gastroenterology 46:371, 1964.

"In our group we are just beginning to have experience with the arterial perfusion of chemotherapeutic agents in treatment of cancer, and are wondering whether the incidence of good results will likely pace the incidence of severe reactions, and also whether factors of age or sex and the grade of malignancy will play any part in the results?"

Reply: In reporting their experience from the Mayo Clinic, Moertel and associates found a significantly greater remission rate in patients with mild to moderate toxicity (judged by degree of leukopenia) when using the FU drugs than in those with no toxicity at all, but they did not observe any advantage associated with severe drug toxicity. There was also no significant relationship between the regression rate and the age or sex of the patients, but patients with lesions of higher grades of malignancy did have a greater rate of objective remission. The total duration of the disease did not appear significantly to influence the regression rate, nor was the degree of toxicity or the regression rate related to the extent of liver function impairment.

Charles G. Moertel, Richard J. Reitemeier and Richard G. Hahn. Fluorinated Pyrimidine Therapy of Advanced Gastrointestinal Cancer. Gastroenterology 46:371, 1964.

"Despite the palliative effects that are sometimes achieved with mechlorethamine (Mustargen) in some types of malignancy, my patients are often made so ill by the drug that I have to abandon it. Will you please state the ameliorative or combative measures that have had most success?"

Reply: Thrombophlebitis: inject via a fast running drip; vomiting: prevent or minimize by 100 mg. promazine (Sparine) orally and 50 mg. promethazine (Phenergan) intramuscularly 1½ hours before treatment; nausea on the day after treatment: oral chlorpromazine (Thorazine), 25–100 mg.

N. L. K. Robson. Nitrogen Mustard in Palliation of Lung and Metastatic Lung Cancer. Brit. J. Dis. Chest 56:194, 1962.

"Cancer chemotherapy is so frustrating because in one case patient A may experience intolerance

before reaching the point of full therapeutic activity whereas patient B will reach both end points more or less simultaneously. Is there no path at all through this wilderness?"

Reply: No. The greatest need in cancer chemotherapy today, with the drugs currently at our disposal, is some sort of test for the patient's toxic threshold for an agent before beginning its use in him.

"Hypercalcemia is often responsible for many symptoms in a wide variety of diseases, including the malignancies. Has satisfactory therapy been devised?"

Reply: At the Boston City Hospital, Goldsmith and Ingbar evaluated the effect of oral or intravenous administration of phosphate in 20 patients with hypercalcemia due to multiple myeloma, lymphoma, carcinoma, hyperparathyroidism and vitamin D overdosage. They were able invariably to induce prompt reduction in serum calcium to normal in 16 individuals and to near normal in the others; relief of symptoms of calcium intoxication usually occurred and in several patients there was improvement in renal function. These investigators did not recognize any deleterious effects of phosphate administration or any contraindications. Inorganic phosphate was given either orally as the disodium or potassium salt or intravenously as 1 liter of a 0.1 M solution of disodium phosphate and monopotassium phosphate (0.081 mole of Na_2HPO_4, plus 0.019 mole of KH_2PO_4 to provide a solution of pH 7.4). The intravenous solution was sterilized and given over a period of 6–8 hours.

Ralph S. Goldsmith and Sidney H. Ingbar. Inorganic Phosphate Treatment of Hypercalcemia of Diverse Etiologies. New England J. Med. 274:1, Jan. 6, 1966.

"What type of patient is considered suitable for arterial perfusion chemotherapy in cancer?"

Reply: Watkins and Sullivan (Lahey Clinic), who reported on the treatment of 136 patients with a variety of neoplasms and a follow-up to 37 months, said that the only patients they considered for this therapy were those with far advanced cancer unsuitable for conventional surgery or roentgen therapy. They further stated that the blood supply of the tumor should be derived from one or at the most two or three arteries, each of which must be perfused. They stated further that tumors receiving blood from multiple segmental sources are usually unsuitable, but they excepted malignant lesions extending over several segments of the trunk supplied by the internal mammary or inferior deep epigastric artery.

Elton Watkins, Jr., and Robert D. Sullivan. Cancer Chemotherapy by Prolonged Arterial Infusion. Surg. Gynec. & Obst. 118:3, 1964.

"What is the rationale of prolonged arterial perfusion with chemotherapeutic agents in cancer; why is it hoped that it will prove to be superior to the more conventional administration of the drugs?"

Reply: This therapeutic approach is based on evidence that in order to be cancerocidally effective the antimetabolite compounds must remain in prolonged contact with tumor cells as they enter an active stage of nucleic acid synthesis. To maintain the necessary concentration throughout the entire body, as would be the case if the drugs were absorbed from the usual administration sites, would be lethal. It must always be remembered in connection with the attack upon cancer with drugs that the agents used are such as interfere with the metabolism of cells, and that this interference is exerted upon normal as well as upon malignant cells. The fact that malignant cells metabolize more rapidly than normal cells is the thing which gives these chemotherapeutic agents such selective action as they have, and the fact that the cells of the gastrointestinal tract and the hematopoietic tissues are the most rapidly metabolizing structures in the body is the factor accountable for the selectively toxic action of the agents in these regions.

"At what rate of infusion of 5-fluorouracil is there least toxicity consistently with achievement of the anticancer effect?"

Reply: In their study, Lemon's group (Omaha) confirmed the experience of others that 50–60% of the patients receiving rapid intravenous injection have moderate to severe toxic manifestations; this was with dosage of 15 mg./kg. But in 52 consecutive patients given 1 Gm., regardless of body weight or surface area, diluted in 1 L. of 5% dextrose in water, the intravenous administration being extended over 8 hours, there were no detectable toxic sequelae in over 80% of the patients and over half of these tolerated an additional 7 Gm. of drug orally during the 2 weeks after intravenous therapy, five infusions having been given during the first week. In another group of 31 patients, in which the slow daily infusions were continued for 7–10 days or until some evidence of mild intoxication occurred, leukopenia became the most important manifestation of intoxication.

Henry M. Lemon, Peter J. Modzen, Rukma Mirchandani, Douglas A. Farmer and John Athans. Decreased Intoxication by Fluorouracil When Slowly Administered in Glucose. J.A.M.A. 185:1012, Sept. 28, 1963.

"A leukemic patient on mercaptopurine (Purinethol) has developed jaundice. Is hepatotoxicity a frequent occurrence with this drug?"

Reply: The occurrence of jaundice during a course of therapy with this drug has not been mentioned often in the literature, though the manufacturers include it in their discussion of the agent. The most frequent of the serious toxic attacks are on the bone marrow: leukopenia, thrombocytopenia, ultimate bleeding.

Morton Einhorn and Israel Davidson (Chicago Medical School). Hepatotoxicity of Mercaptopurine (Purinethol). J.A.M.A. 188:802, June 1, 1964.

"It is all very well to say that the pregnant woman should not be given antineoplastic chemotherapy during the first trimester, but what if she becomes pregnant while on the therapy or is unaware of her pregnancy when the therapy is started?"

Reply: One can only say that the likelihood of her having a malformed infant is somewhat greater than it would otherwise be. However, I have seen reports of several instances in which busulfan (Myleran) was used throughout pregnancy without evidence of serious damage to the fetus. Dennis and Stein, at Hahnemann Medical College, make the point that the danger is lessened in any case in which busulfan is the *only* antineoplastic agent that has been used in the patient.

Lewis H. Dennis and Seymour Stein. Busulfan (Myleran) in Pregnancy: Report of Case. J.A.M.A. 192:715, May 24, 1965.

MALIGNANCY: SOLID TUMORS

"What has been the result of the use of chemotherapeutic agents in solid carcinoma of the various systems?"

Reply: I have seen no more comprehensive cross section of what may be expected in both therapeutic responses and adverse reactions than was supplied by Hurley and Riesch (Marquette University). Patients with involvement of organs other than those of the gastrointestinal tract experience benefit as follows: breast, 60 of 100; soft tissue sarcoma, 6 of 19; bronchogenic carcinoma, 23 of 79; ovarian carcinoma, 6 of 24; tumors of head and neck, 10 of 60; pelvic tumors, 9 of 52. Toxicity of severe degree: alkylating agents alone, 315 patients, leukopenia in 47%, nausea and vomiting in 54%; antimetabolic agents alone (principally 5-FU), 102 patients, nausea and vomiting in 32%, stomatitis and enteritis in 50%, alopecia in 12%; combined drug therapy, 83 patients, leukopenia in 75%, nausea and/or vomiting in 45%, stomatitis or enteritis, 35%, alopecia, 6%.

John D. Hurley and John Riesch. Cancer Chemotherapy of Solid Carcinoma. Wisconsin M. J. 60:297, 1961.

"I have been impressed by the results relayed to me by one of my associates of his treatment of bladder carcinoma by direct instillation of thio-TEPA, but in the 2 cases in which I have tried the measure a rapidly developing bone marrow depression frightened me away from continuation of the treatments. What may I have done incorrectly?"

Reply: I do not know what your dosage or timing were, so I can only tell you how the measure has been employed by Veenema's group (Columbia-Presbyterian Medical Center). Their dosage of thio-TEPA was 60 mg. in 30–60 ml. of saline or water instilled into the bladder for 2 hours retaining. During the 2 hours, the patient lies for 15 minutes on each side, back and abdomen in rotation. In some instances the drug, in 40–60 mg. dosage, was injected directly into the tumors at multiple sites. There were minimal bone marrow depressant effects from this therapy, but when the procedure was employed twice weekly instead of once, the depression presented a problem in continuation of the therapy, just as in your experience. However, there was a considerable leukocyte and platelet fall in all instances, but the blood picture returned to normal in 2–3 weeks after cessation of treatment.

Ralph J. Veenema, Archie L. Dean, Jr., Myron Roberts, Bruno Fingerhut, Binoy K. Chowhury and Hamid Tarassoly. J. Urol. 88:60, 1962.

"In desperation recently, I used corticosteroids in high dosage in a patient with cerebral edema associated with a brain tumor and obtained a remarkable result. How might this be explained, and have others had a similar experience?"

Reply: Precisely how the corticosteroids decrease brain edema I cannot say, but perhaps, as postulated by Galicich and associates at the Universities of Minnesota and Arkansas, they do so by restoring the integrity of the cerebrovascular brain barrier. The Galicich group initiated therapy with 10 mg. dexamethasone phosphate (Decadron PO_4 Injection) intravenously, followed by 4 mg. intramuscularly at 6 hour intervals until the maximum response was obtained. In patients who had surgery the treatment was continued for 2–4 days postoperatively and then gradually tapered off. In 13 of their 14 patients there was dramatic improvement.

Joseph H. Galicich, Lyle A. French (University of Minnesota) and James C. Melby (University of Arkansas). Use of Dexamethasone in Treatment of Cerebral Edema Associated with Brain Tumors. Journal-Lancet 81:46, 1961.

"Does nitrogen mustard administration improve the results attainable with radiotherapy in non-resectable bronchogenic carcinoma?"

Reply: The reports of the Eastern Cooperative Group in Solid Tumor Chemotherapy, and the earlier report of Hughes and Higgins, reporting for the Veterans Administration Surgical Adjuvant Lung Cancer Chemotherapy Study, have seemed rather well to establish that it does not. However, a somewhat more cheering note has come from the University of Wisconsin, where Gollin and associates produced results suggesting that the survival time of patients with inoperable bronchogenic carcinoma after roentgen therapy is significantly increased with 5-fluorouracil added in toxic or near toxic dosage.

Eastern Cooperative Group in Solid Tumor Chemotherapy. Comparative Trial of Chemotherapy and Radiotherapy in Patients with Nonresectable Cancer of the Lung. Am. J. Med. 35:363, 1963. Felix A. Hughes (Memphis, Tennessee) and George Higgins (Washington, D.C.). Veterans Administration Surgical Adjuvant Lung Cancer Chemotherapy Study: Present Status. J. Thoracic & Cardio. Surg. 44:295, 1962. F. F. Gollin, F. J. Ansfield and H. Vermund. Clinical Studies of Combined Chemotherapy and Irradiation in Inoperable Bronchogenic Carcinoma. Am. J. Roentgenol. 92:88, 1964.

"In the light of accumulated experience, is one justified in using the quite toxic agent, mechlorethamine (Mustargen) in advanced metastatic lung cancer?"

Reply: Certainly no substantial change in the primary tumor is to be expected, even with high dosage, but the considerable amelioration of pain that is often accomplished may justify the employment.

"I have a patient with carcinoid tumors in the terminal ileum, mesenteric lymph nodes and liver who has failed to improve after surgical procedures. Is there any drug that might be helpful in controlling the steatorrhea?"

Reply: At the National Institutes of Health, Kenneth Melmon and associates have reported that the serotonin antagonist, methysergide (Sansert), has been more effective in alleviating diarrhea than paregoric in their small series of cases. In 2 patients there was malabsorption, which was also alleviated.

Kenneth L. Melmon, Albert Sjoerdsma, John A. Oates and Leonard Laster. Treatment of Malabsorption and Diarrhea of Carcinoid Syndrome with Methysergide (Sansert). Gastroenterology 48:18, 1965.

"I have a patient with metastatic bronchial carcinoid who has severe, prolonged flushing. Has any drug been effective?"

Reply: At the National Institutes of Health, Sjoerdsma and Melmon reported 2 cases that responded dramatically to corticosteroid therapy. One of the patients was free from attacks for 1½ years at the time of their report, therapy being prednisone (Meticorten, etc.) 10–20 mg. daily.

Albert Sjoerdsma and Kenneth L. Melmon. Severe Flushing Reactions Responsive to Steroids in Patients with Bronchial Carcinoid. Lancet 2:791, Oct. 10, 1964.

"Has pregnancy ever followed chemotherapy in a patient with choriocarcinoma?"

Reply: Yes, it has. At the University of Minnesota, William Spellacy and associates described a patient who had three successful gestations after methotrexate treatment of a widely disseminated choriocarcinoma, and there have been a few other similar reports.

William N. Spellacy, Henry C. Meeker and John L. McKelvey. Three Successful Pregnancies in Patient Treated for Choriocarcinoma with Methotrexate: Report of Case and Review of Literature. Obst. & Gynec. 25:607, 1965.

"I have given a single course of amethopterin (methotrexate) therapy, 20 mg. daily for 5 consecutive days, to a patient with metastatic choriocarcinoma and obtained a surprisingly good remission. Might spontaneous regression have accounted for this result?"

Reply: This is extremely doubtful. According to Hertz and associates (National Institutes of Health), Park reported that of 158 patients with choriocarcinoma and pulmonary metastases, only 3 were known to have survived, and he identified only 20 cases in the world literature that were known to have regressed. Brewer is also said to have reported 5 year survival in only 6 of 103 patients. In Hertz's own series of 63 patients, it appeared that the survival rate was raised by such treatment as you describe from a probable 6% to 48%. In Manila, Manahan and associates obtained remission for as long as 3 years in 41% of a smaller series of cases.

Roy Hertz, John Lewis, Jr., and M. B. Lipsett. Five Years' Experience with Chemotherapy of Metastatic Choriocarcinoma and Related Trophoblastic Tumors in Women. Am. J. Obst. & Gynec. 82:631, 1961. Constantino P. Manahan, Isidro Benitez and Felipe Estrella. Amethopterin (Methotrexate) in Treatment of Trophoblastic Tumors. Am. J. Obst. & Gynec. 82:641, 1961.

"We have become discouraged with our results in the chemotherapy of trophoblastic tumors; what has been the experience of others?"

Reply: K. D. Bagshawe (Charing Cross Hospital Medical School, London) has reported rather favorably on the use of amethopterin (methotrexate) and mercaptopurine (Purinethol), other agents being much less effective. In the 23 patients, there were 17 remissions lasting from 3 months to 4¾ years at the time of the report. In 9 patients, normal menstrual function had returned and there had been one successful normal pregnancy. However, pulmonary embolism occurred in several patients, and there were several instances in which patients with extensive pulmonary metastatic disease became more dyspneic on the therapy.

At Northwestern University, J. I. Brewer's group performed a study which suggests strongly that chemotherapy is a valuable method of treatment of patients with trophoblastic disease and that it provides better results than hysterectomy; furthermore, that hysterectomy performed in conjunction with chemotherapy does not increase the remission rate above that obtained by chemotherapy alone. It must be carefully noted, however, that the findings in all of these series have been too recent to permit of dogmatic conclusions. The Northwestern group used methotrexate orally each day for 5 days, the total dose being about 125–130 mg., based upon the calculation of 2.5 mg./kg.; dactinomycin (actinomycin D), 10 μg./kg. daily for 5 days, was injected into the tubing of a flowing intravenous infusion; and in some cases triple therapy consisted of daily oral administration of 5 mg. of methotrexate and 10 mg. of chlorambucil (Leukeran) and the injection of 0.5 mg. (not to exceed 10 μg./kg.) of actinomycin D into the tube of a running intravenous infusion. Repeat courses of these agents were not given until all evidence of toxicity had subsided except that of alopecia.

K. D. Bagshawe. Trophoblastic Tumors: Chemotherapy and Developments. Brit. M. J. 2:1303, Nov. 23, 1963. J. I. Brewer, A. B. Gerbie, R. E. Dolkart, J. H. Skom, R. G. Nagle, and E. E. Torok. Chemotherapy in Trophoblastic Diseases. Am. J. Obst. & Gynec. 90:566, Nov. 1, 1964.

"What is the present status of progestational therapy in endometrial cancer?"

Reply: At Columbia University, Frick treated 22 patients with recurrent disseminated endometrial carcinoma with the progesterone compound Delalutin in dose levels ranging from 1.5 to 2 Gm./week. There were 4 objective remissions in this group. Best results were achieved in the chest metastases, worst in the abdominal especially if there was ascites. The patients who responded had a lapse of 1–2 years between the primary therapy and recurrence. Two patients with cervical adenocarcinoma, 1 with endocervical carcinoma, 1 with vaginal epidermoid carcinoma, 2 with ovarian adenocarcinoma, 1 with uterine leio-myosarcoma and 2 with endometrial stromal sarcomas did not obtain objective changes under the drug. Two patients were being maintained at the time of the report on Provera after regressions were produced by Delalutin for 6 months and 1 year, respectively. So you see some little has been gained by the use of these agents, and it is surprising that they were not employed earlier. Actually, the first report of their use in treatment of carcinoma of the endometrium was that of Kelley and Baker in 1961, which was at least a decade after it became known that results are achievable in mammary and prostatic carcinoma through hormonal therapy.

Henry Clay Frick, II. Progestational Drugs in Management of Endometrial Cancer. Metabolism 14: (Part 2)348, 1965. Rita M. Kelley and William H. Baker. Progestational Agents in Treatment of Carcinoma of Endometrium. New England J. Med. 264:216, Feb. 2, 1961.

"With the palliative, though quite limited, value of 5-fluorouracil (5-FU) in advanced and hopeless gastrointestinal carcinoma pretty well established, in what type of case are best results to be expected?"

Reply: Hurley and associates (Marquette University) in reporting a favorable response in cancer of the colon in 35 of 104 patients, stated that individuals with local, regional or peritoneal recurrence were more benefited than those with large hepatic metastases or icterus. In the series of Moertel and Reitemeier (Mayo Clinic), in which therapy could be evaluated in 112 patients with all types of gastrointestinal malignancy, no significant difference was observed in the rates of objective remission among the major groups— gastric, colonic, pancreatic, adenocarcinoma of unknown origin usually presumed to be pancreatic carcinoma. There were remissions in individuals with high-grade or low-grade malignancy, in those with rapidly advancing or indolent disease, in those with and without significant liver function impairment and in those with malignant involvement of any of the common sites of metastasis. But among the 112 patients who could be evaluated, there was objective improvement in only 19% and symptomatic improvement in 37%.

Charles G. Moertel and Richard J. Reitemeier. Experience with 5-Fluorouracil (5-FU) in Palliative Management of Advanced Carcinoma of Gastrointestinal Tract. Proc. Staff Meet. Mayo Clin. 37:520, Sept. 26, 1962. John D. Hurley, Edwin H. Ellison and Larry C. Carey. Treatment of Advanced Cancer of Gastrointestinal Tract with Antitumor Agents. Gastroenterology 41:557, 1961.

"In the hideous situation that often develops in a patient with head and neck cancer, what can I do to relieve the pain? I will settle for practically anything if there is a chance that it will afford even a modicum of relief."

Reply: Your word "hideous" is well chosen; certainly euthanasia has a place here if anywhere. Hanna's group (University of Pittsburgh) reported the treatment of about 100 patients with intra-arterial chemicals, nitrogen mustard being the agent of choice. In 70% of cases the superficial temporal artery was used, next commonest the superior thyroid and facial arteries. The largest possible polyethylene tube was led into the partially transected vessel under local anesthesia and secured, checking the location of the cannula end by x-ray when a cervical vessel was employed. Instillations of 3 mg. nitrogen mustard usually took place daily for 2 weeks. Most patients were reported to have received some degree of relief, but some found the procedure intolerable. There were numerous severe complications, but the attempt seems justifiable upon the basis of a desperate remedy for a desperate situation. See the following reply.

Dwight C. Hanna, John C. Gaisford and Robert M. Goldwyn. Intra-arterial Nitrogen Mustard for Control of Pain in Head and Neck Cancer. Am. J. Surg. 106:783, 1963.

"What is the present status of chemotherapy in cancer of the head and neck?"

Reply: I have the feeling, which indeed was hinted at in the report of Oliver Beahrs and associates at the Mayo Clinic, that the most gained by chemotherapy in this region is to keep one's "hand in" so that when a truly effective drug is developed the techniques will be familiar. At present in order to obtain anything resembling a dramatic response in these tumors it is very often necessary to use dosage that proves fatal to the patient.

Oliver H. Beahrs, Vincent T. Caldarola and Edgar G. Harrison, Jr. Treatment of Cancer of Head and Neck by Chemotherapy. J.A.M.A. 189:765, Sept. 7, 1964.

"In diffuse primary or secondary liver cancer, surgery, radiation therapy and systemic chemotherapy are of little practical value. Has anything more promising been developed?"

Reply: At the Lahey Clinic, Robert Sullivan and Wladyslaw Zurek resorted to protracted infusion of antineoplastic drugs through a plastic catheter inserted directly into the hepatic artery in 73 patients. Objective response was noted in 43, and in patients with advanced metastatic lesions from primary tumors of the colorectum, the average survival was increased from the expected 2.1 month to 9.4 months.

Robert D. Sullivan and Wladyslaw Z. Zurek. Chemotherapy for Liver Cancer by Protracted Ambulatory Infusion. J.A.M.A. 194:481, Nov. 1, 1965.

"I have a patient with liver cancer and would like to know by what criteria I may judge whether he is a suitable candidate for hepatic artery infusion treatment."

Reply: Robert Sullivan and Wladyslaw Zurek (Lahey Clinic), who are vastly experienced in this field, are accepting patients for hepatic artery infusion from the following categories: (1) Patients with primary liver cancer *without* widespread dissemination; (2) those with cancer of the gallbladder and bile ducts *without* distant metastasis; (3) those with metastatic cancer of the liver from the colon and rectum *without* distant metastasis, including stage I, asymptomatic patients, and stages II and III, patients who have early hepatic decompensation and those who have advanced hepatic decompensation, respectively; and (4) those *with* metastatic cancer of the liver from the colon and rectum or other primary sites, when the imminent problem producing disability is hepatic decompensation and the primary site of the cancer or other known metastatic tumor, or both, does not represent a threat to life.

Robert D. Sullivan and Wladyslaw Z. Zurek. Chemotherapy for Liver Cancer by Protracted Ambulatory Infusion. J.A.M.A. 194:481, Nov. 1, 1965.

"I have a patient with advanced hepatic decompensation with extreme jaundice from a diffuse intrahepatic neoplasm, general debility, and very abnormal results of liver function tests. Shall I consider intrahepatic infusion for him?"

Reply: According to Sullivan and Zurek (Lahey Clinic), the type of patient you describe is generally a poor candidate for therapy of this sort.

Robert D. Sullivan and Wladyslaw Z. Zurek. Chemotherapy for Liver Cancer by Protracted Ambulatory Infusion. J.A.M.A. 194:481, Nov. 1, 1965.

"We have learned pretty well what we can do with cyclophosphamide (Cytoxan) in acute leukemias, but have so far not tried it otherwise; what has been the experience in lymphoma and the solid tumors?"

Reply: At Ohio State University, Robert Wall and Fred Conrad reported results in 130 patients treated with this drug, most of whom had failed to respond to other types of treatment. Of the Hodgkin's cases, 10 of the 29 had a good response lasting over 4 months; of 21 patients with generalized lymphosarcoma, 15 had a good response; of 16 patients with multiple myeloma, substantial improvement occurred in 9, including striking improvement in mental attitude; there was improvement in only 1 of 5 patients with reticulum cell sarcoma; there were four good responses in 7

patients with chronic lymphatic leukemia; 2 patients of the 10 with carcinoma of the breast had excellent responses; 1 of 2 patients with severe diffuse mycosis fungoides improved temporarily; and there was no favorable response in 7 patients with carcinoma of the lung and 12 patients with various solid tumors.

Robert L. Wall and Fred G. Conrad. Cyclophosphamide (Cytoxan) Therapy: Its Use in Leukemia, Lymphoma and Solid Tumors. Arch. Int. Med. 108:456, 1961.

"Is chemotherapy worth anything in advanced mammary cancer?"

Reply: You have probably stated your question crassly in order to provoke a definitive yes or no answer, but I cannot oblige. So far we have only partial answers in numerous aspects of the situation, but one thing is certain, namely, that so far the chemotherapist has produced little more than palliative measures and there is not yet in all instances even a clear delineation of the criteria for their use and the results that may be expected. Help from some quarter is needed, however, for the surgeons are not doing too well; witness the authoritative review of Leonard Dobson (Stanford University) of the surgical aspects of mammary cancer: of an annual incidence of 60,000 cases, about 18,000 will be inoperable when first seen, and of the 42,000 operated upon, 60% or more will have recurrences or metastases within 10 years. The following are some observations regarding the status of chemotherapy in widespread and carefully performed studies. The data of John D. Hurley and associates (Milwaukee County General Hospital) indicated that the patient with breast cancer recurrence most likely to respond to chemotherapy is one who had radical mastectomy 4 years earlier, who has responded earlier to endocrine therapy, and is now treated with 5-fluorouracil. B. J. Kennedy (University of Minnesota) observed that massive estrogen dosage in premenopausal women could retard the rate of tumor growth through provoking inhibition of a pituitary factor. Bernard Gardner's group (University of California) found a combined use of Meticorten and Cytomel relatively effective in advanced postmenopausal cases. Richard Kaufman and George Escher (New York) found that one is unlikely to observe rebound regression in advanced cases (objective improvement after cessation of hormonal therapy) after use of corticosteroids and progestins, but that it may be seen after the use of androgens and estrogens. Basil Stoll (Melbourne) reported that the proportion of patients responding to corticosteroid therapy was independent of the patient's previous response to sex hormone manipulation, and also that previous cortico-steroid administration does not appear to complicate the problems of postoperative management. In Cincinnati, Herman Freckman and associates found chlorambucil (Leukeran) the alkylating agent of choice because it is effective orally and can be given continuously for weeks without serious toxic effects, and prednisolone (Hydeltra, etc.) the corticosteroid of choice because it is as effective as the newer agents of this group and more economical. They felt that the data from their series, the A.M.A. Sex Steroid Series and the series reported in the Endocrine Ablation Study of the Joint Committee of the American College of Physicians and the American College of Surgeons, justified the attitude that chlorambucil-prednisolone therapy should be the first measure considered in disseminated breast carcinoma and major ablative surgery the last. In a study carried out by the Surgical Adjuvant Chemotherapy Breast Group, organized under the auspices of the National Institutes of Health, a very large group of patients was treated in various medical centers by the so-called Halstead radical mastectomy, with removal of the breast, pectoral muscles and axillary contents en bloc, and given thio-TEPA on the day of operation and for 2 days postoperatively, the controls receiving no chemotherapy. The results, as reported by Rudolf Noer (Louisville, Kentucky) showed that thio-TEPA was of significant benefit in the incidence of early recurrence and metastasis, especially in patients in the premenopausal group who had positive axillary nodes; complication rates were not significantly affected, however, and the ultimate results of the therapy could not be determined at the time of the report because of the relatively long survival time to be expected in these patients.

Robert T. L. Long and A. McChesney Evans (Ellis Fischel State Cancer Hospital, Columbia, Missouri). Diethylstilbestrol as Chemotherapeutic Agent for Ovarian Carcinoma. Missouri Med. 60:1125, 1963. Basil A. Stoll (Melbourne). Corticosteroids in Therapy of Advanced Mammary Cancer. Brit. M. J. 2:210, July 27, 1963. Herman A. Freckman, Harry L. Fry, Fernando L. Mendez and Elmer R. Maurer. Chlorambucil-Prednisolone (Leukeran-Metacortelone, Etc.) Therapy for Disseminated Breast Carcinoma. J.A.M.A. 189:23, July 6, 1964. Rudolf J. Noer. Adjuvant Chemotherapy: Thio-TEPA with Radical Mastectomy in Treatment of Breast Cancer. Am. J. Surg. 106:405, 1963. Leonard Dobson. Management of Metastatic Breast Carcinoma. Surg. Clin. North America 42:861, 1962. John D. Hurley, David S. Trump, Thomas J. Flatley and John D. Riesch. Method of Selecting Patients for Cancer Chemotherapy. Arch. Surg. 83:611, 1961. B. J. Kennedy. Massive Estrogen Administration in Premenopausal Women with Metastatic Breast Cancer. Cancer 15:641, 1962. Bernard Gardner, Arthur N. Thomas and Gilbert S. Gordan. Antitumor Efficacy of Prednisone (Meticorten, Etc.) and Sodium Liothyronine (Cytomel) in Advanced Breast Cancer. Cancer 15:334, 1962. Richard J. Kaufman and George C. Escher. Rebound Regression in Advanced Mammary Carcinoma. Surg. Gynec. & Obst. 113:635, 1961.

"Is it still the consensus that in the treatment of disseminated mammary carcinoma the use of androgens is to be preferred to estrogens if there is skeletal metastasis?"

Reply: I believe at least that it should not be, for the most thoroughgoing study of the matter that has come to my attention, the retrospective study of 944 patients reported by the Subcommittee on Breast and Genital Cancer of the Committee on Research of the American Medical Association, apparently dispelled that belief. Androgens produced objective regression in 20% of premenopausal and 21% of postmenopausal women; estrogens, whose use was limited to postmenopausal patients, in 36% of the patients. In patients with unisystemic dissemination, the estrogens produced more control in soft tissues at all postmenopausal ages, and they were equal or superior to androgens for skeletal and visceral metastases. In fact, both types of hormone were at their most effective after the 8th postmenopausal year, at which time they had reached a plateau of performance. In reporting the findings of the Cancer Chemotherapy National Service Center (Kennedy), based on a protocol believed to incorporate better methods for clinical evaluation, a significantly better regression rate was revealed for diethylstilbestrol than for testosterone propionate, 29.1 and 10.1, respectively.

Subcommittee on Breast and Genital Cancer of the Committee on Research of the American Medical Association. Androgens and Estrogens in Treatment of Disseminated Mammary Carcinoma: Retrospective Study of 944 Patients. J.A.M.A. 172:1271, Mar. 19, 1960. B. J. Kennedy. Diethystilbestrol Versus Testosterone Propionate Therapy in Advanced Breast Cancer. Surg. Gynec. & Obst. 120:1246, 1965.

"One of my associates has been using triiodothyronine (Cytomel) in the treatment of advanced breast cancer with results that seem to me quite indifferent, but he tells me that good results have been reported. Is this true?"

Reply: No, I believe that he is mistaken. The good results that I have seen attributed to the use of triiodothyronine have been achieved when it was used in combination with a corticosteroid, as in such studies as that of Bernard Gardner's group (University of California), which is referred to elsewhere in these discussions. When Emery and Trotter (University College Hospital, London) used triiodothyronine alone in a double-blind study they were unable to adduce evidence that progression of the disease was in the least delayed.

Bernard Gardner, Arthur N. Thomas and Gilbert S. Gordan. Antitumor Efficacy of Prednisone (Meticorten, Etc.) and Sodium Liothyronine (Cytomel) in Advanced Breast Cancer. Cancer 15:334, 1962. E. W. Emery and W. R. Trotter. Triiodothyronine (Cytomel) in Advanced Breast Cancer. Lancet 1:358, Feb. 16, 1963.

"In a patient with advanced breast carcinoma in whom I want to make a trial of methotrexate, does it matter that she is presently receiving androgens?"

Reply: It appears that this combination might cause some trouble. At least on the basis of an unfortunate experience in 1 case, William Vogler's group, at Emory University, advised that the inital course of methotrexate in a patient who has recently received androgens be reduced to a total of 25 mg.

William R. Vogler, Charles M. Huguley, Jr., and Wilson Kerr. Toxicity and Antitumor Effect of Divided Doses of Methotrexate. Arch. Int. Med. 115:285, 1965.

"In a fairly active service I do not see spontaneous hypercalcemia in metastatic breast cancer as often as the literature leads me to believe that I should. Perhaps I have just been lucky. However, I have recently had a run of 3 cases that responded pretty well to corticosteroids. What has been the experience in the large cities?"

Reply: At the M. D. Anderson Hospital in Houston, Ilse Mannheimer treated 40 patients in 59 spontaneous episodes, i.e., excluding all patients who acquired hypercalcemia as a result of estrogen or androgen therapy. Therapy in vomiting and unconscious patients consisted of 80 mg. of methylprednisolone (Depo-Medrol, etc.) and about 3000 ml. of intravenous fluids daily. Patients tolerating oral medication were given 60–80 mg. prednisone (Meticorten, etc.) daily in divided doses; dosage was reduced cautiously when serum calcium levels returned toward normal, usually achieving a maintenance dose of 15–20 mg. prednisone daily throughout the patient's life. A complete response was considered to have occurred if serum and urinary calcium levels returned to normal after corticosteroid therapy; continued high urinary calcium excretion was considered an incomplete response. Results of the therapy were favorable in 32 of the 40 patients, 46 of the 59 episodes being successfully treated.

Ilse H. Mannheimer. Hypercalcemia of Breast Cancer: Management with Corticosteroids. Cancer 18:679, 1965.

"In 1960, there was a report of the Committee on Research of the American Medical Association showing a regression rate of 21% in advanced breast cancer in postmenopausal women when androgens were used and 36% when estrogens were used, but now I have seen a report from the University of Minnesota in which there was claimed an estrogen result of 29.1% but a testosterone result of only 10.1%. Where does the truth lie?"

Reply: The improvement rate under testosterone in the report of the American Medical Association Committee, being about twice as high as that in the Minnesota report of B. J. Kennedy, is probably attributable to the fact that the Committee report was really a retrospective review of a very large number of patients treated by numerous observers. In any case, both studies leave no doubt of the superiority of estrogens over androgens in the therapy of this lesion.

B. J. Kennedy. Diethylstilbestrol versus Testosterone Propionate Therapy in Advanced Breast Cancer. Surg. Gynec. & Obst. 120:1246, 1965.

"Is regional perfusion a valuable adjunct to excisional therapy in the treatment of melanoma of limbs or even as total therapy when excisional therapy is impractical?"

Reply: Creech and Krementz (New Orleans) have made an affirmative answer to both portions of this question. At the time of their report they had used chemotherapy by perfusion in over 200 patients with this lesion. Of the 182 reported upon, 134 had lower limb and 48 upper limb lesions; in 111 of the cases perfusion was used as an adjunctive measure to excision, in the remaining 71 cases as a single measure. Excluding from the list the patients who had been followed for less than 1 year at the time of the report and those with clinically positive iliac nodes and systemic metastases, there were 118 patients in whom a cure rate of 56% was claimed. Complications were related chiefly to wound healing and to the toxic effects of the agents. Seven patients died as immediate result of perfusion, 1 from the operative procedure and 6 from the toxic effects of the chemotherapy itself.

Oscar Creech, Jr., and Edward T. Krementz. Regional Perfusion in Melanoma of Limbs. J.A.M.A. 188:855, June 8, 1964.

"Has anything come out of the hubbub of cancer chemotherapy research nowadays that promises relief to the unfortunate patient with multiple myeloma?"

Reply: In a study by the Midwest Cooperative Chemotherapy Group of the treatment of myeloma, cyclophosphamide (Cytoxan) was selected as the alkylating agent and it was concluded that the most significant improvement noted in connection with its use was the decrease in pain and an improved performance status of many who showed no other change in the course of their disease nor by objective criteria. Of course if one is able to accomplish nothing else in this terrible malady the relief of pain is of major importance. The dosage regimen with which this was sometimes achieved by these investigators was an initial administration of 2 mg./kg. daily by mouth and subsequent adjustment at the discretion of the investigator. Unfortunately, this drug induces nausea and vomiting as does the disease, and it is not always easy to know which is which. See the following Reply.

Donald R. Korst, George O. Clifford, Willis M. Fowler, John Louis, John Will and Henry E. Wilson. Multiple Myeloma: II. Analysis of Cyclophosphamide (Cytoxan) Therapy in 165 Patients. J.A.M.A. 189:758, Sept. 7, 1964.

"I have had a good remission of about 7 months in a patient with myeloma whom I have treated off and on with cyclophosphamide (Cytoxan) as indicated. What am I to expect?"

Reply: Well, I don't know, but Tourtellotte and Call (Loma Linda University) have reported a case, which is certainly unique, of a patient who had gone 42 months on this therapy and remained well at the time of their writing. Their dosage: 150 mg. daily at a total dose of 6 Gm., stopping when the white blood cell count was 2000/cu. mm. and restarting after 1 month with gradual tapering; 13 Gm. had been given on discontinuance. There was complete remission at this time but 150 mg. daily was resumed for a recurrence and reduced after a good response. Later, while on a maintenance dose of 100 mg. weekly, a relapse occurred, at which time dosage was increased to 200 mg. daily and maintained thus for about a month, then being discontinued because of leukopenia; when later reinstituted a good clinical remission followed. The patient was receiving 150 mg. daily at the time of the report, with normal blood count except for occasional mild leukocytosis.

Charles R. Tourtellotte and Melvin K. Call. Prolonged Remission of Myeloma with Cyclophosphamide (Cytoxan). Arch. Int. Med. 113:758, 1964.

"Intractable neoplastic effusions are often a late complication of malignant disease which considerably adds to the patient's discomfort. What appear currently to be the most effective measures with which to combat this situation?"

Reply: I believe that the use of quinacrine (Atabrine) was pioneered by Ultmann and associates (New York); the drug has been used with considerable success by many others. Ultmann's group instilled an initial dose of 50–100 mg. into the pleural or peritoneal cavity and followed this by 200–400 mg. daily for 4 or 5 days in the case of pleural effusions; in patients with ascites, the trial dose was 100–200 mg. followed by 400–800 mg. daily for 3–5 days. In 23 of their patients there were no side effects of the drug; fever occurred in 31, local pain in 14, atelectasis, ileus and nausea in 2 each and abscess and skin pigmentation in 1 each. Of the 12 patients who responded well to quinacrine therapy who eventually came to necropsy, in each there was obliterative fibro-

sis of the pleural cavity or fibrous tissue deposition on the intestinal serosa, but secondary mechanical obstruction of the bowel did not occur although plastic adhesions of loops of intestine were seen. Groesbeck and Cudmore (San Diego) have expressed the opinion that thio-TEPA should be the drug of choice because it is not usually associated with clinical side effects, is readily available and inexpensive. In pleural effusion cases they have instilled 40–45 mg. in 2–3 ml. water immediately after the effusion had been partially removed; in ascites the usual dose was 60–65 mg. in 4–5 ml. of water, also given after partial removal of fluid. Zelenick's group (Fitzsimons General Hospital) have used chlorambucil (Leukeran) effectively. Average dosage was 8–12 mg. daily, altering by 2 mg. weekly, up or down, to maintain a constant leukocyte count of 3000–4000/cu. mm. and a platelet count of not under 50,000/cu. mm. Mark and associates (Yale University) describe what is probably the method of choice of most men combating malignant pleural effusions, namely the use of mechlorethamine (Mustargen). The drug was instilled via needle after thoracentesis or via an indwelling chest catheter that had drained the chest by suction for 24 hours; dosage was 8–40 mg. based on empiric judgment.

James B. D. Mark, Ira S. Goldenberg and Albert C. W. Montague. Intrapleural Mechlorethamine Hydrochloride (Mustargen) Therapy for Malignant Pleural Effusion. J.A.M.A. 187:858, Mar. 14, 1964. John S. Zelenick, Arnold J. Halpern and Derek W. Williams. Treatment of Neoplastic Effusions with Chlorambucil (Leukeran). Obst. & Gynec. 23:703, 1964. John E. Ultmann, Alfred Gellhorn, Martha Osnos and Erich Hirschberg. Effect of Quinacrine (Atabrine) on Neoplastic Effusions and Certain of Their Enzymes. Cancer 16:283, 1963. H. P. Groesbeck and J. T. P. Cudmore. Intracavitary Thio-TEPA for Malignant Effusions. Am. Surgeon 28:90, 1962.

"At our hospital we have found both alkylating agents and radioisotopes effective in treatment of effusions into the pleural, pericardial and peritoneal cavities due to metastatic tumor. But the alkylating agents frequently cause severe nausea and vomiting necessitating heavy premedication, and sometimes there are also local reactions requiring emergency paracentesis. Radioisotopes have their disadvantages also, in that they are not always available, are expensive, and present a radiation hazard to both patient and personnel. What of 5-fluorouracil; could that be used?"

Reply: Leif Suhrland and Austin Weisberger did try this agent in 55 patients at the Highland View Hospital, in Cleveland. The effectiveness of the compound compared favorably with that of other agents, and it was found easy to administer, inexpensive and readily available. There was also no radiation hazard of course, and serious side effects were not encountered in this series, which contained patients with pleural effusions, ascites and pericardial effusions. In the patients with pleural or peritoneal effusions, most of the fluid was removed and then a single dose of 5-fluorouracil was instilled directly into the cavity, dosage varying from 2 to 3 Gm. with an average of 2.5 Gm./patient. Single injections of 500 mg. and 1000 mg. were given to the 3 patients with pericardial effusion. There was constant ECG monitoring throughout the procedure.

Leif G. Suhrland and Austin S. Weisberger. Intracavity 5-Fluorouracil in Malignant Effusions. Arch. Int. Med. 116:431, 1965.

"The tendency of the highly invasive and infiltrative tumor, neuroblastoma, to become necrotic very early often precipitates an awful situation which fortunately runs its course in a matter of a few months, but in those months whatever possible must be done. I have not had the success with cyclophosphamide (Cytoxan) that I had hoped for; what else may be done?"

Reply: Have you used the dosage of the Southwest Cancer Chemotherapy Study group: 5 mg. cyclophosphamide/kg. intravenously for 10 days, followed by 2.5 mg./kg. orally daily? The only other thing I can offer is to draw your attention to the work of Martin Bodian (Hospital for Sick Children, London) who has been using massive vitamin B_{12} therapy in these cases since 1950. His reasoning has been that since vitamin B_{12} is an essential factor for the normal maturation of hematopoietic cells, it might possibly enhance the maturation of neuroblastic tissue towards ganglioneuroma. The results reported by him are certainly remarkable (but see the immediately following Reply). Dosage: 1 mg. (1000 μg.)/7 kg. body weight on alternate days for at least 3 years whenever survival permits.

W. G. Thurman, D. J. Fernbach and M. P. Sullivan and the Writing Committee of the Pediatric Division of the Southwest Cancer Chemotherapy Study Group (Houston). Cyclophosphamide (Cytoxan) Therapy in Childhood Neuroblastoma. New England J. Med. 270:1336, June 18, 1964. Martin Bodian. Neuroblastoma: Evaluation of Its Natural History and the Effects of Therapy, with Particular. Reference to Treatment by Massive Doses of Vitamin B_{12}. Arch. Dis. Childhood 38:606, 1963.

"I have heard it said that vitamin B_{12} therapy is highly effective in neuroblastoma. Is this true?"

Reply: Here we have quite an anomalous situation. In London, Martin Bodian has been recording good effects with this therapy since 1950, but here in the United States, Arthur Sawitsky and Franklin Desposito canvassed

20 investigators whose results with the vitamin indicated no increase in the remission rate when it was used either alone or in conjunction with other chemotherapeutic agents or x-rays. The subject is too important to be dismissed merely because of this disparity in findings, and it is therefore to be hoped that the two groups of investigators will get together and see what can be made to come of the whole thing.

Arthur Sawitsky and Franklin Desposito. Survey of American Experience with Vitamin B_{12} Therapy of Neuroblastoma. J. Pediat. 67:99, 1965. Martin Bodian. Neuroblastoma: Evaluation of Its Natural History and the Effects of Therapy, with Particular Reference to Treatment by Massive Doses of Vitamin B_{12}. Arch. Dis. Childhood 38:606, 1963.

"I have recently lost a patient in fatal hypercalcemia who was being treated with estrogens for disseminated osteolytic metastases. I am afraid that I was caught a bit off guard by the suddenness of the thing; would peritoneal dialysis have helped, and what should have warned me of the impending occurrence?"

Reply: The literature, for one thing, would have warned you because it has contained repeated reports of such occurrences since the first one that appeared in 1949. In 1 of Kleinfeld's (Columbia-Presbyterian Medical Center) patients, the serum calcium level was reduced from 18 mg. to 14 mg./100 ml. in 30 hours by peritoneal dialysis. In patients with disseminated osteolytic metastases, who are most prone to develop hypercalcemia when treated with estrogens, the development of the state might be indicated by constipation, weakness, mental disorientation or lethargy, but in some instances coma and renal insufficiency supervene very rapidly. At the least suspicious symptom the serum calcium level should be determined, and if it is elevated one must of course stop the estrogen. Corticosteroids may occasionally be helpful.

George Kleinfeld. Acute Fatal Hypercalcemia: Complication in Estrogen Therapy of Metastatic Breast Cancer. J.A.M.A. 181:1137, Sept. 29, 1962. J. B. Hermann and associates. J. Clin. Endrocrinol. 9:1, 1949.

"Recently, to my surprise, I achieved good ameliorative effect with an estrogen in metastatic ovarian carcinoma. What is the record?"

Reply: Long and Evans (Columbia, Missouri) gave 15–30 mg. daily of diethylstilbestrol orally to 14 patients with an advanced lesion of this sort. Of the 14, 5 were not followed before death, but both subjective and objective improvement occurred in 4 of the other 9. It is my impression, however, that this is a considerably better result than is usually achieved, but it does seem that this therapy is more effective if the primary tumor has been removed.

Robert T. L. Long and A. McChesney Evans (Ellis Fischel State Cancer Hospital). Diethylstilbestrol as Chemotherapeutic Agent for Ovarian Carcinoma. Missouri Med. 60:1125, 1963.

"I have a patient with pheochromocytoma in whom salt restriction, oral digoxin and biweekly Mercuhydrin are required for maintenance. Is there any drug that will be helpful in the attempt to get this patient ready for surgery?"

Reply: In a case of this sort with cardiomegaly and progressive congestive heart failure, Engelman and Sjoerdsma, at the National Institutes of Health, obtained excellent results from the administration of phenoxybenzamine (Dibenzyline), 30 mg./day orally. Within 1 week of initiating this therapy, excessive sweating disappeared, the pulse rate slowed and the B.M.R. and fasting plasma free fatty acid fell; within 1 month it was possible to discontinue the diuretics, and a little later the patient's condition stabilized sufficiently so that the pheochromocytoma could be removed.

Karl Engelman and Albert Sjoerdsma. Chronic Medical Therapy for Pheochromocytoma: Report of Four Cases. Ann. Int. Med. 61:229, 1964.

"I have in my practice a case that has been diagnosed and confirmed as reticuloendotheliosis. I have learned that the anti–folic acid compounds and the corticosteroids are strikingly effective in this malady, but also know that high dosage of these agents may lead to undesirable and even dangerous side effects. What would you suggest?"

Reply: Paul Freud (New York Medical College) has rotated these compounds so as to avoid both treatment-free intervals and excessive side effects. Initial therapy of three 4 week periods consists of 2 weeks of corticosteroid administration followed by 2 weeks of anti-folic acid administration. Daily cortisone dosage is 250 mg. for a patient of 9 months, 350 mg. for one of 18 months and 400 mg. for one of 30 months, all given in divided doses. The anti–folic acid compound, aminopterin, is given in 2.5 mg. dosage daily. Maintenance dosage after the initial 4 weeks of therapy is begun with 75 mg. of cortisone on 4 alternating days a week and 2.5 mg. aminopterin on the other 3 days. At the time of Freud's report he had had 2 children on this regimen for 2½ and 4 years and 2 for 13 and 18 months.

Paul Freud. Treatment of Reticuloendotheliosis: Use of Corticosteroids and Anti–folic Acid Compounds. J.A.M.A. 175:82, Jan 14, 1961.

"I have a case of reticulum cell sarcoma in my practice, in which I am tempted to use potassium para-aminobenzoic acid (Potaba) on the basis of the case report of Zarafonetis a few years ago. Am I likely to get into any trouble with this agent?"

Reply: Excessive dosage may cause gastrointestinal symptoms, pruritus, rash and fever and possibly even liver damage, but in the case to which you refer the drug was used in dosage of 18–24 Gm. daily off and on for a period of several years without the occurrence of any of these reactions.

Chris J. D. Zarafonetis. Temple University. Reticulum Cell Sarcoma Complicating Atopic Dermatitis: Prolonged Remission Following Potaba (Potassium Para-Aminobenzoic Acid) Therapy. Cancer 14:5, 1961.

"I have heard that retinoblastoma is being treated somewhere without enucleation; can you tell me where and how?"

Reply: At Tulane University, Krementz's group has expressed willingness to treat moderately advanced unilateral disease by combined fractional irradiation with fractional intra-arterial administration of triethylenemelamine (TEM) through an indwelling polyethylene tube inserted in the internal carotid artery. With the provision that they discontinue if the white cell count falls to or below 2500/cu. mm., they give a dose of 0.03 mg./kg. in 2–3 ml. normal saline daily for 7–10 days before irradiation (0.08–0.1 mg./kg. for a single injection). The single intramuscular dose is 0.15 mg./kg. Of their 15 patients, 10 were reported as having no evidence of disease and useful vision in one eye; 3 living without vision, 2 of them with recurrent disease; 2 dead with metastatic retinoblastoma. This result is somewhat better than the 7 alive, 6 with useful vision, of 19 patients treated by other methods.

Edward T. Krementz, Joseph V. Schlosser, Joseph P. Rumage and Ladene Herring. Retinoblastoma: Behavior and Treatment with Fractional Irradiation and Intraarterial Triethylenemelamine (TEM). Ann. New York Acad. Sc. 114 (Art. 2):963, 1964.

"Do we know precisely where we stand in the therapy of metastatic Wilms' tumor; i.e., has a comparative trial been made of vincristine (Oncovin), actinomycin D and radiotherapy?"

Reply: Not to my knowledge, though such a study is much to be desired.

"It has been rumored that chloroquine (Aralen) is an effective prophylactic agent in patients prone to develop basal cell epitheliomas or squamous cell carcinomas. Is there reliable evidence of this?"

Reply: I believe that the routine administration of chloroquine for the prevention of such lesions is not justified in the present state of our knowledge. At Baylor University, Knox and Freeman felt, with some reservations, that such treatment had a moderate suppressive effect on spontaneous carcinogenesis but that the findings were not of sufficient magnitude to justify the prolonged use of a drug that in itself may produce serious side effects. The fact is that, although antimalarial drugs have been tried in a large number of dermatologic maladies since their introduction in this field by Page in 1951, their success has been quite moderate in only a very small number of entities.

John M. Knox and Robert G. Freeman. Prophylactic Use of Chloroquine to Prevent Skin Cancer. Arch. Dermat. 87:315, 1963. F. Page. Treatment of Lupus Erythematosus with Mepacrine. Lancet 2:755, 1951.

MECONIUM PLUG SYNDROME

"In a newborn with the meconium plug syndrome, what is one to do if enemas have not reduced the obstruction?"

Reply: I believe the enema that is usually employed is one part 3% hydrogen peroxide to three parts normal saline. If this is not effective, I suppose that laparotomy has usually to be resorted to. But you would do well to remember that the patient may actually have Hirschsprung's disease. Indeed, Gillis and Grantmyre, at Dalhousie University, have reported 2 cases illustrating the association between Hirschsprung's disease and the meconium plug syndrome.

D. A. Gillis and Edward B. Grantmyre. Meconium-Plug Syndrome and Hirschsprung's Disease. Canad. M. A. J. 92:225, Jan 30, 1965.

MÉNIÈRE'S DISEASE

"I have in my practice a case of Ménière's disease that has resisted all drug therapy. Has anything new and promising been introduced?"

Reply: In Stockholm, T. Gejrot gave intravenous Xylocaine to 11 patients on a number of occasions and brought about disappearance of the tinnitus for 20 minutes, nausea for an hour or two, and vomiting generally for good. Nystagmus was unaffected. A 1% solution of Xylocaine without epinephrine was used in dosage of 1 mg./kg., administered at the rate of 6 mg./minute. The drug was given only during attacks and in periods of severe nausea. In Reno, Nevada, Joseph Elia has used betahistine (Serc) with success in all of a small series of cases; independent confirmation will be awaited with interest. Dosage was 1 tablet of 4 mg. four times daily.

T. Gejrot. Intravenous Xylocaine in the Treatment of Attacks of Ménière's Disease. Acta oto-laryng. Supp. 188, p. 190, 1964. Joseph C. Elia. Double-Blind Evaluation of a New Treatment for Ménière's Syndrome. J.A.M.A. 196:187, Apr. 11, 1966.

MENINGITIS

"It is rumored that so much resistance to the sulfonamides has developed in meningococci that these drugs are no longer the agents of choice in the treatment of meningococcal disease. Is there a sound basis for this?"

Reply: Yes, it seems that there is. The most definitive study that I have seen was that of Leedom and associates, reporting from the Los Angeles County General Hospital at the close of 1965. They found that 33% of 106 strains of *Neisseria meningitidis* were considerably resistant to sulfadiazine. These data appear clearly to indicate the abandonment of sulfonamides as primary therapy in meningococcal disease.

John M. Leedom, Daniel Ivler, Allen W. Mathies, Lauri D. Thrupp, Bernard Portnoy and Paul F. Wehrle. Importance of Sulfadiazine Resistance in Meningococcal Disease in Civilians. New England J. Med. 273:1395, Dec. 23, 1965.

"Now that the meningococcus has become sulfonamide-resistant, what is our best therapeutic agent in a meningococcal infection?"

Reply: Fortunately, meningococcal infections are no longer as important in morbidity and mortality statistics as formerly, but they still constitute a serious problem in children under 5 years of age and in military recruits. At Harvard Medical School, Theodore Eickhoff and Maxwell Finland have studied the subject of your question in terms of in vitro sensitivity of 56 recently isolated strains of meningococci, many of which were sulfonamide-resistant. Penicillin G possessed the greatest activity against these organisms. Ampicillin (Polycillin) was next most active but only one fourth as active as penicillin G. Novobiocin (Cathomycin) and erythromycin (Ilotycin, etc.) were next, followed by tetracycline and chloramphenicol (Chloromycetin). Cephalothin (Keflin), cloxacillin (Orbenin) and nafcillin (Unipen) were of intermediate activity, as were gentamicin (Garamycin), kanamycin (Kantrex) and streptomycin. Bacitracin and polymyxin B sulfate (Aerosporin) showed little or no activity. The sulfonamide-resistant and sensitive strains displayed no difference in susceptibility to the antibiotics.

Theodore C. Eickhoff and Maxwell Finland. Changing Susceptibility of Meningococci to Antimicrobial Agents. New England J. Med. 272:395, Feb. 25, 1965.

"In treating a case of acute meningoencephalitis with antibiotics, should one use corticosteroids in addition?"

Reply: The indications are that this is definitely a bad thing to do. At the University of Bergen, Bøe and associates showed in a retrospective study of 346 cases that every group of patients who were not treated with corticosteroids fared better than those who received them. If only comatose patients were considered, to allow for the possibility that corticosteroids were more often given to severely ill patients, mortality was still higher among patients who received corticosteroids, and among the surviving patients who were comatose during acute illness the frequency of neurologic sequelae was distinctly higher among those who had received the drugs.

Johs. Bøe, Claus Ola Solberg and Trygve Saeter. Corticosteroid Treatment for Acute Meningoencephalitis: Retrospective Study of 346 Cases. Brit. M. J. 1:1094, Apr. 24, 1965.

"Since the fatalities and complications of a pyogenic meningitis may be related to inflammatory exudate over the meninges, is it not rational to attempt enzymatic debridement with pancreatic dornase, as has been advocated?"

Reply: The material would have to be used intrathecally of course, and I believe that you would run some risk. At least Richard Parker and associates, at the University of Utah, reported a case in which they felt that the persistence of fever, nuchal rigidity and cerebrospinal fluid protein elevation into the second week of hospitalization was likely the result of the administration of pancreatic dornase by this route.

Richard H. Parker, W. Dean Wilcox and Thomas S. Dietrich. Toxicity of Intrathecally Administered Pancreatic Dornase. J.A.M.A. 192:169, Apr. 12, 1965.

MENOPAUSE

"What menopausal women should have the benefit of estrogen therapy, and what are the potential hazards?"

Reply: Robert Greenblatt, at the Medical College of Georgia, has answered these questions authoritatively. He says that any woman with signs and symptoms of an estrogen deficiency is a candidate for replacement therapy, but that the withholding of such therapy from women with a history of mammary or uterine cancer is good practice. Estrogens and androgens induce salt and water retention, and therefore their use is interdicted in women with cardiac decompensation. They are also contraindicated in women with a recent history of endometriosis unless a progestational agent is added to the estrogen therapy. Androgens, he considers, may be of considerable aid in less than virilizing doses in minimizing menopausal symptoms in women with fibromyomas of the uterus; estrogens, with or without progestins, stimulate further growth of these tumors. As evidences of the need for estrogens he lists complaints due to imbalance of the autonomic nervous system (hot flushes, sexual excesses, sweats, palpitations, spasms and globus hystericus); psychogenic disturbances (apprehension, depression, insomnia, nervousness, headaches and frigidity); and metabolic disorders (bone demineralization, myalgias and skin and mucous-membrane atrophy). As for the hazards, it would seem that the charge against estrogens of promoting mammary carcinoma can hardly be sustained in view of the well established fact that the incidence of this lesion has not materially increased in the past 30 years despite the introduction of estrogens into medical practice. It would appear that the cyclic rather than the continuous type of estrogen administration should be favored since the association of uninterrupted estrogen administration with endometrial cancer remains obscure. An increase in the incidence of cervical carcinoma in association with estrogen therapy has not been established. If there is any reason to suspect that uterine bleeding in association with estrogen therapy is not explainable as simple withdrawal bleeding in the cyclic type of treatment, then of course studies have to be made to assess the situation. Sometimes there is an annoying pelvic congestion, which is usually overcome by dosage adjustment and so too are edema and gain in weight.

Robert B. Greenblatt. Estrogen Therapy for Postmenopausal Females. New England J. Med. 272:305, Feb. 11, 1965.

"Is it true that when the contraceptive pill of the Enovid type is used in management of the menopause it causes an undesirable increase in libido?"

Reply: Depends upon what you call "undesirable." In J. L. Bakke's study of the menopausal use of the pill, 6 women rejected it because they *disliked* the increase in libido while 6 others liked it because they *enjoyed* the increase. There seemed no doubt in this study that an increase had occurred, because none of the placebo group noted any effect on libido.

J. L. Bakke. A Double-Blind Study of a Progestin-Estrogen Combination in the Management of the Menopause. Pacif. Med. & Surg. 73:200, 1965.

MENORRHAGIA

"Has aminocaproic acid (Amicar) been found useful in treatment of profuse menstruation?"

Reply: As you are aware, this drug has only rather recently been released in this country though considerable experience has been had with it abroad. In Sweden, Inga Nilsson and Sven Björkman used it in 24 women with profuse menstrual flow but without any demonstrable gynecological disorder. Eighteen were otherwise healthy but 6 suffered from a hemorrhagic diathesis. In those with a normal coagulation mechanism, 1 was treated during 19 periods, 5 during 5–9 periods and the remaining 12 during 1–4 periods. The drug was said to have invariably reduced the menstrual flow to normal when given orally in dosage of 0.1 Gm./kg. body weight. Bleeding was also normalized in the patients with hemorrhagic diathesis, but higher dosage was required; in 1 of these patients, who went into shock owing to the large blood loss, the response to Amicar was dramatic. No serious side effects were encountered in this study.

Inga Marie Nilsson and Sven Erik Björkman. Experiences with Aminocaproic Acid (Amicar) in the Treatment of Profuse Menstruation. Acta med. scandinav. 117:445, 1965.

METHEMOGLOBINEMIA

"What drugs should one think of in a patient with methemoglobinemia?"

Reply: Acetanilid, phenacetin, nitrites and nitrates, sulfonamides.

MIGRAINE

"In our area, Bellergal and cypropheptadine (Periactin) are much used in the treatment of migraine, and now methysergide (Sansert) is entering the picture. With which of these drugs would you begin the treatment in a case of average severity?"

Reply: Numerous studies have established the very considerable value of Sansert in this malady; it appears undoubtedly to be more effective than the other two drugs you are using, particularly in prophylaxis when the patient suffers frequent attacks. However, side effects occur rather frequently with Sansert, as evidenced in some of the other Replies in this volume, and indeed Curran and Lance summed up a considerable experience with the drug in Australia by saying that, since Bellergal and Periactin have fewer and milder side effects, they should be tried first, with Sansert reserved for unresponsive patients.

D. A. Curran and J. W. Lance. Clinical Trial of Methysergide and Other Preparations in the Management of Migraine. J. Neurol. Neurosurg. & Psychiat. 27:463, 1964.

"We have been using methysergide (Sansert) effectively in the treatment of migraine, but now rumor has reached us that retroperitoneal fibrosis has appeared in some patients taking this drug. Is there truth in this?"

Reply: Yes, these cases are being seen; J. R. Graham and associates, in Boston, have collected the records of 27. I believe that a direct causal relationship between methysergide and retroperitoneal fibrosis has not been established, but the suspicion is certainly high that such a relationship does exist. David Utz and associates, at the Mayo Clinic, feel that the occurrence of these cases should not interdict the use of the drug and also that evidence of parenchymal kidney disease probably should not be considered an absolute contraindication to its use. However, the Graham group includes renal disease among the other contraindications: peripheral vascular disease (including phlebitis), severe hypertension, angina pectoris, coronary and hepatic insufficiency, pregnancy, valvular heart disease, rheumatoid arthritis, chronic pulmonary disease, history of a "collagen-disease diathesis." All observers agree that any patient who has been taking the drug continuously for a year should discontinue for at least 3 months and have a urinalysis, a test of renal function, and excretory urography performed.

David C. Utz, E. Douglas Rooke, John A. Spittell, Jr., and Lloyd G. Bartholomew. Retroperitoneal Fibrosis in Patients Taking Methysergide. J.A.M.A. 191:983, Mar. 22, 1965. J. R. Graham, H. J. Suby, P. R. LeCompte and N. L. Sadowsky. Fibrotic Disorders Associated with Methysergide Therapy for Headache. New England J. Med. 274:359, Feb. 17, 1966.

"I am puzzled in trying to understand the fibrotic disorders that seem to be appearing in connection with the use of methysergide (Sansert). They seem to be the type of syndrome that would be explainable by an excess of serotonin, since serotonin promotes fibrosis in pulmonary tissue, heart valves, endocardium, arterial linings and the retroperitoneal space in animals and man; yet methysergide is allegedly an 'antiserotonin' agent."

Reply: I have heard it speculated that the explanation may lie in the fact that methysergide competes successfully with serotonin for only certain receptor sites and thus leaves certain other sites open for an excessive serotonin effect on their receptors.

"Is it possible that methysergide (Sansert) may produce vascular insufficiency in some individuals?"

Reply: Very definitely this is possible. Charles Rackley's group, in Durham, North Carolina, reported 2 individuals who developed arterial insufficiency of the lower extremities while on the drug, 1 of whom had several bouts of chest pain compatible with coronary insufficiency. And there have been other reports. You should definitely be alerted to the possibility of this sort of thing in using the drug.

Charles E. Rackley, Charles E. Mengel, Marvin Pomerantz and Henry D. McIntosh. Vascular Complications with Use of Methysergide. Arch. Int. Med. 117:265, 1966. Thomas D. Johnson. Severe Peripheral Arterial Constriction, Acute Ischemia of Lower Extremity with Use of Methysergide and Ergotamine. Arch. Int. Med. 117:237, 1966.

"When a patient with migraine is taking methysergide (Sansert) as a prophylactic measure, is it safe to prescribe ergotamine tartrate for the treatment of a 'breakthrough' headache?"

Reply: In his report on the use of methysergide in 500 patients, John Graham (Harvard Medical School) said that if this is done the ergotamine tartrate dosage should be considerably reduced to avoid undesirable synergistic effects. It must be remembered that methysergide and ergotamine are chemically related compounds.

John R. Graham. Methysergide (Sansert) for Prevention of Headache: Experience in 500 Patients Over Three Years. New England J. Med. 270:67, Jan. 9, 1964.

"What are the reactions to be expected and the contraindications to the use of ergotamine in the treatment of migraine?"

Reply: Probably the most frequently occurring side effects when one is using the drug in migraine therapy are: (1) nausea and vomiting; (2) coronary spasm; (3) muscular cramp in neck and thigh (probably due to vascular spasm, ischemia, or both); (4) a wide variety of vascular symptoms ranging from thrombophlebitis to acute arterial occlusion. Ergotism, which is characterized in its preliminary stage by numbness, cyanosis and paresthesias in the extremities and in the final stage by gangrene, is rare. Actually, this type of toxic response to the drug may require a predisposing factor such as liver disease, sepsis or peripheral vascular disease, but it appears

that pruritus also invites it. Anginoid discomfort is by no means a rare occurrence, and death has occurred in association with the administration of the ergotamines in individuals with coronary disease. It may be well to bear in mind that the ergot compounds sometimes appear to potentiate the adrenergic drugs of the epinephrine group.

Friedman and associates listed the following contraindications to the use of ergotamine: peripheral vascular diseases, angina pectoris, impaired hepatic or renal function, thyrotoxicosis, cachexia, avitaminosis, septic states associated with intravascular diseases, pregnancy. These same observers, however, reported the case of a man who, in the absence of any contraindications, had been taking the drug daily for over 18 years without any reported or observed side effects.

Sodium nicotinate, 140 mg. intravenously, has been used with good effect to reverse the vasoconstrictive action of ergotamine. The hypodermic injection of 0.6 mg. of atropine sulfate will sometimes check the gastrointestinal distress, and the slow intravenous administration of 10 ml. of 10% calcium gluconate diminishes the muscular pains.

A. P. Friedman, T. J. C. von Storch and S. Araki. Ergotamine Tartrate: Its History, Action and Proper Use in the Treatment of Migraine. New York State J. Med. 59:2359, 1959.

MONGOLISM

"Great pressure is being brought to bear upon me by the family of a child with mongolism to institute thyroid therapy. Is this really a valuable therapeutic measure?"

Reply: It has certainly been used a great deal since its recommendation a number of years ago, but no one has convincingly shown it to be effective, and now we finally have a carefully performed study which has proven that it is worthless therapy. At the Children's Hospital of Los Angeles, Richard Koch and associates used liothyronine (Cytomel) in 73 children with a placebo and a control group. Dosage was 12.5 μg./day to age 1 year, 25 μg./day to age 2 years, 50 μg./day to age 3 years, and 75 μg./day thereafter. Using all the modern assessment methods, it was impossible to show significant differences between the groups that were thyroid treated, placebo treated and control treated. The conclusion was, therefore, that Cytomel has no effect on development, growth, height or general clinical condition of infants or children with mongolism.

Richard Koch, Jack Share and Betty Graliker. Effects of Cytomel on Young Children with Down's Syndrome (Mongolism): Double-Blind Longitudinal Study. J. Pediat. 66:764, 1965.

MOTION SICKNESS

"With the increased use of jet planes it seems to me that the amount of motion sickness has decreased considerably; nevertheless, I do occasionally have to prescribe for an individual and would be grateful for a listing, with dosages, of the agents that are in principal use nowadays."

Reply: Scopolamine hydrobromide (also known as hyoscine) is used in initial dosage of 0.6–1.2 mg., with subsequent doses of 0.3 mg. at 6 hour intervals as needed. Unless it has been recently changed, the Army Motion Sickness Preventive Tablet contains 0.4 mg. of scopolamine, 130 mg. of amobarbital and 0.3 mg. of atropine. For short air journeys it is frequently advisable to give 0.3 mg. of scopolamine 4 hours before starting the flight and another dose of the same size as the flight begins; on long air journeys doses may be taken at 4 hour intervals. Some dryness of the mouth and occasionally visual impairment are usually the only side actions. Among the antihistaminics, dimenhydrinate's (Dramamine) adult oral preventive dosage is usually 50 mg. one-half hour before embarking, and this dosage may be repeated before meals and on retiring if considered necessary. Dosage of 100 mg. every 4 hours may be required to control established symptoms. Rectal dosage is the same as oral. Recommended dosage two or three times daily for children of 5–8 years is 12.5–25 mg.; 8–12 years, 25–50 mg.

Meclizine (Bonamine) adult dosage is 25–50 mg. 1 hour prior to embarkation, children one-half this amount. A single dose daily usually suffices thereafter for continued prevention or in treatment, but the drug may be given as often as three times daily if indicated.

Cyclizine (Marezine) adult dosage is 50 mg. 1 hour before embarkation and 50 mg. three times daily thereafter if indicated; children of 6–10 years, one-half this, under 6 years, one-fourth. Intramuscular and rectal dosages are the same as oral.

Promethazine (Phenergan) dosage of 12.5–25 mg. once daily may suffice, but the drug may be given three times daily if needed.

MULTIPLE SCLEROSIS

"If multiple sclerosis is a peculiar auto-immune disease related to the myelin of the brain, it would seem reasonable to expect that corticosteroids would favorably alter the course of the disease. Has this been put to the test?"

Reply: Yes, at the University of Michigan, Tourtellotte and Haerer closely followed 76 outpatients for 18 months while they were receiving either cyanocobalamin (vitamin B_{12}) or methylprednisolone (Medrol) tablets in a double-blind study. Historically and by examination, the patients on the corticosteroid fared somewhat better than those on the vitamin, but only a few statistically significant differences were found to support this. The observers therefore hesitantly concluded that the corticosteroid might have some value in the malady.

Wallace W. Tourtellotte and Armin F. Haerer. Use of an Oral Corticosteroid in the Treatment of Multiple Sclerosis. Arch. Neurol. 12:536, 1965.

"I have heard it rumored that the *intrathecal* administration of corticosteroids has some efficacy in multiple sclerosis; can you substantiate this?"

Reply: I have seen three reports in which successful palliative effect was claimed from intrathecal corticosteroid administration. In the most recent of these, Van Buskirk's group (University of Maryland) described the giving of weekly intrathecal injections of methylprednisolone acetate (Depo-Medrol) to 20 patients who had had the disease for at least a year. Dosage progressed from 20 to 80 mg., using suspensions of 40 mg./ml. When four weekly injections of 20, 40, 60 and 80 mg. had been given, 80–100 mg. was injected monthly. The patients who benefited were those having a prominent spastic component in their illness. A local effect on the lumbar and sacral roots, which was not specific for a multiple sclerosis lesion, was suggested by these investigators in explanation of the corticosteroid action.

Charles Van Buskirk, Arthur L. Poffenbarger, Luis F. Capriles and Braulio V. Idea. Treatment of Multiple Sclerosis with Intrathecal Steroids. Neurology 14:595, 1964.

"In reviewing the recent literature of multiple sclerosis I have come upon a report of the trial of tolbutamide (Orinase) in the malady, the trial failing of course. How silly can you be?"

Reply: Well, my friend, I do not know about yourself, but as for me I am inclined not to look down my nose too hastily. Serendipity has mightily befriended medicine from time to time; perhaps more planned "accidental findings" might not be amiss in these hectic days when research groups are practically promising "breakthroughs" if only they are given money enough to pursue their undeviating line of investigation.

MUMPS

"What about mumps nowadays? Is there any evidence that the corticosteroids are of specific usefulness or that the estrogens prevent orchitis?"

Reply: No, none that is incontrovertible. The corticosteroids sometimes unquestionably lessen the pain and tenderness of the complicating orchitis, but any prophylactic effect of estrogens on the subsequent testicular atrophy has still to be demonstrated conclusively. Have you heard of the relief of the symptoms of orchitis that is allegedly provided by anesthetic block of the spermatic cord?

Richards P. Lyon and Henry B. Bruyn. Mumps Epididymo-Orchitis: Treatment by Anesthetic Block of the Spermatic Cord. J.A.M.A. 196:736, May 23, 1966.

MUSCULAR DYSTROPHIES

"Are there any specific or near-specific drug therapies in any of the muscular dystrophies?"

Reply: Let us list them: myotonia atrophica, amyotonia congenita, progressive muscular dystrophy, myotonia congenita. And the answer is no.

MUSCULOSKELETAL AND SPASTIC DISORDERS

"It seems to me that I am nowadays encountering disabling pain associated with skeletal muscle spasm of one sort or another much more often than formerly, or is it only because the drugs with alleged skeletal muscle relaxant properties are brought more prominently to one's attention? All of the following have been promoted to me: methocarbamol (Robaxin), chlorzoxazone (Paraflex), styramate (Sinaxar), carisoprodol (Rela, Soma), metaxalone (Skelaxin), phenyramidol (Analexin), chlorphenesin carbamate (Maolate). Is this the lot, and in what types of muscle spasm are they really useful?"

Reply: You have certainly named the principal ones (unless we are to include, as some observers do, the three important tranquilizers, meprobamate [Miltown, Equanil], chlordiazepoxide [Librium] and diazepam [Valium]), with the exception of mephenesin (Tolserol, etc.), which is the original and prototype of them all. The latter agent, however, is more difficult to use than the others because of the relative inefficacy of the oral carbamate preparation (Tolseram) and the rather frequent occurrence of toxic manifestations associated with intravenous administration of mephenesin. Most practice nowadays is therefore confined to the use of one or the other of those preparations you have listed. As for comparison of these drugs, one with another, in the relief of skeletal muscle spasm, I do not know of any study in which this has been convincingly accomplished. As for the types of disability in which drugs of the group exhibit such efficacy as they have, this can best be answered by grouping the spasms into related types and then indicating those groups in which the drugs appear to be most useful. First, there is the muscle spasm that appears as a concomitant of the arthritides, fibrositis, myositis, bursitis and spondylitis (perhaps it would be admissible to place the "stiff-man syndrome" here also). Trial of the relaxant drugs is indicated in all of these entities. Second, then, spasm associated with dislocations and fractures, strains and sprains and traumatized ligaments and tendons. Here, too, the drugs may be useful. Third is the group of spastic states, and fourth, the maladies that reflect neuronal damage. In both of these groups some relief can sometimes be attained through the use of these skeletal muscle relaxants as adjunctive therapy, but the incidence of good results is probably quite low. Spastic states: cerebral palsy, hemaplegia, paraplegia, decerebrate rigidity, dystonias, torticollis. States of neuronal damage: poliomyelitis, amyotrophic lateral sclerosis, muscular dystrophy, parkinsonism, multiple sclerosis.

"I have heard that quinine is useful in the treatment of leg cramps. How would one use it?"

Reply: It is usual to prescribe 200 mg. of quinine sulfate to be taken after the evening meal by an individual prone to have these cramps at night and then have a similar dose taken at bedtime. It may take several nights for this therapy to be effective, but sometimes the spasms do not return after the drug is discontinued. Quinine has a slight curare-like action on skeletal muscle.

"One of my associates recently used magnesium sulfate intravenously very effectively in a case of spider bite, and I know that obstetricians use this drug in the treatment of eclampsia. Does it have ability to relax musculature under any other circumstances?"

Reply: Parenterally administered magnesium sulfate is effective in relaxing uterine tetany resulting from overdosage of oxytocin (Pitocin), or from excessive response to it, and it is also sometimes able to overcome the spasmodic uterine contraction known as constriction ring dystocia. These are the uterine muscle relaxant employments. For relaxation of striated muscle it is employed in eclampsia; in the treatment of spider bite, in which it usually overcomes not only the boardlike abdominal rigidity but also relieves the hypertension and pain; and in tetanus, in which it will act analgesically by lessening the severity of the muscular spasms. For its depressant effect on cardiac muscle, which involves action on the conduction mechanisms as well as on the myocardium itself, it is used in recalcitrant cases of paroxysmal atrial tachycardia and even occasionally in ventricular tachycardia. And when used in the therapy of eclampsia there is some evidence of a direct relaxing effect on arterial smooth muscle. The relaxing effect on smooth muscle in general is also the reason for the employment as an antidote to the excessive action of a cholinergic drug such as carbachol (Carcholin). Finally, magnesium sulfate may be used for simultaneous relaxant effects upon all types of musculature in cases of barium poisoning.

The central nervous system depressant action is one of the reasons for employing the drug in eclampsia and the principal reason for its use in the convulsive syndrome in acute nephritis in childhood, the element of cerebral edema in the latter being also combated by the "depleting" effect of the compound which withdraws water from the tissue cells that it is unable to enter.

In acute situations usual adult intravenous dosage is 20 ml. of 20% solution. The effect of such injections usually lasts only about half an hour. Intramuscular dosage of the 20% solution for children is figured at 0.1–0.2 ml./kg.

The bugaboo of parenteral magnesium sulfate administration is the possibility of respiratory depression; there is no doubt that the drug may have this effect to a fatal degree in rare instances. But despite this fact one may use it with perfect safety provided two things obtain: one, that someone is in constant attendance on the patient after the injection is given; and the other, that a 10% solution of calcium gluconate is at hand for intravenous administration as antidote. Calcium counteracts instantaneously both the central and peripheral actions of magnesium through mechanisms that are not understood—actually there is nothing more dramatic than the way in which calcium injection will cause a rabbit that has been completely depressed by magnesium to jump up and resume normal activities, and the same thing occurs in man.

"Have you heard anything of the subarachnoid use of phenolglycerin in cases of spasticity?"

Reply: Yes, the British introduced this method a few years ago, and I cite the recent Swedish report for details if you wish to make a trial of these intrathecal injections. This is certainly not a measure to be entered upon lightly, for it is unsuitable for persons with preserved gait, its suitability in cases of severe inhibited neurogenic bladder insusceptible to medical treatment has not yet been determined, and impairment of the sphincteric and vesicle functions may be effected by the therapy itself.

Ejner Pedersen and Palle Juul-Jensen. Treatment of Spasticity by Subarachnoid Phenolglycerin. Neurology 15: 256, 1965.

"I have in my practice a 9-year-old boy with congenital cerebral spastic infantile paraplegia of unknown origin, who has never shown any tendency toward improvement though my associates and I have tried everything known to us. With so much else to be done one cannot always follow all of the literature; has anything promising been developed recently in this area?"

Reply: The most remarkable report that I have seen in recent times is that of Berman's group (Willowbrook State School, Staten Island, New York) who used chlorzoxazone (Paraflex) in 29 severely spastic children with really impressive results in about half of them. Initial oral dosage was 750 mg. and later 1000 mg. daily, with treatment continued for 8 weeks. The drug was reported to have relieved painful muscle tone and reduced the incidence of muscle spasms and to facilitate passive and active exercises and thus prevent muscle waste and contractures. But its greatest achievement was to make the children sufficiently cooperative for adequate nursing management and food intake. In some instances drooling and skin disorders ceased. It was said that side effects were rare, mild and reversible. Have you tried emylcamate (Striatran) which has also been the subject of a fairly recent favorable report? Charles Carter (Sunland Training Center, Orlando, Florida) used a wide range of starting dosage of 300–4800 mg. daily, and this dosage range was also necessary for maintenance. Significant improvement was reported in 72.7% of his 234 mentally retarded spastic patients and in 91% of the 34 patients with athetosis and spasticity.

Harold H. Berman, Ossy Noe and Florence Goodfield. Relief of Severe Spasticity with Chlorzoxazone (Paraflex). Dis. Nerv. System 25:430, 1964. Charles H. Carter. Emylcamate (Striatran) in Hospitalized Mentally Retarded Spastic Patients. Dis. Nerv. System 23:211, 1962.

"I have had moderate success in relieving spasm in some paraplegics and quadriplegics but have not been able to effect improvement in muscle strength. What has been the experience of others?"

Reply: At the VA Hospital in Portland, Oregon, Everill Fowlks and associates used diazepam (Valium) in 33 adults with major neurologic disorders complicated by severe spasticity, and, like yourself, they found that muscle strength remained unaltered when relief of spasm was achieved.

Everill W. Fowlks, Donald A. Strickland and George A. Perrson. Control of Spastic States in Neurologic Patients with Diazepam. Am. J. Phys. Med. 44:9, 1965.

"I find it very difficult to evaluate drug therapy in cerebral-palsied children because the degree of their responsiveness varies greatly from day to day. Can you discuss an acceptable method of drug study under these circumstances?"

Reply: The best that I can do is call your attention to the report of Henry Marsh, at the Institute of Logopedics, in Wichita, Kans., who studied 9 girls and 17 boys, with an average age of 10½ years, including 24 quadriplegics, 1 hemiplegic and 1 paraplegic (6 were very severely disabled, 9 severely so, 10 moderately and 1 mildly disabled). Diazepam (Valium) or placebo were issued every 2 weeks, to be taken orally for an average period of 20 weeks, dosage varying from 1 mg. twice daily to 5 mg. four times daily. There was a variable duration of placebo administration, and frequent crossovers were made. The final assessment of functional improvement reflected progress in performance during the active drug and placebo therapies. Ten patients were found to have improved under the drug; all were quadriplegics and 9 were severely disabled. Six of 14 athetoids and 3 of 11 spastics improved. There was also some improvement in some instances in response to physical therapy and in articulation and attention span.

Henry O. Marsh. Diazepam in Incapacitated Cerebral-Palsied Children. J.A.M.A. 191:797, Mar. 8, 1965.

MYASTHENIA GRAVIS

"How is edrophonium (Tensilon) used in the diagnosis of myasthenia gravis?"

Reply: Use of edrophonium for diagnostic purpose in suspected myasthenia gravis results usually in a striking increase in muscle strength without fasciculation, whereas the same dosage is provocative of considerable fasciculation in a normal individual. The recommended dose is 2 mg. to be followed 30 seconds later by an additional 8 mg. if the first dose has not elicited a reaction.

Edrophonium should be used with extreme caution if at all in persons with cardiovascular disease or bronchial asthma because, while its action is predominantly specialized for exertion at myoneural junctions in skeletal musculature, there is some element of generalized cholinergic action also, and this may sometimes be manifested as bradycardia, arrhythmias, hypotension and bronchiolar spasm. Other occurrences of an expected type have also been seen: excessive perspiration and lacrimation, disturbances in visual accommodation, increased gastrointestinal motility, etc.

"How is neostigmine (Prostigmin) used in the diagnostic test for myasthenia gravis?"

Reply: The conventional dose here is 1.5 mg. intramuscularly, but 0.5 mg. intravenously may also be used to produce more rapid, clear-cut and complete improvement in even the mildest cases, thus enabling the observer to use objective diagnostic criteria alone. When the drug is given intravenously, 1 ml. of a 1 : 2000 solution of neostigmine methylsulfate (0.5 mg.) is injected during 1 minute. Improvement in a true case of myasthenia gravis often begins before the needle can be withdrawn and is usually maximal in 5 minutes at most. Performance tests given before administration of the drug should be repeated 5 minutes after its administration, and the degree of objective improvement reported, subjective improvement being disregarded. If the response is doubtful in a very mild case the test should be repeated on the following day with 1 mg. of the drug if there have been no untoward reactions to the 0.5 mg. dose. Atropine sulfate, 0.6 mg., should be at hand for subcutaneous injection whenever side effects become manifest, but it should never be injected with the neostigmine. Pronounced side effects from neostigmine almost disprove the diagnosis of myasthenia gravis.

"What is the present position of the cholinesterase inhibiting agents in the treatment of myasthenia gravis?"

Reply: Whether the myasthenic symptoms reflect the presence of cholinesterase in excessive amounts (which seems unlikely), or inadequate acetylcholine activation, or the presence of a curare-like toxic substance that opposes acetylcholine action (which seems not unlikely in view of the transient myasthenia seen at times in the newborn infant of a myasthenic mother), or whether there is actually anatomic abnormality of the myoneural junction and the muscle itself (for which there is tentative evidence), is not known. However, be the cause what it may, the cholinesterase inhibiting agents are definitely effective in combating the symptoms.

Neostigmine (Prostigmin) is the classic drug, oral administration sufficing in about

85% of instances. Average dosage is perhaps 1 or 2 of the 15 mg. tablets three to five times daily, but the treatment has to be highly individualized. Some patients can use the prolonged-action tablets quite effectively and are enabled thereby to avoid dosing during the night. In severe cases, neostigmine methylsulfate must be given hypodermically along with the oral dosage, and in crises it will be necessary to inject intravenously, perhaps in hourly doses. Bowman reported that intramuscular injection of 0.02 mg./kg. body weight effected improvement within 15 minutes in 3 cases of myasthenia in children 3–8 years of age. If there are annoying overactions, which is unusual, one must try to offset them with the belladonna drugs as used in parkinsonism. Note should be made of the three disadvantages that detract from the usefulness of Prostigmin. One is that it may occasionally be absorbed so rapidly from the gastrointestinal tract as to cause smooth muscle cramps and diarrhea; another is that in some instances the desired action at the skeletal muscle effector site becomes excessive and leads to muscle paralysis; and the third is that the use of atropine to counteract the excessive effects may, through this action, mask the warning signs of overdosage.

Pyridostigmine (Mestinon). According to Schwab, this compound, which is an analogue of neostigmine, has approximately an equivalent effect in 60 mg. dosage to that of neostigmine in 15 mg. dosage. It has the disadvantage of not causing the gastrointestinal discomfort with slight overdosage that characterizes neostigmine and serves as a warning; but some patients who cannot obtain relief from their myasthenic symptoms without intolerable gastrointestinal disturbance can satisfactorily substitute this new drug.

Ambenonium (Mytelase) resembles two molecules of neostigmine or of pyridostigmine, linked together in the middle. According to Schwab, ambenonium has a slightly longer period of action than either of the other two drugs and has less gastrointestinal effect on overdosage than neostigmine, but the action appears to be not quite so benign in this respect as that of pyridostigmine. Individual requirements of patients for this drug vary considerably, but perhaps 10 mg. is the average.

Some myasthenic patients learn to obtain best effects by "blending" the three drugs, with suitable dosage adjustments of each.

J. R. Bowman. Myasthenia Gravis in Young Children; Report of Three Cases—One Congenital. Pediatrics 1: 472, 1948. R. S. Schwab. The Pharmacologic Basis of the Treatment of Myasthenia Gravis. Clin. Pharmacol. & Therap. 1:319, 1960.

"I have a patient with myasthenia gravis in whom I have been able to maintain an amount of muscular power compatible with a practicable amount of activity in the extremities but there is persistent ocular weakness. What can be done in such a case?"

Reply: At the University of Michigan, Conrad Giles and Martha Westerberg used physostigmine (Eserine) locally with good effect in a fair proportion of their small number of cases. All 10 patients had ptosis, 7 had diplopia and 4 had blurring; 5 tolerated the drug and improved, 2 improved but did not tolerate the therapy. Neither age nor duration of the malady appeared to be of significance in prognosis. Physostigmine was used in 0.25% strength.

Conrad L. Giles and Martha R. Westerberg. Clinical Evaluation of Local Ocular Anticholinesterase Agents in Myasthenia Gravis. Am. J. Ophth. 52:331, 1961.

MYCOSES

"I have a patient with classical actinomycosis, involving the jaw principally, who has not responded to 1,000,000 units of penicillin daily as well as I thought she would. I hesitate to change the therapy but am wondering whether the addition of a sulfonamide would be advantageous?"

Reply: In 20 patients at the Charity Hospital in New Orleans, Seabury and Dascomb did not find it so, but they concluded that minimal penicillin dosage should be 1,000,000–2,000,000 units daily with a minimal duration of therapy of about 1 month. In fact, they felt that in extensive infections the daily dose should be larger and more prolonged. Penicillin sensitive patients were treated by them effectively with tetracyclines or erythromycin in the dose of about 2 Gm. daily.

John H. Seabury and Harry E. Dascomb (Louisiana State Univ.). Results of Treatment of Systemic Mycoses. J.A.M.A. 188:509, May 11, 1964.

"I have a patient with blastomycosis who has not responded as well as I thought he would on a course of hydroxystilbamidine totaling 5 Gm. Has my dosage been faulty or did I use the wrong drug?"

Reply: The right drug, yes, but perhaps the wrong dosage. At the Charity Hospital in New Orleans, where there is unusually rich opportunity to observe systemic mycotic infections, Seabury and Dascomb have found the minimal desirable total dose of hydroxystilbamidine in blastomycosis to be about 8 Gm. Four of the 20 patients relapsed after receiving 5.5 Gm. or an equivalent amount of stilbamidine. Dosage: intravenously 225 mg. daily for the first 21 days, repeating the therapy on an alternate day basis.

John H. Seabury and Harry E. Dascomb (Louisiana State Univ.). Results of Treatment of Systemic Mycoses. J.A.M.A. 188:509, May 11, 1964:

"Candida tropicalis is generally regarded as a nonpathogenic commensal organism, but I have an infant in whom systemic infection with the organism has induced very severe illness. What drug has been most effective?"

Reply: In such a case, Shurtleff and associates (University of Washington) used amphotericin B in the hope that its antifungal action would outweigh its nephrotoxicity. An initial dose of 0.75 mg./kg. was given intravenously and gradually increased to 1.5 mg./kg. The patient had had a blood urea nitrogen of 84 mg./100 ml., and this fell rapidly under treatment with the blood picture improving at the same time. The patient, who had been in coma, regained consciousness, and by the twelfth day of therapy the blood cultures were negative. Cerebrospinal fluid cultures became negative after an addition of intrathecal amphotericin therapy. Therapy was discontinued but had to be resumed, and it was stopped only after 6 weeks. Then it had to be reinstated when urine cultures became positive. After considerable outpatient treatment during a number of months, the situation was pretty well in hand at the end of the year.

David B. Shurtleff, Wilbur Peterson and John C. Sherris. Systemic Candida Tropicalis Infection Treated with Amphotericin. New England J. Med. 269:1112, Nov. 21, 1963.

"I have a case of coccidioidomycosis in my practice in which all of the involved areas appear to have cleared under amphotericin B therapy except for lesions on the palmar surface of one hand, which persist. Is there record of effective local therapy in a situation of this sort?"

Reply: In a bold maneuver in a case precisely like this, Fonkalsrud and associates (University of California Medical Center, Los Angeles) resorted to isolated perfusion of the arm much as in the treatment of a peripheral neoplasm. The extremity was perfused for 1 hour with heparinized blood and 30 mg. of amphotericin B. Subsequently there was slight edema of the arm, considerable erythema and hypersensitivity about the lesions and a transient low fever, but blood urea nitrogen did not become elevated. Several months after perfusion, biopsy showed scarring without spherules, and culture grew no organisms. The patient became and remained asymptomatic, but a residual coccidioidal infection continued to be manifested by a complement fixation titer of 1 : 256 about 1 year after perfusion.

Eric W. Fonkalsrud, Joyce Shiner, Robert Haan, Samuel A. Marable, Victor Newcomer and Donald B. Rochlin. Experimental Studies and Clinical Experience with Isolated Limb Perfusion of Fungicidal Drugs. Surg. Gynec. & Obst. 113:306, 1961.

"One of my associates is being charged with having induced the dissemination of a primary pulmonary coccidioidomycosis through administration of a corticosteroid to the patient. Is this a likely occurrence?"

Reply: In Phoenix, Arizona, Bernard Lipschultz and Howard Liston have seen 2 cases which they reported as "steroid-induced" disseminated coccidioidomycosis, but I felt that all their evidence was presumptive since both patients had chronic severe maladies—chronic lymphocytic leukemia in one instance and sarcoidosis in the other—and they were residents in an area in which disseminated coccidioidomycosis is a much more frequently encountered malady than in most other parts of the country.

Bernard M. Lipschultz and Howard E. Liston. Steroid-Induced Disseminated Coccidioidomycosis. Dis. Chest 46: 355, 1964.

"We have a lot of coccidioidomycosis in my part of the country and treatment with amphotericin B has not always yielded the results expected. Is there anything new in therapy?"

Reply: A thing of very considerable value that emerged from the study of Holeman and Einstein (Bakersfield, Calif.) was that the assumption of potassium deficiency can probably be safely made in all cases of disseminated coccidioidomycosis. Muscular cramps, weakness and insatiable appetite for fruits and fruit juices arouse the suspicion of hypokalemia. Evidences of nephrotoxicity are frequent when amphotericin B is being used, but in the 6 patients of Holeman and Einstein who died, all of whom showed renal tubule damage, none died in renal failure.

Charles W. Holeman, Jr., and Hans Einstein. Toxic Effects of Amphotericin B in Man. California Med. 99:90, 1963.

"We have just diagnosed a case of pulmonary cryptococcosis in an asymptomatic patient. Should we treat this case with amphotericin B?"

Reply: At the Mayo Clinic, Joseph Geraci and associates decided that patients with focal or localized nonprogressive nodular lesions without pulmonary or systemic symptoms or positive cultures, and those with indeterminate and doubtful infections, are not to be treated. But patients who require amphotericin B therapy should receive at least 1.5–2.5 Gm. over 1–2 months.

Joseph E. Geraci, F. Edmund Donoghue, F. Henry Ellis, Jr., David M. Witten and Lyle A. Weed. Focal Pulmonary Cryptococcosis: Evaluation of Necessity of Amphotericin B Therapy. Mayo Clin. Proc. 40:552, 1965.

"What shall I do in a case of meningeal cryptococcosis when intravenous and intrathecal amphotericin B therapy has failed?"

Reply: At Johns Hopkins Hospital, Kress and Cantrell performed bilateral occipital trephines and injected 5 mg. of amphotericin B into the left lateral cerebral ventricle. The course thereafter was certainly stormy, but the patient, who was 45 years old, eventually came out of the episode pretty well. At the Bowman Gray School of Medicine, Siewers and Cramblett obtained a remarkable result in this disease with 2 years of sulfadiazine therapy in a child of 2 years at the beginning of the treatment. Besides blood transfusions because of anemia, and gamma globulin injections for the prevention of rubeola, the child did not receive any other medication of specific anti-infective nature.

Milton B. Kress and James R. Cantrell. Pulmonary and Meningeal Cryptococcosis: Successful Treatment of Meningitis with Lateral Cerebral Intraventricular Injection of Amphotericin B. Arch. Int. Med. 112:386, 1963. C. M. F. Siewers and Henry G. Cramblett. Cryptococcosis (Torulosis) in Children: Report of Four Cases. Pediatrics 34:393, 1964.

"I have a patient with histoplasmosis who tolerates amphotericin B very badly. What shall I do?"

Reply: John P. Utz, Chief of the Infectious Disease Service at the Clinical Center of the National Institutes of Health, has made the authoritative statement that the use of amphotericin B should be persisted in when life is threatened, unless the patient absolutely refuses to continue treatment, because the alternative (resort to a sulfonamide) will be of value only occasionally.

John P. Utz. Systemic Fungal Infections Amenable to Chemotherapy. Disease-A-Month, Sept. 1963, p. 22.

"A diabetic patient in our practice developed a fulminating mucormycosis (phycomycosis) cellulitis involving the nasal, oral and orbital tissues that was unresponsive to any of the familiar antibiotics and quickly led to a fatal termination. Is there any drug that might have been helpful in this fortunately rare infection?"

Reply: J. D. Mc. Gass reported 2 cases a few years ago in which amphotericin B appeared to effect cure, and there have been a few single case reports of the same sort.

J. D. Mc. Gass. Acute Orbital Mucormycosis: Report of Two Cases. Arch. Ophth. 65:214, 1961.

"I have a case of nocardiosis (diagnosed only through having asked the pathologist particularly to look for nocardia) that has responded dramatically to sulfadiazine therapy after a number of antibiotics had failed to be effective. Is this unusual?"

Reply: It certainly is, but in Australia, G. V. Hall has reported just such a case. You are to be congratulated on having made the diagnosis, because this organism grows more slowly than many, and culture plates are sometimes discarded after 48 hours.

G. V. Hall. Case of Pulmonary Nocardiosis with Apparent Cure with Sulfadiazine. M. J. Australia 2:455, Sept. 19, 1964.

"I have a patient in whom the diagnosis of pulmonary aspergilloma has been made, but in a review of the limited literature available to me I have been unable to find record of well-established efficacy for any remedial agent. Can you suggest anything?"

Reply: I believe it is the consensus that treatment is unnecessary in an asymptomatic patient without hemoptysis, since most of these lesions remain stable for many years. However, it is sometimes considered necessary to eliminate the lesion by pulmonary resection. A few years ago, J. P. Utz and associates reported that in 2 cases they had cleared *Aspergillus* from sputum and lung tissue or abscess drainage material following large doses of potassium iodide, but in a patient of Hideo Ikemoto, in Tokyo, such dosage induced fever, anorexia and hemoptysis. However, in this patient of Ikemoto's, intrabronchial instillation of amphotericin B (Fungizone) was associated with expectoration of many fragments of fungus ball, the fungus ball subsequently disappearing almost completely on the chest roentgenograms.

Hideo Ikemoto. Treatment of Pulmonary Aspergilloma with Amphotericin B. Arch. Int. Med. 115:598, 1965. J. P. Utz and associates. Pulmonary Aspergillosis with Cavitation: Iodide Therapy Associated with Unusual Electrolyte Disturbance. New England J. Med. 260:264, 1959.

"I have been using rather high dosage of potassium iodide in a pregnant woman with sporotrichosis, and now one of my associates has asked whether I do not fear an adverse effect on the infant. Should I?"

Reply: Many years ago, on orders from the Attending in a hospital where I was interning, I gave quite enormous doses of sodium iodide daily for several months to a young pregnant woman with actinomycosis, without damage to either mother or infant; but that single experience proves nothing, for there have been instances of goiter in the newborn as a result of iodide therapy in the mother during pregnancy. Galina's group, in New York, for instance, has reported two neonatal deaths with large goiters when the mothers had taken 234 Gm. and 324 Gm., respectively, of potassium iodide during their pregnancies. Much iodide is taken in the form of proprietary asthma mixtures, whose use should probably be forbidden during pregnancy.

Morton P. Galina, Norman L. Avnet and Arnold Einhorn. Iodides During Pregnancy: Apparent Cause of Neonatal Death. New England J. Med. 267:1124, Nov. 29, 1962.

"What is the preferred antibiotic nowadays in the treatment of oral candidiasis (thrush)?"

Reply: Nystatin (Mycostatin) is used in the form of a suspension of 100,000 units/ml. In infants, 1 ml. of this is given to be swallowed four times daily; the adult sloshes a teaspoonful of the suspension around in the mouth before swallowing it, also four times daily.

"I have a patient who is asymptomatic but has bilateral pulmonary infiltrates, and C. neoformans can be grown from the sputum and bronchial aspirate cultures. He has no fever, night sweats, hemoptysis or cough, and he is well developed, well nourished and shows no evidence of weight loss. There is no hepatomegaly, splenomegaly or lymphadenopathy. Should this patient be treated with amphotericin B?"

Reply: I should not like to risk a categorical "no" at this time, but I can direct your attention to the report of Houk and Moser, at the U.S. Naval Hospital, in Bethesda, of 6 patients with pulmonary cryptococcosis in whom the drug was not used. All have remained well and asymptomatic, 2 of the patients having been followed up in excess of 10 years, 2 in excess of 6 years. The experience of these observers, coupled with the increasing recognition of the pulmonary form of the disease, suggests that routine administration of amphotericin B may not be necessary in cases that offer the characteristics of your case. There are reasons to suspect that pulmonary involvement occurs much more frequently in this malady than the literature suggests; indeed Littman and Zimmerman have estimated that between 5000 and 15,000 cases of subclinical or clinical pulmonary cryptococcosis exist each year in New York City alone.

V. N. Houk and K. M. Moser. Pulmonary Cryptococcosis: Must All Receive Amphotericin B? Ann. Int. Med. 63: 583, 1965. M. L. Littman and L. E. Zimmerman. Cryptococcus neoformans in Pigeon Excretion in New York City. Am. J. Hyg. 69:49, 1959.

"Are any of the newer drugs superior to potassium iodide in the therapy of sporotrichosis?"

Reply: No, it is still the drug of choice, used in a saturated solution of 1 Gr./ml. Initial dosage, according to John Utz, at the University of Virginia, is 1 ml. three times daily. This dose is increased by daily increments of 0.5–1.0 ml. until 9–12 ml. is reached; therapy should then be continued for 2 weeks after all lesions appear to have healed. Acneiform skin eruptions, lacrimation, swelling of the parotid glands, nausea and vomiting are usually easily controlled by stopping the drug for a few days and resuming administration at a somewhat lower dosage.

John P. Utz. Antimicrobial Therapy in Systemic Fungal Infections. Am. J. Med. 39:826, 1965.

MYELOFIBROSIS

"I have a patient with myelofibrosis with myeloid metaplasia, in whom I have used busulfan (Myleran) without satisfaction. Is there any other drug worth trying?"

Reply: Yes, Silver and associates (New York Hospital–Cornell Medical Center) obtained a good response with testosterone in 5 of 10 cases. Erythrocyte, platelet and leukocyte production were all increased, but there was no consistent increase in size of the liver or spleen, and biopsy findings from the posterior iliac crest revealed no consistent increase in hematopoiesis. Dosage of testosterone enanthate: 600 mg. intramuscularly weekly, reducing gradually over several months if possible.

Richard T. Silver, David E. Jenkins, Jr., and Ralph L. Engle, Jr. Use of Testosterone (Delatestryl) and Busulfan (Myleran) in Treatment of Myelofibrosis with Myeloid Metaplasia. Blood 23:341, 1964.

NARCOLEPSY

"What is the best drug to use in combating narcolepsy?"

Reply: The following drugs are used, but I do not know which of them is "best" because no thorough comparative study has been performed: methylphenidate (Ritalin) is used in oral dosage of 10 mg. two or three times daily, usually half an hour before meals (sometimes twice this dosage is required for effect); methamphetamine (Desoxyn, Methedrine) dosage begins with 2.5 mg. two or three times daily, building up slowly (the long-acting preparation, Desoxyn Gradumet, may be given in one dose in the morning with fair expectation that the effect will last all day; beginning dosage 5 or 10 mg.); dextroamphetamine (Dexedrine), dosage ranging from 5 to 30 mg. one or more times daily. Full effectiveness of these drugs may not be developed under several days or even weeks; do not be too quickly discouraged.

NEWBORN

"Are the new synthetic penicillins effective in preventing staphylococci from becoming established in the newborn?"

Reply: This matter was studied by Russell Shaw's group, at the University of Oklahoma, using methicillin (Dimocillin-RT) and oxacillin (Prostaphlin, Resistopen). In their hands the drugs appeared to be effective in preventing establishment of staphylococci but not effective in eradicating staphylococcal nasal colonization once the organisms had become nasopharyngeal residents. The important question of course is whether staphylococcic colonization in newborns is harmful. The investigators' evidence suggested that such colonization is not harmful in nonepidemic situations if the predominant strains are coagulase negative or of low virulence. But if the predominant strains of staphylococcus in the nursery are virulent, and have been demonstrated to produce disease, they proposed the institution of vigorous measures to prevent infants from being colonized.

Russell F. Shaw, Harris D. Riley, Jr., and E. C. Bracken. Influence of Prophylactic Methicillin (Dimocillin-RT) and Oxacillin (Prostaphlin, Resistopen) in Prevention of Staphylococcic Colonization and Subsequent Clinical Infection in Newborn Infants. Clin. Pharmacol. & Therap. 6:492, 1965.

"Is there any drug approaching specific value in the treatment of neonatal idiopathic respiratory distress syndrome?"

Reply: In treating 25 newborns with this malady, Eugene Diamond and Vernon DeYoung used oxygen, water mists, usually with Alevaire, and prophylactic antibiotics. Five of the infants were digitalized and 12 were also given chlorpromazine (Thorazine) through a nasogastric tube—2 mg. as 1 ml. syrup of Thorazine hourly. Of 10 patients treated without chlorpromazine, only 2 lived; of 15 in whom the drug was used, 13 lived.

Eugene F. Diamond (Loyola Univ., Chicago) and Vernon R. DeYoung (Univ. of Ill.). Treatment of Neonatal Idiopathic Respiratory Distress Syndrome with Chlorpromazine (Thorazine). Illinois M. J. 124:538, 1963.

"What is the present status of vitamin K in the prophylaxis of bleeding in the newborn infant?"

Reply: In olden times the incidence of hemorrhagic disease of the newborn was apparently much greater than presently, probably due at least in part to sepsis and trauma. But the syndrome still exists and has not yet been satisfactorily explained, though low levels of prothrombin and stable factor (proconvertin) have been demonstrated, and it is these levels that can be corrected by administration of vitamin K. However, because excessively high dosage of the vitamin has been associated with an increased incidence of hemolytic anemia, hyperbilirubinemia and kernicterus, routine use of the preparation (Hykinone is usually employed) is discouraged by some authorities. But in some hospitals abandonment of the measure has appeared to be responsible for a considerable increase in massive neonatal hemorrhage in the newborn. Such an occurrence at the Parkland Memorial Hospital, Dallas, caused Vietti and associates to investigate the matter. They gave 5 mg. intramuscularly of Hykinone to newborn boys and circumcised them at a mean age of slightly over 24 hours, the total number of patients being 470. Secondary bleeding occurred in 2.5% of those receiving the vitamin and 13.9% of those who did not. Their conclusion was that 1 or 2 mg. of vitamin K soon after delivery will involve a risk of hemolytic anemia and kernicterus that is negligible, while this small dose will be more than sufficient to correct the low prothrombin and proconvertin levels secondary to vitamin K deficiency.

T. J. Vietti, T. P. Murphy, J. A. James and J. A. Pritchard. Observations on Prophylactic Use of Vitamin K in Newborn Infant. J. Pediat. 56:343, 1960.

"To what extent is the newborn of a diabetic mother at greater risk of early death and is there any commendable safeguarding procedure that might be followed?"

Reply: Insulin has not effected a significant reduction in mortality of the newborn of diabetic women. Even under most favorable conditions the risk to the infant is about four times that of the normal, about eight times if the mother has severe complications of pregnancy. The excessive size of the child, or the mother's hyperglycemia, is not an entirely satisfactory explanation for this increased mortality. Some observers have found that such infants may have cardiac hypertrophy and excessive erythropoiesis in the liver, with large numbers of nucleated red blood cells in the peripheral blood during the first days of life. Sometimes these changes are associated with hyperplasia of the islets of Langerhans. Since the blood sugar level may drop to a very low point within an hour after birth, it is the practice of some men to place 10 drops of 50% glucose solution in the back of the baby's mouth with a medicine dropper as soon as it is born, and to repeat this at 30 minute intervals for five doses. Thereafter, 15–30 ml. of glucose solution is given every 2 hours, alternating with the same amount of breast milk. The first 8 hours are believed to be crucial.

"There was a great deal of talk some years ago about the narcotic antagonists in addiction of the newborn. What are the members of this group, and have they found a secure place in practice?"

Reply: The specific narcotic antagonists have indeed been shown to be very useful in combating respiratory depression from overdosage of narcotics and for the prevention of narcotic-induced respiratory depression of the newborn. The two presently available agents are nalorphine (Nalline) and levallorphan (Lorfan). An additional use of these drugs, of a different sort, is in the diagnosis of narcotic addiction. Initial dosage for the treatment of narcotic-induced respiratory depression is 5–15 mg. (100–150 μg./kg.) for nalorphine and 1–2 mg. (20 μg./kg.) for levallorphan. Initial dosage for the diagnosis of narcotic addiction is 1–3 mg., to be followed when necessary by a 3–5 mg. dose and a 5–8 mg. dose at 20 minute intervals. In treating narcotic-induced respiratory depression of the newborn, nalorphine should be given in dosage of 0.2–0.5 mg., or levallorphan in dosage of 0.05–0.1 mg., diluted to 2 ml. with 0.9% saline and injected into the umbilical vein. One-half the initial dosage may be given 5–10 minutes later if the first dose was only partially effective. When injection into the umbilical vein is not feasible intramuscular injection may be made, with or without hyaluronidase (Wydase, etc.), at the upper limit of the recommended umbilical vein dosage.

Francis F. Foldes. The Human Pharmacology and Clinical Use of Narcotic Antagonists. M. Clin. North America 48:421, 1964.

NOSOCOMIAL INFECTIONS

"In our hospital, which is an old municipal institution with open wards housing 30–45 patients, we have long ago given up the administration of antibiotics to patients who do not have convincing evidence of bacterial disease, but when there is acute pulmonary infection or acute exacerbation of chronic pulmonary inflammatory disease, our tendency is to give high dosage of antibacterials in order to prevent spread of these infections. Are we not perhaps inviting superinfection in this way?"

Reply: A definitely positive answer to this question was supplied under similar circumstances at Bellevue Hospital, where Donald Louria and Theresa Kaminski placed patients with such infections on one of four regimens: intramuscular aqueous or procaine penicillin G, 1,200,000–2,400,000 units daily; tetracycline or chloramphenicol, 2 Gm. daily by mouth; penicillin, 1,200,000–2,400,000 units daily, plus streptomycin, 1.5–2.0 Gm. daily intramuscularly; or penicillin, 1,200,000–2,400,000 units daily, plus either tetracycline or chloramphenicol, 2 Gm. per day. The drugs were given for a minimum of 5 days. With penicillin alone, the superinfection rate was 0; 5.4% with tetracycline or chloramphenicol; 19.4% with penicillin plus streptomycin; and 47% with penicillin plus either tetracycline or chloramphenicol. The superinfections appeared solely ascribable to excessive amounts or combinations of the antibiotics that were used; they were not related to sex, age, severity of illness, the presence of underlying disease, or any combination of these factors.

Donald B. Louria and Theresa Kaminski. Effects of Four Antimicrobial Drug Regimens on Sputum Superinfection in Hospitalized Patients. Am. Rev. Resp. Dis. 85:649, 1962.

"Our laboratory people are beginning to tell us that bacteria of the tribe Mimeae are appearing as opportunistic pathogens in hospitalized patients. With what agents can we best hope to combat these nosocomial infections?"

Reply: In Houston, Green and associates studied the matter and found sodium colistimethate (Coly-Mycin Injectable), kanamycin (Kantrex), methenamine mandelate (Mandelamine) and polymyxin B (Aerosporin) to be the most effective therapeutic agents.

G. Sheldon Green, Robert H. Johnson, Jr., and John A. Shively. Mimeae: Opportunistic Pathogens. J.A.M.A. 194:1065, Dec. 6, 1965.

"Has the frequency of hospital-acquired staphylococcic infections decreased and those caused by gram-negative bacilli correspondingly increased since the introduction of penicillinase-resistant penicillins?"

Reply: This does not seem to be precisely what was found by Maxwell Finland's group at the Boston City Hospital. Their survey of the matter in early 1964 indicated that the staphylococcus remained the single most important organism in hospital infection, as it had been shown to be in their study in early 1956, but in 1964 it may be equaled or exceeded numerically by the gram-negative bacilli. However, in some areas, and in some hospitals, the incidence and severity of hospital-acquired staphylococcic infections appears to have declined since its peak in the 1955–57 period. In Seattle, Alfred Bauer ascribes this decline to improvement in hospital housekeeping procedures, work of hospital infection committees in the epidemiologic field, more cautious use of older antibiotics by many practitioners, and the development of other powerful bactericidal antibiotics. And it is of interest that the incidence of staphylococcic resistance does not seem to be increasing outside of hospitals. At least, Bauer was able to show the highest incidence at King County Hospital in his city (Seattle), somewhat lower incidence at University Hospital, and much lower in outside practice at a Group Health Clinic. The two hospitals showed both susceptible and resistant strains, but the Group Health Clinic strains included no such mutants. At least this was true for tests with chloramphenicol, kanamycin and vancomycin, but of 128 strains tested with oxacillin at the Group Health Clinic, 2 were highly resistant, being resistant also to penicillin G though sensitive to all other routinely used antibiotics and to sulfonamides.

It is a very striking fact that vancomycin-resistant staphylococci do not seem to exist although this drug has been in use for at least 7 years.

Jay Ward Kislak, Theodore C. Eickhoff and Maxwell Finland. Hospital-Acquired Infections and Antibiotic Usage in the Boston City Hospital—January, 1964. New England J. Med. 271:834, Oct. 15, 1964. Alfred W. Bauer. Staphylococcic Resistance to Antibiotics: Observations at Two Hospitals and an Independent Clinic. Northwest Med. 64:247, 1965.

"Six days ago a burned patient brought in from another hospital was admitted with a staphylococcus strain that proved to be resistant to penicillin, streptomycin, tetracyclines, kanamycin and neomycin. Today the patient was sent into isolation. What can we expect?"

Reply: Unfortunately nothing very pleasing. In a similar situation in an Australian hospital, Phyllis Rountree and Mary Beard found that on the same day that their patient was isolated the resistant organism, which had not been present in the hospital previously, was isolated from the surgical wound of another patient who had been in the same ward. The infection then spread in succeeding months, and 136 patients experienced sepsis and 67 nasal carriers were detected.

Phyllis M. Rountree and Mary A. Beard. Spread of Neomycin-Resistant Staphylococci in Hospital. M. J. Australia 1:498, Apr. 3, 1965.

OBESITY

"In my limited experience it has seemed that the anorexigenic drugs are without effect in obesity if the patient is taking one of the phenothiazine antipsychotic drugs at the same time. Has this been the experience of others?"

Reply: You pose a question of the sort that is certainly going to arise with increasing frequency as time goes on, for we are now putting all sorts of potent agents into patients without really knowing what effect one drug may have on the other when they are used concomitantly. The specific situation with which you are concerned has been studied by Reid, in Melbourne, who found some evidence indicating that chlorpromazine (Thorazine) does actually block or antagonize the action of phenmetrazine (Preludin), possibly at the hypothalamic level. The mean weight losses for his 10 patients on chlorpromazine and phenmetrazine were 1.03 lb. in 4 weeks; for 12 on chlorpromazine and placebo, 1.7 lb.; for 28 on phenmetrazine alone, 3.43 lb.; and for 26 on placebo alone, 1.15 lb.

A. Arnaud Reid (Plenty Hospital, Melbourne). Pharmacologic Antagonism Between Chlorpromazine and Phenmetrazine in Mental Hospital Patients. M. J. Australia 1:187, Feb. 8, 1964.

"Has a double-blind controlled comparison of the principal anorexiants available nowadays been made by which we may be guided in use of these agents in treating obesity?"

Reply: Not of such nature as to provide a drug of choice in all cases, which is probably what you would like. It is very difficult to make accurate drug comparisons in obesity because individuals vary so much in their attitude toward fatness as well as in the sincerity with which they enter the study. And unless a large group of patients could be brought under segregated conditions with the closest possible surveillance, there would be no way to know how much food is actually consumed. Not all fat people are strictly honest in recording their food consumption, as all of us know. I should say that we are fortunate in having a fairly large number of anorexiants nowadays, not only because we can switch about among them for psychologic reasons, but because we are able to make changes when tolerance to any member of the group appears to be developing.

"I rarely succeed in significantly reducing weight in the long-term treatment of an obese patient. Are there any concomitant signs or symptoms, or any individual characteristics, in fat people that would indicate which one of them will be most likely to be reducible?"

Reply: I think not. At least in the thorough study of Berkowitz and Beck (Hahnemann Medical College), failure or success of a reducing program was found independent of age, sex, duration of obesity, family history, hypertension, carbohydrate metabolism or cholesterol levels. They found the three factors important for failure to be lack of motivation, lack of intelligence and a severe emotional overlay. The emotionally disturbed individuals were severely handicapped by the fact that their headache, nervousness, irritability, dizziness and depression were relieved only by the ingestion of food.

Donald Berkowitz and Nathaniel Beck. Long Term Management of Obesity in Union Health Center: Analysis of Successes and Failures. J.A.M.A. 172:1381, Mar. 26, 1960.

"I always have difficulty in taking weight off a patient whose obesity makes him a relatively bad risk for surgery. Is there anything that is more effective in this situation than the usual anorexigenic drugs?"

Reply: A few years ago Phillip Lebon, in London, reported the treatment of 63 overweight patients with chorionic gonadotropin and a low calorie diet: 125 units chorionic gonadotropin (Antuitrin-S) once daily by deep intragluteal injection, and a 500 calorie, fat-free high-protein diet. The mean weight loss of 44 patients treated for 40 days was 25 pounds; excluding 6 who did not cooperate well the mean weight loss was 28 pounds. In 21 consecutive days of the therapy the average weight loss was 16 pounds in 19 patients. Lebon said that none of the patients felt hungry or weak during treatment or had difficulty carrying out normal activities – which made them quite exceptional individuals, I should say!

Phillip Lebon. Treatment of Overweight Patients with Chorionic Gonadotropin. J. Am. Geriatrics Soc. 9:998, 1961.

"What are the chances of success with anorexigenic drugs in obese psychiatric patients?"

Reply: At the Graylingwell Hospital, in England, L. R. C. Haward found both dietary and drug regimens generally unsatisfactory when applied in isolation from psychological aspects of treatment. Two controlled trials with anorexigenic drugs and placebo on matched samples of 15 obese patients yielded no significant effect except for a trend in the experimental group to increase weight while taking the drugs. He explains the failure partially on the basis of the assumption that in the psychiatric obese patient food is taken for its oral as well as its alimentary satisfaction. I did not find Haward's study entirely

satisfactory because from a psychiatric population that was generally overweight he chose the 15 heaviest individuals, which seems to me unfortunate because everyone knows that the grossly overweight individual in any population is the most difficult to reduce.

L. R. C. Haward. The Inadequacy of Anorexigenic Drugs in the Treatment of Obese Psychiatric Patients. Psychiat. et Neurol. 149:129, 1965.

"We have recently had in our practice a young woman who put herself into a stuporous state through excessive ingestion of ammonium chloride in a 'slimming' attempt. We got her out of it all right, but now are wondering in what type of person ordinary dosage of the drug might be dangerous?"

Reply: The drug should probably be used cautiously in a patient with cardiac failure presenting cerebral manifestations or in one with severe liver impairment. It is very likely to be dangerous, too, in elderly individuals in whom the kidneys are unable to excrete maximally acid urine and produce ammonia. Ammonium chloride poisoning may be differentiated from the low salt hyponatremia syndrome by the high level of plasma chlorides, reflecting increased chloride reabsorption and excessive water loss.

Arnold S. Relman, Palmer F. Shelburne and Armistead Talman (Boston). Profound Acidosis from Excessive Ammonium Chloride in Previously Healthy Subjects: Study of Two Cases. New England J. Med. 264:848, Apr. 27, 1961.

"Some wonderfully colorful advertising is being done nowadays for chlorphentermine (Pre-Sate, Lucofen) in the treatment of obesity. Is the drug really superior?"

Reply: I do not know, because any drug will have an uphill road in this malady and it will take a long time to determine whether patients are going faithfully to stick to its use and get a better effect than with earlier drugs. However, I can cite one study, that of Seaton's group in Edinburgh, that may possibly indicate how the wind is going to blow. In this study the patients were divided into two comparable groups by matching them in pairs according to age, weight and degree of overweight. The active tablets were 75 mg. chlorphentermine in sustained-release form, and the placebo tablets contained lactose and other inactive ingredients. The instruction was to take 1 tablet daily with breakfast. There were 3 defaulters from the study, 19 who received placebos and 20 who received the active drug. The mean loss of the placebo group was 0.42 pounds (191 Gm.) at the end of 12 weeks; 10 patients had lost and 9 had gained weight. The mean weight loss of the patients who had received the active drug was 3.5 pounds (1.6 kg.) after 12 weeks; 13 had lost and 6 had gained weight and 1 was unchanged. Tolerance to the anorexiant effect was said to have developed after an average of 6 weeks' treatment. Summarized, therefore, from the practical standpoint one can say that half as many patients gained as lost weight on the drug, and that this does not differ greatly from what is accomplished with other agents in the appetite-suppressant group. More study is needed, however.

D. A. Seaton, Kathleen Rose and L. J. P. Duncan. Sustained-Action Chlorphentermine in Correction of Refractory Obesity. Practitioner 193:698, 1964.

OBSTRUCTIVE BRONCHIOLITIS

"Sometimes, even though one puts infants with obstructive bronchiolitis in an oxygen-enriched humid atmosphere and gives an antibiotic to limit bacterial infection, they die very quickly and are found at necropsy to have the principal lesion in the bronchioles and peribronchiolar tissue rather than in the alveoli. To a recent infant with only a relatively mild obstruction I gave 400 mg. of hydrocortisone during a period of 16 hours. The signs of obstruction disappeared, but I really do not know whether this was mere coincidence or whether the therapy had true rationale?"

Reply: Murray McGeorge (Dunedin, N.Z., Hospital) did this sort of thing in a group of 26 infants, with practically uniformly good effects, 9 of the patients being in serious condition when admitted. How is one to explain all of the actions of the corticosteroids? Probably in the present instances hydrocortisone would reduce the acute inflammatory reaction in the bronchioles and thus indirectly decrease pulmonary vascular resistance. Febrile, debilitated infants are sometimes helped by a broad-spectrum antibiotic. Bronchodilators, antihistamines, expectorants and sedatives are not effective, exception being the occasional favorable response to an injection of epinephrine.

Murray McGeorge. Severe Obstructive Bronchiolitis in Infancy: Treatment with Hydrocortisone. Clin. Pediat. 3:11, 1964.

OPHTHALMOLOGY

"I have heard that pretty good results can be achieved with corticosteroids in the treatment of inflammatory diseases of the anterior segment of the eye, but this has not been precisely my experience. What could be at fault?"

Reply: I think it is conceded that the corticosteroids are more strikingly effective in acute than in chronic diseases of the anterior segment of the eye. In the experience of Robert Coles and associates (New York University Medical Center), patients with scleritis, episcleritis and keratitis appeared to benefit particularly from the therapy. They used an injection of 0.5 ml. Depo-Medrol (20 mg.), usually injecting into the upper temporal quadrant of the globe, 10–14 mm. from the limbus, after topical anesthesia with tetracaine.

Robert S. Coles, David L. Krohn, Harvey Breslin and Richard Braunstein. Depo-Medrol in Treatment of Inflammatory Diseases of Anterior Segment of the Eye. Am. J. Ophth. 54:407, 1962.

"I have a patient with accommodative esotropia in whom an iris cyst has formed as a complication of echothiophate iodide (Phospholine) therapy. Is there any way to avoid this?"

Reply: N. B. Chin's group of 20 patients were treated in one eye with 0.125% echothiophate iodide and in the other eye with phenylephrine, 10%, 5%, or 2.5%, together with the echothiophate iodide. None of the eyes protected with phenylephrine in any strength developed cysts, but 11 patients developed them after 7–42 days of medication with the echothiophate iodide alone.

N. B. Chin, A. A. Gold and G. B. Breinin. Iris Cysts and Miotics. Arch. Ophth. 71:611, 1964.

"We have found echothiophate iodide (Phospholine) quite effective in the majority of a small group of cases of accommodative esotropia, but not at all in nonaccommodative cases. Has this been the usual experience, and how well is the drug tolerated over a long period?"

Reply: As for the failures in nonaccommodative cases, this agrees with the experience of Abrahamson and Abrahamson, in Cincinnati. As for toleration, the drug was borne very well by their 40 patients, 13 of whom were treated for 6–11 months, 24 for 3–5 months, and 3 for less than 3 months: iris cysts or floccules occurred in three instances, blurred vision in five and a burning sensation for several seconds in four.

Ira A. Abrahamson, Jr., and Ira A. Abrahamson, Sr. Preliminary Report on 0.06% Phospholine (Echothiophate) Iodide in Management of Esotropia. Am. J. Ophth. 57:290, 1964.

"Since the introduction of alpha chymotrypsin in cataract extraction, in 1958, many opinions have been expressed, pro and con, regarding its clinical merit. There appears to be agreement that the zonule is digested and extraction of the lens facilitated, but uncertainty appears to exist as to the residual effects of the measure. Can you cite authoritative opinion?"

Reply: The conclusion of Harold Scheie's group, based on the experience of 3½ years and more than 1200 operations for senile cataract at the Hospital of the University of Pennsylvania, was that the advantages of the therapy greatly outweigh the disadvantages. Shortly after they instituted this therapy, the impression of greater postoperative reaction was gained, though no permanent ill effects resulted. They then studied various dilutions and settled upon 1 : 10,000 solution for routine employment, though occasionally employing 1 : 5000 in individuals under 40 years of age to be certain of maximal effect. These investigators concluded that alpha chymotrypsin is contraindicated when vitreous pressure is high and the incision gaping, for in such eyes, when the zonule is dissolved, support for the lens is lost and there is a great tendency to vitreous loss. They agreed also with the widely held opinion that alpha chymotrypsin should not be used for congenital cataracts, and they avoid its use in patients under 30 years of age. In the latter, even though the zonule may be digested, the ligamentum hyloidea capsulare remains firmly attached to the lens and vitreous is pulled out and lost as the lens is delivered. They found that this can also occur in the 30–40-year-old group and occasionally even in an older individual. No difficulty was noted with wound healing or corneal haze in this series of patients.

At the Massachusetts Eye and Ear Infirmary, Vicente Jocson concluded from study of the matter of aqueous outflow in 16 patients in whom applanation tonometry, tonography and gonioscopy were performed before and 2–4 months after cataracts were extracted with the use of 1 : 5000 alpha chymotrypsin intraocularly, that the drug had no tendency to cause either a persisting detrimental effect or a persisting beneficial effect on the channels for aqueous outflow, either in cataractous normal eyes or in cataractous glaucomatous eyes. However, in Miami, Ralph Kirsch has been studying a transient, often severe, open-angle glaucoma that he and others find occurring in the majority of cases after extraction with alpha chymotrypsin.

Vicente L. Jocson. Tonography and Gonioscopy. Before and After Cataract Extraction with Alpha Chymotrypsin. Am. J. Ophth. 60:318, 1965. Harold G. Scheie, David L. Edwards, Jr., and Myron Yanoff. Clinical and Experimental Observations Using Alpha Chymotrypsin. Am. J. Ophth. 59:469, 1965. Ralph E. Kirsch. Further Studies on Glaucoma Following Cataract Extraction Associated with the Use of Alpha Chymotrypsin. Tr. Am. Acad. Ophth. & Otolaryng., Nov.-Dec., 1965, p. 1011.

"I have had very little success in the treatment of fungous corneal ulcers. What is currently giving the best results?"

Reply: At Duke University, Banks Anderson and Ernest Chick used amphotericin B (Fungizone) and felt it the best available antifungous agent but that the best is still none too good. The intravenous preparation of the drug was dissolved in water or suspended in saline in the usual concentration of 1 mg./ml. but sometimes up to as high as 4 mg./ml.; the solution was refrigerated and used for 1–2 weeks. Initial application was at the rate of 1 drop hourly, but this was lengthened as improvement occurred, and treatment was continued for several weeks after there was re-epithelization. These investigators found that biweekly scrapings under topical anesthesia of the unepithelized central portion of the ulcer was helpful in some instances.

Banks Anderson, Jr., and Ernest W. Chick. Mycokeratitis: Treatment of Fungous Corneal Ulcers with Amphotericin B and Mechanical Debridement. South. M. J. 56:270, 1963.

"Is there any danger connected with the use of corticosteroids topically for an inflammatory or allergic condition of the lids, conjunctiva, cornea or anterior segment of the eye?"

Reply: Yes, there is. These topical steroids may produce a state similar to primary open-angle glaucoma, which, in its early stages, is symptom free and without changes in the optic disc or visual field. This steroid-induced glaucoma is somewhat more resistant to therapy than chronic simple glaucoma. And of course the corticosteroids should be used only with the greatest caution in primary open-angle glaucoma or when there is the suspicion of glaucoma or a family history of the malady. If the drugs must be used, one should be on the alert to control the intraocular pressure with miotics, epinephrine or carbonic anhydrase inhibitors.

Bernard Becker and Donald W. Mills (Washington University). Elevated Intraocular Pressure Following Corticosteroid Eye Drops. J.A.M.A. 185:884, Sept. 14, 1963.

"Although cyclitis is of unknown etiology and follows a progressive course and so far seems to by uninfluenced appreciably by any form of treatment, one cannot nevertheless give up trying to accomplish something in these cases. Is any new therapy available?"

Reply: The only thing that has come to my attention that appears to be worthy of note is the trial of methotrexate (Amethopterin) by Vernon Wong and Evan Hersh in 6 cases at the National Institute of Neurological Diseases and Blindness. After studying the bone marrow and creatinine clearance, a test dose of 25 mg. of methotrexate was given and the patient observed for 1 week. If no excessive clinical or hemotologic sensitivity to the drug occurred, it was then injected intravenously every 4 days for 6 weeks in dosage of 25 mg./M². of body surface area. The drug was dissolved in 10 ml. of water and delivered slowly (1–2 minutes) through the tubing of a 5% dextrose in water infusion. All 6 patients showed improvement, anterior chamber activity decreasing within 1 week and the chamber appearing to be normal a week later. In 2½–3 weeks there was some regression of the peripheral lesions in the fundus; exudative changes flattened and decreased in size, and adjacent vitreous opacities as well as the cellular reaction in the anterior part of the vitreous began to resolve. At the end of the treatment period visual acuity had improved and the visual field defects originally observed in 2 patients had regressed. Hepatotoxic effects of the treatment occurred in 4 of the 6 patients, but returned to normal within 1 month after discontinuance of the therapy. There was minimal hematologic toxicity and only a few instances of anorexia and mild nausea and vomiting. In 1 patient there was transient ulceration of the mucous membrane of the lower lip. The authors of this article, and the authoritative discussant, were able to marshal considerable theoretical basis for expecting methotrexate to influence the course of the uveitis, but there was agreement that a larger series of cases must be studied and that potential toxicities must be carefully weighed against what palliative effect is achieved.

Vernon G. Wong and Evan M. Hersh. Methotrexate (Amethopterin) in the Therapy of Cyclitis. Tr. Am. Acad. Ophth. & Otolaryng. 69:279, Mar.-Apr., 1965.

"I have heard that the much used cycloplegic agent, cyclopentolate (Cyclogyl), sometimes causes schizophrenia-like behavior patterns associated with ataxia. Is the incidence of the reaction significantly high?"

Reply: A few such cases have been reported by Harry Mark (New Haven, Connecticut) and others, but I do not think the evidence so far indicates more than instances of drug idiosyncrasy rather than a specific characteristic of this agent. The belladonna alkaloids themselves will occasionally induce bizarre behavior patterns on ordinary dosage.

Harry H. Mark. Psychotogenic Properties of Cyclopentolate (Cyclogyl). J.A.M.A. 186:430, Oct. 26, 1963.

"I have heard that glycerin is a useful drug in the treatment of acute glaucoma, but do not know anyone who has tried it. Do you know anything about this?"

Reply: Yes, in London, Casey and Trevor-Roper, and in India, Consul and Kukhrestha, have reported the very effective use of glycerin in a dosage of 1.5 Gm./kg. body weight, mixed in fruit juice and carbonated water. The average fall in pressure in patients in Casey and Trevor-Roper's cases with simple open-angle glaucoma was half of its initial level; 1 patient had a fall from 36 to 11 mm. Hg, compared with a fall from 30 to 22 mm. Hg after 500 mg. of oral acetazolamide (Diamox). Since glycerin is easily available at any corner drug store, its use could be looked upon as a very simple emergency measure to relieve the pain and avoid the serious damage that could follow the delay in having the patient admitted to hospital. The 1.5 Gm./kg. dosage is about 2 teaspoonfuls for an individual of 150 pounds; this is considered to be much below toxic levels, although D'Alena and Ferguson, in San Francisco, have thought that in an elderly diabetic such dosage was likely responsible for the ensuing severe acidosis.

T. A. Casey and P. D. Trevor-Roper. Oral Glycerol in Glaucoma. Brit. M. J. 2:851, Oct. 5, 1963. Peter D'Alena and William Ferguson. Adverse Effects After Glycerol Orally and Mannitol Parenterally. Arch. Ophth. 75:201, 1966. B. N. Consul and O. P. Kukhrestha. Oral Glycerin in Glaucoma. Am. J. Ophth. 60:900, 1965.

"I have used intravenous urea in acute glaucoma with excellent effect but would sometimes like to have a more prolonged action than I obtain; for example, in such conditions as pseudotumor cerebri, hyphema with imminent blood staining, central retinal artery occlusion, etc. Is oral use of urea feasible?"

Reply: Yes, it is. At New York Hospital–Cornell Medical Center, Miles Galin and associates found that they obtained reduction in intraocular pressure with oral urea in 2½–3 hours after the ingestion of 1.5 Gm./ kg. The drug, in the form of 50% solution of lyophilized, ammonia-free urea, was dissolved in cherry sirup and cooled with cracked ice; but this is a nasty mixture, of which the 70 kg. (154 lb.) person must drink nearly a tumblerful!

Miles A. Galin, Futaba Aizawa and John M. McLean. Oral Urea as Osmotic Ocular Hypotensive Agent. Arch. Ophth. 62:1099, 1959.

"I understand that corticosteroids are being used locally as a provocative diagnostic test for glaucoma; i.e., patients with glaucoma being said to respond with a higher rise in pressure than nonglaucomatous individuals. May this be a dangerous procedure?"

Reply: It has been considered that the artificially provoked rise in tension is always reversible, but until much more experience has accumulated it would seem to me to be advisable to proceed cautiously with this test because Finn Spiers, in Denmark, has reported the case of a 67-year-old woman who developed a moderate *irreversible* rise in pressure in the exposed eye after instillation of dexamethasone (Decadron, Deronil) into one eye four times daily for 4 weeks. The tension of the control eye was not affected.

Finn Spiers. A Case of Irreversible Steroid-Induced Rise in Intraocular Pressure. Acta ophth. 43:419, 1965.

"Would anything be gained by adding a cardiac glycoside to a carbonic anhydrase inhibitor in the treatment of glaucoma?"

Reply: The introduction of the carbonic anhydrase inhibitor, acetazolamide (Diamox) to decrease intraocular pressure, by Bernard Becker in 1954, was probably one of the true milestones in the therapy of glaucoma. I do not think it has been established that the additional use of a cardiac glycoside will be helpful, though Awasthy and Saxena, in India, have felt that the combination therapy was more effective than acetazolamide alone provided the digoxin was given before the acetazolamide in order to permit it to facilitate the activity of the latter. The reasoning underlying use of the cardiac glycoside was that it allegedly interferes directly with enzyme transport of sodium and potassium, being therefore in its own way an enzyme inhibitor.

P. N. Awasthy and R. B. Saxena. Cardiac Glycosides in Treatment of Glaucoma. J. Internat. Coll. Surgeons 42: 188, 1964. Bernard Becker. Decrease in Intraocular Pressure in Man by a Carbonic Anhydrase Inhibitor, Diamox. Am. J. Ophth. 37:13, 1954.

"So many drugs are being used nowadays for one or another sort of action in the central nervous system; what effects do these agents have on intraocular pressure?"

Reply: Only a few observations have been made and none of them definitive since the number of cases involved was small. Pentobarbital (Nembutal) occasionally causes slight lowering of the pressure; diphenylhydantoin (Dilantin) also lowers it slightly in an occasional patient; primidone (Mysoline), mephenytoin (Mesantoin) and dextroamphetamine (Dexedrine) appear not to have any effect; thiopental (Pentothal) acutely lowers

the pressure when it is used in anesthetic dosage; pressure has been lowered transiently by single doses of chlorpromazine (Thorazine), but the effect is not sustained on repeated administration, and this is true of mephenesin (Tolserol) also; occasionally meprobamate (Miltown, Equanil) can reduce the peaks of diurnal fluctuations in pressure, and reserpine may do so to an insignificant degree also; the only effect of caffeine seems to be occasionally to cause a slight transient rise.

J. D. Peczon and W. M. Grant. Sedatives, Stimulants and Intraocular Pressure in Glaucoma, Arch. Ophth. 72:178, 1964.

"What is the effect of the corticosteroids on intraocular pressure and visual fields?"

Reply: By administering 0.1% dexamethasone (Decadron, Deronil) four times daily to one eye of groups of patients with open-angle glaucoma, glaucoma suspects and normal volunteers, J. P. Nicholas found an elevation of 6.6 mm. Hg and a decrease in facility outflow of 0.06 in the eyes of the normal individuals, 8.6 and 0.03, respectively, in the eyes of the glaucoma patients, and 8.7 and 0.04 in the eyes of the glaucoma suspects. Treatment was discontinued after 24 days and the pressures all returned to pretreatment levels a short time later. In the matter of visual fields, A. E. Kolker and associates found the effects variable, some glaucoma and glaucoma-suspect eyes failing to show fewer changes even when the intraocular pressure was raised to high levels for days to weeks, whereas many patients showed increased field loss when the pressure became elevated with corticosteroid therapy.

J. P. Nicholas. Topical Corticosteroids and Aqueous Humor Dynamics, Arch. Ophth. 72:769, 1964. A. E. Kolker, B. Becker and D. W. Mills. Intraocular Pressure and Visual Fields: Effects of Corticosteroids. Arch. Ophth. 72:772, 1964.

"In glaucomatous eyes in which I cannot get the desired degree of miosis with pilocarpine, I have been using demecarium (Humorsol) with good effect except that sometimes the extreme degree of miosis effected by this drug reduces strikingly the visual acuity of some cataractous eyes. Would it be feasible in such a situation to use a sympathomimetic agent?"

Reply: The effect of phenylephrine (Neo-Synephrine), 10%, on both normal and glaucomatous eyes treated with one of these intensely acting miotics was studied by Bernard Becker's group (Washington University), who found that in both groups the drug dilated the pupils without significantly altering the intraocular pressure or outflow facility.

Bernard Becker, Tracy Gage, Allan E. Kolker and Andrew J. Gay. Effect of Phenylephrine (Neo-Synephrine) Hydrochloride on Miotic-Treated Eye. Am. J. Ophth. 48:313, 1959.

"It has been rumored that guanethidine (Ismelin) is useful in the therapy of glaucoma. Can you cite a study of the matter?"

Reply: At the University Eye Clinic, in Amsterdam, J. A. Oosterhuis applied 2 drops of a 10% guanethidine solution in the conjunctival sac and obtained some degree of miosis that was clearly visible for 3–9 days, though the reaction to light persisted. Frequently there was also narrowing of the palpebral fissure. In 13 of 17 eyes treated (in patients not responding well to other therapy), a drop in intraocular pressure occurred on the first or second day of guanethidine therapy and persisted during the treatment in all but one eye, the decrease ranging up to 15 mm. Hg. Some redness seen after instillation of the drug was not due to irritation but to hyperemia. Bitter taste and nasal stuffiness occasionally occurred, but there were no systemic effects.

J. A. Oosterhuis. Guanethidine (Ismelin) in Ophthalmology: II. Clinical Application in Glaucoma. Arch. Ophth. 67: 802, 1962.

"It appears that in our area echothiophate iodide (Phospholine) is being used increasingly in preference to pilocarpine in the treatment of open-angle glaucoma. What is really the comparative status of these two drugs?"

Reply: Many men still feel that one is not justified in changing to Phospholine if pilocarpine is reasonably effective, but this is not the consensus. At the Bronx Eye and Ear Infirmary at New York, Paul Barsam and Herbert Vogel compared the two agents in a small number of cases. Patients on pilocarpine received 2% of the drug at 12:30, 5:00 and 10:00 p.m. and at 8:00 a.m., and patients on Phospholine, 0.06%, received this drug at 11:00 p.m. only. After recording the tension at 9:00 a.m., the patients were discharged and their medication reversed, then being readmitted after at least 2 weeks of therapy. The average tension from 12:00 noon to 12:00 midnight was compared with the average at 3:00 a.m. and 6:00 a.m., and in both eyes of all patients on Phospholine it fell more or rose less than on pilocarpine during the night as compared with the daytime. In 11 of the 18 eyes, the peak tension during the night on pilocarpine was 25 mm. Hg or more, but 12 mm. Hg or less on Phospholine. In 7 eyes, there was satisfactory night control on both drugs but the Phospholine level was consistently lower. There were no side effects

during the experiment, but H. D. Markman's group, in New York, reported a case of severe diarrhea, nausea and weakness associated with the use of Phospholine. No side effects were reported by Fisher's group in London.

Paul C. Barsam and Herbert P. Vogel. Effect of Phospholine Iodide on Diurnal Variations of Intraocular Pressure in Glaucoma. Am. J. Ophth. 57:241, 1964. H. David Markman, Philip Rosenberg and Wolf D. Dettbarn. Eye Drops and Diarrhea: Diarrhea as First Symptom of Echothiophate Iodide (Phospholine) Toxicity. New England J. Med. 271:197, July 23, 1964. R. Fisher, R. Smith and C. Wheeler. Brit. J. Ophth. 49:369, 1965.

"I have a patient with chronic narrow-angle glaucoma who cannot be controlled with conventional medical therapy and has refused surgery. Is one justified in using echothiophate iodide (Phospholine) therapy in such a case?"

Reply: Many ophthalmologists consider that drugs of this type are contraindicated in this form of glaucoma, but John Sussman (Montefiore Hospital, New York) reported successful use of echothiophate iodide in 14 of 17 eyes of such patients as you mention. He also drew attention to the fact that the frequently encountered opinion in the literature of the contraindication of such drugs as echothiophate iodide is based mainly on the reports of dilute narrow-angle attacks precipitated by isoflurophate (DFP). In his own series each patient received echothiophate iodide in dosage of 0.125 or 0.06% twice daily and was observed for at least 6 months, during which time there was no progression of visual field defects, the gonioscopic appearance of the angles did not change, and no patient experienced an increase of intraocular pressure or an acute attack.

John D. Sussman. Phospholine (Echothiophate) Iodide. Am. J. Ophth. 59:308, 1965.

"I have treated several cases of herpes simplex keratitis with idoxuridine (IDU) without results that were convincing of the efficacy of this therapy. But there have been numerous favorable reports; how explain this disparity?"

Reply: Yes, it is true that there have been numerous rather enthusiastic accounts of this therapy, but the fact is that few controlled studies have been performed, and most of those that have been are open to some suspicion from the standpoint of diagnosis in some instances and of the employment of concomitant measures in others. The most satisfactory study I have seen reported was that of Davidson and Evans, at the Birmingham and Midland Eye Hospital, who compared IDU, gamma globulin and iodization. IDU drops of 0.1% solution were used hourly during the day and

2 hourly at night, with no other therapy than a pad and bandage; gamma globulin drops of 1% were used instead of the IDU drops, and otherwise the treatment was the same; iodization of the affected areas of the cornea was performed with an alcoholic solution of iodine and potassium iodide, together with topical therapy of atropine 1% drops twice daily and chloramphenicol (Chloromycetin) ointment 1%, three times daily, a pad and bandage being also applied in these cases. The patients were randomly allocated to the three groups, and the usual double-blind conditions applied to the study. Of the 25 patients in the IDU group, 8 were rejected as tissue culture was negative for virus; the remaining 17 patients responded to IDU. Of the 25 patients in the gamma globulin group, virus could not be grown in 11; the remaining 14 patients responded to the gamma globulin drops. Of the 25 patients in the iodization group, virus could not be isolated in 5; the remaining 20 patients responded to iodization. When the cases were studied from the standpoint of the most effective healing procedure, iodization obtained first place, IDU second and gamma globulin third. When combining the excellent and good results (corresponding to healing within 1 and 2 weeks respectively) it became apparent that iodization was by far the most efficient procedure. The IDU results were not nearly as good as those reported in some of the other less rigidly controlled studies. The result of this study was the conclusion by the investigators that, because iodization often causes great discomfort to the patient in the first 24 hours following its use, and the eye often remains irritable for several days afterwards, IDU is justifiable first treatment for herpes simplex keratitis, to be followed by iodization only if healing does not occur within 7 days. A note of caution is in order: do not scrub too vigorously when using the iodization technique because there may be a resultant break in Bowman's membrane, leading to a violent chemical keratitis.

Down in Georgia, U.S.A., Ben Jenkins has combined chymotrypsin and corticosteroids with IDU in a small series of cases: 100,000 units of lyophilized chymotrypsin applied with the eye cup once daily for 15 minutes following topical anesthesia, 1 drop of corticosteroid solution three times daily, and 2 drops of the IDU every hour while awake.

S. I. Davidson and P. Jameson Evans. IDU and the Treatment of Herpes Simplex Keratitis. Brit. J. Ophth. 48:678, 1964. Ben H. Jenkins. Successful Combination Therapy in Dendritic Keratitis After Failure with IDU. South. M. J. 58:1122, 1965.

"One of my associates has had the misfortune to have a lesion develop on the cornea in one of his young patients with chicken pox. The outcome was not a very happy one; might the new drug, idoxuridine (IDU) have been helpful?"

Reply: This is of course a rare lesion, but I have seen the report of 1 case in which IDU was successfully used, that of J. E. Cairns, in London.

J. E. Cairns. Varicella of Cornea Treated with 5-Iodo-2′-Deoxyuridine (IDU). Brit. J. Ophth. 48:288, 1964.

"In cases of traumatic hyphema the blood that has entered the anterior chamber of the eye is usually absorbed and vision restored if the patient is put at absolute rest with sedation and both eyes covered, but sometimes there occurs a secondary hyphema several days later, which causes considerable concern because this additional hemorrhage may block the drainage system of the eye and cause sufficient secondary glaucoma to force blood cells into the substance of the cornea. Have any drugs been helpful in this situation?"

Reply: The intravenous use of urea has been recommended by Marvin Kwitko and Frank Costenbader, at Children's Hospital, Washington, D.C. Dosage in their cases was 1 Gm./kg. body weight. In India, Chandra and Gupta found buccal varidase, 1 tablet/6 hours, a useful adjunct in acute intraocular hemorrhage and acute uveitis and in cases of both acute and chronic extraocular orbital disease, but Wright, in Norfolk, Va., failed to find that it influenced very much the rate of absorption of blood from the anterior chamber. In Denmark, Kjeldsen has used mannitol with satisfaction, all patients, regardless of weight, receiving 500 ml. intravenously of a 20% solution, given at a rate of 8–14 ml./minute.

Marvin L. Kwitko and Frank D. Costenbader. Urea Therapy in Glaucoma Due to Secondary Hyphema. Canad. M. J. 86:447, Mar. 10, 1962. D. B. Chandra and L. C. Gupta. Clinical Studies with Buccal Varidase in Some Eye Diseases. Am. J. Ophth. 58:828, 1964. James C. Wright. Hyphema Treated by Buccal Varidase: Double-Blind Study. Am. J. Ophth. 58:479, 1964. Mogens H. Kjeldsen. Treatment of Intraocular Hemorrhages with Mannitol. Acta ophth. 43:128, 1965.

"In the relatively small number of cases of macular degenerative changes in the eye that enter my practice I have been using peripheral vasodilators with what has seemed to me to be some success, but now I have seen the report of animal experimentation indicating that this therapy may not favorably influence the course of the disease. Has the matter been given thorough study?"

Reply: Until about 15 years ago this was looked upon as a hopeless condition. But with increasing acceptance of the theory that at least the senile variety of the disease is essentially vascular in character, some ophthalmologists, but by no means all, have been using vasodilators in therapy. The most extensive recent report I have seen is that of H. Wyatt Laws (Queen Elizabeth Hospital of Montreal) who reported use of these drugs in 203 patients. The agents used were nicotinic acid, 100 mg. three times daily after meals; nicotinyl alcohol (Roniacol), 50 mg. similarly; tolazoline (Priscoline), 25 mg. similarly; and nylidrin (Arlidin), 6 mg. similarly. These appear to be equivalent doses so far as general vasodilator effect is concerned, but the results with nylidrin were sufficiently superior to those with the other agents that this drug was used exclusively in the last several years. There were only a few complaints of lightheadedness, headache, palpitation. No more than clinical impression of the usefulness of vasodilators was derivable from the study, which did not lend itself well to statistical analysis, but Laws thought that the drugs were valuable, particularly in maintaining vision at the level of acuity present when therapy was begun.

H. Wyatt Laws. Peripheral Vasodilators in the Treatment of Macular Degenerative Changes in the Eye. Canad. M. A. J. 91:325, Aug. 15, 1964.

"The powerful miotic agents, such as pilocarpine or physostigmine (eserine), cause considerable postoperative pain through the intense miosis they produce, and I therefore like to avoid them as much as possible. What is the ideal dilution of acetylcholine to accomplish best miosis with it? I understand of course that the action will be more brief than with the other drugs."

Reply: In Bogotá, Colombia, J. I. Barraquer found that all of the dilutions he used, ranging from 1 : 5000 to 1 : 100, showed activity but that the only one that reliably produced sufficient effect to be of value was the 1 : 100. He found that with this concentration, a good pupillary contraction can be expected if the iris is not enclaved and eye in a good state of hypotony. At completion of the operation he allowed the anterior chamber to remain filled with acetylcholine solution or to be filled with air, according to the situation in individual cases.

José I. Barraquer M. Acetylcholine as Miotic Agent for Use in Surgery. Am. J. Ophth. 57:406, 1964.

"In an active ophthalmic service we have recently had a small outbreak of postoperative staphylococcic infections after intraocular procedures. Might prophylactic antibiotic measures have prevented this?"

Reply: At the USPHS Hospital, Staten Island, New York, Robert Aronstam reported a small outbreak of this sort. Four patients had received a subconjunctival injection of 100,000 units of potassium penicillin G and 10 mg. of streptomycin in 0.25 ml. of water; infection occurred in them in 26.5 days, range 21–40 days. In 4 other cases, not so treated, the interval averaged 4.5 days, range 2–7 days. Aronstam suggested that the antibiotic mixture might have delayed the onset of the manifestations of infection and thus clouded the diagnosis and discovery of the type of organism involved, but it is difficult for me to see how this could have been the case since it presupposes the remaining of the mixture in the subconjunctival tissues for an unlikely period of time. In short, then, I cannot give you a definite answer.

Robert H. Aronstam. Pitfalls of Prophylaxis: Alteration of Postoperative Infection by Penicillin-Streptomycin. Am. J. Ophth. 57:312, 1964.

"How long should the prophylactic administration of a cycloplegic be continued in patients with progressive myopia?"

Reply: The optimal length of treatment has apparently not been determined, but Seymour Gostin (Southwestern Medical School) felt that treatment might be stopped at the end of a year and the state of affairs determined at intervals thereafter, reinstituting therapy as indicated. His preferred treatment was 0.25% scopolamine hydrobromide twice daily in each eye, with the use of bifocal glasses for full myopic correction and clip-on absorptive lenses for outdoor use.

Seymour B. Gostin. Prophylactic Management of Progressive Myopia. South. M. J. 55:916, 1962.

"The most effective treatment for the granulomatous uveitis of toxoplasmosis nowadays appears to be the combination of pyrimethamine (Daraprim), a sulfonamide and a corticosteroid. But I have had some unpleasant reactions in a small series of cases. What has been the larger experience?"

Reply: At Henry Ford Hospital, Andrew TenPas and Joseph P. Abraham have reported the cases of 2 patients who developed severe thrombocytopenic purpura and macrocytic anemia attributable to the pyrimethamine in this combination therapy, and 1 showed evidence of myocarditis and a peculiar bronze pigmentation of the skin. At the Wills Eye Hospital, in Philadelphia, Mrinmay Ghosh and associates recorded the complications of this combined therapy in 114 patients. About half of them complained of nausea and vomiting in the initial periods of treatment, which was minimized in all but two instances by use of antiemetics and antacids and giving the drugs after meals. In 1 patient, extreme malaise and a spiking fever necessitated discontinuing pyrimethamine. In 14 patients there was leukopenia, thrombocytopenia and/or anemia; in 5 of these it was necessary to discontinue pyrimethamine, but the other 9 responded to Leucovorin therapy and a temporary decrease or discontinuation of the drug. One patient suffered spontaneous abortion at 12 weeks' gestation together with thrombocytopenia and a blood loss at the time of abortion that necessitated transfusion. A mild diffuse increase in pigmentation of the terminal phalanges of 1 patient receiving pyrimethamine has also been noted by another observer. One patient developed urinary albumin and casts from the sulfonamide, which had to be discontinued; and a few of the patients developed the typical signs of corticosteroid overaction. I certainly think that Conrad Giles, at the National Institutes of Health, is justified in his assertion that until it is confirmed that severe bone marrow depression can be blocked by the use of folinic acid when using the high dosage of pyrimethamine that is necessary in toxoplasmosis, weekly blood counts should be performed in all patients.

Andrew TenPas and Joseph P. Abraham. Hematologic Side Effects of Pyrimethamine (Daraprim) in Treatment of Ocular Toxoplasmosis. Am. J. M. Sc. 249:448, 1965. Mrinmay Ghosh, Phillip Levy and Irving H. Leopold. Therapy of Toxoplasmosis Uveitis. Am. J. Ophth. 59:55, 1965. Conrad L. Giles. Treatment of Toxoplasma Uveitis with Pyrimethamine (Daraprim) and Folinic Acid (Leucovorin). Am. J. Ophth. 58:611, 1964.

"How is chymotrypsin best used in the treatment of dendritic ulcers, and what are the undesirable reactions?"

Reply: As a result of their combined experiences, Ben Jenkins (Newnan, Georgia) and M. N. Stow (Washington, D.C.) concluded that early ulcers are best treated by a drop method, and older lesions that have been previously treated, by an eye bath and lid suturing method until recovery has begun, then changing to the drop method until the lesion heals. *Drop method:* mix 100,000 units of lyophilized chymotrypsin with 10 ml. normal saline or sterile distilled water (solution stable for 4 days), and use 1 or 2 drops in the affected eye every hour while the patient is awake, an antibiotic ointment being used at night and continued at bedtime for 1 week after the ulcer heals. *Eye bath method:* Dissolve 100,000 units of lyophilized chymotrypsin in 3 or 4 ml. normal saline or sterile distilled water, and place in an eye cup, which the patient is then to hold over the involved eye for 5–10 minutes;

the eyelids are then sutured together with 4-0 silk to prevent their action from irritating the ulcer site – inspect after 24 hours and repeat if the ulcer is not completely healed, and when healed use 2 drops of an antibiotic solution in the eye every 2 hours. In 27 of the 403 cases covered in this review, including 140 of the observers' own, the therapy had been discontinued because of burning and itching or scratching, pain, dermatitis of the lids, moderate blepharitis, red and swollen lids, or lack of response. It was felt that some of the nonresponders might have obtained acceptable results if instillation therapy had been discontinued at once after appearance of the untoward symptoms and the daily eye bath substituted.

M. Noel Stow and Ben H. Jenkins. Further Evaluation of Use of Chymotrypsin in Treatment of Dendritic Keratitis. Tr. Am. Acad. Ophth. 67:702, 1963. Ben H. Jenkins and M. Noel Stow. Chymotrypsin in Treatment of Dendritic Ulcers. South. M. J. 56:275, 1963.

"I understand that the corticosteroid preparation, Kenalog Parenteral, that is widely used for intramuscular, intra-articular and intrabursal injection for anti-inflammatory action is now being used subconjunctivally in the treatment of ocular inflammatory conditions. Could you cite someone's experience?"

Reply: At the Mount Sinai Hospital in New York, Robert Sturman's group has reported the satisfactory use of this preparation in 8 categories of ocular inflammation: iridocyclitis; uveitis, posterior; intraocular surgery; keratoconjunctivitis, corneal ulcers, corneal burns; endophthalmitis and panophthalmitis; dendritic keratitis; episcleritis; and optic neuritis and retrobulbar neuritis. In addition to these categories, one of the observers used it subconjunctivally at the conclusion of about 100 routine operations for cataract, corneal grafts and glaucoma. A Kenalog Parenteral suspension containing 40 mg./ml. is injected, usually in the inferotemporal conjunctival fornix, in an amount of 0.5 ml. through a 26-gauge needle after thorough anesthetization of the conjunctiva through application for 4 or 5 minutes of a cotton tipped applicator soaked in 4% Xylocaine or 0.5% Ophthaine. It is said that the corticosteroid begins to act promptly but absorbs slowly so that the duration of action is between 3 and 6 months.

Robert M. Sturman, Joseph Laval and Martin F. Sturman. Subconjunctival Triamcinolone Acetonide. Am. J. Ophth. 61:155, 1966.

"Conflicting reports of the effect on intraocular pressure and pupil size of intramuscular atropine and scopolamine have appeared in the literature. What has been recent experience?"

Reply: The position of atropine has not been determined with satisfaction, so far as I am aware, but in India recently, Mehra and associates, being prompted by the need to find a safe premedication for glaucomatous patients requiring drainage operations under general anesthesia, investigated the effect of scopolamine in 100 patients with normal pupil size and intraocular pressure and 10 patients with glaucoma. When given intramuscular injections of scopolamine hydrobromide, 0.06 mg./14 pounds, it was found in the normal subjects that the pupil size increased by 9%, and the intraocular pressure by 5%; in the 10 glaucomatous patients no changes occurred. The conclusion was that scopolamine affords a safe method of premedication before general anesthesia in glaucomatous patients.

K. S. Mehra, P. Chandra and B. B. Khare. Ocular Manifestations of Parenteral Administration of Scopolamine (Hyoscine). Brit. J. Ophth. 49:557, 1965.

OPTIC NEURITIS

"Is there any worthwhile drug therapy for optic neuritis?"

Reply: If the lesion is secondary to an acute infectious disease, the effective drug therapy is of course that of the primary disease, and if it is in association with diabetes mellitus the drug therapy is equally obvious. Methyl alcohol and nicotine cases are approached prophylactically simply through avoiding these two poisons; therapeutically there is little to do for the methyl alcohol poisoning, but the nicotine-induced affair reverses when the individual stops smoking. The latter type of optic neuritis is rarely seen, however, except in persons who are heavily addicted to both alcohol and tobacco. Vasodilators, corticosteroids and fever therapy are all resorted to in the cases that are not intercurrent in an infectious disease, but the record certainly leaves much to be desired.

ORTHOSTATIC HYPOTENSION, IDIOPATHIC

"I have a patient whose orthostatic hypotension appears to be idiopathic, at least I can uncover nothing that might account for it. Has any drug therapy been found effective in such a situation?"

Reply: At the Mayo Clinic, Alexander Schirger and associates treated 5 patients with idiopathic orthostatic hypotension rather effectively with fludrocortisone (Florinef, F-Cortef), giving 1 mg. twice daily until there was weight gain or a decrease in degree of fall in blood pressure when the patient stood, then reducing to a maintenance dose of 0.5 mg. once or twice daily. I suppose you are sure that your patient does not have diabetes mellitus, in which orthostatic hypotension is sometimes a manifestation of autonomic nervous system involvement in the neuropathy?

Alexander Schirger, Edgar A. Hines, Jr., George D. Molnar and Juergen E. Thomas. Idiopathic Orthostatic Hypotension. J.A.M.A. 181:822, Sept. 8, 1962.

"I have a patient with idiopathic orthostatic hypotension in whom all physical measures to increase venous return, and administration of vasopressor agents, have failed; what other therapy might be resorted to?"

Reply: This uncommon disorder of the autonomic nervous system is thought by some observers to be possibly merely a part of a general degenerative central nervous system disorder. I have nothing to suggest except to point out that in a series of 29 patients in whom all other measures had failed as in your case, Schatz's group (Henry Ford Hospital) effected considerable improvement in 5 individuals through the use of corticosteroids. It is difficult to appreciate what the rationale of such therapy could be.

Irwin J. Schatz, Stephen Podolsky and Boy Frame. Idiopathic Orthostatic Hypotension: Diagnosis and Treatment. J.A.M.A. 186:537, Nov. 9, 1963.

OSTEOARTHRITIS

"Has indomethacin (Indocin) been used effectively in the treatment of osteoarthritis of the hip?"

Reply: I have no personal knowledge of such therapy and have only seen one report of its use, that of Wanka and Dixon, in London, who employed the drug in a double-blind crossover trial of 4 weeks in a dosage of 75–150 mg./day against a placebo. It was said that a significant preference for indomethacin was shown both subjectively as regards effort and rest pain and objectively as regards the range of abduction of the hips.

J. Wanka and A. St. J. Dixon. Treatment of Osteo-Arthritis of the Hip with Indomethacin. Ann. Rheumat. Dis. 24: 288, 1964.

"One of my associates is having a bad time in connection with an injection he made into an osteoarthritic joint. How often have there been serious complications in connection with this procedure?"

Reply: In 1960, Charles Bonner (Boston University) reviewed the literature and found that there had been less than 0.02% of serious complications reported in the 50,757 injections that had been given by various workers during the preceding 5 years. I have seen no more recent statistics. I think, however, that your attention should be drawn to the fact that the relatively painless joints resulting from intra-articular corticosteroid injections may be abused by stoical patients and provoke articular damage more severe than that expected in the natural course of the disease. Alarcón-Segovia and Ward (Mayo Clinic) have reported an instance of this sort resulting in a Charcot-like arthropathy.

Charles D. Bonner. Intra-articular Injections for Osteo-arthritis. Rheumatism 16:84, 1960. D. Alarcón-Segovia and L. Emmerdon Ward. Charcot-like Arthropathy in Rheumatoid Arthritis. J.A.M.A. 193:1052, Sept. 20, 1965.

OSTEOPOROSIS

"One of my associates is using an androgen-estrogen preparation (Dumone), 1 tablet orally once or twice daily, in the treatment of senile osteoporosis. Is this therapy theoretically sound?"

Reply: "Soundness" may possibly be derived from the facts that both male and female hormones promote retention of calcium phosphate and interfere with osteoclastic activity and that male hormone decreases nitrogen excretion. In Dallas, Texas, M. P. Knight used the preparation you refer to with considerable satisfaction in a small series of women with senile osteoporosis. I suggest the additional use of calcium salts and vitamin D in moderate amounts.

M. P. Knight. Treatment of Senile Osteoporosis with Orally Administered Androgen-Estrogen Preparation. J. Am. Geriatrics Soc. 12:395, 1964.

"Since it is reasonable to suppose that a measure substantially increasing bone mass will reverse the course of osteoporosis, would it be logical to use sodium fluoride in therapy?"

Reply: In Seattle, Rich and Ivanovich actually tried such therapy in a man with severe primary osteoporosis, giving 40–50 mg. of fluoride ion daily for 122 weeks. They were able to show significant and increasingly great retention of calcium during this treatment and radiographic measurements of bone density showed increase from subnormal to low-normal values, the most striking changes being in the metaphyses of the bones examined. For the first 34 weeks the dosage was 110 mg. of sodium fluoride in enteric coated tablets and thereafter 88 mg. daily. No important toxic action of the fluoride was encountered. Such a result has not been obtained in all instances, however, and it must always be borne in mind not only that osteoporosis has several causes but also that in some patients the disorder appears to wax and wane spontaneously. Adams and Jowsey have very well emphasized that much more experimental work needs to be done before sodium fluoride can be recommended as safe and useful in treatment of bone diseases.

Clayton Rich and Peter Ivanovich. Response to Sodium Fluoride in Severe Primary Osteoporosis. Ann. Int. Med. 63:1069, 1965. Peter H. Adams and Jenifer Jowsey. Sodium Fluoride in the Treatment of Osteoporosis and Other Bone Diseases. Ann. Int. Med. 63:1151, 1965.

OTORHINOLARYNGOLOGY

"I have not had much success with the oral administration of estrogens in atrophic rhinitis. What of this?"

Reply: Try the new method of administration reported by Michael Zeman (University of Louisville). He dissolves 20 mg. Premarin in 30 ml. of sterile distilled water and has the patient spray this from a sterile plastic nasal spray bottle directly into the nose three times daily. Excellent results were reported in all of his 44 patients after 3 weeks' continuous treatment.

Michael S. Zeman. Use of Premarin as Topical Agent in Treatment of Atrophic Rhinitis: Clinical and Histologic Study. Laryngoscope 73:1219, 1963.

"I have recently lost a patient with cavernous sinus thrombosis in spite of everything we could do for him. This is of course not surprising since the mortality in this entity was practically 100% prior to the introduction of antibiotics and is even now very high, but I would like to know what you would think would be ideal therapy in this malady?"

Reply: The difficulty here is that the high mortality and morbidity is due to the fact that the infection is in a vital area that is inaccessible to surgical drainage. Since in most instances the offending organism will be a gram-positive one, usually *Staphylococcus aureus*, and since there is a high incidence of resistance to penicillin G in hospital strains of this organism, the rational thing is to institute therapy with one of the newer semisynthetic penicillins. You want to use a penicillin if possible because of its bactericidal properties, but it is advisable to combine with it a broad-spectrum antibiotic as well. Of course as soon as the result of culture studies is available the choice of an antibiotic can be modified in accordance with these findings. The recommendation of Leonard Vinnick's group, consequent upon their fortunate result in a case stemming from a dental surgical procedure, was that a combination of 10 million units of penicillin G and 12 Gm. of methicillin (Dimocillin-RT, Staphcillin) be given daily by the intravenous route and that a broad-spectrum antibiotic should also be used because of the rare case caused by a gram-negative organism.

Leonard Vinnick, Everett B. Cooper and Edwin L. Overholt. Cavernous Sinus Thrombosis. Arch. Otolaryng. 82:303, 1965.

"I have heard promethazine (Phenergan) praised as a nasal decongestant, but in my practice it has not worked well at all. What could be at fault?"

Reply: According to the observations of J. W. McLaurin and associates (Tulane University), it is the choice of Phenergan preparations that is important. They found that the preparation known as "Phenergan Expectorant" caused significant nasal congestion in about 50% of individuals, while "Phenergan Expectorant with phenylephrine" produced a significant decongestant effect. In their experience, Phenergan syrup alone was an effective decongestant when the congestion was secondary to an allergic state but not in other conditions. The "Phenergan Expectorant solution" contains fluidextract ipecac, potassium guaiacolsulfonate, chloroform, citric acid, sodium citrate and alcohol. They found that ipecac alone, or in combination with chloroform, appeared to be causative of, or at least contributed to, the congestant effect of the mixture.

J. W. McLaurin, H. Komet and J. Avegno. Evaluation of Decongestant Properties by Nasal Rhinometry: Phenergan (Promethazine), Phenergan Expectorant and Phenergan Expectorant Plus Phenylephrine. Laryngoscope 73:1496, 1963.

"In a relatively limited experience I have been unable to decide which of the several available decongestants is most effective; can you cite a significant study?"

Reply: At the Massachusetts Eye and Ear Infirmary, Pullen and Montgomery compared three sustained-action preparations in 246 patients with symptoms of upper respiratory mucosal congestion: Dimetapp Extentabs (parabromdylamine maleate 12 mg., phenylephrine hydrochloride 15 mg. and phenylpropanolamine 15 mg.), Disophrol Chronotab tablets (dexbrompheniramine 6 mg. and d-isophedrine sulfate 120 mg.) and Triaminic tablets (phenylpropanolamine hydrochloride 50 mg., pheniramine maleate 25 mg. and pyrilamine maleate 25 mg.). One tablet of Triaminic was given every 8 hours and 1 tablet every 12 hours of Dimetapp Extentabs and Disophrol Chronotabs. Excellent responses were obtained as follows: Disophrol, 74%, Triaminic, 59%, and Dimetapp, 57%. The incidence of side effects was 11.5% with Triaminic, 6.4% with Disophrol, and 5.3% with Dimetapp; drowsiness principally, but never severe enough to cause discontinuance of the treatment.

Fredric W. Pullen, II, and William W. Montgomery. Comparative Evaluation of Oral Decongestants: Controlled Clinical Study. Arch. Otolaryng. 77:10, 1963.

"Many acute laryngologic disorders are accompanied by the typical signs and symptoms of inflammation even though they are noninfectious in origin. Do you know of any drug that is of aid in reducing the things which delay the healing process and cause needless pain and disability — such as swelling, redness, heat and cellular infiltration — without disturbing the desirable responses that enable the body to localize the offending agent and hasten tissue repair?"

Reply: The corticosteroids will reduce the entire inflammatory process and certainly not fulfill your requirements; aspirin, too, will relieve the discomfort but nothing else. L. H. Teitel and associates claimed to have accomplished pretty well what you want through the use of oxyphenbutazone (Tandearil), which they evaluated in a double-blind study in 104 office patients with acute otolaryngologic disorders of various sorts. The dosage was 600 mg. for 2 days and 300 mg. for 5 additional days, in divided doses. It did not seem to me that their report really revealed the things that they claimed for the drug; about two thirds of the patients received an antibiotic or a sulfonamide in addition to the oxyphenbutazone, and there was a considerable disparity in numbers of those treated with the active drug and with the placebo.

L. H. Teitel, S. B. Harris, E. A. Thompson and B. W. Billow. Oxyphenbutazone (Tandearil): New Anti-inflammatory Agent in Treatment of Acute Otolaryngologic Disorders. Arch. Otolaryng. 78:91, 1963.

"I have a patient who is threatened with the loss of his job as a life guard because of acute otitis externa which resists therapy that I have used successfully in other cases. My usual treatment is to identify the organism by smear and culture, clear the canal of debris and cleanse it with irrigation, and then insert carefully into the canal a cotton wick moistened with 4–8 drops of Cresatin, as antiseptic, and 1% thymol, as analgesic. After 10 minutes, I remove the wick and clear the canal of all debris. But in this case the thing has not worked satisfactorily. Can you suggest anything else?"

Reply: John Holland (Margate City, New

Jersey), after doing precisely as you do, inserts a second wick moistened with 5 8 drops of 5% solution of glacial acetic acid in 95% ethyl alcohol. This is left in for 24 hours and kept moist with VoSol Drops (propanediol diacetate, acetic acid and benzethonium in propylene glycol). He also uses concurrently, as you probably do, intensive oral therapy with antibiotics as indicated by the smear and culture procedure.

John W. Holland. Acute Otitis Externa: Etiology, Diagnosis and Management. J. M. Soc. New Jersey 59:506, 1962.

"I have a patient with otitis externa with contiguous dermatitis that is worsening despite trial of practically all of the otic medications that are currently in vogue. What do I do?"

Reply: The experience of Owen Jensen's group, at Letterman General Hospital, strikingly revealed that neomycin sensitivity is involved in many of these cases since this antibiotic is a constituent of so many of the preparations that are now in use. They were successful in handling their cases by taking the patients off of all previous medication and applying antibiotic-free corticosteroid creams and lotions.

Owen C. Jensen, Harold J. Allen and Lindley R. Mordecai. Neomycin Contact Dermatitis Superimposed on Otitis Externa. J.A.M.A. 195:131, Jan. 10, 1966.

"I have heard that pancreatic dornase has been effectively used in the treatment of otitis media. Can you cite the experience?"

Reply: Yes, as a matter of fact, Walter and Mary Loch (Johns Hopkins University), found this agent, which they used as Dornavac, more effective than antibiotic therapy, the pancreatic dornase treatment being effective in 80% of 75 patients, whereas there was only 32% success in 75 patients treated with antibiotics. Method: From 10,000 to 20,000 units of the stock solution (100,000 units in 2 ml. saline solution) were applied with a dropper or syringe into the middle ear, and after 2–3 minutes the solution and liquefied pus were removed. Best results were obtained when treatment was carried out every day or every other day.

Walter E. Loch and Mary H. Loch. Enzyme Treatment of Ear Infections: Local Use of Pancreatic Dornase. Laryngoscope 72:598, 1962.

"What drug therapy has been most effective in the treatment of acute otitis media in children?"

Reply: Of the many published studies, I like best the clear-cut one of Mark Rubenstein and associates, at the Mayo Clinic. They analyzed the treatment of 462 episodes in 449 children, most of whom had bilateral involvements. The treatments compared were penicillin alone; penicillin plus pseudoephedrine; penicillin plus triple sulfonamide; penicillin, triple sulfonamide and pseudoephedrine; tetracycline alone; tetracycline plus pseudoephedrine. The addition of pseudoephedrine had no effect on the rate of failure, recurrence or residual effects. Failures occurred in 5.8% of the children treated with penicillin, 2.7% of those treated with penicillin and triple sulfonamide, and 10.2% of those treated with tetracycline. Penicillin coupled with triple sulfonamide was therefore considered the most effective of the therapies.

Mark M. Rubenstein, James B. McBean, LeRoy D. Hedgecock and Gunnar B. Stickler. Treatment of Acute Otitis Media in Children: III. Third Clinical Trial. Am. J. Dis. Child. 109:308, 1965.

"In the postadenotonsillectomy state vomiting is a frightening and sometimes hazardous experience for a child. Has the use of antiemetic drugs been found useful and harmless?"

Reply: In 30 children undergoing adenotonsillectomy, Philip Marcus and Max Ettenberg, Boston City Hospital, gave 2 ml. (200 mg.) of trimethobenzamide (Tigan) intramuscularly immediately after induction of anesthesia, controlling the study with placebos and the double-blind method. Of the 30 children receiving the placebo 14 had symptoms of nausea and/or vomiting. Of the 30 who received the active medication, 1 had nausea but no vomiting, another had mild nausea and vomiting, and a third had marked nausea and vomiting. There were no objectionable side effects from use of the drug. So at least in this study, and with this drug, it appeared that antiemetic prophylaxis was worthwhile.

Phillip S. Marcus and Max Ettenberg. Antiemetic Prophylaxis in Adenotonsillectomies. J.A.M.A. 189:695, Aug. 31, 1964.

"In treating vertigo as an otolaryngologist, I usually have more success with antihistaminic preparations in patients who come to me on their own rather than in those who are referred by internists or general practitioners. Why is this?"

Reply: It is general experience that better results are had in patients with vertigo who also exhibit nystagmus or abnormalities of the audiogram and caloric test than in those who have no objective changes. Furthermore, you have to reckon with the fact that the placebo effect of the doctor, as doctor, is worn thin by the time the referred patient reaches you.

Adriaan J. Philipszoon (Univ. of Amsterdam). Influence of

Cinnarizine (Mitronal) on Labyrinth and on Vertigo. Clin. Pharmacol. & Therap. 3:184, 1962.

PAGET'S DISEASE OF BONE

"I have a patient with Paget's disease of the bone (osteitis deformans). Since the patient is not yet confined to bed, I felt justified in using a high calcium diet with vitamin D, but nothing has come of this. Is there any new drug that might be helpful?"

Reply: Not new, to be sure, but Peter Maurice's group, at Seton Hall College of Medicine, has obtained surprisingly good effects in a small series of patients from the use of good old aspirin in dosage of 3–6 Gm. daily for periods of 3 days to 8 months. There was said to have been a prompt and significant decrease in serum, urinary and fecal calcium, serum phosphorus and urinary and fecal magnesium. When aspirin was stopped, all values slowly returned toward control levels. In some of the patients prolonged aspirin treatment resulted in relief from bone pain and general clinical improvement, and in a patient with an advanced form of the disease involving the entire skull (with a serum alkaline phosphatase of 15 Bodansky units), a skull biopsy 3 weeks after beginning the use of 4.8 Gm. of aspirin daily showed no osteoclasts, less numerous and less active osteoblasts and less cellular marrow and the reappearance of fat cells. In explaining this rather surprising result of therapy with a drug so familiar as aspirin, the authors felt justified in returning to Paget's original thesis that osteitis deformans represents an inflammatory or perhaps an auto-immune disease of bone.

Peter F. Maurice, Theodore N. Lynch, Charles H. Bastomsky, Theodore A. Dull, Louis V. Avioli and Philip H. Henneman. Metabolic Evidence for Suppression of Paget's Disease of Bone by Aspirin. Tr. A. Am. Physicians 75:208, 1962.

PAIN

"In my practice it has seemed that anileridine (Leritine) and meperidine (Demerol) are about the same in analgesic effect, but I cannot make up my mind which is the more sedative. What has been the usual experience?"

Reply: Just what yours has been. But do not overlook the fact that both Leritine and Demerol are drugs of addiction.

"All of us are frequently asked by patients to recommend the best of the 'pain killer' preparations that they can buy in the drug store without prescription. Which of them *is* the best?"

Reply: In Baltimore, Thomas DeKornfeld and associates compared five widely advertised analgesic preparations in the following types of patient: 298 postpartums, 9 arthritics, and a group of 60 elderly patients, the latter being used only for an investigation of the amount of gastric upset caused by the drugs. The study revealed no important differences between the preparations in rapidity of onset or degree or duration of analgesia, but it did offer some evidence of a slightly higher incidence of gastric upset from Excedrin and Anacin than from Bayer aspirin, St. Joseph's aspirin or Bufferin. Bayer aspirin and St. Joseph's aspirin each contain simply the drug designated; Bufferin contains 5 gr. aspirin, 0.75 gr. aluminum glycinate and 1.5 gr. magnesium carbonate; Excedrin contains 2.25 gr. aspirin, 2.25 gr. acetophenetidin (Phenacetin) and 1 gr. caffeine; and Anacin contains 3.25 gr. aspirin, 3 gr. acetophenetidin (Phenacetin) and 0.235 gr. caffeine. The price of these preparations probably varies in different areas, but in the light of this study it appears that the cheapest would be the best.

T. J. DeKornfeld, L. Lasagna and T. M. Frazier. Comparative Study of Five Proprietary Analgesic Compounds. J.A.M.A. 182:1315, 1962.

"Several men in our hospital use phenylbutazone (Butazolidin) freely and do not seem to get into trouble with it, but is this not a fairly toxic drug?"

Reply: Side actions occur in about 40% of patients, causing discontinuance of the drug in 15%. Since some of these reactions are serious, the drug is one that cannot be used without painstaking contact with the progress of events in the individual patient. The most frequently occurring reactions in order of incidence are nausea, edema from sodium chloride retention, rash, epigastric pain, vertigo and stomatitis. The most serious reactions are reactivation of peptic ulcer, agranulocytosis, purpura, exfoliative dermatitis, psychosis, hypertension and toxic hepatitis. Other side effects, whose incidence has so far not been high, are visual disturbances; general central nervous system stimulation or the opposite, lethargy; aptyalism; fever; cardiac arrhythmia; diarrhea or stubborn constipation; megaloblastic anemia. Interestingly, more women than men have been more or less seriously affected by this drug.

E. F. Mauer. The Toxic Effects of Phenylbutazone (Butazolidin); Review of the Literature and Report of the 23rd Death Following Its Use. New England J. Med. 253:404, 1955.

"Would you kindly list the opium alkaloids and related synthetic analgesic compounds and state which of them are addictive?"

Reply: The potentially addicting ones are opium itself, morphine, codeine, Pantopon, levorphanol (Levo-Dromoran), oxymorphone (Numorphan), meperidine (Demerol, etc.), methadone (Dolophine, etc.), anileridine (Leritine), alphaprodine (Nisentil), hydromorphone (Dilaudid, Hymorphan), phenazocine (Prinadol), priminodine (Alvodine).

Those that are not potentially addicting are: dihydrocodeine (Paracodin, Drocade), dextromethorphan (Romilar, Methorate), hydrocodone (Codone, Hycodan, Dicodid), levallorphan (Lorfan) and nalorphine (Nalline).

"How do the drugs that have been introduced from time to time as substitutes for morphine in the relief of pain actually compare with it?"

Reply: First let me list the principal of these agents: meperidine (Demerol), dihydromorphinone (Dilaudid), methadone (Dolophine), levorphanol (Levo-Dromoran), anileridine (Leritine), priminodine (Alvodine), opium alkaloids (Pantopon), phenazocine (Prinadol), alphaprodine (Nisentil), oxymorphone (Numorphan). And then let me say that I am not aware of convincing evidence supporting the claims made for the striking reduction in nausea, vomiting, bronchial or biliary spasm or urinary retention that are made. An important point, which unfortunately is too little observed in connection with any of our newer drugs, is that these agents are more expensive than the classical drug. Of course if an individual has an idiosyncrasy for morphine it is very nice to know that one of these newer drugs can be substituted with full effectiveness. But it must not be forgotten that these, too, are addictive agents.

"What advantage does oxymorphone (Numorphan) have over morphine as an analgesic agent?"

Reply: None that I can see, really, unless it may be that it causes slightly less vomiting and constipation. It is probably advisable to consider it fully as addictive as morphine, though M. L. Samuels (M. D. Anderson Hospital, Houston) did report that in one of their patients, in whom they suddenly dropped dosage from 200 to 30 mg. daily, there were no severe withdrawal symptoms.

M. L. Samuels, John S. Stehlin, Sebron C. Dale and Clifton D. Howe. Critical Evaluation of Numorphan: New Synthetic Morphine-Like Alkaloid. South. M. J. 52:207, 1959.

"Recently an associate of mine was pounded by the attorney in a court case with the contention that one could not justify a single use of morphine other than for the relief of pain. Is this true?"

Reply: Morphine is certainly used almost exclusively for its analgesic action, the subsequent sleep being accepted usually as an additional beneficent action and the respiratory depression as an unavoidable and not always desirable concomitant. Occasionally, however, the drug is used primarily for the advantages bestowed by the psychic and respiratory depressions. Perhaps the best example of such employment is in the case of the pulmonary crisis of paroxysmal cardiac dyspnea, in which the slowing and deepening of respiration effected by morphine, plus its relief of the patient's excessive anxiety, are often extremely useful in the emergency. When morphine is used in preanesthetic medication, which is routine in many hospitals, it is also desired to take full advantage of the psychic and respiratory depressant actions. In the treatment of a severe acute diarrhea it is traditional to use opium in the form of its tincture or of paregoric; the morphine content of these preparations is low, to be sure, but nevertheless the constipative action is due to the morphine, and so one must list this as another nonanalgesic use of the drug.

"A patient of mine recently experienced an asthmatic type of reaction shortly after the nurse had administered a dose of morphine. Is there such a thing as true morphine allergy?"

Reply: The fact that some individuals are allergic to morphine is often disregarded with risk. Persons, such as nurses, who have developed dermatitis from frequent contact with the drug should be given it therapeutically with great caution. Some of the systemic reactions are of the asthmatic type, some manifest as circulatory collapse; in others there are hay fever–like symptoms or urticaria. In some individuals a flare of lymphangitis extends up the arm from the site of injection; this is probably evidence of local sensitiveness and does not indicate systemic allergy. Some patients faint shortly after they have been given morphine, particularly if they sit up suddenly. This also is probably not an allergic reaction but merely a reflection of greater than usual vasodilatation.

In many of the lower animals – the horse family, the cats and bears, the cow, the pig, sheep and goats – morphine is excitant instead of depressant to the central nervous system to such extent that these animals become hyperactive under its influence and may finally become delirious and go into generalized convulsions. This sort of thing is rarely but spectacularly seen in man also as a true manifestation of drug idiosyncrasy, and should not be considered to be an allergic reaction, which it is not.

"A patient with a severe head injury that has not caused unconsciousness is often very apprehensive and sometimes in considerable pain, yet one hears that morphine should not be used to give him relief; is this anything more than an old wives' tale?"

Reply: Morphine is contraindicated in head injury cases for several reasons: (1) the respiratory center is already much depressed, even though the case is one of only simple concussion, and morphine will depress it more; (2) morphine causes a slight rise in spinal fluid pressure in the normal individual and a very considerable one in the patient with a head injury (we do not know why), and increased spinal fluid pressure itself depresses the respiratory center; (3) the drug may increase the tendency toward convulsions through its stimulating action on the spinal cord; and (4) its effects on the pupils and the sensorium might mask symptoms and interfere with diagnosis. Quite an indictment!

"In a recent case of black widow spider poisoning, I found opiates very little effective in relieving the pain. The episode finally wore itself out, but what other drug might I have used with some hope of success?"

Reply: Magnesium sulfate, given intravenously in dosage of 20 ml. of 10% solution, repeated as necessary to overcome spasticity and hypertension, has been repeatedly reported upon favorably. Earlier claims of the therapeutic effectiveness of intravenously administered calcium salts do not seem to have been borne out by recent experience. The agonizing pain in this malady is principally due to generalized muscle spasm and very often a boardlike rigidity of the abdominal wall. This being the case, resort to the skeletal muscle relaxant drugs, that are discussed elsewhere in these Replies, is rational. A good many years ago J. E. Bell, Jr., and J. A. Boone reported the case of a patient who experienced quick relief from the intramuscular injection of 2 ml. of 1 : 2000 prostigmine methylsulfate and 1/150 gr. (0.4 mg.) of atropine sulfate.

Jon R. Li (Louise Obici Memorial Hospital, Suffolk, Virginia). Methocarbamol (Robaxin) in Treatment of Black Widow Spider Poisoning: Report of Case. J.A.M.A. 173:662, June 11, 1960. J. E. Bell, Jr., and J. A. Boone. Spider Bite. J.A.M.A. 129:1016, 1945.

"I have just seen the report of a fatality in an individual who had consumed, every 2 or 3 days for more than a decade, a 100 tablet bottle of a proprietary analgesic preparation containing 200 mg. per tablet of phenacetin, and I hear that there have been a few other such cases. I have not heretofore looked upon phenacetin as a dangerous drug; what about this?"

Reply: I look upon phenacetin as a valuable nonopiate analgesic agent that carries no threat of kidney damage at all to its casual user. All the individuals involved in the newly discovered nephrotoxic action of the drug have been phenacetin addicts, i.e., individuals who have been taking inordinately large amounts of the drug during a long period of time. With all of the new drugs that are coming into use, we will soon be in a sorry state if we condemn each one of them that causes trouble when it is abused. It seems to me ridiculous to be stirring up trouble for the manufacturers of proprietary preparations containing phenacetin merely because there are people who take these preparations in inordinate amounts. To be consistent, we should also attack aspirin, for this is likewise a lethal drug in overdosage. And what about alcohol, which is sanctioned and consumed excessively by some of our youth right on university campuses? We need to calm down in this country, and not ban or prohibit but educate.

"I have heard it rumored that the old familiar analgesic drug, phenacetin, may not only cause severe kidney damage but hemolytic anemia as well. Is there any truth in this?"

Reply: The only report of this sort of thing that I have seen was that of H. E. Hutchinson's group, in Glasgow, who were able to present 3 patients in whom ingestion of the drug had apparently induced hemolytic anemia. But in these cases, as in all of the cases involving kidney damage, the individuals had ingested large amounts of the drug that had no relationship to therapeutic dosage.

H. E. Hutchinson, J. M. Jackson and Patricia Cassidy. Phenacetin-Induced Hemolytic Anemia. Lancet 2:1022, Nov. 17, 1962.

"Like many of my associates, I abandoned the use of aminopyrine as analgesic many years ago because of the numerous cases of agranulocytosis that were associated with its use at that time. Now dipyrone, a drug that I understand is chemically closely related to aminopyrine, seems to be used increasingly in our area. Is this not also a dangerous drug?"

Reply: It seems to me that the answer was clearly supplied by the Ad Hoc Committee of the Food and Drug Administration, on December 1, 1964, when it delivered the opinion that the only conditions in which aminopyrine or dipyrone may possibly be indicated are febrile convulsions in children where a parenteral antipyretic may be needed; in rare instances of Hodgkin's disease; and in similar malignant diseases in which the fever cannot be controlled by any other means. It does truly seem that aminopyrine, and presumably this would be true of dipyrone also, is more effectively antipyretic than other drugs in the patient with Hodgkin's disease, whose fever sometimes incapacitates him though he is otherwise under fair control with radiation or chemotherapy; this was first shown by Paul W. Spear, at the Downstate Medical Center, in Brooklyn, in 1962. Some of the brands of aminopyrine and Dipyrone that are prescribed in the United States are the following, as listed by Charles Huguley at Emory University: *Aminopyrine*: Aminopyrine (Lilly), Amytal with aminopyrine (Lilly), Cibalgine (aminopyrine-allobarbital) (Ciba), Pyramidon (Winthrop). *Dipyrone*: Dipralon Forte (Arnar-Stone), Fevonil (Carrtone), Key-Pyrone (Key), Migesic (Misemer), Narone (Ulmer), Novaldin (Winthrop), Pydirone (Breon), Pyralgin (Savage).

Charles M. Huguley, Jr. Agranulocytosis Induced by Dipyrone, a Hazardous Antipyretic and Analgesic. J.A.M.A. 189:938, Sept. 21, 1964. Paul W. Spear. Use of Aminopyrine To Control Fever in Hodgkin's Disease. J.A.M.A. 180:970, June 16, 1962.

"Even after long years of practice I am still surprised at the different reactions of individuals to pain and the different responses I obtain through analgesic drugs. Has anyone proposed a reasonable explanation for these things?"

Reply: Apropos the part played by "circumstances" in the appreciation of pain, H. K. Beecher at Harvard has cogently remarked that the reactions to painful stimulation usually fall into one of three general groups: (a) responses of skeletal muscles; (b) reactions mediated by the autonomic nervous system; and (c) the unconscious processing of the original stimulation by the central nervous system. It is this third element, the "processing," that is most important of all because it is the intimate part of the pain experience that can really determine the presence or absence of suffering. One may assume that for a given stimulus the discharge from the sensory receptors and the afferent course of the stimulus is the same for all individuals, but the secondary response, i.e., the processing of the sensation after it reaches the brain, may be different for each individual. And it appears necessary, in the very reasonable view presented by Beecher, to face the fact that processing doubtless begins before awareness has been achieved. Once this premise is accepted it follows with complete logic that the psychic reaction, the mental process set up by the original stimulation, will depend entirely upon the individual's concept of the significance, importance and seriousness of the sensation within the framework of the moment. Past experience, memory, judgment, current distraction, all will enter into the appreciation of this "pain."

H. K. Beecher. Measurement of Subjective States. *In* (D. R. Lawrence, ed.) Quantitative Methods in Human Pharmacology & Therapeutics. N. Y., Pergamon Press, 1959, p. 98.

"I have obtained a significant pain relief in 2 cases of epididymitis through administration of 100 mg. four times daily of oxyphenbutazone (Tandearil). There have been no side effects other than mild nausea and vomiting in 1 patient. Have I just been lucky or is the drug really no more toxic than this?"

Reply: There has been a pretty high incidence of side effects when the drug is used in the treatment of rheumatic disorders and some of them have been quite serious. In R. G. Robinson's 129 patients, in Sydney, side effects occurred in 39.5% and were severe enough to warrant discontinuing the therapy in 14.7%. However, his dosage was 600 mg. daily instead of the 400 you have been using. When using your dosage, Gerald Schwarz (Portland, Oregon) observed side effects in 14% of 300 patients.

Gerald R. Schwarz. Long Term Evaluation of Oxyphenbutazone (Tandearil) in Rheumatic Disorders. Northwest Med. 61:927, 1962. R. G. Robinson. Oxyphenbutazone (Tandearil) in Rheumatic Disease. M. J. Australia 2:49, July 14, 1962.

"I have a patient in whom it seems that aspirin in ordinary dosage induces symptoms of hypoglycemia. Has such a thing been noted by others?"

Reply: Yes, this fact has been known for many years. Indeed, one should be cautious in using high salicylate dosage in diabetics for this reason. Shortly before his untimely death, Reid had been able to show that a short intensive course of aspirin lowers fasting blood sugar and leads to a disappearance of glycosuria and reduction of ketonuria in mild to moderately severe diabetes, clinical remission coinciding with biochemical improvement. Unfortunately, the diabetic symptoms are replaced by the annoying and often prohibitive side effects that develop with the serum salicylate levels required to control blood sugar.

George A. Limbech, Rogelio H. A. Ruvalcaba, Ellis Samols and Vincent C. Kelley. Salicylates and Hypoglycemia. Am. J. Dis. Child. 109:165, 1965. J. Reid and T. D. Lightbody. The Insulin Equivalence of Salicylate. Brit. M. J. 1:897, 1959.

"Salicylates are well known to produce tinnitus, hearing loss and vertigo when they are taken in excessive dosage. Has the hearing loss ever been known to persist after the drug is discontinued?"

Reply: The occurrence must be extremely rare. In the only report of such an instance that I have seen, that of Kapur in India, a 13-year-old boy developed hearing difficulty on the very day he took 2 tablets of aspirin, which was borne out by the history of the patient, by the parents and by the school teacher. The case was interesting in that there were no signs of idiosyncrasy to the drug other than the hearing loss and dizziness for 2 days; and the hearing loss persisted in moderately severe degree.

Y. P. Kapur. Ototoxicity of Acetylsalicylic Acid. Arch. Otolaryng. 81:134, 1965.

"A very simple question: What dosage of aspirin should be prescribed for relief of the common headache of the stress, fatigue or 'toxic' type?"

Reply: I think that nothing should be done to disabuse the lay mind of the belief that 10 gr. is the upper limit of aspirin dosage that should be taken, since many undisciplined individuals take a second or third dose ("a couple of aspirins") an hour or so after the first dose if they do not quickly obtain a complete disappearance of the pain, or may even take a third dose. But actually it is doubtful that 10 gr. is really the ideal dosage for common analgesic effect. We give 15 or 20 gr. for analgesic and antiphlogistic action in the rheumatic disorders, and I see no reason why we should not do so for the relief of less specific discomfort; but we must prescribe the drug as acetylsalicylic acid when doing this and have the prescription clearly marked "not to be repeated under 4 hours."

"In my practice I have been using phenylazodiamino-pyridine (Pyridium) freely as an analgesic in pain associated with infection in the urinary tract and have never encountered any difficulty with it. Could it be that there is trouble just around the corner?"

Reply: Until a short time ago I would have answered in the negative, but now I have seen two reports of hemolytic anemia associated with use of the drug, so this should engender caution.

E. Peter Gabor, Louis Lowenstein and Nannie K. M. de Leeuw (McGill Univ.). Hemolytic Anemia Induced by Phenylazodiamino-Pyridine (Pyridium). Canad. M. A. J. 91:756, Oct. 3, 1964. Mortimer S. Greenberg and Helena Wong. (Harvard Med. School) Methemoglobinemia and Heinz Body Hemolytic Anemia Due to Phenazopyridine Hydro-Chloride (Pyridium). New England. J. Med. 271: 431, Aug. 27, 1964.

"One of my associates has been using Dolonil effectively for relief of urinary distress after instrumentation or removal of an indwelling catheter. Was not this preparation discarded some years ago because of toxicity?"

Reply: No, that is not correct. One of its ingredients, Pyridium, was displaced some time ago as a urinary antiseptic by the sulfonamides and antibiotics; it has been revived recently as an analgesic, however, and that explains its presence in this mixture. The other ingredients in Dolonil are l-hyoscyamine and butabarbital; the latter of course may be habit forming, but not likely under the circumstances in which your colleague is using the preparation. Hyoscyamine overdosage would be manifested by belladonna-like symptoms. It is recommended that Dolonil be not used if there is renal and hepatic disease, glaucoma, bladder neck obstruction or of course known sensitivities to either the belladonna drugs or the barbiturates. The urine will be colored orange-red by the preparation.

"What is the comparative analgesic effectiveness of aspirin and salicylamide?"

Reply: In New York, Alfred Vignec and Mary Gasparik compared the two drugs in 512 pediatric patients whose initial temperatures were over 101° F. and whose physical findings justified an initial trial of antipyretic measures alone. They were unable to determine any qualitative difference between the two drugs, but this report has been somewhat severely criticized; and as a matter of fact the earlier literature was rather conflicting. In any case, the oral preparations, Dropsprin and Liquiprin, are superior to aspirin in ease of administration, acceptability and control of dosage in children. There is some evidence, however, that the rapidity of absorption and elimination of salicylamide make it more difficult to maintain at an effective therapeutic level than aspirin. A report which caught my eye a few years ago, that of L. J. Boyd and associates, was to the effect that 250 mg. of salicylamide and 100 mg. of phenacetin together form an effective hypnotic combination. Their series of patients was small, and I have heard nothing further of this, but Frank Berger (Wallace Laboratories) had earlier reported a similar unexpected finding in mice.

Alfred J. Vignec and Mary Gasparik. Antipyretic Effectiveness of Salicylamide and Acetylsalicylic Acid in Infants: Comparative Study. J.A.M.A. 167:1821, Aug. 9, 1958. L. J. Boyd, W. Gittinger and J. Schwimmer. Sleep Induction with Combined Administration of Salicylamide and

Acetophenetidin. New York J. Med. 57:924, 1957. F. M. Berger. Hypnotic Action Resulting from Combined Administration of Salicylamide and Acetophenetidin. Proc. Soc. Exper. Biol. & Med. 87:449, 1954.

"I am confused in the matter of aspirin's role in the causation of gastrointestinal bleeding and anemia. Could you sketch the record?"

Reply: Evidence has been piling up steadily through the years since Douthwaite, in 1938, first drew attention to the matter, that there is a likely association of salicylate ingestion with gastric hemorrhage. Of Muir and Cossar's (England) 106 patients hospitalized with gastroduodenal hemorrhage, 53% admitted having taken aspirin within 48 hours of their initial bleeding, whereas only 17% of another group of the same size who were without hemorrhage had done so. At the Central Middlesex Hospital, London, Alvarez and Summerskill were able to incriminate salicylates in over 40% of the 103 consecutive patients hospitalized with hematemesis and/or melena associated with peptic ulcer. But the lesion induced by salicylate was difficult to define at gastroscopy or at partial gastrectomy. The clinical history, with findings at emergency partial gastrectomy, indicated that acute erosions in the stomach (and possibly lower in the gastrointestinal tract) were sometimes responsible, although activation of a pre-existing chronic peptic ulcer seemed likely in many instances. In about 50% of patients there was some occult blood loss in the stools when they were taking salicylates whether or not they had a peptic ulcer or an x-ray negative dyspepsia; but the more prone to massive hemorrhage were patients with previous history of dyspepsia. In contrast, nonsalicylate analgesics did not influence the stool occult blood content. This aspirin-promoted bleeding is quite apart from the drug's prothrombin-lowering action. Perhaps a third of the patients given sufficiently high aspirin dosage to accomplish a plasma titer of 30–35 mg./100 ml. experience a drop of prothrombin concentration below 75% of normal, but a fall to the dangerously low level of 20% of normal occurs very rarely and is probably due to hypersensitivity when it does. The nature of this action is undetermined; it is not elicited in vitro and appears to be associated with blockage of vitamin K utilization. Routine employment of vitamin K when aspirin is used for ordinary analgesic purposes is devoid of rationale, but when surgical procedures are proposed in individuals on high salicylate dosage, it is probably advisable to give 1 mg. of vitamin K/Gm. of salicylate; of course if there is liver damage much higher vitamin K dosage will be required.

The above evidence is all pretty "scary," and has caused some men to become rather reluctant to prescribe aspirin, at least as freely as they did formerly. However, I think it only fair to call to your attention the study of Baragar and Duthie (Edinburgh), who reported that patients with rheumatoid arthritis can tolerate regular aspirin without an increase in anemia. They felt that the dangers of causing peptic ulceration or precipitating gastrointestinal hemorrhage with aspirin appear to have been greatly exaggerated. I do think, however, that one should never fail to investigate the matter of aspirin ingestion in a patient who presents with melena.

F. D. Baragar and J. J. R. Duthie. Importance of Aspirin as Cause of Anemia and Peptic Ulcer in Rheumatoid Arthritis. Brit. M. J. 1:1106, Apr. 9, 1960. F. Norman Vickers and Malcolm M. Stanley. Aspirin Gastritis: Gastroduodenoscopic Observations – Four Case Reports. Gastroenterology 44:419, 1963. John R. Kiser. Chronic Gastric Ulcer Associated with Aspirin Ingestion: Report of Five Cases and Review of Literature. Am. J. Digest. Dis. 8:856, 1963. Norman Pomerantz, Julian B. Hyman, Margaret S. N. Lai and Robert Wallach. Hemorrhagic Diathesis Due to Salicylate-Induced Hypoprothrombinemia. New York J. Med. 64:795, Mar. 15, 1964. A. S. Alvarez and W. H. J. Summerskill. Gastrointestinal Hemorrhage and Salicylates. Lancet 2:920, Nov. 1, 1958. A. Muir and I. A. Cossar. Aspirin and Gastric Haemorrhage. Lancet 1:539, 1959.

"Here is a simple question. When you want to avail yourself of the analgesic effect of a salicylate what drug do you use?"

Reply: The simple answer is aspirin of couse. The alleged superiority of none of the newer preparations is convincingly established and they are more expensive. If you suspect that aspirin is causing some gastrointestinal bleeding, then have it taken immediately after meals or with a large amount of water. And if your patient does not like or really cannot swallow the tablet he can easily place the latter in the bowl of a spoon and crush it under the bowl of another spoon and mix it with his jam or honey.

"What is acceptable analgesic and antipyretic dosage of aspirin for children?"

Reply: Average child of 15 pounds at 6 months, four doses of 150 mg. (2½ grains) to total 0.6 Gm. (10 grains) during the 24 hours; for the average 1 year old of 20 pounds, four doses of 200 mg. (3 grains) to total 0.8 Gm. (12 grains); for the average 2 year old of 26 pounds, four doses of 250 mg. (4 grains) to total 1 Gm. (16 grains); for the average 3 year old of about 30 pounds, four doses of 300 mg. (5 grains) to total 1.3 Gm. (20 grains); and for the average 7 year old of about 50 pounds, four doses of 500 mg. (7½ grains) to total 2.0 Gm. (30 grains).

"Sometimes in dermatologic practice we encounter very distressful situations, such as the neurogenic type of pain in herpes zoster and the severe itching, burning pain and paresthesia in extensive dermatoses, in which we need to give the patient rest from his suffering but do not dare to use the opiates, and unfortunately the non-opiate analgesics are usually ineffective under these circumstances. Can you suggest anything?"

Reply: Try tetraethylammonium chloride (Etamon) in dosage up to 20 mg./kg., injecting half into each buttock and giving two or three injections daily. Procaine solution, 1 ml. of 2%, may be added to lessen the pain of intramuscular injection. But be careful. A precipitous drop in blood pressure may occur, especially in a hypertensive individual, with accompanying nausea, vomiting, sweating, pallor and temporary peripheral circulatory collapse. Caution is also advisable in nonhypertensives with an excessively labile sympathetic nervous system. Elderly individuals are prone to develop delayed blood pressure falls of a secondary nature. Patients often notice a metallic taste and disturbances in visual accommodation. In those with peptic ulcer history, typical ulcer pain may be caused, probably as an expression of imbalance in the two portions of the autonomic nervous system. Sometimes the injections cause weakness, sleepiness, dyspnea, lightheadedness, difficulty in performing voluntary movements and in urinating, and fasciculation of muscles. Neostigmine (Prostigmin), in dosage of 1–2 ml. of 1 : 2000 solution is a logical antidote to this drug rather than epinephrine, levarterenol (Levophed) and metaraminol (Aramine) because the compensatory reflexes available to combat the acute rise in blood pressure induced by these adrenergic agents are blocked by the Etamon.

"A dermatologist in our office building has been using hydroxyzine (Vistaril) intravenously for some time instead of procaine to produce a certain measure of local anesthesia, at least to allay the patient's anxiety and apprehension and reduce hypermotility, when performing simple office procedures that are painful. Is this an entirely safe practice?"

Reply: "Entirely safe" is of course a great deal to say of any therapeutic measure, and in the present instance I should think that the patient should be warned against possible sleepiness and the consequent undesirability of driving his car for a few hours after the dose has been injected. However, Theodore Cornbleet (University of Illinois) says that his patients leave the office within 30–60 minutes, apparently without drowsiness. He injects slowly intravenously a solution of 25–50 mg. hydroxyzine in two to three times as much saline or water; for children aged 3–4 years, 10 mg.; 15 mg. for a child aged 12. He finds his patient relaxed and ready for simple dermatologic procedures within 10 minutes.

Theodore Cornbleet. Use of Intravenously Given Hydroxyzine (Vistaril) for Simple Pain-Producing Office Procedures. J.A.M.A. 172:56, Jan. 2, 1960.

"Could one hope to gain anything through giving morphine by continuous intravenous drip rather than intermittent injections in an individual with terminal malignancy?"

Reply: Yes, one could. As long ago as 1941, Neuhoff ascribed remarkable analgesic action to a continuous intravenous drip of morphine and said that there was almost complete absence of the other and objectionable effects of the drug; but for some reason the method has not been given much trial. Morphine sulfate, in an amount of 40 mg., is added to 1000 ml. of physiologic saline solution, and 100 ml. of this solution (containing 4 mg. of morphine) is given intravenously/hour continuously; of course for a patient already addicted the dosage would doubtless have to be raised considerably.

H. Neuhoff. The Continuous Intravenous Administration of Morphine After Operation. J. Mt. Sinai Hosp. 7:601, 1941.

"Would you kindly make a brief statement of opinion of some of the trade-named nonopiate analgesics that are considerably prescribed in some practices?"

Reply: *Darvon* (dextropropoxyphene) appears to have analgesic properties lying somewhere between those of aspirin and codeine and certainly has the advantage over the latter of not requiring compliance with the antinarcotic laws in prescribing it. It is available alone and in combinations with other analgesics and with tranquilizers (*Darvon Compound* has propoxyphene [a tranquilizer], aspirin, phenacetin and caffeine; in Darvon Compound-65 there is also codeine). *Dipralon Forte* contains two established analgesics, salicylamide and acetaminophen; there is also some ascorbic acid and dipyrone. The presence of the latter agent makes the preparation unacceptable to me because dipyrone is sufficiently closely related to aminopyrine to make one think of the possibility of inducing agranulocytosis when the mixture is used. *Equagesic* is promoted for treatment of pain accompanied by anxiety and tension. The patient should be instructed to take no more than 2 tablets at a time, because if you double the amount of meprobamate (Miltown, Equanil) and aspirin that the preparation contains you will still be within safe therapeutic limits, but doubling the content of ethoheptazine (Zactane), the other ingredient, would give a dosage higher than that usually recommended for this agent when it is used alone. *Ropad* is proposed for treatment of fibrositis, neuritis, bursitis, gout and allied conditions; in addition to aluminum hydroxide and ascorbic acid it contains aspirin and dexamethasone (Decadron, etc.). Certainly* the full corticosteroid precautions and contraindications should be in mind when using the mixture. Salicylamide, which is available as *Dropsprin, Liquiprin*, etc., has been found by manufacturers to be a good aspirin substitute because, being less reactive than aspirin, it can be combined with numerous other agents and offered in very palatable preparations. The drug's side actions and toxicities probably differ little from those of aspirin but there does not seem to be aspirin's effect on prothrombin time, though such effect appears even with aspirin usually only in high dosage. I do not think that the ability to substitute salicylamide for aspirin in all situations has been fully established, though it is true that individuals who are sensitized to aspirin can sometimes take the new drug with safety. Sodium gentisate, which is available as *Gensalate, Gentasol, Gentisan, Na-Gent* and *Casate*, is a salt of a metabolite of the salicylates. It is a very acceptable analgesic that is often well tolerated for months, but a thing that appears to have militated against its general acceptance is the fact that it is so rapidly eliminated that more frequent administration is necessary than is usually acceptable. Choline salicylate (*Actasal, Arthropan* and calcium acetylsalicylate carbamide (*Calurin*) are aspirin substitutes which are alleged to provide the doubtful advantage of a few minutes quicker onset of action through more rapid absorption than the classical drug. To me they simply pose the question of whether you want your patient to pay more for his aspirin or not. *Soma Compound* is a mixture of carisoprodol (Soma, Rela), phenacetin, caffeine and codeine, for use where pain is somewhat compounded by skeletal muscle tension; of course it carries the slight toxic potentialities of each of its ingredients. *Trancoprin* and *Trancogesic* are tablets containing the tranquilizer, chlormezanone (Trancopal) and aspirin, a logical combination when pain is aggravated by skeletal muscle tension (*if* Trancopal really has the muscle-relaxant properties that have been claimed for it). Acetaminophen is simply the analgesic metabolite of phenacetin; it is currently enjoying some vogue as *Dialog*, in which it is combined with a barbiturate to provide the relaxing properties it lacks. Two preparations having heavy advertising play just now are *Fiorinal* and *Phenaphen with Codeine*. The former contains a barbiturate, aspirin, phenacetin and caffeine, and is probably just about as effective as the other combinations of these ingredients. The latter replaces the caffeine with hyoscyamine, and its contained codeine would surely give it greater analgesic potency but at the price of course of requiring narcotic prescription.

PANCREATITIS

"In a case of acute pancreatitis, should I use anticholinergic agents such as propantheline (Pro-Banthine), etc.?"

Reply: Well, since the essence of the therapy in this severe malady is to promote in every way possible a state of quiescence in the pancreas, the three most logical therapeutic approaches are to allay the anxiety of the patient through the use of sedatives (and of course analgesics to diminish the pain as much as possible), the use of continuous suction to prevent accumulation of acid in the stomach and thus reduce secretin release, and the inhibition of pancreatic secretion through direct drug action as nearly as that can be accomplished. Nothing will promote this latter objective any better than the anticholinergic agents, but the best is none too good. The trouble is that the high dosage necessary to produce a really effective blocking of secretions is likely to introduce very objectionable side actions of this group of drugs. Of course if the patient is really seriously affected, i.e., if the attack of pancreatitis is a very fulminating one, he will be in shock and that will require prompt and full treatment as well.

"Most of the reviews of therapy in acute pancreatitis have come from University-affiliated hospitals in which there have been planned programs of therapy under evaluation, but such findings are not always applicable to the conditions of private practice. Are you aware of a study of the use of corticosteroids in private hospitals?"

Reply: Yes, Kaplan's group has reviewed the use of corticosteroids in 15 patients at Touro Infirmary, in New Orleans, who had failed to respond to routine therapy. In each of these cases there was a dramatic response to steroid therapy. In general, 100–200 mg. hydrocortisone was given intravenously every 6–8 hours for 2–3 days or until the acute illness subsided. Dosage was then reduced and gradually withdrawn over 10 days or longer. ACTH was used in conjunction with corticosteroids in 2 of the patients. The only survivors from hemorrhagic pancreatitis were steroid-treated patients; 4 of the 9 in this group survived. Indications for corticosteroid therapy were felt to be: hemorrhagic pancreatitis, postoperative cases and patients with acute edematous pancreatitis who do not respond within 12–24 hours to routine management. Adequate fluid and blood replacement and other supportive measures should of course be included in the regimen. Myself, I would use corticosteroids only in desperation, for these agents can themselves cause pancreatitis.

Murrel H. Kaplan, Alvin M. Cotlar and Samuel J. Stagg. Acute Pancreatitis: Six-Year Survey with Evaluation of Steroid Therapy. Am. J. Surg. 108:24, 1964.

"I have a patient with chronic relapsing pancreatitis, who requires meperidine (Demerol) to accomplish at least partial control of his pain. But he has now developed hallucinations, which I have not heretofore experienced as a reaction to this drug. Could the occurrence be a manifestation of the disease itself?"

Reply: Yes, it could. Marvin Schuster and Frank Iber, Baltimore City Hospital, found transient hallucinations appearing more frequently in their 30 patients with relapsing pancreatitis than any of the commonly accepted complications, such as diabetes, pancreatic insufficiency and pancreatic calcifications.

Marvin M. Schuster and Frank L. Iber. Psychosis with Pancreatitis. Arch. Int. Med. 116:228, 1965.

"I have a patient with chronic pancreatitis whose steatorrhea is being treated with restriction of dietary fat and use of pancreatic enzymes. Which of the latter preparations is most likely to be effective?"

Reply: I have seen no published study that would supply a convincing answer to your question. The principal preparations available are pancreatin (Panopsin, Stamyl), Cotazym, Enzypan, Festal, Panteric and Viokase. Enzypan and Festal contain bile salts in addition to the pancreatic enzymes, amylase, trypsin and lipase, which may sometimes relieve the bloating. On principle, I should avoid the enteric-coated among these preparations because some of these may pass through the intestinal tract without dissolution.

"A few years ago oxyphenbutazone (Tandearil) was found very beneficial in experimentally induced pancreatitis in dogs. Has this been put to the test in man?"

Reply: Yes, in Richmond, Virginia, Benjamin Weisiger and Albert Wasserman gave the drug a sufficiently extensive double-blind trial and found it to be not in the least helpful.

Benjamin B. Weisiger and Albert J. Wasserman. Oxyphenbutazone in Pancreatitis. J.A.M.A. 195:121, Jan. 3, 1966.

PARKINSONISM

"In my cases of parkinsonism I have used trihexyphenidyl (Artane) with good results in most instances, but control with the drug always decreases after a while. Has the newer drug, orphenadrine (Disipal) been found any more satisfactory?"

Reply: In Stockholm, R. R. Strang made comparative trial of the two drugs in 43 geriatric parkinsonism patients. Twenty-three patients considered that the overall results of orphenadrine were superior, 9 preferred trihexyphenidyl and 11 were unable to differentiate. Of the latter, 5 stated that neither drug was effective and 6 said both were equally so. Artane caused side effects sufficient to discontinue the drug, or produced less than an optimal clinical effect, in 40% of the patients while orphenadrine did so in only 12%. However, the development of tolerance to orphenadrine, as in the case of trihexyphenidyl, may be expected to occur in most cases after 2 or 3 years.

R. R. Strang. A Comparative Study of Trihexyphenidyl (Artane) and Orphenadrine (Disipal) in the Treatment of Geriatric Parkinsonism. J. Am. Geriatrics Soc. 13:756, 1965.

"I have heard that the antihypertensive drugs are to some extent effective in relieving the symptoms of parkinsonism, but I have not succeeded with them myself. Do you know anything of this?"

Reply: I do not know of any claim for the antihypertensives as a group, but I have seen the report of Marsh and associates (London) who, in a double-blind trial in a small group of patients, found methyldopa (Aldomet) in daily dosage of 1–1.5 Gm. for 1 week useful in diminishing tremor in most patients. There was no effect on rigidity, and the drowsiness and depression that were the main side effects of the therapy could of course be undesirable in this malady. There is, however, fairly sound basis for trial of this agent because it inhibits dopamine and 5-hydroxytryptamine, and the latter produces tremor in cats under experimental conditions; and in mice such tremor has been inhibited by pretreatment with α-methyldopa. The effect on tremor in human parkinsonism is quite interesting since it is the opposite of what is achieved with the principally used compounds, namely the anticholinergics, whose effect is principally on rigidity.

D. O. Marsh, H. Schnieden and John Marshall. Controlled Clinical Trial of α-Methyldopa in Parkinsonian Tremor. J. Neurol. Neurosurg. & Psychiat. 26:505, 1963.

"Of course we do not have specific therapy in parkinsonism, but there is a large number of drugs that provide symptomatic relief of some degree in many cases. However, one sometimes wonders in the individual case whether one is making full use of all that is available, and would be grateful for a compact list of the drugs that may be tried in their several categories. Is such a list available?"

Reply: There have been many such listings, but they all manage to get themselves lost somehow with the passage of time. The following is the compilation I prepared for the 1962–63 Year Book of Drug Therapy; it is still up-to-date.

Belladonna alkaloids: atropine; tinctures of belladonna, stramonium and hyoscyamus; Bellabulgara; Vinobel; Bellafoline; Bellal; Donna Extentabs; Novadonna solution; scopolamine; stramonium; Rabellon (hyoscyamine, atropine and scopolamine); Prydon Spansules (atropine, scopolamine and hyoscyamine).

Synthetic belladonna substitutes: trihexyphenidyl (Artane); caramiphen (Panparnit); ethopropazine (Parsidol); cycrimine (Pagitane); benztropine (Cogentin); procyclidine (Kemadrin); biperiden (Akineton).

Antihistaminics: principally used have been diphenhydramine (Benadryl); phenindamine (Thephorin); orphenadrine (Disipal); chlorphenoxamine (Phenoxene).

"We have recently had a patient in our clinic who developed an acute brain syndrome while on standard antiparkinsonism therapy with the addition of diphenylhydantoin (Dilantin), the symptoms disappearing within 48 hours when all therapy was withdrawn. I am aware that the antiparkinsonism agents might themselves have been responsible for the observed reaction, but could diphenylhydantoin have contributed?"

Reply: In New York, Bernard Swerdlow has reported 2 cases, in at least 1 of which it appeared that diphenylhydantoin alone was responsible for an acute brain syndrome.

Bernard Swerdlow. Am. J. Psychiat. 122:100, 1965.

PAROXYSMAL NOCTURNAL HEMOGLOBINURIA

"I have a patient with paroxysmal nocturnal hemoglobinuria in whom it appears that parenteral iron therapy has increased hemolysis. Has such a thing actually been recorded?"

Reply: Yes, at Duke University, Charles Mengel's group reported 4 patients in which this appeared to be the case. It is felt by students of the subject that in this malady, which is characterized by accelerated intravascular hemolysis during sleep, the defect is probably an abnormal red blood cell stroma. Mengel feels that in this situation the administration of iron might initiate lysis of erythrocytes that may contain increased amounts of arachidonic and pentanoic acids and reduced amounts of oleic acid. Not a real explanation of course but an interesting hypothesis.

Charles E. Mengel, Herbert E. Kann, Jr., and Bert W. O'Malley. Increased Hemolysis after Intramuscular Iron Administration in Patients with Paroxysmal Nocturnal Hemoglobinuria: Report of Six Occurrences in Four Patients and Speculations on Possible Mechanism. Blood 26:74, 1965.

PEMPHIGUS

"One is accustomed to obtaining fairly good results in selected cases of pemphigus through use of corticosteroids, but it is practically always necessary to raise the dosage to the point of inducing typical cushingoid symptoms. Is there any remedy for this?"

Reply: In Hungary, Imre Csoka and Elisabeth Vadasz reported that in 2 out of 5 cases of pemphigus they were able to reduce the required dose of prednisolone and ACTH though the daily intramuscular administration of 10 mg. of desoxycorticosterone acetate (DOCA).

Imre E. Csoka and Elisabeth K. Vadasz. The Use of Desoxycorticosterone Acetate (DOCA) in the Management of Pemphigus. Acta dermat-1 venereol. 45:59, 1965.

PEPTIC ULCER

"Would you please discuss the rationale of using the anticholinergic agents in the treatment of peptic ulcer?"

Reply: Since physiologists hold that pain fibers in the gastrointestinal tract are insensitive to chemical stimuli, and the introduction of acid into the stomach of ulcer patients nevertheless causes pain though it arouses no sensation in normal individuals, it must be conceded that pain in peptic ulcer results from stimulation by acid of afferent nerves in the ulcer base — unless, however, the stimulation of these nerves by acid initiates motor activity reflexly, and the motor activity causes the pain. Palmer's group performed a study of the matter in active peptic ulcer cases which caused them to deny the latter possibility and to postulate that the only circumstance in which cholinergic blocking drugs may be expected to relieve pain is when they decrease the rate of gastric emptying. Thus there could be hope of effecting relief with such drugs only in duodenal, but never in gastric, ulcer. This viewpoint has gained rather general clinical acceptance, except that many physicians would like to look upon the relief sometimes associated with the use of atropine in ulcer as due to prolongation of gastric emptying time *and* reduction of the volume of gastric secretion. In the experimental animal — the dog is used almost universally in this work — stomach motility and gastric secretory responses of all types are depressed fairly uniformly, but the necessary dosage is usually above what might be considered therapeutic.

W. L. Palmer, F. Vansteenhuyse and J. B. Kirsner. Peptic Ulcer: Effect of Anticholinergic Drugs on Mechanism of Pain. Am. J. M. Sc. 224:603, 1952.

"May one construe the effect sometimes achieved with the anticholinergic agents in peptic ulcer as truly effecting actual healing of the ulcers?"

Reply: Certainly not. Indeed, several years ago Clarence W. Legerton (Charleston, South Carolina) rather cogently made the point, citing representative cases, that these drugs may sometimes be harmful through reducing the distress and episodes that might otherwise have demanded more definitive remedial attention.

Clarence W. Legerton, Jr. Anticholinergic Anesthesia. South. M. J. 52:927, 1959.

"I think that most of us use anticholinergic agents in many of our cases of peptic ulcer, but the profusion of these preparations made available by the pharmaceutical houses, and their rather pleading promotion in the advertising pages, make one wonder about the true worth of the compounds. What is your opinion of their value in this therapy?"

Reply: The last time I made count of the synthetic anticholinergics officially available there were 28 of them, and several have been added since that time. This fact alone should make one skeptical of their value; at least it may be taken to mean that the competing manufacturers are endeavoring to win acceptance for the product which they feel is superior to all the others. Now since these drugs are all actually effective inhibitors of acid secretion, the thing for which their promotors are vying must be something else. And it is, namely, lesser toxicity. For the hitch in all of this is that these compounds are all atropine-like in their action and share with atropine the toxic proclivities of anticholinergic action. One sometimes sees the opinion expressed in reviews that none of the synthetic compounds is superior to the belladonna alkaloids in inhibiting either basal secretion of gastric acid or reducing the mean acidity of the gastric contents after the taking of food, but I think it doubtful that such a viewpoint is entirely justified, for some of them do seem to perform a bit better in these respects. But they have their toxic side actions. Many of us remember the great stir that was made by methantheline (Banthine) when it came upon the market some years ago, but now one very rarely hears the horn being blown for it in competition with the newer congeners. Are they better? I doubt it. It seems to me that they are just newer and that one can expect to have the same experience with all of them, namely, that the patient will be helped by their use if he is not made too uncomfortable by their overactions.

Robert D. Mitchell, J. N. Hunt and Morton I. Grossman (Los Angeles). Inhibition of Basal and Postprandial Gastric Secretion by Poldine (Nacton) and Atropine in Patients with Peptic Ulcer. Gastroenterology 43:400, 1962.

"I have a patient with duodenal ulcer in whom I should like to try the effect of prolonged achlorhydria, but I do not seem able to accomplish this with oral anticholinergic drugs. Has there been favorable experience with intramuscular injection?"

Reply: At Lenox Hill Hospital (New York), Kasich and associates tried several of the synthetic anticholinergics intramuscularly and did accomplish a prolonged period of achlorhydria. Injections were made at 6 hour intervals; this would hardly be practicable, I should think, under most circumstances. There is available a 30 mg. ampule of propantheline bromide (Pro-Banthine), which is the dose that was used by these investigators.

Anthony M. Kasich, Harry D. Fein, Austin P. Boleman, Jr., and Lestra Carpe. Prolonged Achlorhydria in Duodenal Ulcer from Intramuscular Administration of Anticholinergic Drugs. Am. J. Digest. Dis. 7:886, 1962.

"Numerous drugs available nowadays, and much prescribed, contain silicates. Has any harm come from putting so much silicon as this into the body economy?"

Reply: I have seen only one report, that of a kidney stone composed of pure silicon dioxide in a patient who, for 2 or 3 years, had been taking 30–35 tablets daily of a preparation containing 0.5 Gm. magnesium trisilicate and 0.25 Gm. aluminum hydroxide. It is surprising that enough of the "nonabsorbable" magnesium trisilicate could have gotten into the system to produce this stone, but apparently that was the case.

John R. Herman and Aaron S. Goldberg (Albert Einstein College of Medicine). New Type of Urinary Calculus Caused by Antacid Therapy. J.A.M.A. 174:1206, Oct. 29, 1960.

"There are so many antacids available nowadays that I have lost my way among them. Will you please give me a statement of their respective merits and demerits?"

Reply: SODIUM BICARBONATE, the laymen's beloved baking soda, is really not a very good antacid. The effect is not long lasting and therefore usual dosage is 1–2 Gm. to take care of the acid present at the moment and that to accumulate shortly. The result of such dosage is evolution of considerable carbon dioxide, which may be dangerous. Furthermore, the likelihood is great that some of the agent will be absorbed and provoke systemic alkalosis, and the patient's pain may be aggravated, after the period of initial relief, by the physiologic acid rebound provoked by such a strongly alkaline agent. Sodium bicarbonate in large doses also alkalinizes the urine and occasionally causes precipitation of crystalline phosphates in the pelvis of the kidney, the ureter and the bladder.

MAGNESIUM OXIDE. In 1 Gm. dosage this agent is more effective than sodium bicarbonate in neutralizing acid, but it is likely to be cathartic and there is some release of carbon dioxide. Systemic alkalosis is not caused by this drug.

MILK OF MAGNESIA. This preparation is an approximately 8% aqueous suspension of magnesium hydroxide. It is less effective as antacid than magnesium oxide and likely to be cathartic in dosage greater than 1 teaspoonful. It does not cause systemic alkalinization.

MAGNESIUM TRISILICATE. This drug, slower and more prolonged in action than sodium bicarbonate, neutralizes slightly more acid than the latter in the same dosage. Furthermore, a gelatinous compound, silicon dioxide, is formed which protectively coats the ulcer crater to some extent and also has absorbent properties. Dosage is 1–4 Gm. before meals. Carbon dioxide liberation does not occur nor is there absorption to cause systemic alkalinization; catharsis is caused only by very high dosage usually. This compound is much used together with aluminum hydroxide, in such preparations as *Gelusil, Trisogel* and many others that are available in suspension and tablet formulations.

CALCIUM CARBONATE reacts with hydrochloric acid to form calcium or magnesium chloride, carbon dioxide and water. Average dosage is 1 Gm. In a comparative study of biochemical and economic considerations with regard to antacids, Brody and Bachrach concluded that calcium carbonate is the antacid of choice if care is taken to prevent constipation, and if there is no predisposition to alkalosis, depression of renal function or development of renal lithiasis. This drug is much prescribed as *Titralac*, in both tablet and liquid forms, in which there are present other ingredients to protect against constipation; *Alkets Tablet* is a somewhat similar preparation.

ALUMINUM HYDROXIDE (AMPHOJEL; CREAMALIN, ETC.), MAGNESIUM ALUMINUM HYDROXIDE (MAALOX) AND ALUMINUM PHOSPHATE (PHOSPHALJEL) are preparations with a high acid-combining power, some astringency (constriction of the mucosa), some ability to coat the ulcer surface, some adsorptive power and actually some inhibiting action on pepsin. Unlike the carbonates, they do not liberate large quantities of carbon dioxide and they are not laxative as magnesium trisilicate tends to be; indeed, aluminum hydroxide is even constipating, but the phosphate gel is less so and the magnesium aluminum hydroxide perhaps not at all. They are not absorbed into the systemic circulation and they do not cause acid rebound in the stomach or significantly affect the absorption of nutrients; but they do interfere strikingly with the absorption of tetracycline antibiotics. The effects of these agents, which are often successfully employed when others have failed, are more slowly achieved than are those of sodium bicarbonate.

Dosage is 1–2 teaspoonfuls stirred up in half a glass of water or milk at 2 hour intervals throughout the day and three times as much at bedtime, or the equivalent in tablets. The patient who has severe night pain associated with continuous night secretion may have his bedtime dose repeated at midnight and again at 3 a.m. In some instances one or other of the compounds, in 1% suspension, is continuously instilled through a nasal gastric tube at the rate of 15 drops per minute, day and night, for an average period of 10 days.

The phosphate is preferred to the hydroxide preparation by some men because dog studies have shown that hydroxide interferes with phosphate absorption over long periods. However, it is not proved that the ulcer patient maintained on a phosphorus-rich diet (considerable milk and cheese) experiences phosphorus deficiency when taking aluminum hydroxide. Absorption of amino acids, ascorbic acid, vitamin A, glucose or neutral fat from the intestinal tract is also apparently not disturbed.

When aluminum hydroxide gel is given by mouth, an equal quantity of magnesium oxide is sometimes added to the evening dose to prevent constipation.

DIHYDROXYALUMINUM AMINOACETATE (ROBALATE, ETC.). The properties of this compound that are serviceable in states of hyperacidity are probably quite similar to those of aluminum hydroxide; dosage is 0.5–1.0 Gm. after meals and at bedtime or as needed.

GASTRIC MUCIN. This product, which precipitates when the mucosal lining of hog stomach is digested with hydrochloric acid and pepsin and the supernatant treated with 60% alcohol, has limited buffering properties but was logically introduced into antacid therapy as the result of gastroscopic observation that the coating action of the aluminum preparations and magnesium trisilicate occurs only when sufficient gastric mucus is present to allow the agents to diffuse through it and cling to the stomach wall. It is considerably used alone in granular form and in such preparations as *Mucotin*, in which aluminum hydroxide and magnesium trisilicate are also present.

POLYAMINE-METHYLENE RESIN (RESINAT, ETC.) adsorbs acid anions through giving up others in exchange and also acts as coating agent. Pepsin is inactivated as the result of the acid removal as well as through direct action. *Resinat* is available in 250 mg. capsules; *Resmicon* in tablets containing 50 mg. of resin with some gastric mucin. Average dosage is 1 or 2 capsules or tablets every 2 hours from 7 a.m. to 9 p.m. A large-scale definitive comparison of resins, aluminum compounds and alkalis has not been reported, to my knowledge. The resins cause some nausea and belching, but they do not interfere with absorptive processes and cause neither constipation nor diarrhea.

PROTEIN HYDROLYSATES (AMINONAT, ETC.). In some practices the use of hydrolysate is considered the treatment of choice when continuous intragastric drip is desirable, when a duodenal ulcer is causing persistent pain, in the esophageal ulcer, and in gastric ulcer when a rapid response to medical management may swing the decision against surgery. Hydrolysate solutions are felt to be unsatisfactory when the ulcer is marginal and the material is promptly dumped into the jejunum, with resultant abdominal cramps or diarrhea.

A method of administration frequently employed is to give 30 Gm. of a hydrolysate and 30 Gm. of Dextro-Maltose in 150 ml. of water hourly during 14 hours of the day, possibly supplementing with atropine or one of its substitutes in resistant cases. Sometimes the same mixture is started as an intragastric drip, beginning 1 hour after a bland meal and continuing until 1 hour before the next meal, and then throughout the night; or in milder cases the drip is used only at night.

The protein hydrolysate mixtures are expensive, and the ones for oral use, such as *Caminoids*, etc., unpalatable (a possible advantage of this is lessening of the psychically stimulated flow of gastric juice), and are likely to cause flatulence and diarrhea and, ultimately, vomiting. Occasionally edema results from sodium retention. There is no convincing evidence that the patient with uncomplicated peptic ulcer cannot digest whole protein and requires to have it administered in this hydrolyzed form.

"What drugs may worsen the symptoms in a patient with peptic ulcer?"

Reply: Aspirin will sometimes do it and so also will phenylbutazone (Butazolidin), though the related drug, oxyphenbutazone (Tandearil) appears much less capable; any of the corticosteroids; and any of the rauwolfias (such drugs as Harmonyl, Moderil, Raudixin, Rauserpa, Reserpoid, Serpasil, Singoserp, Rauwiloid, Rauval, Rauloydin, Raurine, Rau-Sed, Sandril, Serfin, Serpate, Vio-Serpine).

"I have a patient who has undergone resection and bilateral truncal vagotomy for recurrent ulcer symptoms after a previous gastrectomy, and now I have a full-blown 'dumping syndrome' to deal with—weakness, dizziness, pallor, tachycardia, sweating, palpitation and a desire to lie down. Now these symptoms are really evidence of a vasomotor component in this syndrome, and I am therefore much tempted to try a serotonin antagonist in treatment. Has this ever been done?"

Reply: Yes, it has and with reportedly good results. At the University of Pennsylvania, Gerald Peskin and Leonard Miller, after preliminary animal experimentation, gave 200 ml. of 50% glucose orally to 8 patients with severe dumping and were able strikingly to diminish or even abolish the symptoms by pretreatment with 2 mg. of methysergide (Sansert) three times daily. The symptoms returned when the drug was stopped and diminished again when its use was resumed, and there was placebo confirmation of the effectiveness. There was also the change to a normal stool habit in the 3 patients who had diarrhea, but they continued to have the other intestinal components of the syndrome.

Gerald W. Peskin and Leonard D. Miller. Use of Serotonin Antagonists in Postgastrectomy Syndromes. Am. J. Surg. 109:7, 1965.

"As an internist, I find some of my surgical friends inclined to leave their postprandial dumping syndrome after a gastrectomy problem with me. Of course, conventional therapy fails as much in my hands as in theirs, so what am I to do?"

Reply: In England a few years ago, Hobsley and Le Quane reported the effective use of insulin given before the intake of food in the dumping syndrome. The sulfonylureas might be expected, in theory at least, to be useful also since they cause the release of insulin from the pancreas. Then, too, the trial of a serotonin antagonist became logical after the observations of Johnson and associates suggested that a humoral agent recoverable by them from the portal blood of dogs after a glucose meal might be serotonin. All of this was put together upon a practical basis by Sullivan and Patton (Medical College of Alabama), who found that the characteristic vasomotor and gastrointestinal symptoms of the syndrome were significantly decreased in 29 of their 33 patients by administering tolbutamide (Orinase), or cyproheptadine (Periactin), or a combination of the two drugs. Dosages were, tolbutamide 0.25–0.5 Gm., 5–10 minutes before meals; cyproheptadine, 4–8 mg., 30 minutes before meals.

M. Bruce Sullivan, Jr., and Thomas B. Patton. Insulin, Tolbutamide, Serotonin and Dumping Reaction. Ann. Surg. 159:742, 1964. M. Hobsley and L. P. Le Quane. The Dumping Syndrome. Brit. M. J. 1:247, 1960. Floyd P. Johnson, Richard D. Sloop and John E. Jusseph. Treatment of Dumping with Serotonin Antagonists: Preliminary Report. J.A.M.A. 180:493, May 12, 1962.

PERIARTERITIS (POLYARTERITIS) NODOSA

"An associate of mine has produced what appears to be a remission in a case of polyarteritis nodosa through use of anticoagulants. What is to be expected?"

Reply: In selected cases the attempt to arrest the thromboses through use of anticoagulants is probably rational, but there is nevertheless considerable risk in this because of the vascular involvement with microaneurysms and perivascular hematomas.

David E. Dines (Rochester, Minn.). Polyarteritis Nodosa: Report of Patient Receiving Long-Term Anticoagulant Therapy. J.A.M.A. 189, July 13, 1964.

"I have a case of polyarteritis nodosa occurring in a hypertensive patient under treatment with guanethidine (Ismelin). Has such a thing been reported?"

Reply: Yes, a case has been reported in England by Dewar and Peaston in which there was suspicious association with this drug, but this is the only report that I have seen. This lesion has allegedly occurred, however, in connection with use of all the following drugs (and the list is very likely not complete): barbiturates, bismuth, chloramphenicol, chlorpromazine, corticosteroids, gold, hydantoin derivatives, hydralazine, iodides, organic arsenicals, penicillin, phenylbutazone, quinidine, streptomycin, sulfonamides.

H. A. Dewar and M. J. T. Peaston. Three Cases Resembling Polyarteritis Nodosa Arising During Treatment with Guanethidine. Brit. M. J. 2:609, Sept. 5, 1964.

"I have a case of polyarteritis nodosa in which there has been a very prompt response to the corticosteroids. What am I to expect?"

Reply: I should say a temporary effect only, because when the arteritis is healed the vessels are occluded, and then there is infarction.

PERICARDITIS

"What is the best drug therapy for acute pericarditis?"

Reply: Acute pericarditis can hardly be considered a disease sui generis, for it occurs merely as a complication of some other primary malady in nearly all instances. Therefore the therapy, so far as drugs are concerned, is that of the underlying disease.

"What is the preferred drug therapy in chronic constrictive pericarditis?"

Reply: As was said in the preceding Reply, the treatment, so far as drugs are concerned, is that of the underlying disorder. But the diuretics, used as in the treatment of congestive heart failure, are of value in the majority of instances, and their use may suffice so far as drug therapy directed toward alleviation of the circulatory embarrassment is concerned. Many men would list pericarditis of this sort as a contraindication to the use of digitalis, though the opinion is not unanimous that it is so. Nowadays of course surgery is offering much help to these patients.

"I have a patient who has developed acute pericarditis, cause unknown. In the hands of another physician he has been taking several drugs whose identity he does not know. Is there such a thing as a drug-induced pericarditis?"

Reply: Yes, pericarditis as part of an allergic reaction to drugs has been reported; the drugs involved: hydralazine (Apresoline), anticoagulants (hemorrhagic, of course), phenylbutazone (Butazolidin), streptomycin, tetracycline, (Achromycin, etc.), methylthiouracil (Muracil, etc.), an experimental cytotoxic agent used in far-advanced cancer, and in a recent instance penicillin.

Arthur H. Schoenwetter and Earl N. Silber. Penicillin Hypersensitivity, Acute Pericarditis and Eosinophilia. J.A.M.A. 191:672, Feb. 22, 1965. J. Shafar. Phenylbutazone-Induced Pericarditis. Brit. M. J. 2:795, 1965.

PERIODIC PARALYSIS

"I have a patient with long-standing periodic paralysis whose severe intermittent attacks have so far always been controllable through potassium administration. Would it be rational to look upon the malady as an intermittent hyperaldosteronism and treat accordingly?"

Reply: Such a thing was suggested several years ago by Conn and associates, but both Jones' group and Rowley and Kliman found such an association to be inconstant. However, Poskanzer and Kerr (Newcastle-upon-Tyne) have reported the successful treatment of a case with spironolactone (Aldactone). The drug was given orally in two courses for 10 and 9 days, respectively, 200 mg. twice daily in the first course and 100 mg. twice daily in the second. Both courses resulted in striking improvement in muscle strength and performance. At the time of their report, maintenance therapy at 100 mg. twice daily had controlled the situation for 8 months.

David C. Poskanzer and David N. S. Kerr. Periodic Paralysis with Response to Spironolactone (Aldactone). Lancet 2:511, Sept. 2, 1961. J. W. Conn, S. S. Fagans, L. H. Louis, D. H. P. Streeten and R. D. Johnson. Intermittent Aldosteronism in Periodic Paralysis. Lancet 1:802, 1957. P. T. Rowley and B. Kliman. The Effect of Sodium Loading and Depletion on Muscle Strength and Aldosterone Excretion in Familial Periodic Paralysis. Am. J. Med. 28:376, 1960. R. V. Jones, R. R. McSwiney and R. V. Brooks. Periodic Paralysis: Sodium Metabolism and Aldosterone Output in Two Cases. Lancet 1:177, 1959.

PERIPHERAL VASCULAR DISORDERS

"In treating patients with peripheral vascular diseases with phenoxybenzamine (Dibenzyline) I have experienced so much nasal stuffiness, tachycardia and excessive hypotension that I have finally abandoned the drug. Could you give me a quick run-down of the other drugs that are used in these situations?"

Reply: First let me say that if you experienced only the symptoms you enumerate in your use of phenoxybenzamine you have been lucky because sometimes there is also severe nausea and vomiting; failure of ejaculation in the male has also been reported; and there have been rare instances of central nervous system stimulation, disorientation and convulsions as well as temporary visual impairment and loss of bladder control.

Best effects have been achieved with tolazoline (Priscoline) in Raynaud's disease, least in thromboangiitis obliterans (Buerger's disease). Benefit is not to be expected in advanced arteriosclerotic lesions.

Injection into the femoral artery in 25–50 mg. dosage produces amazing peripheral dilation of about 2 hours' duration, the extremities becoming intensely red, hot and burning. Effect can be had with the same dosage in 2 minutes from intravenous injection and in 10 minutes from intramuscular injection. Such injections are sometimes given four times daily, but the most practicable method of administration in nonhospitalized patients is to give 25 mg. tablets orally: 1 tablet after breakfast and supper for 3 days; 1 after three meals for the next 4 days; 1 after three meals and at bedtime during the next week; then have the patient report back for check-up and dosage readjustment. Effect is had within 30 minutes of oral administration and lasts 3–8 hours.

Occasional side effects of tolazoline are hypertension or orthostatic hypotension, excessive tachycardia with arrhythmia, palpitation and substernal discomfort, nausea, abdominal pain, diarrhea, exaggeration of peptic ulcer symptoms, coldness, prickly sensations along the spine, and goose flesh. Use of the drug should probably be considered to be contraindicated in individuals with coronary disease or peptic ulcer and certainly in those in a state of collapse or shock.

Favorable findings are sometimes reported with azapetine (Ilidar) in such peripheral vascular entities as acrocyanosis, acroparesthesias, Raynaud's syndrome and causalgia; but I believe that little is accomplished when there are peripheral arteriosclerotic or thrombotic lesions. Usual dosage is 25 mg. three times daily, gradually increasing to three times this amount. The drug has also been employed intravenously in dosage of 1 mg./kg in 250 ml. of saline with slow injection.

When Green and DuBose several years ago purposely pushed their patients to tolerance, the principal symptoms experienced were dizziness, nausea and weakness with an occasional patient complaining of drowsiness. In 2 patients the occurrence of nervousness, weakness, palpitation and sweating suggested a hypoglycemic reaction, and in 1 of these cases the ingestion of food seemed to be helpful.

Diarrhea appeared in 3 cases and reactivation of previously diagnosed peptic ulcer in 2. Only once did the drug appear to aggravate the symptoms for whose relief it had been given.

Nylidrin (Arlidin) has been useful at times in Raynaud's disease and acrocyanosis but the claims made for it in other peripheral vascular disorders have not been impressive. Average beginning dosage of 6 mg. three times daily is sometimes cautiously increased. Dizziness, palpitation, tachycardia and hypotension have been reported as side actions.

Isoxsuprine (Vasodilan) has been to some extent useful in acrocyanosis and Raynaud's disease and some favorable findings have been reported in arteriosclerotic peripheral disorders, one of the latter indeed, that of Samuels and Shaftel, being quite favorable. Oral dosage in the series just referred to was 10–20 mg. three times daily. No troublesome side effects or toxicities except for occasional dizziness and palpitation, nausea and vomiting and weakness have been reported to my knowledge.

Cyclandelate (Cyclospasmol) has been used favorably in acrocyanosis and in Raynaud's disease and there are some favorable reports in cases of peripheral thrombosis and arteriosclerotic disorders. Average dosage has been 100 mg. three or four times daily. Associated side effects have been flushing, tingling, dizziness, sweating, nausea and headache, but the incidence has been relatively low.

S. S. Samuels and H. E. Shaftel. Use of a New Vasodilator Agent in Management of Peripheral Arterial Insufficiency. J.A.M.A. 171:142, 1959. H. D. Green and H. H. DuBose. Clinical Trial of Ilidar, a New Dibenzazepine Adrenergic Blocking Drug, in the Treatment of Peripheral Vascular Diseases and Miscellaneous Complaints. Circulation 10:374, 1954.

"Occasionally I see a patient with an edema of local origin and have had very little success with diuretic agents. Has there been recorded experience in this area?"

Reply: Not very much. At the Mayo Clinic, Nelson Barker and associates used chlorothiazide (Diuril) with striking effects in 4 patients with chronic lymphedema, variable effects in 8 patients with edema of chronic venous insufficiency and in 8 with idiopathic sedentary edema.

Nelson W. Barker, Beverly Carey and William Brough. Effect of Chlorothiazide (Diuril) on Patients with Edema of Lower Extremities of Local Origin. Minnesota Med. 42:227, 1959.

"Magnesium sulfate has been described as a drug that, when used parenterally, depresses 'all types of muscle.' It is used to relax uterine tetany, in eclampsia, in the treatment of spider bites, in tetanus; and even for its depressant

effect on cardiac muscle. Since 'all types of muscle' certainly must include the smooth musculature of arteries and arterioles, why do we not use this drug to combat peripheral vascular disorders?"

Reply: Actually it has been done. An Englishman, S. E. Browne, used a 50% magnesium sulfate solution to treat peripheral vascular diseases of various types, and reported marked, prolonged vasodilator action in each instance. There were patients with incipient gangrene, chronic leg ulceration, Raynaud's disease, acrocyanosis, chilblains, intermittent claudication, etc. He even used the agent in individuals with effort dyspnea and a history of coronary thrombosis and in a few with angina pectoris and threatened myocardial infarction. Typical dosage, as used in intermittent claudication for example, was 6 ml. of the 50% solution intramuscularly three times weekly and then maintenance dosage of 4 or 6 ml. weekly or every 2 weeks. Browne's results were so suggestive in all categories that I certainly think a large scale study under carefully controlled conditions is in order.

S. E. Browne. Parenteral Magnesium Sulfate in Arterial Disease. Practitioner 192:791, 1964.

"Erythromelalgia is a rare syndrome of unknown etiology in which we are so helpless. Has any promising drug therapy been proposed lately?"

Reply: B. N. Catchpole (St. Bartholomew's Hospital, London) has reported a case in which the symptoms were controlled with methysergide (Sansert) after failure with all of the following: chlorpheniramine (Chlor-Trimeton) 4 mg. three times daily; atropine sulfate 0.65 mg. three times daily; phenoxybenzamine (Dibenzyline), 20 mg. three times daily. The Sansert dosage was 2 mg. three times daily, and the symptoms appeared to be relieved completely without untoward side effects. And then we have the amazing report of Samuel Bloom, in Brooklyn, whose patient obtained complete relief from 0.6 Gm. dosage of aspirin at 4 hour intervals. This aspirin therapy is so simple, and the drug so well known to everyone, that one wonders whether many cases of erythromelalgia may never be seen professionally because the patients quickly find the remedy for themselves. There has been recent evidence that this malady may provide a clue to early diagnosis of hematologic disorders, particularly polycythemia vera; have you been aware of this?

B. N. Catchpole. Erythromelalgia. Lancet 1:909, Apr. 25, 1964. Samuel Bloom. Erythromelalgia. New York J. Med. 64:2470, Oct. 1, 1964. D. Alarcón-Segovia, R. R. Babb, J. F. Fairbairn, II, and A. B. Hagedorn. Erythromelalgia: A Clue to Early Diagnosis of Myeloproliferative Disorders. Arch. Int. Med. 117:511, 1966.

"I saw a report a few years ago on the favorable use of tolbutamide (Orinase) in thromboangiitis obliterans. Has the matter been studied since?"

Reply: Yes, Jejurikar and associates, in India, from which country the original report had come, looked into the matter, using tolbutamide, 0.5 Gm. three times daily, usually for 2–3 weeks, and withholding other vasodilator drugs and analgesics. The results in 23 patients did not seem to justify extension of the experiment.

D. A. Jejurikar, V. Marwah and M. L. Gandhe (Med. College Hosp., Aurangabad, India). Treatment of Obliterative Vascular Disease with Tolbutamide. Indian J. Surg. 25: 606, 1963.

"I have 2 patients with peripheral arterial insufficiency who suffer considerably from pain in the extremities when at rest or in bed at night. Are there agents other than the potent analgesics that might bring them some relief?"

Reply: Isoxsuprine (Vasodilan), in dosage of 10–20 mg. three times daily, has often been found not only to increase walking capacity in such individuals but also to lessen their resting discomfort. Kaindle and associates, in Austria, have particularly stressed the amount of subjective improvement in patients under this drug. I think that I should add, however, that in the experience of most men the vasodilator drugs have not been very effective in the relief of intermittent claudication, either subjectively or objectively. It is a confusing field in which to investigate because the malady itself manifests such wide variations in severity from time to time. To relieve rest pain the drugs should increase blood flow down to the feet; to relieve claudication, there must be an increase of muscle blood flow in the calf. Furthermore, the vasodilator effect must be localized through the diseased site else there will be a hypotensive response to a generalized action. At the University of St. Andrews, J. A. Gillespie studied a number of these drugs quite thoroughly, though isoxsuprine was not actually among them. His conclusions were quite skeptical regarding the potential and actual value of the group.

Saul S. Samuels and Herbert E. Shaftel (Stuyvesant Polyclinic, New York). Use of New Vasodilator Agent in Management of Peripheral Arterial Insufficiency. J.A.M.A. 171:142, Sept. 12, 1959. F. Kaindle et al. Wien. klin. Wchnschr. 68:186, 1956. J. A. Gillespie. Case Against Vasodilator Drugs in Occlusive Vascular Disease of Legs. Lancet 2:995, Dec. 5, 1959.

"I want so badly, as we all do, to be able to help my patients with arteriosclerosis obliterans, but can never be sure that I have done so other than through the impressions I gain. Is there any way to measure this sort of thing with exactness?"

Reply: No, there does not seem to be. For example, Rudolph Fremont (VA Hospital, Brooklyn) studied the effects of cyclandelate (Cyclospasmol) in 19 patients with obliterative arteriosclerosis of the lower extremities, using serial plethysmographic tracings to check on his clinical findings. What happened was that plethysmographic evidence of improvement was much less frequent than the actual improvement in walking ability: 80% of the patients improved to the extent of at least a 50% increase in claudication distance, while the plethysmograph recorded improvement in only 50% of them. But from the practical, clinical standpoint isn't this all right? The fellow can walk better, and that is what he wants. Again from the practical standpoint only, in a group of patients whose predominant complaint was leg cramps, Chesrow's group (Oak Forest, Ill., Hospital) reported that over a period of 6 weeks of therapy with carisoprodol (Soma), 350 mg. four times daily, they obtained definite improvement in 81% of their 26 patients.

Rudolph E. Fremont. Clinical Plethysmographic Observations on use of Cyclandelate (Cyclospasmol) in Arteriosclerosis Obliterans. Am. J. M. Sc. 247:182, 1964. Eugene J. Chesrow, Sherman E. Kaplitz, John T. Breme and Helga Vetra. Use of Carisoprodol (Soma) for Treatment of Leg Cramps Associated with Vascular, Neurologic or Arthritic Disease. J. Am. Geriatrics Soc. 11:1014, 1963.

PERITONITIS

"In a case of peritonitis in which it appears that all continuing sources of infection have been eliminated, and the patient is one who initially was not cachectic and could have been expected to have adequate resistance — in such a case when therapy is failing to save the patient, what could be at fault?"

Reply: At the Lahey Clinic, Frank Foster has said that under these circumstances the failure is likely the result of incorrect use of antibiotics. He points out that bacteria responsible for most cases of peritonitis that continue to be threatening in spite of treatment require the most potent, most toxic and least familiar antibiotics for their treatment; namely kanamycin (Kantrex), neomycin, polymyxin (Aerosporin), colistin (Coly-Mycin), chloramphenicol (Chloromycetin) and tetracycline in high dosage. He says that for *Pseudomonas* infection just two antibiotics, polymyxin and colistin, are effective, and that both are definitely nephrotoxic and mildly neurotoxic. For *Proteus, var. mirabilis,* penicillin is effective in high dosage; for all other varieties of *Proteus,* neomycin or kanamycin are the drugs of first choice, both being nephrotoxic and may cause deafness; and the alternative drug, chloramphenicol, may damage the bone marrow. *E. coli* responds best to kanamycin or neomycin, with chloramphenicol the drug of second choice and polymyxin the third; each of these drugs is toxic. For *Aerobacter* infections, tetracycline is the drug of choice, but it must be given parenterally in high dosage with the possibility of severe diarrhea, secondary yeast infection and liver damage as complications; chloramphenicol is the alternative drug.

Frank P. Foster. Peritonitis: A Plan When Treatment Fails. M. Clin. North America 50:551, 1966.

PHOTOSENSITIZING DRUGS

"Can you provide a list of drugs that induce photosensitivity reactions?"

Reply: In a very brief but enlightening article on photosensitivity induced by drugs, Rudolf Baer and Leonard Harber (New York University) have provided such a list, which I herewith reproduce with the kind permission of Dr. Baer. Coal tar derivatives (anthracene, acridine, phenanthrene, pyridine); antiseptics (bithionol [Bisphenol], tetrachlorsalicylanilide [Impregon]); diuretics (thiazides and related sulfonamide components); tranquilizers (chlorpromazine [Thorazine]); antibiotics (demethylchlortetracycline hydrochloride [Declomycin]); sunscreening agents (digalloyl trioleate [Neo-A-Fil], aminobenzoic acid); antifungals (griseofulvin [Fulvicin, Fulvicin U/F, Grifulvin, Grifulvin V, Grisactin, Griseofulvin], N-butyl-4 chlorosalicylamide [Jadit]); antihistamines (promethazine hydrochloride [Phenergan Hydrochloride]); antibacterials (sulfonamides); oral hypoglycemic agents (chlorpropamide [Diabinese], tolbutamide [Orinase]; miscellaneous agents (furocoumarins).

Rudolf L. Baer and Leonard C. Harber. Photosensitivity Induced by Drugs. J.A.M.A. 192:989, June 14, 1965.

PICA

"I am using iron therapy in a child with pica and obtaining good results, at least presently. What is the prognosis?"

Reply: In Cape Town, Robert McDonald and Sheila Marshall injected an iron preparation in 13 patients and saline solution in 12. At 3 or 4 months after administration of iron began, nearly all of the treated children had lost their pica, but after 5 or 6 months there was no difference between the treated children and the controls. These observers felt that the ultimate failure was due to a subsequent fall in hemoglobin, but it does not seem to me that they adequately explained this fall in all instances. It certainly does not appear at the present time that iron administration is the absolutely reliable remedy for this aberration.

Robert McDonald and Sheila R. Marshall. Value of Iron Therapy in Pica. Pediatrics 34:558, 1964.

PITYRIASIS RUBRA PILARIS

"Pityriasis rubra pilaris is a relatively rare skin disease, still one does occasionally encounter a case. What is there to do?"

Reply: That there is nothing of truly specific value is evident, I believe, in the long list of agents that have been tried: organic and inorganic arsenic, vitamin A, vitamin B complex, carotene, pituitary extract, corticosteroids, ACTH, thyroid preparations, tar preparations, starch baths, antituberculosis agents, hyperthermia, grenz rays, x-rays.

PLAGUE

"Plague is not such an 'exotic' disease as we like to think; there have been a few cases here in the United States in recent times. Is there a specific drug therapy nowadays?"

Reply: Yes, both streptomycin and chloramphenicol (Chloromycetin) are quite effective if they are given *very early* in the bubonic cases. In the pneumonic cases even this early therapy is not often successful. The tetracyclines may also be effective in the bubonic cases.

PNEUMONIA

"What is to be expected of the antibiotics or the chemotherapeutic agents in the viral pneumonias?"

Reply: In the adenoviral and other so-called "viral" pneumonias there is nothing to be expected of specific treatment, but in Eaton-agent pneumonia, which is now known to be due to a pleuropneumonia-like organism and not a true virus, the tetracyclines may be to some extent effective. In none of the other viral pneumonias, such as those secondary to smallpox, measles, chickenpox, etc., is there any response to these specific agents.

"Some years ago we used tetracycline in the treatment of our pneumococcus pneumonias and then abandoned it for more efficient drugs. Recently, we returned to it on an experimental basis and found to our surprise that some of the cases were resistant. Have these tetracycline-resistant pneumococci been around for a long time?"

Reply: No, such cases have apparently just begun to emerge after at least a decade of employment of the drug, and I do not know why this should be the case. The first report of this sort to reach the literature was that of Evans and Hansman, in Australia in 1963.

W. Evans and D. Hansman. Tetracycline-Resistant Pneumococcus. Lancet 1:451, 1963. G. C. Turner (Liverpool). Tetracycline-Resistant Pneumococci in a General Hospital. Lancet 2:659, Sept. 28, 1963.

"In a patient with a pneumococcus infection, who is hypersensitive to penicillin, what is the antibiotic of choice?"

Reply: At the Boston City Hospital, J. Kislak and associates tested the in vitro susceptibility of recently isolated pneumococci to nine antibiotics and found the order of effectiveness of the drugs to be: erythromycin, penicillin G, cephaloridine, ampicillin, nafcillin, oxacillin, cephalothin, cloxacillin and tetracycline. They felt that penicillin G remains the drug of choice in infections due to the pneumococcus, unless the patient is allergic to this drug, and that in such instances erythromycin would be the drug of choice. It appears that pneumococci resistant to penicillin G or to erythromycin have never been encountered.

Jay Ward Kislak, Lawrence M. B. Razavi, A. Kathleen Daly and Maxwell Finland. Susceptibility of Pneumococci to Nine Antibiotics. Am. J. M. Sc. 53:261, 1965.

POISON IVY DERMATITIS

"After all the studies, promotion and publicity, what is really left us of value in the treatment of poison ivy dermatitis?"

Reply: I only know of four things that have actual proven worth. One, is to wash the exposed areas as quickly as possible with hot water and soap. Two, is to dab very hot water onto the affected patches with a wash cloth in order to relieve itching. Three, is to try compresses of U.S.P. Calamine Lotion for the same purpose. And four, is to give a corticosteroid orally, which may quite considerably lessen the itching (sometimes simple aspirin will do this too).

POLYCYTHEMIA RUBRA VERA

"For several reasons I have become dissatisfied with the results that I have been achieving with radiophosphorus in polycythemia. Is there any satisfactory alternative treatment available nowadays?"

Reply: At the Middlesex Hospital in London, Jones and Jelliffe followed up the earlier favorable report by others on the use of pyrimethamine (Daraprim). They used this antimalarial agent in 22 cases in daily dosage not exceeding 25 mg. Control blood counts were done at 4–6 week intervals. Satisfactory results were achieved in 16 patients, with maintenance of the packed cell volume at or below 50%, and development of no other hematologic abnormalities. Symptoms were rapidly relieved and the spleen became impalpable. Minor symptoms, not preventing continuation of the treatment, appeared in 5 persons: sore mouth, scrotal irritation in hot weather, folic acid deficiency and an irritating rash on the hands. In another patient, a skin eruption required withdrawal of the drug after 15 months. Six patients were untreatable with the drug because of severe skin sensitization in 1 and marked thrombopenia in the other 5.

J. S. P. Jones and A. M. Jelliffe. Pyrimethamine: Alternative to Radiophosphorus in Treatment of Polycythemia Rubra Vera. Clin. Radiol. 14:424, 1963.

POLYMYOSITIS

"Polymyositis is a rather frequently occurring primary myopathy in which it is felt that the corticosteroids are the most useful form of treatment, but the details of such therapy are not presented in the literature available to me. Could you supply them?"

Reply: In Cleveland, Paul Vignos and associates studied this matter carefully in 38 patients of whom 16 made significant improvement under corticosteroid therapy. Analysis of their results indicated to them that successful treatment is dependent upon: (1) initiation of early treatment preferably within 3 months of onset; (2) initial high corticosteroid dosage, the equivalent of prednisone (Meticorten, etc.), 40–60 mg. daily; (3) rational titration of corticosteroid dosage guided by serial determinates of muscle strength and laboratory indices; and (4) continuation of treatment for sufficiently long periods (i.e., an average of at least 1 year in their series). Patients with polymyositis not treated with corticosteroids do not often spontaneously improve to a significant degree.

Paul J. Vignos, Jr., Gerald F. Bowling and Mary P. Watkins. Polymyositis. Arch. Int. Med. 114:263, 1964.

PORPHYRIA

"I have a patient in whom a diagnosis of hepatic porphyria is being entertained. Is much to be expected of chelating agents, and what other measures are advisable to be taken in the therapy of the malady?"

Reply: As to the chelating agents, one can

cite the experience of Peters's group (University of Wisconsin), who treated 26 patients with BAL only, 7 with BAL combined with intravenous ethylenediamine tetra-acetic acid (EDTA), and 4 with EDTA alone. BAL dosage was from 50 to 1200 mg. in divided doses/24 hours of a 10% solution in 20% benzyl benzoate in peanut oil. EDTA, 1–10 Gm./24 hours, was given in 5% glucose in water in a ratio of 2.5 : 5 Gm. EDTA/1000 ml. BAL was given in individual instances from 4–6 consecutive days, and EDTA during 2–4 hours, usually for 2–5 consecutive days. Occasionally oral EDTA, 1–3 0.5 Gm. tablets, was used in subacute phases. Results were favorable in 31 of the patients, equivocal in 3 and negative in 3. Regarding other measures, one should provide maximum nursing care and physical therapy when indicated, and should avoid the use of barbiturates, alcohol, heavy metals, sulfonamides, exposure to oil-based paints and solvents and sunbathing.

Henry A. Peters, Peter L. Eichman and Hans H. Reese. Therapy of Acute, Chronic and Mixed Hepatic Porphyria Patients with Chelating Agents. Neurology 8:621, 1958.

"I have a patient with acute intermittent porphyria whose attacks are precipitated by menstruation. Would the use of an oral contraceptive pill be rational therapy?"

Reply: In 3 cases of this sort reported by Mark Perlroth and associates at the National Institutes of Health, the cyclical use of the contraceptive pill was successful in preventing the appearance of symptoms. Perhaps it would be apropos to add here the list of drugs that have been presumptively associated with porphyria in a causative role, as compiled by Zarowitz and Newhouse: barbiturates, sulfonamides, alcohol, chloroquine (Aralen), allylisopropylacetyl carbamide (Sedormid), fungicides and related chemicals, tolbutamide (Orinase), chlorpropamide (Diabinese).

Harold Zarowitz and Stanley Newhouse. Coproporphyrinuria with a Cutaneous Reaction Induced by Chlorpropamide. New York J. Med. 65:2385, Sept. 15, 1965.
Mark G. Perlroth, Harvey S. Marver and Donald P. Tschudy. Oral Contraceptive Agents and the Management of Acute Intermittent Porphyria. J.A.M.A. 194:1037, Dec. 6, 1965.

"In a patient with acute intermittent porphyria I have tried to relieve the severe pain with corticosteroids; imipramine (Tofranil) as monoamine oxidase inhibitor; methysergide (Sansert) as serotonin antagonist; and meperidine (Demerol) as opiate analgesic; all without effect. To what shall I turn?"

Reply: Try chlorpromazine (Thorazine). Alfred Taylor, at the Cleveland Clinic, effected complete relief with this drug in a severe case,

but was obliged to increase dosage to 50 mg. every 6 hours in order to attain it.

Alfred M. Taylor. Acute Intermittent Porphyria—Relief of Severe Pain After Treatment with Chlorpromazine Hydrochloride (Thorazine): Report of a Case. Cleveland Clin. Quart. 29:204, 1962.

PORTAL HYPERTENSION

"Just how does vasopressin (Pitressin) reduce portal pressure in cases of portal hypertension, and what precautions should be taken in using the drug?"

Reply: The cessation of hemorrhage presumably results from the temporary drop in portal blood pressure that is a reflection of the increased splanchnic resistance and lowered hepatic blood flow resulting from splanchnic vasoconstriction effected by the drug. The patient usually experiences colicky discomfort and evacuation of the bowel and has facial pallor, and since vasopressin is a smooth muscle and coronary artery constrictor, a preliminary electrocardiogram should be taken before it is given to determine whether there is a contraindicating myocardial ischemia. Sheila Sheilock's dosage and method: vasopressin (20 units/ml.), diluted with 100 ml. of 5% dextrose, is given intravenously during 10 minutes, the stomach being aspirated every 30 minutes.

Sheila Sheilock. Management of Portal Hypertension and its Consequences. Disease-A-Month, March, 1966.

POSTHERPETIC NEURALGIA

"I have an elderly patient with postherpetic neuralgia that is responding to none of the feasible analgesics, and both she and I are becoming rather desperate. Can you suggest anything promising?"

Reply: One must of course be skeptical regarding the therapeutic claims made for any agent in this malady because it is difficult to assess the quality and degree of pain in the individual and the disorder itself runs a very variable clinical course. However, I can draw your attention to the 9 patients in whom H. J. Roberts, West Palm Beach, Florida, observed a remission of pain associated with the administration of nandrolone phenpropionate (Durabolin), injected intramuscularly at intervals of 3–7 days and in dosage ranging between 12.5 and 37.5 mg. (0.5–1.5 ml.). This is the latest "effective" remedy that has come to my attention, but I would remind you that there is a considerable graveyard of other remedial measures that have all been highly praised in their time in this malady.

H. J. Roberts. Observations on the Treatment of Postherpetic Neuralgia with Nandrolone. J. Am. Geriatrics Soc. 13:166, 1965.

POST–LUMBAR PUNCTURE SYNDROME

"None of my associates seem any more aware than I am of how effectively to treat the post-lumbar puncture syndrome, defining this as a state in which there is headache intensified in the erect position, with or without accompanying stiff neck, nausea, vomiting or lightheadedness; back pain; pain on neck flexion or straight leg raising. Have there been helpful recent studies?"

Reply: At the Mount Sinai Hospital, New York, Stephen Kulick divided 200 patients receiving lumbar punctures in an acute neurology service into four groups of even size. In the first group, routine lumbar puncture was followed by intrathecal instillation of 10 ml. of 0.9% saline; in the second group there was instillation of 40 mg. of methylprednisolone acetate with polyglycol vehicle in 10 ml. of 0.9% saline; in the third group there was instillation of 1 ml. of polyglycol vehicle in 10 ml. of 0.9% saline; and in the fourth group there was merely the lumbar puncture without any subsequent intrathecal instillations. Examination at 8–24 hours and even longer after lumbar puncture revealed a statistically significantly diminished incidence of post–lumbar puncture symptoms in the group receiving methylprednisolone acetate as compared to the other groups.

Stephen A. Kulick. The Clinical Use of Intrathecal Methylprednisolone Acetate Following Lumbar Puncture. J. Mount Sinai Hosp. 32:75, 1965.

POSTOPERATIVE ILEUS

"When it appears necessary in a case of postoperative ileus to supplement the use of Wangensteen suction, intravenous replacement of fluids and electrolytes (and the use of antibiotics if there is peritonitis) with the use of bethanechol (Urecholine), from what type of administration may I expect best results?"

Reply: Administration of bethanechol may be sublingual, oral or subcutaneous, but dosage has to be individualized since patients vary considerably in their response. By the sublingual route, 10 mg. three times daily, beginning the day after surgery, perhaps succeeds in most patients, though sometimes twice this dosage is necessary. Oral administration is generally less reliable. The subcutaneous administration of 5 mg. will often produce passage of flatus and stool within 5 minutes, but such administration is more likely to be accompanied by disagreeable side actions.

"A few years ago there was a flurry of interest in dexpanthenol (Cozyme, Ilopan, Motilyn) for the treatment of paralytic ileus, but I've heard nothing of this lately. Has the worth of the drug been established?"

Reply: This drug, d-pantothenyl alcohol, converts to panthothenic acid, which in turn combines with some protein moiety to form coenzyme A, which in turn produces acetylcholine. And acetylcholine is the substance responsible for stimulation of peristalsis when liberated at the endings of the postganglionic parasympathetic fibers in the gut. Thus the use of the drug is rational unless the ileus is due to obstruction or to potassium deficiency, but I do not believe one can say its worth has been truly established. M. L. Stone et al. (New York Medical College) and J. W. Frazer et al. (Duke University), T. A. Lamphier (Boston) and G. L. Nardi and G. D. Zuidema (Harvard Medical School), among others, have reported somewhat favorably. But, more recently, we have two unfavorable reports, those of Robert Salerno and José Ferrer (Columbia-Presbyterian Medical Center) and Alvin Watne et al. (Roswell Park Memorial Institute, Buffalo). So, to repeat, the value of the drug is controversial.

Robert A. Salerno and José M. Ferrer, Jr. Trial of d-Pantothenyl Alcohol (Ilopan) in Treatment and Prevention of Paralytic Ileus and Urinary Retention. Surg. Gynec. & Obst. 114:614, 1962. Alvin L. Watne, Catalino Mendoza, Robert Rosen, Sigmund Nadler and Robert Case. Role of Dexpanthenol (Cozyme, Ilopan, Motilyn) in Postoperative Ileus. J.A.M.A. 181:827, Sept. 8, 1962. George L. Nardi and George D. Zuidema. Postoperative Use of Dextro Pantothenyl Alcohol (Cozyme). Surg. Gynec. & Obst. 112:526, 1961. Timothy A. Lamphier. Appraisal of Routine Postoperative Use of Pantothenyl Alcohol (Cozyme) for Prevention of Intestinal Atony. Am. Surgeon 26:350, 1960. Joe W. Frazer, Benjamin H. Flowe and William G. Anlyan. d-Pantothenyl Alcohol in Management of Paralytic Ileus. J.A.M.A. 169:1047, Mar. 7, 1959.

POSTOPERATIVE NAUSEA AND VOMITING

"The number of antiemetic drugs available nowadays is rather large and one is puzzled how to choose among them since the relatively limited experience in any one practice cannot really be definitive. Can you cite the report of any large scale study?"

Reply: The largest authoritative assessment of these drugs that comes to mind is that of Bellville and associates (Sloan-Kettering Institute). These people carried out a double-blind study of the four principal drugs in use at that time in preventing postoperative nausea and vomiting. Of 3454 patients, 1114 received nothing, 367 a placebo, 754 received 7.5, 15 or 30 mg. triflupromazine (Vesprin), 537 received 50 or 100 mg. cyclizine (Marezine), 442 received 4 or 8 mg. fluphenazine (Prolixin) and 240 received 12.5 or 25 mg. promethazine (Phenergan). Fluphenazine and promethazine appeared to come out best in the study, being somewhat more antiemetic and associated with less side effect. So here we have the preference being given to drugs of the phenothiazine group. Other agents of this group that have a potent antiemetic component are chlorpromazine (Thorazine), fluphenazine (Prolixin, Permitil), perphenazine (Trilafon), promazine (Sparine), promethazine (Phenergan), prochlorperazine (Compazine), trifluoperazine (Stelazine), thiethylperazine (Torecan) and triflupromazine (Vesprin). These phenothiazine compounds, as you will doubtless recognize, belong to the group of major tranquilizers that are used in the treatment of the psychoses, and as such may of course produce all the well known side actions and toxicities of the group. However, the likelihood of occurrence of serious reactions is considerably less in the brief period of their use in postoperative vomiting than when they are employed on a long-haul basis in the treatment of psychotic individuals.

The following are the principal nonphenothiazine agents that are in considerable use as antiemetics nowadays: cyclizine (Marezine), hydroxyzine (Atarax, Vistaril), meclizine (Bonine), trimethobenzamide (Tigan), pipamazine (Mornidine), cinnarizine (Mitronal), dimenhydrinate (Dramamine) and diphenhydramine (Benadryl). I have not seen report of a full-scale comparison of all these agents, but at the Massachusetts Eye and Ear Infirmary, John Snow found hydroxyzine (Atarax, Vistaril) superior to prochlorperazine (Compazine) of the phenothiazine group.

J. Weldon Bellville, Irwin D. J. Bross and William S. Howland. Antiemetic Efficacy of Cyclizine (Marezine) and Triflupromazine (Vesprin). Anesthesiology 20:761, 1959. John C. Snow. Hydroxyzine for Post-Operative Nausea and Vomiting Following Ophthalmic Surgery. Anesth. & Analg. 44:487, 1965.

POSTOPERATIVE PAIN

"Some of our residents are pushing for the elimination of postoperative narcotics, saying that Benson Roe has shown this to be feasible in his hospital in California. What about this?"

Reply: Well, they had better know precisely the conditions under which Roe restricted the postoperative use of narcotics. The patient must be told the following things:

that the incision, having been securely closed, cannot be disrupted by his moving or coughing; that he can expect pain as a consequence of his operation but that this is not an abnormal thing; that an essential for safe and rapid convalescence is early mobility and ventilation. And in connection with the latter point, each patient is taught deep breathing and coughing before operation, and there is a demonstration of the positive pressure breathing apparatus that is routinely used. In a patient so "prepared," it is considered that restlessness is an indication for narcotics only when it can be ruled out as a sign of hypoxia. If reassurance or other supportive measures cannot assuage what appears to be genuine pain, the patient is given a narcotic intravenously at 10–30 minute intervals only to the point of relieving the discomfort. It was said that in 5 years of this policy, applied to more than 600 patients, the consumption of morphine was reduced from 50–100 mg. of morphine per surgical case to an average of less than 4 mg., many patients receiving no narcotic at all. The attending, resident and nursing staffs voted in favor of this narcotic restriction by a considerable majority. So much for Roe's study and his evidence. As for myself, the only thing that would convince me that this sort of thing is worth doing would be proof that the mortality figures were considerably improved and the bed occupancy lessened, though, with regard to the last point, it is not inconceivable that a certain number of patients would want to escape as quickly as possible from any hospital in which such radical narcotic restriction was practiced. I am simply unable to believe that a frightened and highly sensitive individual can be properly cared for on such a program, and I do not see the point of making the attempt. But of course I am very old-fashioned and do not want to suffer pain needlessly myself.

Benson B. Roe (University of California). Are Postoperative Narcotics Necessary? Arch. Surg. 87:50, 1963.

POSTOPERATIVE URINARY RETENTION

"Since the parasympathetic nerve supply to the urinary bladder relaxes the sphincter and contracts the detrusor muscle, I like to use the cholinergic drug, bethanechol (Urecholine), to combat postoperative urinary retention since this appears to be a neurogenic disorder. However, I am not satisfied that I obtain the best effects possible with this drug. Would you like to describe a method of using it that has been effective in the hands of other men?"

Reply: Perhaps the most effective method

of using it in these cases is to inject 5 mg. subcutaneously at 30 minute intervals postoperatively three times, omitting the dose or doses after the patient voids satisfactorily. If the third injection does not produce urination, catheterization is probably in order, the drug trials being resumed in 8–10 hours if there is discomfort or desire to void without being able to do so.

POSTOPERATIVE VAGINAL DISCHARGE

"None of us in our group (including the patients!) have felt that we are very successful in dealing with the odorous discharge from the vagina that so frequently occurs postoperatively in patients who have had total abdominal hysterectomy or one of several vaginal operations. The discharge and foul odor emanate from collections of blood, bacteria and necrotic material in the vaginal vault. Is anyone handling this situation effectively?"

Reply: Yes, a good many men have had success with the treatment introduced by William ReMine and Thomas Murphy at the Mayo Clinic, who used the streptodornase-streptokinase mixture, Varidase, in the form of a thin jelly administered by syringe through a catheter in the vagina. Proper consistency is obtained by mixing one vial of Varidase in 20 ml. of water and adjusting viscosity in the syringe by adding standard hospital lubricant jelly. The patient lies flat in bed for 30 minutes after the instillation, treatment beginning on the fifth or sixth postoperative day and continuing 2 or 3 days thereafter. In 87 of ReMine and Murphy's 100 patients, the foul-smelling discharge was completely eliminated and considerably decreased in 8 others. No more than three instillations, and usually only two, were required, and there were no complications.

William H. ReMine and Thomas R. Murphy. Streptokinase and Streptodornase in Treatment of Postoperative Vaginal Discharge. Proc. Staff Meet. Mayo Clin. 34:459, 1959.

POSTPARTUM BREAST ENGORGEMENT

"One of the men at our hospital is using synthetic oxytocin (Syntocinon) for prevention and relief of postpartum breast discomfort and claiming good results; but I have tried it a few times and cannot confirm him. What has been the result of a careful study?"

Reply: At the Boston Lying-in Hospital, George Ryan and Dick Brown studied this matter in a double-blind experiment, patients being given a nasal spray inhaler containing Syntocinon, 40 I.U./ml., or a spray containing the vehicle only, within 24 hours after leaving the recovery room. They were asked to begin medication when breast discomfort began and to use it at 20 minute intervals until relief or until the supply of medication was exhausted. Whether each nostril was sprayed only once or twice, there was no appreciable difference between results obtained with the drug and with the placebo. These investigators very pertinently drew attention to the fact that about one third of the patients did not have sufficient breast discomfort to require medication, and that, had medication been given to all starting immediately after delivery, these individuals would have been categorized as having an excellent result.

George M. Ryan, Jr., and Dick A. J. Brown. Intranasal Syntocinon and Postpartum Breast Engorgement. Obst. & Gynec. 20:582, 1962.

POSTPARTUM CERVICAL EROSIONS

"I have been using nitrofurazone (Furacin) vaginal suppositories in the attempt to reduce the frequency of cervical erosions found at the initial postpartum examination. But I have not had the success that I have heard claimed for it. Where does this matter stand?"

Reply: Your experience seems precisely like that of Stewart and Lammert (Cleveland Clinic) who, after a careful double-blind study, were unable to recommend that such suppositories be prescribed routinely to reduce the incidence of postpartum cervical infection. Each of their patients received 14 suppositories with the instruction to use one each night, beginning on the seventh postpartum day. Now I hold no brief for this drug, but I do wonder whether it was given fair trial in such a study, for how is one to know that the suppositories have actually been used by all patients just as prescribed?

Steele F. Stewart, Jr., and Albert C. Lammert. Postpartum Use of Nitrofurazone (Furacin) Vaginal Suppositories: Double-Blind Study. Am. J. Obst. & Gynec. 85:532, 1963.

POSTPARTUM ENEMA

"For a long period of time we have been using a phosphate-type enema of 4 ounces for postpartum evacuation; it is effective but not very acceptable to the patient or convenient for the nursing staff. Has anything 'neater' been devised?"

Reply: At New York Hospital, William Sweeney has used with considerable satisfaction a new hypertonic microenema available as a 6 ml. disposable unit, in comparison with a 4 ounce phosphate-type enema and a 4 ounce tap-water enema. Each was administered by hospital personnel on the second postpartum day, and note was made of the relative quality of the results, the presence of side actions and the patient's acceptance. In more than 90% of patients there was adequate response within one-half hour, which was fairly closely comparable with the effect of the phosphate-type enema, but somewhat superior to the tap-water enema. There were 4 side actions with the microenema (2 of abdominal cramps and 2 of rectal burning) and 2 with the tap-water enema (abdominal cramps). The most important quality of the new preparation was its acceptance by the patient; only 3 of the 92 patients disliked the microenema, whereas 10 complained about the tap-water and 7 about the phosphate enema. It was therefore concluded that the compactness, rapidity of use and patient acceptance of the microenema attested to its usefulness for postpartum bowel evacuation. Each 1 ml. of this preparation contains 90 mg. of sodium citrate, 9 mg. of sodium lauryl sulfoacetate, 625 mg. of sorbitol, 1 mg. of sorbic acid and 125 mg. of glycerin, formulated in an aqueous vehicle.

William J. Sweeney, III. Postpartum Use of a New Microenema Preparation. Obst. & Gynec. 26:426, 1965.

POSTPARTUM PAIN

"The leading investigator of pain, H. K. Beecher, has told how the soldier recently injured in combat feels very little pain because his wound symbolizes to him his path to safety and comfort for awhile. Why should not the woman who has just passed through the travail of labor be considered to be in a comparable state of tremendous generalized relief? Does she really need the postpartum dose of aspirin and codeine that is usually given? Has anyone studied this?"

Reply: Yes, J. R. Bruni and R. E. Holt have done so at a small community hospital in Niles, Michigan. On breaking the code in their double-blind study they found that 182 women had received ethoheptazine plus aspirin (Zactirin), 189 codeine plus aspirin, 191 aspirin, 195 placebo, and 219 had requested no medication whatever. Delivery had been spontaneous in the great majority in each group, episiotomies had been similar, and lacerations were considered to have been responsible for a like degree of discomfort. None of the active medications differed significantly in their effects from the others, but all were significantly superior to placebo for the first two doses (4 hour intervals), aspirin not being significantly different from placebo on the third and

fourth doses. Since placebo was relatively potent, the investigators felt that postpartum pain is usually mild and does not justify the routine use of narcotics. They felt also that ethoheptazine with aspirin was an effective substitute for codeine with aspirin when analgesic medication is called for.

J. R. Bruni and R. E. Holt. Controlled Double-Blind Evaluation of Three Analgesic Medications for Postpartum Discomfort. Obst. & Gynec. 25:76, 1965.

"In our group we have given oral trypsins a trial for the prophylaxis of episiotomy pain but abandoned it because of poor results. Other observers, however, seem to have done better with it; where may we have been at fault?"

Reply: The use of trypsin in these circumstances cannot be looked upon as a truly analgesic measure but one which may only hasten the physiologic restorative process by relieving congestion after the traumatic insult; its use may therefore be considered only on the basis of increased comfort. It may be that you did not use the enzyme early enough. In a recently reported favorable experience of Bare and Fine (Methodist Hospital, Philadelphia), patients scheduled for induction were given trypsin tablets or placebo tablets, starting about 14 hours before amniotomy. Ten tablets were given before and 14 after delivery. It was said that pain at the episiotomy site, pain on walking and perineal edema were all substantially less in the enzyme-treated group than in the placebo group, 38 in the former and 36 in the latter. Another Philadelphia group used chymotrypsin effectively, 2 tablets four times daily for the first 3 postoperative days.

Wesley W. Bare and Edward S. Fine. Prophylaxis of Episiotomy Pain: Controlled Study of Oral Trypsins on Postpartum Course. Am. J. Obst. & Gynec. 87:268, Sept. 15, 1963. H. D. Bumgardner and G. I. Zatuchni. Prevention of Episiotomy Pain with Oral Chymotrypsin. Am. J. Obst. & Gynec. 92:514, 1965.

PREMATURITY

"Is anything to be gained by prescribing thyroid for a premature infant?"

Reply: No. Stevenson and associates showed that routine administration of thyroid to premature infants is without observable benefit and sometimes harmful.

S. S. Stevenson, P. Wirth, R. Bastiani and T. S. Danowski. Some Effects of Exogenous Thyroid or Thyroxin on Premature Infants. Pediatrics 12:263, 1953.

"At very infrequent intervals in a large obstetrical practice one sees salt and water retention in a premature infant that is being artificially fed.

Would it be advisable to use diuretics in these cases?"

Reply: P. Verger and associates, at the Center for Prematures, in Bordeaux, described the use of diuretics in the following dosage: chlorothiazide (Diuril), 62–125 mg./day for 3–4 days; spironolactone (Aldactone), 25–50 mg./day for 3 days. However, Sydney Gellis, in Boston, says that he would be reluctant to resort to diuretics in these cases and would be content to wait out the spontaneous disappearance of the edema or, at most, offer a low sodium intake. Breast feeding is certainly the best safeguard against the occurrence of this problem.

P. Verger, Cl. Martin and J.-P. Carcanade. Late Edemas of Prematures. Arch. franç. pédiat. 21:441, 1964. Sydney S. Gellis. 1965–66 Year Book of Pediatrics, p. 23.

PREMENSTRUAL TENSION

"In approaching premenstrual tension as an aberration in the electrolyte and water balance, in what sort of dosage is ammonium chloride effectively used to prevent retention of sodium in the tissues?"

Reply: Dosage of 1 Gm. three times daily, starting 14 days before the expected period, is often found effective. The patient is asked to refrain from using table salt or sodium bicarbonate-containing preparations during the treatment; this of course makes the regimen rather rugged.

"I have several patients with premenstrual tension in whom I have been using Cytran tablets quite effectively, but now I have heard that this preparation may cause myopia. Is this so?"

Reply: Yes, but I believe it is nothing to worry about. The ingredients of the Cytran tablet are a progesterone compound, mild tranquilizing agent and ethoxzolamide (Cardrase). It is the last of these ingredients, a carbonic anhydrase inhibitor, which has caused the transient myopia. But the cases, at least the reported ones, have been very few.

Frank J. Beasley (Fort Lauderdale, Florida). Transient Myopia and Retinal Edema During Ethoxzolamide (Cardrase) Therapy. Arch. Ophth. 68:490, 1962.

"In our area the use of diuretics in the treatment of premenstrual tension has its advocates, but I have not been as successful as I would have liked. What may be wrong?"

Reply: I think it is the consensus that promotion of diuresis to achieve adequate dehydration and consequent relief from symptoms associated with fluid accumulation in this situation is the most rewarding of all the treatments devised to date; but there do seem to be some instances in which progesterone deficiency plays a part in causation of the aberration. As example of this, E. H. Shabanah (Royal Victoria Hospital, Montreal) performed cervical and nasal smears over two or three menstrual cycles for each of his patients and determined the need for hormone therapy and for a diuretic on the basis of these smears. Of the 50 patients treated, 16 were given supplementary hormone injections; single injections of 125–250 mg. Delalutin were usually used, although a few patients received chorionic gonadotropin instead. All patients also received benzydroflumethiazide (Naturetin) as diuretic, usually in a daily dosage of 5–15 mg. Medication was started 4–9 days before anticipated onset of menstrual flow and discontinued with appearance of the discharge. This combined type of attack was highly successful in Shabanah's hands, and I think the approach was a more rational one than that employed by Barfield and associates, of Greenblatt's group at the Medical College of Georgia, who used Cytran, a combination of a progestin, a diuretic and a tranquilizer in one tablet, which was given routinely to all patients without preliminary determination of the need for progestin supplementation.

E. H. Shabanah. Treatment of Premenstrual Tension. Obst. & Gynec. 21:49, 1963. William E. Barfield, Edwin C. Jungck and Robert B. Greenblatt. Premenstrual Tension Syndrome: Comprehensive Approach to Treatment with a Progestin-Diuretic-Tranquilizer Combination. South. M. J. 55:1139, 1962.

PREOPERATIVE SKIN DISINFECTION

"In our hospital povidone-iodine (Betadine) is very much used for preoperative skin disinfection. Is this procedure likely to influence the subsequent PBI determinations?"

Reply: In Toronto, H. P. Higgins and associates studied this matter and found no evidence that the PBI determinations are disturbed when Betadine is used in the manner recommended by the manufacturer.

H. P. Higgins, G. H. Hawks, M. O'Sullivan and M. Shaw. Effect of Providone-Iodine (Betadine) on Serum Protein-Bound Iodine, When Used as Surgical Preparation on Intact Skin. Canad. M. A. J. 90:1298, June 6, 1964.

PROCTALGIA FUGAX

"At all times I have several patients in my practice who suffer frequent spasms of the anal pain variously designated proctalgia fugax, coccygodynia and proctodynia. I have been able to do very little to relieve the attacks; what success have others had?"

Reply: Your experience is certainly not unique, but I think best results are being achieved nowadays with agents that combine a skeletal muscle relaxant effect with some degree of tranquilizing action; such drugs as carisoprodol (Soma, Rela) and diazepam (Valium). Many years ago a patient of mine rid himself of these excruciating attacks by stopping smoking.

John Q. McGivney and Benny R. Cleveland (Galveston). The Levator Syndrome and Its Treatment. South. M. J. 58:505, 1965.

PROPHYLACTIC ANTIBIOTICS IN SURGERY

"Despite the abandonment of prophylactic use of antibiotics after 'clean' operative procedures by many surgeons, it appears that the practice has been resumed by some teams during open-heart operations. Can you tell me what their results have been?"

Reply: At the New York Hospital–Cornell Medical Center, George Holswade and associates used various antibiotics and combinations of antibiotics prophylactically for approximately 1 week postoperatively in 300 consecutive open-heart operations. There were wound infections in 3 patients, blood stream infections in 2, urinary tract infections in 23, atelectasis in 7, pneumonia in 7. Infection was either the cause of death or a strong contributing factor in 6 patients. One patient incurred severe thrombopenia as a result of antibiotic treatment, 8 a minor rash, and 7 a *Monilia* infection. The investigators concluded to continue the use of methicillin prophylactically in dosage of 1 Gm./6 hours.

George R. Holswade, Peter Dineen, S. Frank Redo and Edward I. Goldsmith. Arch. Surg. 89:970, 1964.

"In our hospital we have the impression, which admittedly is not based upon careful statistical study, that patients undergoing extensive radical cancer procedures develop more postoperative infection than do other surgical patients. If this is truly the case, is the staphylococcus carrier more liable to such infection than the noncarrier, and has anyone studied the effectiveness of prophylactic antibiotic measures in this particular situation?"

Reply: The matter has been investigated by A. S. Ketcham and his group at the National Institutes of Health, and two answers were obtained. A survey of 506 consecutive patients of the type you describe showed that those who were preoperative carriers, usually asymptomatic, of staphylococci ran a greater risk of postoperative infection than the non-carriers; the rates among the carriers were 35.3% and among the noncarriers 12%. The infections in 57 of the 65 carriers were of staphylococcic origin, 54 of the same type organism that the patient carried. Regarding antibiotic prophylaxis, the study compared the postoperative infection rate in 45 patients treated with chloramphenicol (Chloromycetin) 3 days before and 7 days after operation with that in 46 controls receiving a placebo for like periods, dosage being 2 Gm. every 6 hours. Extensive cancer surgery was done in 77 individuals (10 of these admitted with severe infectious processes) and less extensive surgery in 14. The postoperative infection rates were 8.9% in the chloramphenicol group and 17.4% in the placebo group, but it appeared that it was only the postoperative and not the preoperative treatment that accounted for the difference. I do not think that these findings should be interpreted as a blanket endorsement of "antibiotic" prophylaxis since only one drug of that group of compounds, chloramphenicol, was used in the study.

A. S. Ketcham, J. E. Lieberman and J. T. West. Antibiotic Prophylaxis in Cancer Surgery and Its Value in Staphylococcic Carrier Patients. Surg. Gynec. & Obst. 117:1, 1963.

"If the abdominal operation I am about to perform is likely to involve incision of organs potentially contaminated by bacteria, shall I use prophylactic antibiotics or not?"

Reply: There is not yet agreement on the subject, but Harvey Bernard and William Cole, studying the matter thoroughly at Barnes Hospital, St. Louis, felt that their findings did not justify the prophylactic administration of the agents in all cases. They felt, however, that they did suggest use of the drugs in patients undergoing serious operations with the likelihood of contamination by significant numbers of virulent organisms, especially if the resistance of the host is lowered because of the nature of his illness or the nature of the operation. There was much discussion of Bernard and Cole's paper when it was read, and I was particularly impressed by the expressed feeling that if an antibiotic is to be given it should be during the operation, as was indeed the case in Bernard and Cole's series, rather than postoperatively when the nurse gets around to it during or subsequent to the recovery room procedures. It certainly seems rational to have the drug in the dead tissue before the bacteria begin to multiply there.

Harvey R. Bernard and William R. Cole. Prophylaxis of Surgical Infection: Effect of Prophylactic Antimicrobial

Drugs on Incidence of Infection Following Potentially Contaminated Operations. Surgery 56:151, 1964.

"What is the present status of the bacteriologic preparation for colonic operations?"

Reply: This subject, as you undoubtedly know, has been tossed about a good deal, and it is certain that the last word has not yet been pronounced. A few years ago, Isidore Cohn, Jr., (Louisiana State University) concluded from a 5 year study of the quantitative effect on the fecal flora of over 30 different drugs, combinations and dosages, that the advantages of intestinal antisepsis outweigh the disadvantages, and that it should, therefore, be used for all elective operations on the colon. But then Russel Grant and Anthony Barbara (Hackensack, New Jersey, Hospital), studying the records of 469 patients who underwent procedures requiring colotomy with closure, closure of colostomy or one-stage colonic resection during a period of about 8 years, felt that preoperative antibiotic administration in intestinal surgery of this sort is not only of doubtful value but may even contribute to increased morbidity. And there have been many other pro and con expressions of opinion. Decidedly, the subject is still a controversial one.

Russel Burnett Grant and Anthony Carl Barbara. Preoperative and Postoperative Antibiotic Therapy in Surgery of Colon. Am. J. Surg. 107:810, 1964. Isidore Cohn, Jr. Bacteriologic Preparation for Colonic Operations. S. Clin. North America 42:1277, 1962; Controversy in Internal Medicine (F. J. Ingelfinger, A. S. Relman and M. Finland, eds.), Phila., W. B. Saunders Co., 1966, p. 605.

"In our Surgery Department we have decided, after careful consideration, to retain 'bowel preparation' before colonic surgery, but are wondering whether we are using the best procedure. Would you care to discuss this?"

Reply: The procedure that has probably been most used is that popularized by Poth's group:
1. *Nonobstructed*
   Castor oil 60 ml. at 1 p.m.
   Neomycin 1 Gm. and phthalylsulfathiazole (Sulfathalidine) 1.5 Gm. at 1 p.m., 2 p.m., 3 p.m., 4 p.m., 8 p.m., 12 midnight, 4 a.m. and 8 a.m.
   Operation at 9 a.m.
2. *Partial bowel obstruction*
   Gastric suction (decompression)
   When bowel movements have begun, give neomycin 1 Gm. and phthalylsulfathiazole 1.5 Gm. every 4 hours for 3–4 days.
3. *Postoperatively*
   If the bowel has been sutured, neomycin

1 Gm. and phthalylsulfathiazole 1.5 Gm. p.o. every 4 hours as soon as peristalsis has resumed. Discontinue neomycin on the ninth postoperative day, and phthalylsulfathiazole on the eleventh postoperative day.

Recently, however, there has been increasing realization that preoperative preparation of this sort may suppress the sensitive bacteria but permit the colonization of the bowel with virulent strains of *Staphylococcus aureus* with the possible development of enterocolitis or postoperative wound infections. Actually the additional administration systemically of penicillin and a broad-spectrum antibiotic to the scheme seems to accentuate the trend toward superinfection. So numerous new methods are being tried. Herewith the schema of Altemeier and Hummel, based on their experience at the University of Cincinnati.
1. *Two days preoperative*
   Castor oil, 30 ml.
   Phthalylsulfathiazole (Sulfathalidine), 1.5 Gm. every 4 hours
   Low residue diet
   Saline enema in the afternoon
2. *One day preoperative*
   Phthalylsulfathiazole, 1.5 Gm. every 4 hours
   Full liquid diet
   Saline enema in the afternoon
3. *Postoperatively*
   If the bowel has been transected or resected:
   Penicillin, 3,000,000 units ⎫
   Tetracycline ⎬ I.V. each 24 hours
   or ⎪ for 48–72 hours.
   Chloramphenicol, 0.75–1.5 Gm. ⎭

W. A. Altemeier and R. P. Hummel. Antibiotic Agents in Colon Surgery. S. Clin. North America 45:1087, 1965. E. J. Poth, S. M. Fromm, R. G. Martin and C. M. Hsiang. Neomycin: An Adjunct in Abdominal Surgery. South. M. J. 44:226, 1961.

"In view of the fact that penicillin prophylaxis might increase the incidence of penicillin-resistant organisms in a hospital, has it ever been shown that there is advantage in so using the drug? I have thoracic surgery particularly in mind."

Reply: Since the staphylococci in most hospitals are already resistant to moderate amounts of penicillin, this phase of the subject is hardly of paramount importance. The usefulness of the measure, therefore, should probably depend principally upon evidence for or against its efficacy in reducing postoperative mortality when the drug was used in very high dosage. There have been few controlled studies in this area, but a rather impressive one was that of Citron, in London, though it is unfortunate that there were only 96 patients in the control group and 80 in the penicillin group. But the patients were allocated to the two groups at random and the penicillin group was given 2,000,000 units of crystalline penicillin twice daily starting on the day before operation and continuing to include the fourteenth postoperative day. All patients were then observed for wound infection, pleural space infection and lung infection. Postoperative infections of one sort or another occurred in 27 of the 96 control patients and in 9 of the 80 prophylactically-treated patients, *Staphylococcus aureus* being the organism most often isolated. There were 14 deaths in the control group and 3 in the penicillin group.

K. M. Citron. Controlled Trial of Prophylactic Penicillin in Thoracic Surgery. Thorax 20:18, 1965.

PROPHYLACTIC ANTICOAGULANTS IN SURGERY

"Why is it that orthopedic surgeons are less inclined to anticoagulate their immobilized patients than are other surgeons?"

Reply: While fully realizing that the immobilized individual is prone to develop thromboembolic phenomena, I think that the orthopedic patient is often not anticoagulated because of the surgeon's fear of hemorrhage into the fracture site. However, in Springfield, Missouri, Leo Neu and associates studied the value of routine prophylactic warfarin sodium (Coumadin) anticoagulation in a consecutive series of patients who suffered trauma of the pelvis and lower extremities. There were no thromboembolic episodes in the 50 anticoagulated patients and 10 such episodes in the 50 nonanticoagulated individuals. They concluded that it is not safe to rely on a minor thrombophlebitis to herald the onset of further embolic phenomena before beginning prophylactic anticoagulation.

Leo T. Neu, Jr., Jim R. Waterfield and Charles J. Ash. Prophylactic Anticoagulant Therapy in the Orthopedic Patient. Ann. Int. Med. 62:463, 1965.

"At our hospital we are engaged in a hassle over the question of anticoagulant prophylaxis of postoperative thromboembolism. While willing to grant that the anticoagulationists have many points in their favor, I nevertheless feel strongly that other things are of importance too. Would you kindly supply a list of these matters so that we may be assured that we are fully meeting our obligation all along the line irrespective of the use of the drugs?"

Reply: I shall tersely summarize the listing of these things recently provided by James Breneman (Galesburg, Michigan) in a searching study of the subject. Reduce the overweight patient; do not immobilize preoperatively for "study," x-ray diagnosis, or for a rest; reduce the duration of anesthesia and postoperative immobilization as much as possible; have the surgeon operate with "cautious haste" and the anesthetist calculate the anesthetic duration accordingly; institute early postoperative ambulation, and if this is impossible remember that 10% elevation of the legs on pillows will double the rate of venous return; prevent intra-abdominal pressure due to ileus, ascites, too tight closures of large herniae, etc.; do rectal and genitourinary surgery in the lithotomy position with the feet higher than the knees; discourage prolonged use of tourniquets and avoid prolonged intravenous administration in the lower legs; correct cardiac decompensation, dehydration, plethora and sickling crises to optimal; whenever possible allow several weeks of ambulation between operations, and do not follow cystoscopy, dilatation and curettage, colostomy and other diagnostic procedures requiring an anesthetic immediately by another operation; use appropriate preventive measures such as saphenous ligation, femoral ligation, or mechanical pulsating equipment to the lower extremities; be aware that postoperative complications urgently requiring another anesthesia, such as hemorrhage, wound dehiscence, abscess drainage and bile duct or ureteral repair, add to the hazard.

James C. Breneman. Postoperative Thromboembolic Disease. J.A.M.A. 193:576, Aug. 16, 1965.

PROPHYLACTIC DIGITALIS IN SURGERY

"Since cardiac complications, principally atrial fibrillation, atrial flutter and congestive heart failure, are fairly common occurrences after pulmonary tissue resection in elderly individuals, would it not be rational to digitalize such patients preoperatively rather than waiting for the appearance of the arrhythmias postoperatively in order to institute the specific therapy?"

Reply: At Barnes Hospital, St. Louis, Myron Wheat and Thomas Burford investigated this matter and derived an affirmative answer. Of 439 patients aged 55 years or older undergoing chest operations, 137 were given digitalis, usually preoperatively but always before the development of any cardiac complications. There were 68 cardiac complications in the 302 patients not digitalized, an incidence of 23%, and only 16 such complications in the 137 who were digitalized (an incidence of 12%). This difference was declared to be statistically significant, though I would feel more comfortable about it had the numbers of the treated and nontreated patients been more nearly comparable. At any rate these investigators concluded that withholding digitalis until the classic indications appear is no longer justified, and that one should routinely digitalize all patients over 60 before major surgery. Nevertheless, I think that one should bear in mind the fact that the aging patient is the most likely candidate for digitalis toxicity.

Myron W. Wheat, Jr., and Thomas H. Burford. Digitalis in Surgery: Extension of Classic Indications. J. Thoracic & Cardiovas. Surg. 41:162, 1961.

"Is it advisable to digitalize the patient undergoing cardiac surgery?"

Reply: The prophylactic use of digitalis in cardiac surgery has come about as a result of recent animal experimentation indicating, contrary to earlier opinion, that the drug increases the force of contraction of the normal as well as the abnormal heart. There have been a number of reports favorable to this procedure in man, but in a careful analysis of all the considerations, pro and con, Arthur Selzer's group, of the Presbyterian Medical Center in San Francisco, in whose hospital more than 1000 open-heart operations were performed during the period used for analysis, decided that after balancing the high toxic potential of digitalis against benefits suggested by experimental studies but unproved under clinical conditions, the conclusion was justified that at the present time neither the routine use of digitalis in open-heart surgery nor its prophylactic use in general is justified.

Arthur Selzer, John J. Kelly, Jr., Frank Gerbode, William J. Kerth, John J. Osborn and Robert W. Popper. Case Against Routine Use of Digitalis in Patients Undergoing Cardiac Surgery. J.A.M.A. 195:549, Feb. 14, 1966.

PROSTATISM AND PROSTATECTOMY

"I have thought that attempts at endocrine therapy for benign prostatic hypertrophy with estrogen or androgen or both had all ended in failure, but recently I have heard that progesterone is being used with some success. Is this correct?"

Reply: Therapy of this sort has been based on the hypothesis that altered secretion of testicular steroids is a factor in the production of this malady, and you are certainly correct in saying that this has usually failed. But at Albert Einstein College of Medicine, Jack Geller's group has tried it again, being intrigued by the fact that benign prostatic hypertrophy is rare or absent in eunuchs and patients

with hypopituitarism, and that prostatic atrophy occurs following castration. They used hydroxyprogesterone caproate (Delalutin) in dosage of 3 Gm./week for 1½–14 consecutive months. In 2 patients with chronic urinary retention, spontaneous ability to void and normal residual urine volumes occurred after 2 months of therapy; in 1 patient an elevated residual urine volume returned to normal in the same period of time and remained so; in the remaining patients, who had normal residual urine volumes before therapy, there was sustained clinical improvement after 3–6 months of use of the drug, which was supported by microscopic evidences of glandular atrophy. Real proof of the efficacy of this therapy, however, could only be obtained through a well-controlled study of a large number of patients through a period of at least 5 years.

Jack Geller, Raif Bora, Theophilus Roberts, Harry Newman, Albert Lin and Robert Silva. Treatment of Benign Prostatic Hypertrophy with Hydroxyprogesterone Caproate. J.A.M.A. 193:121, July 12, 1965.

"During my time in practice I have seen the mortality after prostatectomy drop from about 20% to 5% or even somewhat less, due to greatly improved evaluation of patients, advances in anesthesia, blood replacement, and of course the use of antibiotics. But there is still a relatively high morbidity rate after the operation, and the question I should now like to have answered is whether prophylactic broad-spectrum antibiotic therapy is justified as a routine measure after prostatic surgery. It is a procedure that is widely employed, but is it justified?"

Reply: At New York University, Peter Bogdan performed a double-blind study of prophylaxis *after* surgery in 67 elderly men with benign prostatic hyperplasia, 34 being given a 100 mg. dose of tetracycline intramuscularly immediately after operation and every 12 hours for a total of four doses, and then 250 mg. orally every 6 hours for 9 days; the other 33 patients received a suitable placebo. Significant febrile reactions and the major and minor complications of prostatectomy were observed to occur twice as often in the placebo group as in the tetracycline group. As for prophylactic measures *before* surgery, Miller's group, at Baylor University, produced findings indicating that this is of no value if the patient has a sterile urine, but that intravenous nitrofurantoin (Furadantin) might help in preventing significant postoperative fever. They found also that antibiotics are of no value in the prophylaxis of epididymitis as a complication of prostatectomy except when given postoperatively. However, in a limited but controlled study of prophylaxis before and after transurethral prostatectomy, Kudinoff's group, in Los Angeles, observed that the incidence of bacteriuria was reduced with methenamine–mandelic acid but not with kanamycin (Kantrex); indeed, use of the latter was associated with a high incidence of post-treatment *P. aeruginosa* and *S. aureus* infections.

Peter E. Bogdan. The Value of Prophylactic Tetracycline Therapy after Prostatic Surgery: Interim Report of a Double-Blind Study. J. Am. Geriatrics Soc. 12:977, 1964. A. Lamar Miller, Jr., F. Brantley Scott and Russell Scott, Jr. Evaluation of Antibiotics Prior to Prostatectomy. J. Urol. 92:711, 1964. James F. Reeves, Russell Scott, Jr., and F. Brantley Scott. Prevention of Epididymitis After Prostatectomy by Prophylactic Antibiotics and Partial Vasectomy. J. Urol. 92:528, 1964. Zoya Kudinoff, Sydney M. Finegold, George M. Kalmanson and Lucien B. Gaze. Use of Kanamycin or Urinary Acidification for Prophylactic Chemotherapy in Transurethral Prostatectomy. Am. J. M. Sc. 251:70, 1966.

"If one is to use antibiotics routinely as a prophylactic measure immediately after prostatectomy, will the organisms cultured from the urine before operation serve as a guide to the choice of the agent to be used?"

Reply: In the experience of Peter Bogdan, at Bellevue Hospital, the organisms cultured from the urine collected before operation frequently were not the same as those found after operation, which indicates the value of postoperative urine cultures. His own experience was that tetracycline served satisfactorily to reduce significant febrile reactions and the major and minor complications of the procedure.

Peter E. Bogdan. The Value of Prophylactic Tetracycline Therapy After Prostatic Surgery: Interim Report of a Double-Blind Study. J. Am. Geriatrics Soc. 12:977, 1964.

"Sometimes in an elderly patient after prostatectomy there is a period of disorientation apparently resulting from the antidiuresis and consequent mild water intoxication resulting from operative trauma. Has intravenous urea been used as a diuretic to relieve this situation?"

Reply: Yes, and quite effectively. At the Stirling, Scotland, Royal Infirmary, G. B. McKelvie gave 4% urea in 5% dextrose intravenously to 161 patients, of whom 110 received 3000 ml. every 24 hours during the first 72 hours, 3 had 4000 ml. at the same intervals and period, and 48, 3000 ml. every 24 hours for only 48 hours. The lowest urinary output in the first 24 hours after operation was 2300 ml., in 146 patients it was over 3000 ml., and it was over 3000 ml. during the second and third days in all patients. Diuresis was achieved even in patients with impaired renal function and in those with congestive heart failure. The measure ap-

peared helpful also in preventing urinary infection, and it was felt that the simple closed drainage system employed reduced postoperative nursing problems. Furthermore, the high urine outflow was looked upon as preventing clot formation by diluting blood that oozed from the prostatic cavity.

G. B. McKelvie. Intravenous Urea as Diuretic in Prostatectomy. Brit. M. J. 2:1711, Dec. 29, 1962.

PRURITUS

"We all have cases of more or less severe pruritus that are quite protracted and difficult to influence. Can you cite a study of some of the newer drugs in the treatment of this disturbing symptom?"

Reply: In a recent review, Arnold Gould and Edward Neary (Georgetown University Medical School) dealt with a number of these newer drugs in the relief of itching. Trimeprazine (Temaril) is a phenothiazine compound that does not have as much antiemetic, hypotensive and hypnotic-potentiating action as some of the other members of that group but does have considerable antihistaminic action and is recommended as an antipruritic in dosage of 2.5 mg. four times daily, or 5 mg. (as a sustained-release capsule) every 12 hours. Drowsiness appears to be the most frequently encountered side effect, which often disappears as therapy proceeds, but one must always bear in mind liver toxicity and blood dyscrasias when any phenothiazine compound is used. This drug has been favorably reported upon as an antipruritic in several studies. Dexbrompheniramine (Disomer) and dexchlorpheniramine (Polaramine) are antihistaminics from which some antipruritic effect might be expected, though a specific study of this type of action does not seem to have been published. Adult dosage of either drug is 2 mg. four times daily or 4–6 mg. twice daily if the prolonged-action tablet is used. There seem to be very few side effects other than mild sedation. Methdilazine (Tacaryl) is another phenothiazine compound which has a long-acting antihistaminic effect. Double-blind controlled studies with this drug have shown it to have considerable efficacy in chronic pruritus in both allergic and non-allergic skin disorders. Dosage is 8 mg. twice daily, and drowsiness is the most frequent side effect. But again, this is a phenothiazine and one should be on guard. Dimethindene (Forhistal) is an antihistaminic that has been shown to be an effective antipruritic, but it appears that double-blind studies of this action of the drug have not been reported. Dosage is 1–2 mg. one to three times daily, or 2.5 mg. of the long-acting tablet twice daily. As with the other antihistamines, sedation is the most frequent side action. Cyproheptadine (Periactin) has been shown to relieve pruritus in allergic skin disorders like the other antihistaminics, but not in very critical studies, it seems. Adult dosage is 4 mg. three to four times daily.

Arnold H. Gould and Edward R. Neary. Newer Developments in Oral Antipruritics. M. Clin. North America 48: 411, 1964.

"One of our group, returning from a meeting, reports the use of guanethidine (Ismelin) in the treatment of pruritus. What about this?"

Reply: It is true that Lawrence Solomon (University of Pennsylvania) has reported effective use of the drug (though others have not always been so favorably impressed), the underlying hypothesis being that atopic dermatitis may reflect in part a cutaneous affinity for noradrenaline, which would be counteracted by the inhibiting action of guanethidine on noradrenaline at the postganglionic level and its consequent depletion in the affected tissues. Divided dosage in a daily total of 0.75–1.25 mg./kg. was given for 5–30 days. All but 10 of the 30 patients obtained substantial relief. Topical application of guanethidine-containing ointments was ineffective. As a new approach this is very interesting, but I should hesitate to employ it until more investigative studies have been performed. Guanethidine is potentially an agent of considerable toxicity.

Lawrence M. Solomon. Observations on Antipruritic Effect of Guanethidine in Atopic Dermatitis. Canad. M. A. J. 90:644, Mar. 17, 1964. Kristian Thomsen and Poul E. Osmundsen. Guanethidine in the Treatment of Atopic Dermatitis. Arch. Dermat. 92:418, 1965.

"I know that there is a good deal of question about the physiologic versus psychologic results from using antipruritic drugs, but in my occasional case I seem to be getting very good effect with trimeprazine (Temaril) and I intend to continue using it. Am I likely to encounter trouble from serious side effects?"

Reply: In 1960, R. B. Pittelkow (Milwaukee) reported that 87% of his 572 cases had experienced complete or at least satisfactory relief of daytime or night-time itching and that none of the patients were disturbed by side effects. Frank Ayd and associates (Baltimore) found side effects related to dosage, usually occurring when over 10 mg./day was given: weakness or fatigue, dryness of the mouth, dizziness, gastric distress, disturbing dreams, and syncope without hypotension.

Frank J. Ayd, Jr., Emidio A. Bianco and Leonard M. Zullo (Franklin Square Hosp., Baltimore). Trimeprazine (Temaril) Therapy for Physiologic and Psychologic Pruritus. South M. J. 52:1554, 1959. R. B. Pittelkow. An Evaluation of Trimeprazine in Pruritus. Wisconsin M. J. 59:367, 1960.

"Word has gone around of the use of griseofulvin (Fulvicin, etc.) in cases of intractable pruritus vulvae and ani. Is this safe therapy?"

Reply: I think that one need not be particularly concerned about its safety, and as a matter of fact Alan Rubin (University of Pennsylvania) has reported the effective use of the drug in a small number of patients, giving 500 mg. three times daily for several months when necessary. But there are so many factors entering into the etiology and responsiveness of this type of pruritus that I am inclined to be somewhat skeptical of the worth of any newly proposed agent until there has been long trial of it in the hands of a good many people. It is so difficult to study the subject under controlled conditions. Analyzing 25 reports on antipruritic drugs during a 15 year period, Cormia and Dougherty found that the number of patients compared in the studies, the use of a double-blind method, control of adjunctive therapy and associated variables, and statistical elimination of chance variables had been quite inadequate in most instances.

Alan Rubin. New Treatment for Intractable Pruritus Vulvae and Ani. Obst. & Gynec. 24:669, 1964. F. E. Cormia and J. W. Dougherty. Clinical Evaluation of Antipruritic Drugs. Arch. Dermat. 79:172, 1959.

"I have heard that the corticosteroids are effectively used in the treatment of pruritus ani. How are they employed?"

Reply: In making his rather remarkable claim that he has succeeded in controlling the symptoms of itching and causing a regression of skin changes in 90% of over 1000 cases of this malady by the use of prednisolone (Meticortelone, etc.), Sidney Copland, in Dayton, offers the following method: Oral administration of prednisolone during a 16 day period as follows: day 1–4, 5 mg. four times daily (after meals and on retiring); day 5–8, 2.5 mg. four times daily; day 9–12, 2.5 mg. twice daily (after breakfast and supper); day 13–16, 2.5 mg./day (after breakfast only). The drug is simultaneously used locally in strength of 1% (most commercial preparations contain 0.25 or 0.5%) ointment, which is rubbed into the affected area for 1 full minute twice daily. When the skin changes are widespread, a spray of steroid solution is employed due to ease of application. Copland says that the oral therapy can be repeated after 6–8 weeks, and that the local therapy is continuous for 2–3 months.

Sidney M. Copland. Management of Pruritus Ani. J.A.M.A. 194:184, Oct. 11, 1965.

PSITTACOSIS

"Is there an agent of choice among the antibiotics for the treatment of psittacosis?"

Reply: Yes, the tetracyclines are definitely the preferred agents, with chloramphenicol perhaps being in the second place, though it is said that penicillin in very high dosage is equally effective. Do not discontinue treatment under 10 days even though the symptoms may recede earlier.

PSORIASIS

"What is the Ingram method of treating psoriasis?"

Reply: This is a method of treating psoriasis without the use of either corticosteroids or antimitotic agents. The technique comprises incorporating anthralin in stiff Lassar's paste with 2% salicylic acid and then covering the lesions with a semiocclusive dressing. The method has been much used on the Continent and in England but not so far to any great extent here in the United States. As described by Stanley Comaish, of Newcastle-upon-Tyne, the steps involved are first the bathing of the patient in a coal-tar bath (liquor carbonis detergens, 4 oz. to 20 gal.) gently scrubbing the affected skin, and then exposing the lesions to ultraviolet radiation starting at low dosage and steadily increasing to a mild erythemal dose. Then the paste, containing 0.4% anthralin and 2% salicylic acid, is accurately applied to each plaque of psoriasis, talcum powder is then sprinkled over the paste and rolls of stockinet are rolled onto the limbs and trunk, taking care to avoid smearing. A complete suit can be made in this way and the patient can put on his street clothes over it. The entire regimen is repeated daily and is said to have no side effects. Comaish says that with this treatment 95% of the patients are completely cleared clinically in between 2 and 3 weeks, many within 10 days.

Stanley Comaish. Ingram Method of Treating Psoriasis. Arch Derm. 92:56, 1965.

"In our part of the world we use a great deal of vitamin B$_{12}$ in treating psoriasis on the basis of clinical impression that the drug is helpful. Is it really?"

Reply: You should stop this. In England several years ago, Baker and Comaish studied the use of this drug in 73 patients with uncomplicated psoriasis, using double-blind controlled methods. There was no identifiable advantage of vitamin B$_{12}$ treatment in either sex, in any age group, or in any severity group.

Harvey Baker and J. S. Comaish. Is Vitamin B$_{12}$ of Value in Psoriasis? Brit. M. J. 2:1729, Dec. 29, 1962.

"In my general practice I have several psoriasis patients in whom I am getting just about the usual results. I would like to try the new occlusive dressing type of treatment in one of them if the risk is not too great. What is the consensus?"

Reply: I do not believe that one can speak of consensus as yet for the thing is still so new that authoritative opinion has not yet crystallized. It seems to me, however, that we still need more careful observation to determine with certainty that the likelihood of the development of intercurrent infections under the dressings is not going to assume the proportions of a major deterrent. In England, Stevenson and Whittingham treated 27 patients with extensive, long-standing psoriasis by applying a fluocinolone acetonide (Synalar) 0.025% ointment thinly to all the psoriatic lesions and then covering practically the entire body with polyethylene sheeting held in place with stockinet and adhesive tape. Polyethylene gloves were used on the hands and the facial lesions were treated with the ointment without occlusion. This "suit" was worn for 3 days and a bath was then taken and treatment repeated. Therapy was continued until the patient was either clear of lesions or for a maximum of 21 days. Folliculitis occurred in 8 of the first 11 patients; for the remaining 16, 2% chlorhexidine dihydrochloride was added to the ointment. In 6 of the 7 failures to respond the fault was laid at the door of the folliculitis. The infecting organism in the folliculitis cases was a staphylococcus of the same phage type cultured from a patient on the ward with a chronic varicose ulcer. Other complications included a sweat-retention type of rash in 5 patients, purpura of the extremities in 3 and an eczematous eruption in 1.

C. J. Stevenson and G. E. Whittingham. Psoriasis Treated with Topical Fluocinolone Acetonide (Synalar) and Occlusive Dressings. Brit. M. J. 1:1450, June 1, 1963.

"I can often dramatically control an extensive psoriasis with corticosteroids, but the manifestations return very quickly when effective dosage is reduced, and if I don't reduce dosage I have a case of Cushing's syndrome on my hands. Would I fare any better with methotrexate?"

Reply: This drug, amethopterin or methotrexate, is also a two-edged sword since folic acid antagonists can quickly produce dire results in the toxic dosage that is required in psoriasis. However, in a case in which internist, dermatologist, orthopedist, physiatrist and physical and occupational therapist all worked together as a team, Robert Cress and Nell Deaver, in Durham, North Carolina, were able to produce quite astonishing results through use of this drug in a severe case of psoriasis and arthritis. The drug, which as I have said constituted only a part of the treatment, was given in dosage of 0.25 mg./kg. intravenously at 10–14 day intervals.

Robert H. Cress and Nell L. Deaver. Methotrexate in Management of Severe Psoriasis and Arthritis: Report of a Case. South. M. J. 57:1088, 1964. T. J. Ryan, H. R. Vickers, S. N. Salem, S. T. Callender and J. Badenoch (England). Treatment of Psoriasis with Folic Acid Antagonists. Brit. J. Dermat. 76:555, 1964.

"In our hospital the Committee on Chemotherapy in Malignancy is very circumspect in employing the antineoplastic agents in each candidate case, but I hear some of the dermatologists speaking rather glibly of their use of these drugs in such a relatively benign malady as psoriasis. Can you reconcile these attitudes sufficiently so that I may feel at ease in a psoriatic patient for whom I would like to do everything that is conservatively possible?"

Reply: I believe that Hamilton and Elion's study of the distribution and metabolism of 6-mercaptopurine (Purinethol) in man initiated the use of these drugs in psoriasis, but aminopterin and amethopterin (Methotrexate) are now more popular. These drugs are being recommended for use only when all local therapy has failed, but that does not seem to me a truly satisfactory criterion because local therapy ultimately fails in all cases of psoriasis, at least fails to prevent recurrent attacks. The protagonists of this sort of treatment speak of its relative safety because of their use of low dosage, but it seems to me that they are treading pretty close to something highly risky when, as in William Dobes's 65 patients, the drug had to be discontinued in 12 because of ulceration of the mouth; there was also mild stomatitis or burning of the mouth and tongue in 29 patients, who usually tolerated the drug again, however, after a rest period. In 3 patients the drug had to be discontinued because of hair loss and in 1 because of esophageal swelling and intestinal bleeding. Dobes's regimen: adults received one 0.5 mg. aminopterin tablet daily for 16 days, during which 16 mg. triamcinolone (Aristocort, Kenacort) was given daily for 2 days, 12 mg. daily for 2 days, 8 mg. daily for 2 days, and 4 mg. daily for 2 days. With considerable improvement of the psoriatic process, 4–8 mg. of triamcinolone was given daily for another 8 days; if clearing

was only slight or moderate, the higher dosage schedule was repeated during the second 8 days. After 16 days, the corticosteroid was discontinued but aminopterin was given every 2 days for 2–4 weeks, depending on tolerance and clearing of lesions. At the Queen Elizabeth Hospital, Adelaide, where Hunter preferred amethopterin (Methotrexate), the routine dosage was 1 tablet daily for 7 days, repeated after 1 week of rest; if there was no response and no side effects, the dosage was raised to 2 tablets daily, but rarely exceeded. In the preliminary report of their experience at the Cleveland Clinic, Roenigk and associates said that they felt a single weekly oral dose of 25 mg. of Methotrexate provided an effective method of treating selected cases of psoriasis.

William L. Dobes (Atlanta, Georgia). Use of Folic Acid Antagonists and Steroids in Treatment of Psoriasis. South. M. J. 56:187, 1963. G. A. Hunter. Use of Methotrexate in Treatment of Psoriasis. Australian J. Dermat. 6:248, 1962. Henry H. Roenigk, John R. Haserick and George H. Curtis. Methotrexate for Psoriasis. Cleveland Clin. Quart. 32:211, 1965. L. Hamilton and G. B. Elion. The Fate of 6-Mercaptopurine in Man. Ann. New York Acad. Sc. 60:304, 1954.

PSYCHOSES AND NEUROSES

"I find it very confusing that we are using entirely different types of drugs in the treatment of psychoses and psychoneuroses and yet are calling them all 'tranquilizers.' Could you provide a clear statement of what is accomplished by the drugs in these two classes of maladies and perhaps suggest some distinctive designations for the two types of drugs?"

Reply: The suggestion has already been made by Frank Berger, and it seems to me that it is a very good one, that those drugs now called "major" tranquilizers because they are used in the treatment of the true psychoses be hereafter designated "antipsychotic" drugs or "neuroleptic" agents and that the term "tranquilizers" be allowed to apply only to those drugs that are used in the treatment of the psychoneuroses and the psychosomatic conditions. The pioneers among the first type, or antipsychotic drugs, were the *Rauwolfia* compounds, but they are very little used for their original purpose nowadays not only because they tend to cause serious depressions but principally because the phenothiazine derivatives are fully as effective, act much more rapidly, and are infrequently followed by depression. I shall therefore make a statement of what has been accomplished with the *phenothiazine derivative compounds* in the true psychoses, using *chlorpromazine (Thorazine)* as the typical as it was the first of these agents, and defining the psychotic individual as one in whom the very core of the personality has disintegrated so that the patient is no longer himself, i.e., he has lost touch with reality.

It is in the hospitalized, hyperactive, assaultive, destructive, noisy, incontinent and frequently nude psychotic patient that chlorpromazine has exhibited its therapeutic efficacy most dramatically. Deming has given expression to an experience that has been had in mental hospitals throughout the world in pointing out that one can now tour the wards of a state hospital and see curtains, plants and other signs of domestic living where previously there had been nothing but bare walls for fear that the patients would destroy everything in sight. And those patients who in the past ran around naked and screaming are now neatly dressed, no longer incontinent, and either quietly idle or engaged in occupational therapy. Not infrequently patients of this sort can actually be discharged under influence of the drug. Tuteur and associates, reviewing experience at the Elgin State Hospital, stated that of 822 patients treated, 258 were discharged and that of the 77 who returned only 26 represented relapses while taking the drug diligently.

Not only is the need for electroconvulsive and surgical types of therapy being considerably reduced by this new type of treatment, but there is also a great diminution in the amount of restraint, seclusion, hydrotherapy and even simple sedation that is being employed in the new era. Many patients are being made amenable to psychotherapy, thus lightening the task of the psychiatrist through significantly reducing the number of psychotherapeutic interviews required; and the greater tidiness and reduced destructiveness of patients has much facilitated nursing care, thus freeing the staff from custodial to rehabilitative activities. In senile psychoses, the response has been much better in irritable, quarrelsome and apprehensive individuals than in those manifesting predominantly depression, negativism, apathy and withdrawal.

The excitement and hyperactivity of acute alcoholic hallucinosis and delirium tremens are also effectively controlled, but it is the universal experience that the severely deteriorated, withdrawn, vegetating type of chronic hospital patient does not respond at all well to the drug. Nonhospitalized patients of the most susceptible group do not respond as well either as those in the hospital, principally because of lack of discipline, but actually most of the patients who comprise the most responsive group are in hospital to begin with.

As for the *true tranquilizing agents*, using the classic *meprobamate (Miltown, Equanil)* as typical of the group, and defining an individual with a psychoneurosis as one in whom the personality is maladjusted but has retained its organization, it may be said that this drug is not in the least competitive with the phenothiazine derivatives in the true psychoses, though it is sometimes helpful in senile psychoses when there is agitation and angry resistance to nursing procedures. Its tranquilizing properties are principally demonstrable in treating the irrational fears and dreads characterizing the anxiety state in psychoneurotic individuals, and in lessening the bodily tensions, irritability and difficulty in concentration experienced by such persons. Although not itself an analgesic, meprobamate appears to contribute toward the relief of intractable pain through its tranquilizing action. Likewise it induces sleep when desired through allowing the patient to drift into a quiet, unworried, receptive state. It is also said to be helpful in treating premenstrual tension, in the sobering-up phase of acute alcoholism and the abstemious periods in chronic alcoholics, and as an aid to the stutterer. The many other uses to which the drug and the other members of the tranquilizing group have been put, principally as a result of their relaxing effect on skeletal muscle, do not enter into the present enumeration of clinical effects.

Q. Deming. Tranquilizing Drugs. Am. J. Med. 27:767, 1959. W. Tuteur, R. Stiller and J. Glotzer. Chlorpromazine—Four Years Later. Illinois M. J. 116:9, 1959. Frank M. Berger. Major and Minor Tranquilizers. J.A.M.A. 194: 681, Nov. 8, 1965.

"What is this I hear about the tranquilizers not being any better than phenobarbital?"

Reply: What you hear is nonsense. I am not at all impressed by the rigidly controlled studies of these drugs by experts in research hospitals. How often does a practicing physician hospitalize a patient primarily for a neurotic condition? And when he does, in order to study the case better, does he not expect that the patient will be more influenced by attitudes of other patients and the total environment than by drugs? The true measurement of response to therapy in a neurosis can be made only when the patient is living under the circumstances that are provoking his malady. And it is only when the patient's awareness, and that of his associates, of an alteration in his state, combined with the physician's impressions, give evidence of progress or the lack of same that we can know where we stand in an individual case.

Harry Beckman. Requirements in Clinical Evaluation of Tranquilizers. J. Neuropsychiat. 5:464, 1964.

"Despite the contrary opinion of some of my associates, I am convinced that several of the tranquilizers are superior to phenobarbital if merely tranquilization and not hypnosis is desired. But what of the respective toxicities of the two groups?"

Reply: The barbiturates appear to be a considerably more toxic group than the tranquilizers. Ingestion of 5–15 times the hypnotic dose of the former may be lethal, whereas ingestion of 50 or more doses of the tranquilizers is usually survived. A substantiating fact is that despite the much greater sale of tranquilizers than barbiturates in this country nowadays, the incidence of suicide with the former is very much less than with the latter.

F. M. Berger. The Role of Drugs in Suicide. Symposium on Suicide, George Washington University School of Medicine, Oct. 14, 1965.

"I am becoming increasingly suspicious that many failures in the outpatient care of psychiatric patients with drugs is due to the fact that these people simply do not take the prescribed medicines. Has the matter been studied?"

Reply: Yes, in England, Willcox and associates made tests on 125 psychiatric outpatients to learn whether they were taking the chlorpromazine (Thorazine) or imipramine (Tofranil) that had been prescribed, and found that 48% of them were not doing so. The failure rate was not found to be associated with age, sex, intelligence or drug side effects. Men living alone defaulted more often than those living with their wives, which suggests a beneficial influence of supervision.

D. R. C. Willcox, R. Gillan and E. H. Hare. Do Psychiatric Out-Patients Take Their Drugs? Brit. M. J. 2:790, Oct. 2, 1965.

"I have a patient who was always made drowsy by the amount of tranquilizer spaced throughout the day that was necessary to relieve her anxiety and tension; so I withdrew the daytime medication, gave her a whopping big dose at night, and controlled the situation beautifully. My associates now poke a bit of fun at me, but was this not a rational procedure? These people frequently need a good night's sleep as much as anything else, and if the next day's hangover is not excessive but just holds down their jitteriness, what is wrong with that?"

Reply: Nothing at all that I can see.

"I have heard it rumored that a study, in the New York area, of the prevention of psychiatric hospitalization through use of phenothiazines has shown the drugs to be of no value since after 1 year of therapy the patients treated with them were still being hospitalized whereas this was no longer true of the placebo-treated group. What of this?"

Reply: The explanation of course (I think your question probably relates to the study of David Engelhardt's group at the Downstate Medical Center in Brooklyn) is that the placebo-treated individuals who were going to be hospitalized at all had achieved that goal very much earlier.

David M. Engelhardt, Norbert Freedman, Bernard Rosen, David Mann and Reuben Margolis. Phenothiazines in Prevention of Psychiatric Hospitalization: III. Delay or Prevention of Hospitalization. Arch. Gen. Psychiat. 11: 162, 1964.

"Is it advantageous or disadvantageous and dangerous to use phenothiazines and reserpine in combination with electroshock therapy?"

Reply: After reviewing the literature since 1955, John Gonzalez and John Imahara, at Louisiana State University, concluded that use of electroshock therapy and reserpine is potentially quite dangerous and should be avoided. They then reviewed the records of 240 patients treated with a combination of electroshock and phenothiazines and concluded that this procedure was quite safe and indeed that the combination can be more useful than electroshock alone or the phenothiazines alone in producing a more rapid remission, a smoother treatment course and a higher overall remission rate. I am inclined to believe, however, that Stanley Lesse, of Columbia University, perhaps more nearly expressed the feeling many workers experienced in this field when he stated that he was unwilling to recommend the routine use of combined therapy because he found it had no advantage over shock therapy alone, except in a few specific instances, such as in the more agitated or manic patients in intervals between electroshock treatments during the first few days of therapy. Of course he admitted that the drugs may help calm the agitation during an electroshock series and the agitation and restlessness during the postelectroshock treatment of organic psychoses.

John R. Gonzalez and John K. Imahara. Electroshock Therapy with Phenothiazines and Reserpine: Survey and Report. Am. J. Psychiat. 121:253, 1964. Stanley Lesse. Electroshock Therapy and Tranquilizing Drugs. J.A.M.A. 170:1791, Aug. 8, 1959.

"Would you kindly list the principal phenothiazine agents (i.e., the true antipsychotics) used in treatment of the psychoses and indicate the drug of choice?"

Reply: Acetophenazine (Tindal), carphenazine (Proketazine), chlorpromazine (Thorazine), fluphenazine (Permitil, Prolixin), mepazine (Pacatal), perphenazine (Trilafon), prochlorperazine (Compazine), promazine

(Sparine), thiopropazate (Dartal), thioridazine (Mellaril), trifluoperazine (Stelazine), triflupromazine (Vesprin). I do not think anyone can say truthfully of the phenothiazine compounds that have appeared in the wake of chlorpromazine (Thorazine) that this or that one is superior for clearly discernible reasons. The absence of enough well controlled double-blind studies simply makes it impossible. I believe it is quite generally agreed, however, that chlorpromazine itself is still to be preferred in the most seriously involved patients and that competition among the other drugs is with each other and not with chlorpromazine in this type of case. One must remember always that a great many more doses of chlorpromazine have been given than of any of the others and that this may give the newer drugs an advantage regarding relative freedom from toxicity that is more apparent than real. But see the immediately following Reply.

"There are so many phenothiazines available now for the treatment of schizophrenia and considerable argument among the practitioners with whom I am associated about which is the best of the lot. Could you cite one clearcut study of the matter?"

Reply: As convincing a study as any that has come to my attention, in which the several drugs of this group are compared with each other, was that conducted by Adelson and Epstein at the University of California in 1962. In a well controlled and evaluated double-blind study, employing 288 patients and chlorpromazine (Thorazine), perphenazine (Trilafon), prochlorperazine (Compazine), triflupromazine (Vesprin), and an active placebo containing scopolamine and chlorprophenpyridamine maleate, and an inactive lactose placebo, they found the group as a whole acquitting themselves nobly (bringing up for discharge about seven times as many patients as did the mere passage of time, i.e., the placebo-treated group), and any one of the drugs was as good as any other.

Daniel Adelson and Leon J. Epstein. Study of Phenothiazines with Male and Female Chronically Ill Schizophrenic Patients. J. Nerv. & Ment. Dis. 134:543, 1962.

"That great drug, chlorpromazine (Thorazine), which I still feel to be superior to any of the newer agents that have been introduced as substitutes for it in psychiatric practice, has other useful employments as well but I do not know what all of them are. Would you kindly list these additional uses briefly?"

Reply: Chlorpromazine is very valuable in potentiating the *analgesic and sedative* action of the narcotics of the morphine group in individuals with advanced malignant lesions or other types of severe pain. The drug appears not only to make possible at times a reduction in opiate dosage but also to enable patients to view their pain somewhat as an objective phenomenon. If potent narcotic analgesics are used together with chlorpromazine they should be given in only one-fourth to one-half dosage. Numerous observations in both obstetric and surgical services have established the fact that the pharmacologic attributes of chlorpromazine together with its actual performance in the operating room secure a place for it as adjuvant to the classic drugs—the opiates, barbiturates and belladonna group—in *preanesthetic medication.* The aspects of its multifaceted action that are important here are its contribution to the relaxation of the patient through its tranquilizing action, its potentiation of the analgesic and hypnotic drugs, its checking effect on salivary and gastric secretions, its reduction of alarm responses and reflex respiratory reactions and its lightening of the postoperative management load through depressing nausea and vomiting. Some protection is afforded by the drug against epinephrine-induced arrhythmias during general anesthesia, but the fact that patients who become hypotensive during surgical procedures do not respond to vasopressor drugs in usual doses while under the influence of chlorpromazine is undoubtedly a disadvantage that must be realized and reckoned with.

The use of chlorpromazine in the "lytic cocktail" method of *inducing hypothermia* is not as much in fashion now as formerly. This method employs three drugs, chlorpromazine (Thorazine), promethazine (Phenergan) and meperidine (Demerol). The attempt is made with these agents to block the autonomic nervous system because the body's defensive mechanisms against alterations in the internal environment are largely mediated through this system and its hypothalamic connections with the cerebrum. The fall in temperature, which may be to 94°F. (34°C.) or even lower, is the desirable thing but it is accomplished when these drugs are given only as an expression of the fact that the patient is not reacting in any "defensive" way to the surgical stress. It is now the consensus that the active constituent of the cocktail is chlorpromazine, that meperidine decreases shivering somewhat while contributing very little to the fall in temperature, and that promethazine practically does not enter into the action. The matter of shivering comprises a major roadblock in the accomplishment of hypothermia by this method and is therefore usually combated by the use of a curariform drug in addition to the cocktail. The chief hazard in hypothermia is the occurrence of ventricular fibrillation.

Chlorpromazine is highly effective in *combating nausea and vomiting* of most diverse causation; indeed, it has replaced practically all other antiemetic drugs in most varieties of this malady, such as those associated with the following states: uremia, brain tumor, radiation sickness, carcinomatosis, the post-anesthetic state, hyperemesis gravidarum, parturition, high dosages of the morphine group of drugs, the tetracyclines, the nitrogen mustards and the folic acid antagonists. The vomiting in gastroenteritis and that associated with obstructive gastrointestinal lesions is less affected than most other types, and it is a very disconcerting fact that motion sickness (seasickness and airsickness) is almost completely resistant to chlorpromazine.

Chlorpromazine has proved to be by far the most effective agent ever introduced into the therapy of intractable *hiccup.*

It has been alleged that chlorpromazine is the most effective remedial agent thus far employed to combat the pain and nervous manifestations of *porphyria.* It is often successful in *pruritus* when other measures have failed. It is sometimes effectively used in combination with the classic bronchodilator agents in the therapy of *paroxysms of bronchial asthma.* Its use has sometimes made the management of *tetanus* cases much easier. Combined with hyperventilation it is used as a method of *activation in the encephalographic study of epileptic patients.* There has been a report, based on a considerable experience in India, that it is helpful in *cataract surgery* through reducing the number of cases of vitreous prolapse and postoperative iris prolapse. There is sometimes a considerable *diuretic effect* when used in patients with congestive heart failure of various etiologies. There is some evidence of intensification of the *muscle relaxing action* of drugs of the curare group, but it is doubtful that the action is anything more than a reflection of the centrally produced generalized hypotonicity that is characteristic of the drug. Effective use in *Ménière's syndrome,* at least to the extent of lessening the vertigo component, has been reported.

"The psychiatrist in our group is able occasionally to show a good result from the use of an androgenic steroid in schizophrenia. How would one rationalize such therapy?"

Reply: A truly rational explanation might be a bit difficult to achieve, but I think we all recognize that the schizophrenic characteristically lacks stamina in practically all re-

spects. A few years ago, Leonard Lapinsohn (VA Hospital, Coral Gables, Florida) reported that in his hands methandrostenolone (Dianabol) had decided clinical value in treatment of many patients with schizophrenia, but I have heard nothing further of this. He suggested that the increased appetite and subsequent increased caloric protein intake may aid in bringing about improved reaction to stress and improved adrenal response.

Leonard I. Lapinsohn. Use of Δ¹,17-α-Methyl Testosterone (Dianabol) as Adjuvant in the Treatment of Schizophrenic Reactions. Dis. Nerv. System 22:443, 1961.

"It is not always easy to keep the schizophrenic patient rigidly on his therapy when he is not living under rigid control conditions. In fact, some individuals do not seem to be greatly harmed by a period without drugs, while others quickly deteriorate. Is there any predictability in this situation?"

Reply: At the Anoka, Minn., State Hospital, Olson and Peterson found that sudden interruption of chemotherapy did not adversely affect chronic patients immediately, and indeed that most of them could remain drug-free for several months without distress. Diamond and Marks, at the VA Hospital, American Lake, Washington, reported substantially the same thing, and so too did Martin Gross, at the Springfield State Hospital, Sykesville, Maryland, but the latter showed that it is nevertheless necessary for the patient who has been discharged on the drugs to continue their use in order to remain in the non-hospitalized community. As for predictability, Blackburn and Allen (VA Hospital, Lebanon, Pennsylvania) found no basis for determining which patients will deteriorate and which will remain relatively unchanged when medication is interrupted. They also observed that significant deterioration was unrelated to initial adjustment level, type of drug, drug dosage, age or length of current hospitalization.

H. L. Blackburn and J. L. Allen. Behavioral Effects of Interrupting and Resuming Tranquilizing Medication Among Schizophrenics. J. Nerv. & Ment. Dis. 133:303, 1961. Gordon W. Olson and Donald B. Peterson. Sudden Removal of Tranquilizing Drugs from Chronic Psychiatric Patients. J. Nerv. & Ment. Dis. 131:252, 1960. Leon S. Diamond and John B. Marks. Discontinuance of Tranquilizers Among Chronic Schizophrenic Patients Receiving Maintenance Dosage. J. Nerv. & Ment. Dis. 131: 247, 1960. Martin Gross. Impact of Ataractic Drugs on Mental Hospital Outpatient Clinic. Am. J. Psychiat. 117: 444, 1960.

"There appears to be a burgeoning tendency in psychiatry to place a drug on test in a widely scattered group of hospitals, with the conditions of the experiment laid down in some distant office, and then present the aggregate findings as having acquired significance through the large number of patients that was involved in the total study. Is this sort of thing truly admissible?"

Reply: Admissible, well who shall say? With the Food and Drug Administration nowadays requiring that the therapeutic efficacy of a drug be established before its use in practice is permitted, it is difficult to see how else the thing can be done since larger numbers of cases are required than can usually be obtained in the population of one or a small number of hospitals. And theoretically the method is sound: the conditions under which the drug is to be administered are carefully prescribed, the determinants of successful employment fully delineated, the methods of data accumulation and recording clearly established, and the processing and computerizing exhaustively done in the home office. And yet my old-fashioned mind fails to chortle happily at the prospect of all our drugs gaining access to practice along such a route in the future. Quantitation cannot truly be an acceptable substitute for sophistication in any of the affairs of mankind. In an approach of this kind, which I analyzed from the armchair several years ago, there were 512 patients initially incorporated in the study in 32 hospitals. Simple division would derive the figure of 16 patients per hospital, but of course this would be a fallacious figure since there must surely have been many more than that in some hospitals and very probably many fewer in some others. The report, however, did not supply figures on this head. And nothing that was really enlightening was said about the personnel involved in the performance of the investigation—would one be unfair in wanting to know something about the shifts that occurred among all the psychologists, psychiatrists, nurses and nursing assistants who were involved in the study in the various hospitals? How many of them were truly dedicated or even cared about the matter at all; can we really believe that the stipulations emanating from the sponsoring organization were carried out with equal interest and integrity in all of the institutions? Anyone who is engaged in clinical research in a single hospital knows how difficult it is in any experiment that extends beyond a very brief period to hold the undivided, nonprejudiced and wholly objective interest of a small and initially dedicated group. So I am skeptical, and I also believe that we have reached an impasse. The incursion of public, i.e., political, influence into the conduct of medical investigation is bound to impose standards that I suppose we shall have to learn to accept, but let's not do it resignedly. I for one protest that study methods are not bound to be successful in medicine simply because they have been productive of results in industrial operations. The loading of freight cars, the manipulations involved in the making of steel, the processing of pulp in paper manufacture—these things may probably all be standardized and nationally studied and controlled. But patients and their doctors and nurses are people. People are individuals, no two alike, and the most difficult things in the world to study.

"The phenothiazine derivatives have certainly been tremendously useful in the therapy of mental disorders, but their use is undeniably accompanied by a considerable amount of toxicity. I am sure that in specialized institutions this is all taken in stride; for a private practitioner like myself, who does not very frequently have occasion to use one of these drugs, have any signposts been devised to warn of impending trouble?"

Reply: The list of toxic manifestations of these drugs is certainly a long one, but they are usually reversible if the drug is omitted and therefore not particularly serious affairs if considered in relation to the very dour situations in which the drugs are justifiably employed. Fortunately the most serious of these reactions, agranulocytosis, is the least common. From experience gained in 18 instances of this reaction at the Milwaukee County Hospital, Anthony Pisciotta concluded that weekly leukocyte counts are essential, especially between the second and tenth week of treatment; also that monthly counts be made thereafter as long as the patient continues to receive the drug; and that sore throat, stomatitis, fever, malaise, chills or other evidences of infection be reported promptly. In his series the total cumulative dose that induced the reaction ranged from 2 to 112 Gm., and the time required for leukopenia to develop from 10 to 400 days. However, in most patients a drop in the leukocyte count was recognized after 20 to 45 days of therapy, but it was impossible to predict when a sudden drop in the count would occur.

Anthony V. Pisciotta. Hematologic Safeguards During Treatment with Phenothiazine Derivatives. J.A.M.A. 170:662, June 6, 1959.

"Would you not be surprised if a patient on a low dose of a phenothiazine derivative developed such extrapyramidal side effects as tremor, rigidity, trismus, dystonic movements, sialorrhea, etc.?"

Reply: These things do occur from ordinary dosage, you know, but relatively rarely, to be sure. I would be inclined to suspect that the patient was taking higher dosage than you recommended. They will do it when they do not get early relief from the symptoms for which the drug was prescribed, or when the pressure from the job or some troubles at home push them increasingly.

Glenn A. Bacon (Racine, Wisconsin). Compounding of Symptoms with Prochlorperazine (Compazine). Wisconsin M. J. 63:475, 1964.

"I have a patient with chronic undifferentiated schizophrenic reaction who has been receiving phenothiazine therapy for 4 years, and I have now found faint, almost transparent lenticular opacities on ophthalmoscopic study. On slit-lamp examination, pigmentary deposits may be seen in the anterior lens cortex near the capsule. There is no corneal involvement and no disturbance in visual acuity or increase in intraocular tension or other changes. Is this sort of thing characteristic of long-term phenothiazine administration?"

Reply: The association of pigmentary lenticular deposits and cutaneous pigmentation has been documented as a complication of chlorpromazine (Thorazine) therapy, and, at the University of California, Lester Margolis and John Goble have reported a study demonstrating that ventricular opacities may be induced by trifluoperazine (Stelazine), and they postulate that the capacity for producing such changes may be a potential property of any phenothiazine derivative. Regarding skin pigmentation, the experience of L. W. C. Massey, in Ontario, indicates the advisability of maintaining daily dosage of chlorpromazine at 500 mg. or below when the patient is exposed to sunlight, for his patient did not pigment at that dosage though she did so previously on higher dosage.

Lester H. Margolis and John L. Goble. Lenticular Opacities with Prolonged Phenothiazine Therapy: Potential Hazard with All Phenothiazine Derivatives. J.A.M.A. 193:7, July 5, 1965. L. W. C. Massey. Skin Pigmentation, Corneal and Lens Opacities with Prolonged Chlorpromazine Treatment. Canad. M. A. J. 92:186, Jan. 23, 1965.

"Some of my associates feel that the appearance of extrapyramidal system disturbance is a wholly undesirable occurrence when using the phenothiazine tranquilizers, and therefore use the drugs in slowly increasing amounts in the attempt to accomplish maximal improvement with a minimal amount of this side action; but others feel that this type of disturbance is a sine qua non for improvement, and therefore push the drugs from the beginning. Where does the truth lie?"

Reply: I think it has not really been determined, but in their limited study at the Rockland State Hospital, Orangeburg, New York, George Simpson and associates failed to find a correlation between the severity of parkinsonian manifestations and general improvement in their patients.

George M. Simpson, Dominick Amuso, John H. Blair and Tibor Farkas. Phenothiazine-Produced Extrapyramidal System Disturbance. Arch. Gen. Psychiat. 10:199, 1964.

"I have a patient on chlorpromazine who has developed spontaneous galactorrhea which is persistent despite regular menses. Could this be attributable to the drug?"

Reply: Yes, this reaction has been reported with both chlorpromazine and reserpine and most recently with imipramine (Tofranil). In the latter instance the lactation ceased 3 weeks after the drug was stopped and resumed 2 weeks after the drug was prescribed again; then it again ceased when the drug was discontinued.

Jerome J. Klein, Robert Lloyd Segal and Richard R. Pichel Warner. Galactorrhea Due to Imipramine. New England J. Med. 271:510, Sept. 3, 1964.

"I have recently had a patient die suddenly from a cause that could not be ascribable to anything but the phenothiazine derivative medication that he was taking. Could it be possible that the drug was really responsible?"

Reply: I do not know, though Leo Hollister and Jon Kosek, in Palo Alto, have taken the position that drugs of this group possibly cause ventricular fibrillation more often than they cause such feared complications as agranulocytosis and toxic attack on the liver. They reported 6 cases in their own experience in which there was an abrupt syncopal or seizure-like attack followed immediately by death, with necropsy findings that were inadequate to explain the culmination. Certainly the subject merits renewed attention, but I feel that before ascribing too many of these occurrences to the use of the drugs in question we should fully take into account the fact that many sudden unexpected deaths are not traceable to drug ingestion. Alan R. Moritz and Norman Zamcheck recorded that among 40,000 necropsies of soldiers dying in World War II, 1000 sudden deaths were encountered, 140 of which could not be readily explained.

Leo E. Hollister and Jon C. Kosek. Sudden Death During Treatment with Phenothiazine Derivatives. J.A.M.A. 192:1035, June 21, 1965. Alan R. Moritz and N. Zamcheck. Sudden and Unexpected Deaths of Young Soldiers. Arch. Path. 42:459, 1946.

"Will sudden withdrawal of chlorpromazine (Thorazine) from a patient who has been receiving the drug for some time cause gastrointestinal disturbances? I ask this because I am wondering whether perhaps the nausea and vomiting I am attributing to another cause in a present patient may actually be due to the fact that since hospitalization she has been deprived of the chlor-promazine that she had been taking."

Reply: Yes, chlorpromazine withdrawal can cause gastrointestinal disturbances, and indeed the study of Philip Haden, in Ontario, indicates that some of the other phenothiazine drugs may do this also. He gave chlorpromazine (Thorazine), thioridazine (Mellaril), perphenazine (Trilafon) or chlorprothixene (Taractan) to groups of 10 patients, and then suddenly withdrew the medications. Three patients receiving chlorpromazine developed gastrointestinal symptoms, 3 who had received thioridazine, 1 who had received chlorprothixene, and none who had received perphenazine. Actually, perphenazine is used as an antiemetic and it is not surprising that it did not cause nausea and vomiting as the others did upon withdrawal. I think your point, that symptoms attributed to other drugs or to some development in the malady under treatment may actually be due to the withdrawal of a drug that had been chronically used by the patient, is one that does not receive the consideration that it should. We are certainly still in comparative ignorance of the potentialities of all these new drugs that are crowding in upon us nowadays.

Philip Haden. Gastrointestinal Disturbances Associated with Withdrawal of Ataractic Drugs. Canad. M. A. J. 91: 974, Oct. 31, 1964.

"I have recently had the experience of seeing a patient display marked trismus after a very small dose of one of the phenothiazine compounds. Is there any antidote for this?"

Reply: Peter Gott, at St. Luke's Hospital Center in New York, says that an intravenous injection of 50 mg. of diphenhydramine (Benadryl) will allay these symptoms in a few seconds. In Racine, Glenn Bacon found intravenous injection of 2 mg. benztropine (Cogentin) provided dramatic relief in a patient who had many other extrapyramidal side effects of the drug in addition to trismus.

Peter H. Gott. Drug Reaction Simulating Tetanus. New England J. Med. 274:167, 1966. Glenn A. Bacon. Compounding of Symptoms with Prochlorperazine (Compazine). Wisconsin M. J. 63:475, 1964.

"I have a psychiatric patient who has to be frequently rehospitalized because when discharged on what appears to be satisfactory maintenance dosage of a phenothiazine compound he invariably gets into trouble and has to be brought back. What shall I do?"

Reply: Keep him snowed under! There is a great tendency among us to forget that the suitable dose of any drug in any situation is that which causes greatest effect without intolerable side effects. And we simply have to develop this dosage experimentally in the individual patient. In discussing a situation such as yours, Fred Forrest and associates, in Palo Alto, have said that in discharged chronic mental patients on maintenance doses of 600–1200 mg. chlorpromazine or equivalent doses of other phenothiazines, most side effects can be controlled by regular administration of antiparkinsonian drugs. If there is a prevalent feeling of fatigue during the day, 1200 mg. can be divided into 200 mg. three times a day with meals and 600 mg. at bedtime. I think that these investigators have made a very important point when they say that chronic mental illness should be treated as a metabolic disease, and that a "compensated" patient should not be "decompensated" for other than stringent medical reasons.

Fred M. Forrest, Clyde W. Geiter, Harold L. Snow and Meyer Steinbach. Drug Maintenance Problems of Rehabilitated Mental Patients: The Current Drug Dosage "Merry-Go-Round." Am. J. Psychiat. 121:33, 1964.

"It is rumored that in Scandinavia effective use is being made of thyroid drugs in the treatment of schizophrenia. Is this true?"

Reply: A study of this matter was published by Karl Lochner and associates a few years ago, but I am not acquainted with any subsequent investigation. Lochner found in a small, controlled study in which the treated patients received 50 μg. of liothyronine (Cytomel) orally twice daily, doubled after 1 week and then 200 μg. daily for the next 6 weeks, that in some instances favorable changes are produced in the mental state and ward behavior of chronic schizophrenics. It has never been possible through the years to establish a relationship of thyroid deficiency to schizophrenia, but that failure is of no importance in relation to Lochner's experience because none of his patients had been shown to be thyroid deficient prior to the initiation of therapy. There is certainly no present indication that thyroid therapy may be expected to compete successfully with the potent antipsychotic drugs.

Karl H. Lochner, Marilyn R. Scheuing and Frederic F. Flach. Effect of L-Triiodothyronine (Cytomel) on Chronic Schizophrenic Patients. Acta psychiat. scandinav. 39: 413, 1963.

"I find that in my service in a big-city teaching-research psychiatric clinic I am tending to use drugs more frequently than formerly and cutting down on intensive psychotherapy. Am I doing injustice to my patients in this?"

Reply: In Philadelphia, Blaine McLaughlin

considered precisely such a situation in the case of borderline personalities on the ragged edge of requiring hospital care, and concluded that they can often be maintained as outpatients through the use of tranquilizing drugs and a reduction in the amount of time earlier devoted to psychotherapy alone. When the drugs were used in only moderate dosage no *decisive* changes occurred in the patients' adjustment, but they were kept out of hospital and in a more comfortable state through short-term control of their anxiety symptoms, and a great deal of clinic time was saved. He found that under these circumstances it was often advantageous to switch about among the drugs and that the amount of enthusiasm shown by the physician for a given drug often had a favorable influence upon both the degree and extent of time in which the agent was effective.

Blaine E. McLaughlin. Long-Term Therapy with Neurotropic Drugs in Psychiatric Outpatients. GP 30:99, 1964.

"Recently when using succinylcholine (Anectine, etc.) as a 'softening' agent in convulsive therapy we experienced a frightening period of apnea and were helpless to deal with it other than through artificial respiration and the administration of oxygen. What antidotal drugs should we have been familiar with?"

Reply: There are no specific antidotal drugs for this skeletal muscle relaxant which effects its paralysis through preventing the repolarization of the endplate. In the case of curare paralysis it is rational to attempt antidotal action through employing agents to promote piling up of acetylcholine, but the use of these agents—such drugs as physostigmine, neostigmine (Prostigmin) and edrophonium (Tensilon)—would only worsen matters in the case of overaction from succinylcholine.

"I have a patient with Huntington's chorea in whom I have been able to effect some slight diminution in the choreic movements through the use of phenothiazine-derivative tranquilizers, but the other symptoms have not been affected. Is there anything that can be recommended?"

Reply: Unfortunately the emotional disturbances and personality deterioration, that characterize this hereditary malady together with the chorea, have so far resisted all types of therapy. It is perhaps a fortunate fact that in all age groups the life expectancy of the individual with Huntington's chorea is only half that of the nonchoreic person.

"In the senile patient, often referred to euphemistically as having the 'chronic brain syndrome,'

there is sometimes a state of agitated depression which would appear to call for the use of both tranquilizing and antidepression measures. Is there any drug which combines both of these properties?"

Reply: There is a fairly new drug, tybamate (Solacen), which has not yet had its position fully established though there have been some favorable reports of its use in such situations as those you have in mind. For example, in the study of 87 institutionalized male geriatric patients suffering from chronic brain syndrome, Eugene Chesrow and associates, in Oak Forest, Illinois, found that the 44 patients given this drug in a placebo-controlled, double-blind study were significantly more improved than the 43 control patients in such matters as insomnia, agitation, restlessness and tension, anxiety, depression and behavioral disorders. In Philadelphia, Francis Stern made a double-blind crossover comparison of meprobamate (Miltown, Equanil) and tybamate (Solacen) and found the newer drug more beneficial and less soporific than meprobamate, which is an important quality in the treatment of aged patients.

Eugene J. Chesrow, Sherman E. Kaplitz, Raoul Sabatini, Helga Vetra and Gilbert H. Marquardt. A New Psychotherapeutic Agent Effective in Management of Geriatric Anxiety, Depression and Behavioral Reactions. J. Am. Geriatrics Soc. 13:449, 1965. Francis H. Stern. New Drug, Tybamate, Effective in Management of Chronic Brain Syndrome. J. Am. Geriatrics Soc. 12:1066, 1964.

"Do we really have clear-cut evidence that some of our drugs are specifically effective only in the treatment of depressions and others only in the treatment of schizophrenic reactions?"

Reply: It is certainly the consensus that this is true but the opinion is not unanimous. I shall cite the experience of John Overall and associates, in Palo Alto, who randomly assigned one or the other type of drug to newly hospitalized patients diagnosed as having either schizophrenic or depressive reactions, the nature and the assignment of treatments being unknown to both physicians and patients. The agents compared were imipramine (Tofranil) in the antidepressant class and thioridazine (Mellaril) in the phenothiazine class. It was found that thioridazine was significantly superior to imipramine in some schizophrenic patients. There were essentially no significant differences between the drugs in depressive patients, although the observed mean differences tended to favor thioridazine. Summing across both patient samples, thioridazine was said to have been significantly superior to imipramine in a number of symptom areas, whereas imipramine was superior only in reducing motor retardation. This study therefore did not confirm the specificity of action ordinarily attributed to drugs in these two classes, and the investigators expressed the feeling that this lack of clear distinction suggests that pharmacologic screening tests for antipsychotic and antidepressant drugs need re-evaluation. Unfortunately, I do not find this evidence as convincing as could be wished because the work was not done in one hospital but spread out among 68 schizophrenic patients in four Veterans Administration hospitals and 77 depressed patients in seven Veterans Administration hospitals. Might not this rather thin spread have meant that very few observations were made in some of these stations?

John E. Overall, Leo E. Hollister, Fred Meyer, Isham Kimbell, Jr., and Jack Shelton. Imipramine (Tofranil) and Thioridazine (Mellaril) in Depressed and Schizophrenic Patients: Are There Specific Antidepressant Drugs? J.A.M.A. 189:605, Aug. 24, 1964.

"Though I have heard expression of contrary opinion, it is my own observation that the antidepressant drugs, such as imipramine (Tofranil) and amitriptyline (Elavil) and the newer agent, desipramine (Norpramin, Pertofrane), are really effective in relieving depression. But recently I have been puzzled by the fact that when I use one of these drugs together with a phenothiazine such as chlorpromazine (Thorazine), I obtain more satisfactory response in a schizophrenic than with a phenothiazine alone even though depression was not a prominent symptom in the case. Have others observed this sort of thing?"

Reply: Yes, there have been reports of such observations but all so far on a small scale, so that one does not yet know to what extent the antidepressants may be accepted as potentiators of the action of the phenothiazines.

"When I have a depressed patient in my practice, which is not at all a rare occurrence, I put him or her on an antidepressant agent if careful study indicates that the use of such a drug may be desirable, and then watch for signs of improvement. But as I read the psychiatric literature it seems to me that I cannot determine what results I am getting unless I use at least three or four tests with such resounding eponymous titles as the Minnesota Multiphasic Personality Inventory, the Clyde Mood Scale, the Wechsler Adult Intelligence Scale, the Numerical Ability subtest of the Differential Aptitude Tests, the Standard Interview, the Maudsley personality inventory, the Hildreth feeling scale, the Mill Hill vocabulary scale, the Brengelmann picture-recognition test, the Babcock-Levy error-free speed test, etc., etc. What of this; do I or do I not know whether my patient is getting better?"

Reply: I know nothing about the performance or value of these tests, save what I read in the literature, and I am going to condemn nothing out of hand. *But*, if a patient says he is feeling better and behaves as though he is, and his family and associates say that he is better, and you too find him much less depressed—then he is better, isn't he? Myself, I would like Clinical Impression to have capitals too!

"I have several people on tranylcypromine (Parnate), but I am a bit worried because I do not precisely understand the 'cheese syndrome' in connection with the use of this drug. Would you kindly explain?"

Reply: In the summer of 1963, reports appeared in the British literature describing a "cheese hypertension" in individuals who were being treated with monoamine oxidase inhibitors. It was actually the husband of one of B. Blackwell's patients who suggested that the diets of the patients involved be studied. When this was done it was found that 8 of the 10 patients had eaten cheese within 2 hours of the onset of their acute hypertensive attack. At this point, A. M. Asatoor and associates, attracted to the study by the fact that cheese contains amines produced by bacterial action on the amino acids of casein, analyzed cheeses of various sorts and found that all of them contained tyramines. Thus the "cheese syndrome" came into being, predicated upon the belief that the normal degradation by monoamine oxidases of the tyramine in cheese is prevented by the inhibitors of these enzymes when administered as drugs. At the National Institutes of Health, Horwitz's group put the matter to the test experimentally by administering tyramine hydrochloride intravenously during several hours to patients before and during treatment with a monoamine oxidase inhibitor. Only one-tenth to one-hundredth as much tyramine was required to effect a systolic pressure response during the monoamine oxidase inhibitor administration as when the inhibitor was not being given. It is therefore not only your Parnate that may involve the patient in a situation of this sort but any other monoamine oxidase inhibitor as well. The following are the principal drugs of this group: Eutonyl, Marplan, Niamid, Nardil and Parnate. At the University of Witwatersrand, J. Mendels found that pre-existing hypertension apparently does not predispose individuals to one of these hypertensive episodes.

B. Blackwell. Tranylcypromine. Lancet 2:414, 1963. A. M. Asatoor, A. J. Levi, M. D. Milne. Tranylcypromine and Cheese. Lancet 2:733, 1963. David Horwitz, Walter Lovenberg, Karl Engelman and Albert Sjoerdsma. Monoamine Oxidase Inhibitors, Tyramine and Cheese. J.A.M.A. 188:1108, June 29, 1964. Herbert F. R. Plass. Monoamine

Oxidase Inhibitor Reactions Simulating Pheochromocytoma Attacks. Ann. Int. Med. 61:924, 1964. J. Mendels. Side Effects of Tranylcypromine. South African M. J. 39:175, 1965.

"I find the antidepressant drugs associated with so much disagreeable side action, such as dryness of the mouth, constipation, weight gain, difficulty in micturition and postural hypotension, that many patients refuse to continue taking them. Is there any remedy for this?"

Reply: In New York City, John Prutting successfully used pilocarpine nitrate in dosage of 2.5–5 mg. once to four times daily in overcoming these objectionable reactions to imipramine (Tofranil) and amitriptyline (Elavil) in a small group of patients. There were no unpleasant side effects from the drug except that in 1 patient there was slightly excessive perspiration until dosage was reduced. However, this antidotal measure should probably not be employed if there is gastrointestinal irritability or hyperacidity or if the patient is asthmatic.

John Prutting. Pilocarpine Nitrate and Psychostimulants: Antagonistic Agent to Anticholinergic Effects. J.A.M.A. 193:236, July 19, 1965.

"Would you please provide a list of the principal antidepressant drugs currently in use and make some suggestions regarding choice among them?"

Reply: Nowadays we find ourselves in possession of a scientifically devised and legitimate group of central nervous system stimulants that had as well be designated "psychomotor stimulants" as "antidepressants." It is important for us to be aware, however, that a number of these drugs, unlike the "tonics" of an earlier period and the current trumpery nostrums of the newspaper advertisements, are potent agents with great potentialities for harm if improperly used or if they sensitize the patient, and also that their use does not abrogate the claim the patient has upon us for the exercise of our psychotherapeutic acumen and our guidance in rehabilitative measures.

The drugs are used to combat depressive symptoms in both the psychoses and the neuroses. In the former, the opportunity for objective determination of improvement is considerable and therefore measurement of drug efficacy can be accomplished with reasonable facility. But in the neuroses the opportunities for controlled study are meager; this, coupled with the intangible placebo effect of the physician's attention and prescription plus the transient nature of many of these depressions, should make one chary of accepting at face value all the rosy claims for success that are made for these drugs.

Since these agents are quite the vogue at present a number of reviews of them by psychiatrists have appeared; but I find most of them quite wordy and not very useful from a practical standpoint. However, at the end of 1965 Dale Friend, who is an internist and not a psychiatrist, summarized the respective merits of the compounds quite tersely and satisfactorily.

The monoamine oxidase inhibitors comprise isocarboxazid, nialamide, phenelzine, pargyline and tranylcypromine. Isocarboxazid (Marplan) dosage is 10 mg. three times daily with maintenance dosage of 10–20 mg. daily, adjusting always for the individual patient's needs. The drug appears to be a useful one if the depression is of mild degree; i.e., it is much less effective than imipramine (Tofranil) and considerably more toxic. Nialamide (Niamid) dosage is 25–50 mg. four times daily, adjusted to the patient's needs. Maintenance dosage may be as little as 12.5 mg. on alternate days. This drug is probably about as effective as isocarboxazid. Phenelzine (Nardil) dosage is 15 mg. three or four times daily and possibly at bedtime if needed, with maintenance dosage perhaps as low as 15 mg. every second day. It appears to be agreed that this drug is more effective usually than either of the preceding ones but not as effective as imipramine (Tofranil). Tranylcypromine (Parnate) dosage is 10 mg. twice daily with attempt to obtain maintenance on 5 or 10 mg. every other day. This appears to be the most useful of the monoamine oxidase inhibitors, being in fact probably as effective as imipramine (Tofranil). Pargyline (Eutonyl) dosage is 25–50 mg. daily and increased until effect is reached or toxicity occurs; maintenance dosage has to be worked out individually of course but one should strive for 25 mg. daily or every other day. The efficacy of this drug is somewhat doubtful though it appears almost certainly to be a less potent agent than tranylcypromine.

Since one or more of these side actions have occurred with some of the monoamine oxidase inhibitors it is advisable to consider that such reactions may occur with any of them: a feeling of fullness in the head, weakness, dizziness, blurred vision, mouth dryness, constipation (even adynamic ileus), rashes, postural hypotension, hallucinations, overstimulation, inhibiton of ejaculation, anemia, leukopenia and rarely toxic hepatitis. All these effects are reversible when the drug is discontinued. The drugs of this group have a tendency to potentiate the action of certain other drugs, which makes it inadvisable to use them together with the sympathomimetic amines of the amphetamine type, aminopyrine, barbiturates, acetanilid, cocaine and procaine, meperidine, insulin, opiates, antihypertensive agents, alcohol, ether. Since severe fulminating hypertension has occurred when one of the drugs of this group, tranylcypromine (Parnate), is used in an individual who is eating cheese, it is advisable to consider that the eating of cheese should be interdicted in patients who are being treated with any of these drugs.

Another group of antidepressant agents, the iminodibenzyl or so-called tricyclic compounds, has the following as its principal members: imipramine, desipramine, amitriptyline and nortriptyline. These drugs are often quite effective antidepressants, particularly in the neuroses, and they are certainly in the main much less toxic than the monoamine oxidase inhibitors. However, the list of side actions and true toxic reactions recorded in connection with the use of imipramine is quite large, and I think it advisable to be alert to the potentiality of any of these occurrences in the other drugs of the group as well: generalized tremor, fainting, falling suddenly without premonitory signs, hallucinations, urinary retention, dryness of the mouth, tachycardia, excitement, orthostatic hypotension, Parkinson syndrome, enhancement of intraocular pressure, constipation, disturbances of accommodation, sweating, skin rashes, jaundice, pruritus, angioneurotic edema, leukopenia, agranulocytosis. The suggestion has been made that sodium and water retention may be promoted, arrhythmias induced and the convulsive threshold lowered. Insomnia is of course a not unlikely occurrence, though it appears that in the case of amitriptyline the more frequent occurrence is sedation; this drug also upon occasion causes gastrointestinal distress.

Imipramine (Tofranil) dosage usually begins with 100 mg. daily and may be cautiously increased to 250 or 300 mg. unless the patient is an adolescent or elderly; gradual reduction to 50–150 mg. daily is striven for. Desipramine (Norpramin, Pertofrane) dosage is 25–50 mg. three times daily, increasing to 200 mg. daily when necessary. Amitriptyline (Elavil) dosage is 25 mg. three times daily, increasing to 150 or even 300 mg. daily if necessary, though one should be very cautious in adolescents and the elderly. Nortriptyline (Aventyl) dosage ranges widely from 10 to 300 mg. daily according to need, but one should certainly be cautious with the upper range of such dosage.

Dale G. Friend. Anti-Depressant Drug Therapy. Clin. Pharmacol. & Therap. 6:805, 1965.

"How do the several antidepressant drugs compare in speed of action?"

Reply: At the University of California,

Harvey Widroe rates them as follows in this regard. Possible improvement within hours: dextroamphetamine and amobarbital (Dexamyl); methylphenidate (Ritalin); methamphetamine (Desoxyn); dextroamphetamine (Dexedrine). A lag of several days before improvement: imipramine (Tofranil); amitriptyline (Elavil). A lag of at least 1 week before improvement: phenelzine (Nardil); nialamide (Niamid); isocarboxazid (Marplan). He has made the point that to change from one of the quickest acting drugs to one of the intermediate group one should wait 24 hours after discontinuing the first drug; to change from a drug of the intermediate group to one of the slowest group, wait 4 days; to change to any drug after discontinuing a drug of the slowest group, wait 10 days.

Harvey J. Widroe. A Schema for the Use of Antidepressant Drugs. Am. J. Psychiat. 121:1111, 1965.

"What is the present position of the amphetamines (Benzedrine, Dexedrine) in the treatment of depression?"

Reply: Use of the amphetamines in depressed states is still widespread when it is felt that the condition is psychosomatically oriented and not the expression of a true psychosis or deep-seated neurosis. In such patients the improvement in mood throughout the day under influence of the drug will often outweigh the inability to sleep at night of which they so frequently complain. The drugs may also make chronic illness more bearable, lighten the despondency of the aged, smooth out some postpartum and menopausal difficulties, aid convalescence if not used in excessive dosage, and relieve fatigue during a period of mandatory overwork. Narcolepsy is much alleviated, dextroamphetamine (Dexedrine) being apparently more effective than amphetamine (Benzedrine), and in an occasional case the same drug is astonishingly helpful in mental retardation. Alcoholics frequently find that these drugs only serve to increase their general shakiness and restlessness between drinking bouts rather than give them the mood lift they want, but in some individuals they appear to have a quieting effect during an acute drinking bout. The amphetamines—dextroamphetamine (Dexedrine) especially—are occasionally helpful in behavior problems in children and in mental retardation, tending to lessen quarrelsomeness in the overactive and bring the withdrawn out of their retreats; but this helpfulness does not extend to alleviation of the true psychoses in children any more than in adults.

There appears to be very little danger of serious habituation with these drugs, but the following side actions, none of them usually serious, may occur: dryness of the mouth, headache, temporary exhilaration with a sense of intoxication that may last for a few days, insomnia if taken too late in the day, constipation. Some physicians feel that the only way they can use these drugs with reasonable assurance that they will not raise the blood pressure is to employ them in combination with a barbiturate. When using the amphetamines in pregnancy one should bear in mind this possibility of effect on the blood pressure and also the fact that the patient should not be allowed to lose appetite sufficiently to cause disturbances due to malnutrition in either herself or the infant.

Excessive dosage of amphetamine is associated with severe symptoms: hyperirritability, apprehension and perhaps even acute psychosis, profuse perspiration, tachycardia, tachypnea, weakness and often a severe headache; there is usually a striking blood pressure rise and cerebral hemorrhage may occur. Fatalities have been recorded. Treatment is supportive and sedative, and cautious administration of an adrenergic blocking agent may be indicated in selected cases.

"There have been fatalities attributed to the combined use of an antidepressant drug and a monoamine oxidase inhibitor in treating a depression, and serious warnings have been issued about use of such combinations. But I know several men who are using them in their practices with apparent impunity. What is the true state of affairs?"

Reply: This is a difficult question to answer. Certainly it would appear advisable to heed the warnings, at least under usual circumstances. Nevertheless, there have been several reports of beneficial effects from the use of such combinations without the occurrence of serious side effects. I shall cite the experience of D. R. Gander (St. Thomas' Hospital, London). In Gander's clinic 45 patients were treated with phenelzine (Nardil) and amitriptyline (Elavil); 18 with isocarboxazid (Marplan) with amitriptyline; 12 with iproniazid (Marsilid) with amitriptyline; 2 with nortriptyline with phenelzine; and 13 with combinations of imipramine (Tofranil) or desipramine (Pertofrane, Norpramin) with an amine oxidase inhibitor. The average length of treatment was 7.05 months except in 7 cases when side effects necessitated stopping the therapy after 2 weeks or less. The dosage prescribed with combined medication was usually slightly lower for each drug than would have been prescribed had the individual drugs been used alone. And dosage was gradually reduced as the patient improved and eventually the medication was stopped. There was improvement in 62 of the 83 patients. All had

received previous treatment including electroconvulsive therapy, single antidepressants, and psychotherapy, some for many months and some for more than 2 years, but with insignificant benefit. Patients with weight loss, anorexia, anxiety and somatic symptoms did particularly well with combined drugs. Side effects were said to have been identical in nature and similar in frequency to those seen when single antidepressant drugs were used, the only exception being weight increase, which occurred in 52% of the patients on combined therapy. None of the serious side effects previously reported, such as muscular twitching, hyperpyrexia or loss of consciousness, was seen. This investigator suggested that antidepressants should not be given parenterally when combined, and that amitriptyline may be safer than imipramine when used in combination with a monoamine oxidase inhibitor.

D. R. Gander. Treatment of Depressive Illnesses with Combined Antidepressants. Lancet 2:107, July 17, 1965.

"The drug deanol (Deaner) has performed pretty well for me in the treatment of behavior problems in children, but since it is generally considered contraindicated in epileptics I sometimes wonder whether I am not subjecting a child to some risk when I place him on dosage of 50 mg. in the morning and 25 mg. in the evening without having previously made EEG studies to divulge a possible dysrhythmia?"

Reply: There is definitely a risk involved here; for example, in the study of Bostock and Shackleton (University of Queensland), such therapy caused aggravation of symptoms in 7 children, all of whom had the EEG pattern of cerebral dysrhythmia, among 33 treated. But to perform EEG studies on every child before instituting therapy with the drug would seem to me rather excessive action. I certainly think that its use without such tests is entirely justified and would stand up in court.

John Bostock and Marjorie Shackleton. Use of DMAE (Deaner) in Behavior States. M. J. Australia 2:337, Sept. 1, 1962.

"In my pediatric practice I sometimes have a 'disturbed' child of the type that the psychiatrists say may be successfully treated with antidepressant drugs in what they style an 'open setting.' So far as I am concerned, this means treating the patient in the home, and my results have not been good. What can be at fault?"

Reply: "The fault, dear Brutus, is not in our stars, but in ourselves." Meaning that it is precarious to transfer the findings of a group, who have studied their cases in institutions where there is a full complement of specialized personnel and equipment, into the environmental situation of the home. In a hospital study of the sort, for example, carried out by Conners and Eisenberg (Johns Hopkins University), the results of therapy are assessed by technical personnel using such things as the Wechsler Intelligence Scale, the Children's Manifest Anxiety Scale, etc., and the verdict can be a truly objective one with all the conditions controlled as nearly as possible. But in the home you are handicapped in your treatment by all the adverse factors which probably to a considerable extent engendered the child's state in the first place. This seems to me to be a situation in which not much is to be hoped for from drugs.

C. Keith Conners and Leon Eisenberg. Effects of Methylphenidate (Ritalin) on Symptomatology and Learning in Disturbed Children. Am. J. Psychiat. 120:458, 1963.

"A patient who is obliged to spend most of his time in a wheelchair has now developed a reactive type of depression. May I safely use one of the new antidepressant drugs in such an individual?"

Reply: This question has been considered by Rosen and Martorano, at the New York University Medical Center, who list the following side effects of the antidepressant drugs that may be of particular significance in a disabled person: orthostatic hypotension, tachycardia, an atropine-like disturbance of visual accommodation, urinary retention, visceral and peripheral paresthesias, incoordination and muscular weakness, occasional epileptic seizures, and the precipitation of acute hypomanic and manic states in psychotic patients. Because of these side effects there should certainly be increased surveillance of a physically handicapped patient when placed on an antidepressant drug. Orthostatic hypotension, for example, may present much more of a problem for the individual who has difficulty in leaving his wheelchair than for the ordinary patient, and so too with disturbances of visual accommodation or a bout of muscular weakness. Certainly such patients should be fully informed of all the possible side effects that may be expected. One should watch, too, for signs of urinary retention and stasis in an individual with lower motor neuron and spinal cord injury; in such a case it may be necessary to use a parasympathetic agent such as bethanechol (Urecholine) to stimulate the bladder musculature in addition to reducing the dosage of the antidepressive agent. And of course if the patient has a motor impairment he is much more liable to fall and be injured if he becomes dizzy or experiences a postural hypotension than is the nonhandicapped person.

Sidney Rosen and Joseph Martorano. Clinical Application of the Antidepressant Agents in Disabled and Rehabilitation Patients. Arch. Phys. Med. & Rehabil. 61:739, 1965.

"What have been the principal types of adverse reaction associated with use of the true antipsychotics, such drugs as Thorazine, Compazine, etc.?"

Reply: Extrapyramidal reactions (parkinsonism-like, dyskinetic); hepatitis with obstructive jaundice; blood dyscrasias; orthostatic hypotension; anticholinergic reactions (warning: glaucoma, prostatism), constipation, urinary retention, blurred vision, dry mouth; menstrual disturbances; photosensitivity.

"What are the principal types of reaction associated with the use of the true tranquilizers, such drugs as Miltown (Equanil), Librium and Valium?"

Reply: Gastrointestinal discomfort, dryness of mouth, rashes, chills and fever (other signs of hypersensitization, as well as liver, kidney and blood dyscrasias, have been rare).

"Would you kindly list the principal tranquilizing agents that are used in the neuroses and the psychosomatic conditions (i.e., the true 'tranquilizers'), and indicate the drug of choice among them?"

Reply: Meprobamate (Miltown, Equanil), chlordiazepoxide (Librium), diazepam (Valium), chlormezanone (Trancopal), emylcamate (Striatran), hydroxyphenamate (Listica), mephenoxalone (Trepidone, Lenetran), oxanamide (Quiactin), hydroxyzine (Atarax, Vistaril), buclizine (Softran), benactyzine (Suavitil), ectylurea (Nostyn, Levanil), phenaglycodol (Ultran), phenyltoloxamine (Bristamine), oxazepam (Serax), tybamate (Solacen). Certainly the three members of this large group that are in principal use are meprobamate, chlordiazepoxide and diazepam. The two latter members of this triumvirate, chlordiazepoxide and diazepam, are "Johnny-come-lately's," and the evidence that they are superior to meprobamate has not been impressive.

PULMONARY ALVEOLAR PROTEINOSIS

"I have a case of pulmonary alveolar proteinosis in my practice. Is there any effective drug therapy?"

Reply: In most records of improvement or recovery the patient has been given potassium iodide, but it is far from certain that this drug really contributed effectively, since spontaneous recovery is also reported. A type of local drug therapy has been described by Jose Ramirez-R and Guy D. Campbell, who use endobronchial infusions of 0.9% saline solution containing 50–75 units/ml. of heparin and 1 or 5% acetylcysteine, the infusions being administered unilaterally for 7–30 days. Improvement was described in 4 cases so treated.

Cedric L. Mather and Giles B. Hamlin. Pulmonary Alveolar Proteinosis. New England J. Med. 272:1156, June 3, 1965. Jose Ramirez-R and Guy D. Campbell. Pulmonary Alveolar Proteinosis. Ann. Int. Med. 63:429, 1965.

PULMONARY EDEMA

"In the acute emergency of pulmonary edema even the most potent of the standard diuretic drugs often produce a disappointing response because of the decreased cardiac output and reduced glomerular filtration rate. Has anything new developed in this area?"

Reply: Stuart Fine and Robert Levy, at the Sinai Hospital of Baltimore, have reported the occurrence of a significant diuresis after the administration of ethacrynic acid in 5 patients. Urine flow and sodium excretion began to increase promptly after the start of the infusion and reached a peak on the average of 30 minutes after the drug was given. They dissolved 50 mg. of ethacrynic acid in 70 ml. of 5% dextrose in water and infused this intravenously over a period of 30–50 minutes. At Maimonides Hospital, in Brooklyn, Rosenberg's group has also reported favorably.

Stuart L. Fine and Robert I. Levy. Ethacrynic Acid in Acute Pulmonary Edema. New England J. Med. 273:583, Sept. 9, 1965. Benjamin Rosenberg, Gerald Dobkin and Richard Rubin. The Intravenous Use of Ethacrynic Acid in the Management of Acute Pulmonary Edema. Am. Heart J. 70:333, 1965.

"One of my associates has recently had a case of pulmonary edema that, so far as he could determine, was associated with the inordinate ingestion of aspirin during several preceding weeks in the attempt to control a painful situation. This patient had no history of previous cardiac disease or cardiorespiratory disorder, but the occurrence raises the question of advisability of discontinuing the use of salicylates when treating pulmonary edema in patients with or without heart disease. Correct?"

Reply: I have seen only two reports of pulmonary edema in salicylate intoxication of a patient with a normal heart, the most recent

being that of Saul Greenstein (Newington, Connecticut). Most episodes of this sort have occurred in persons with heart disease or cardiac abnormalities, but I certainly think that your point is well taken.

Saul M. Greenstein. Pulmonary Edema Due to Salicylate Intoxication: Report of Case. Dis. Chest 44:552, 1963.

PULMONARY EMBOLISM

"What is the most useful drug therapy in pulmonary embolism?"

Reply: The *only* truly useful drug therapy in pulmonary embolism is heparin. Give intravenously in dosage of 50–100 mg. and repeat at 4 hour intervals for at least the first 2 days. You may of course institute oral anticoagulant drug administration also at once if you wish, to be maintained for several weeks after recovery from the acute episode, as appears indicated in the individual case. Animal experimentation has shown that there occurs during pulmonary embolism a widespread radiation of autonomic reflexes affecting the heart, the pulmonary vascular tree, the bronchi and the gastrointestinal tract; these reflexes being predominantly vagal, the use of atropine is rationally indicated. Unfortunately, however, the clinical results of its use have not been impressive. Similarly, the use of papaverine as a vasodilator is certainly rational, but this drug is very rapidly affixed to plasma proteins and thus rendered ineffective, and so not much is to be expected from its use. If one were to give it in rectal suppository after the acute situation is passed, as I have described elsewhere in these Replies, papaverine might be effective.

"Is it acceptable to use morphine or atropine in a patient with pulmonary embolism?"

Reply: Morphine is dangerous when there is some degree of hypoxia; for example, in cases of impaired respiration associated with chest wounds, bulbar poliomyelitis, pneumothorax, hemothorax, pleural effusion and pulmonary edema, as well as in states of circulatory impairment or in the patient with a head wound. Some of us feel that the drug is also contraindicated in pulmonary embolism because it sensitizes the vagus centrally, and animal experimentation has shown that a widespread radiation of autonomic reflexes affecting the heart, the pulmonary vascular tree, the bronchi and the gastrointestinal tract occurs during an embolic episode. These reflexes being predominantly vagal, the use of atropine but not morphine is rationally indicated.

"I have just used Thrombolysin in a case of pulmonary embolism without effecting any relief at all. What has been the general experience?"

Reply: From their experience at Edgewater Hospital in Chicago, M. S. Mazel and associates drew two conclusions: first, that early use of the agent is mandatory if even a fair degree of success is to be attained because a lapse of 6–8 hours results in damage to vital structures, and that for best results it must be given intra-arterially rather than intravenously for treatment of arterial clots.

M. S. Mazel, Houck E. Bolton and Rogelio Riera. Thrombolysin Treatment of Pulmonary Embolism Following Surgery: Report of Two Cases. Angiology 15:171, 1964.

"We at our hospital, as at other hospitals everywhere, are agitated over the question of the advisability of routine anticoagulation of patients in certain categories. It seems to me, however, that resolution of this question would be immensely facilitated through exact knowledge of the incidence of the pulmonary thromboembolism that we are trying to prevent. Just what *is* the magnitude of the problem of pulmonary embolism?"

Reply: The various answers supplied vary somewhat with the sources. In hospitals in which necropsies on medical patients predominate, or where many of the patients have been older individuals suffering from chronic heart disease, the figures may run as high as 30% or even slightly higher; but the average incidence of pulmonary embolism in routinely performed adult necropsies is usually listed at about 10%. However, when the matter is looked into more minutely, these figures are very consideraly raised. At the Beth Israel Hospital (Boston), David Freiman and associates found that careful examination of the pulmonary arteries in a series of 61 consecutive adult necropsies reasonably representative of the total autopsy population at their hospital, revealed the presence of old or recent thromboemboli in 64% of the cases. This high figure was in large part due to the inclusion of organized and organizing traces usually overlooked unless extreme care is taken and, most importantly, the index of suspicion is high. Granting that many of these episodes are multiple and of little clinical significance, attesting to the efficiency of the disposal mechanisms, the investigators nevertheless felt that even more severe episodes are frequently unrecognized during life.

David G. Freiman, Joe Suyemoto, and Stanford Wessler. Frequency of Pulmonary Thromboembolism in Man. New England J. Med. 272:1278, June 17, 1965.

"I recently lost a patient who suffered a fat embolism after fracture despite supportive meas-

ures such as maintenance of the airway, resuscitation from shock, and the parenteral administration of fluids. Are there any drugs that might have contributed effectively to the therapy?"

Reply: Charles Evarts (Cleveland Clinic) commends small intravenous injections of 10–50 mg. of sodium heparin every 6–8 hours to achieve a chylolytic effect without the risk of hemorrhage. It is said also that intravascular administration of 500 ml. of Dextran-40 every 12 hours will reduce intravascular aggregation of red blood cells, increase the fluidity of blood, improve capillary flow, increase tissue perfusion and exert a siliconizing effect on injured walls of blood vessels. The efficacy of Dextran used in this way in cases of fat embolism has been reported by S. E. Bergentz, in Scandinavia.

Charles M. Evarts. Diagnosis and Treatment of Fat Embolism. J.A.M.A. 194:899, Nov. 22, 1965. S. E. Bergentz. Studies on the Genesis of Posttraumatic Fat Embolism. Acta chir. scandinav. Suppl. 282:1, 1961.

PURPURA

"What has been the effect of corticosteroid therapy in the treatment of idiopathic thrombocytopenic purpura?"

Reply: At the University of Illinois, Irving Schulman said that if these drugs are used early in the disease, complete and permanent remission will occur in 20–25% of cases, and a temporary rise in the platelet count in about another 40%. He said, however, that there is no apparent correlation between response to the therapy and ultimate prognosis, and that continued use of the drugs in high dosage may suppress platelet formation and prevent a remission. It seems that the corticosteroids decrease the bleeding tendency through a direct effect on vascular permeability that is independent of the effect on platelets. Schulman begins therapy with 1 ml. of prednisone (Meticorten, etc.)/kg. for the maximum of 3 weeks, and then tapers dosage and discontinues in the fourth week. A second course, again limited to 4 weeks, is given if thrombocytopenia persists beyond 3 months. Incidentally, Schulman is not anxious to do splenectomies in purpuric children and defers the operation somewhat more than a year if the symptoms are minimal. Ironically, the corticosteroids sometimes induce the purpuric state themselves.

Irving Schulman. Diagnosis and Treatment: Management of Idiopathic Thrombocytopenic Purpura. Pediatrics 33: 979, 1964.

"What is the value of the flavonoids, as present together with ascorbic acid in such a preparation as C.V.P., that is promoted to increase capillary resistance and decrease fragility?"

Reply: In 1957, W. N. Pearson reported his conclusion to the American Medical Association Councils on Foods and Nutrition and on Drugs that the flavonoids are of little or no value in the treatment of disease, and I have seen no subsequent reports in authoritative contradiction of his statement. It seems to me therefore that in any of the rutin combinations that are on the market you are paying for at lease one ingredient whose value has not been fully established.

W. N. Pearson. Flavonoids in Human Nutrition and Medicine. J.A.M.A. 164:1675, 1957.

"A patient has just come into my practice, in whom the diagnosis of idiopathic thrombocytopenic purpura was made elsewhere about 6 months ago. I am tempted to undertake the treatment with corticosteroids; has success been attained in cases as long-standing as this?"

Reply: In the 71 patients of Meyers (University of Michigan), in each of whom therapy was initiated with corticosteroids or ACTH, no sustained remissions were attained in cases of more than 4 months' duration before initiation of therapy.

Muriel C. Meyers. Results of Treatment in 71 Patients with Idiopathic Thrombocytopenic Purpura. Am. J. M. Sc. 242:295, 1961.

"I have a patient with the serious vascular disorder, purpura fulminans, who has not responded to antibiotics, corticosteroids or heparinization. I am at my wit's end. What is there to do?"

Reply: There has been a report by Joseph Patterson and associates (Emory University) of the use of clinical dextran (6% in saline solution) in a dosage of 500 mg./kg. every 3 days, with production of what was described as a remarkable response with apparent recovery. It was felt that the agent acted not only by preventing sludging of the blood but also by coating the formed elements, including platelets, and the walls of the vessels.

Joseph H. Patterson, Robert B. Pierce, J. Richard Amerson and W. Lorraine Watkins. Dextran Therapy of Purpura Fulminans. New England J. Med. 273:734, Sept. 30, 1965.

"When a patient presents with purpura, what drugs should be thought of in the possible causative role?"

Reply: I surely do not know all of them, but the following have come to my attention (I am not including such drugs as meprobamate [Miltown, Equanil], heparin, digitalis, phenacemide [Phenurone], stibophen [Fuadin], the carbonic anhydrase inhibitors, penicillin and streptomycin for the reason that the instances associated with their use have been very rare and not always fully documented): sulfonamides, phenylbutazone (Butazolidin), chloramphenicol (Chloromycetin), novobiocin (Albamycin, etc.), ristocetin (Spontin), diphenylhydantoin (Dilantin), sodium thiocyanate, quinine, quinidine, nitrogen mustards, mercaptopurine (Purinethol), PAS, corticosteroids, thiazide-derivative diuretics, gold salts, penicillamine (Cuprimine), acetazolamide (Diamox), chlorpropamide (Diabinese), tolbutamide (Orinase).

PYLOROSPASM

"I have an infant with pylorospasm in whom atropine has not been effective even when I have increased the dosage up to the point of causing considerable flushing. Is there any better drug?"

Reply: Unfortunately the cholinergic blocking action of atropine is not as reliably obtained at the pylorus as would be desirable. Sometimes a better effect is obtained by using Donnatal Elixir, which contains hyoscyamine, hyoscine, atropine and phenobarbital; 10 drop dosage of this elixir one-half hour before feedings may be adjusted up or down. Or you might try atropine methylnitrate (Eumydrin, Harvatrate, etc.); sometimes this salt of the alkaloid is more effective than the familiar sulfate.

PYODERMA GANGRENOSUM

"I have a case of the rare dermatologic lesion, pyoderma gangrenosum, on my hands, in which neither antibiotics nor chemotherapeutic agents have been effective. What have others done?"

Reply: At Wayne State University, Jus Altman and Colman Mopper have described the successful use of sulfones (the drugs that are used in the treatment of leprosy) in 2 cases of this malady. They used dapsone (Avlosulfon) in dosage of 100 mg. twice daily, and later 50 mg. twice daily, with supplemental iron salts. I do not understand the action of the drug, because this lesion has never been shown to be primarily bacterial or infectious in nature.

Jus Altman and Colman Mopper. Minnesota Med. 49:22, 1966.

RADIATION SICKNESS

"Have any drugs stood the test of time in the treatment of the gastrointestinal component of radiation sickness?"

Reply: I do not know how long a time-test may be, but it does appear that there is merit in using some of the tranquilizing agents as well as pyridoxine in treatment of this malady. In Melbourne, Basil Stoll used a large number of agents in 1042 trials in patients with radiation sickness, assessing separately the response of nausea, vomiting, anorexia and listlessness. The drugs were randomized and used in a sequential method, but the weak point of the study was that they were not made up into tablets of equal appearance; therefore it may be assumed that there was some patient bias entering into the findings. However, he found that what he called "newer tranquilizers," i.e., trifluoperazine (Stelazine), 1 mg. three times daily, and haloperidol (which he used in a form combined with an antihistaminic), 2 mg. three times daily, relieved the nausea in about 90% of instances. They relieved the listlessness and vomiting also, but were less effective than pyridoxine and what he called the "older phenothiazines" (such drugs as chlorpromazine, prochlorperazine, thiopropazate, etc.) in the control of anorexia. His pyridoxine dosage was 10 mg. four times daily. In New Zealand, E. M. Johnson has recently reported the favorable use of thiethylperazine (Torecan); dosage was 20 mg. three times daily, cut in half after 48 hours, with injections or suppositories being superior to oral medication.

Basil A. Stoll. Radiation Sickness: Analysis of Over 1,000 Controlled Drug Trials. Brit. M. J. 2:507, Aug. 25, 1962. E. M. Johnson. Control of Radiation Sickness with Thiethylperazine (Torecan). New Zealand M. J. 64:649, 1965.

RAT-BITE FEVER

"Unfortunately there are still shameful areas in this country in which the poor can be bitten by rats while they sleep. What drugs are effective in rat-bite fever?"

Reply: In the most common type of this disease, that known as sodoku, penicillin has superseded all other agents in treatment. But it is advisable to give it in the form either of a large dose of a long-acting preparation or oral dosage at frequent intervals for about a week. The next most effective agent is probably streptomycin with tetracycline in third place. In the much more rare form of the disease, Haverhill fever, penicillin is also the agent of choice.

RECTAL PROCIDENTIA

"I have a patient with rectal procidentia who is a poor risk for major abdominal surgery and whose life expectancy is rather short. Is there any drug therapy that might be helpful?"

Reply: No systemic therapy at all, but Atkinson and McAmmond, in Vancouver, have described the local use of sclerosing agents. I suggest that you resort to their original article for description of their technique.

K. G. Atkinson and E. N. C. McAmmond. Treatment of Rectal Procidentia by Sclerosing Agents. Dis. Colon & Rectum 8:319, 1965.

REFLUX ESOPHAGITIS

"In reflux esophagitis the only benefit usually obtained from conventional oral administration of antacids is momentary relief since these preparations are in the esophagus for only a matter of seconds. Has any improvement in method been devised?"

Reply: Yes, Ivan Beck's group, in Montreal, has successfully instituted a constant intraesophageal antacid drip. They suspend at 3 or 4 feet above the bed a bottle containing one part of such an antacid as Gelusil to nine parts of water, connect to this a thin polyethylene tube and introduce it through the nostril into the midesophagus at a distance of 25–30 cm. The drip is set at about 30–40 drops per minute and not more than 2000 ml. is introduced daily. Their success with 15 patients was very good.

Ivan T. Beck, Marcel Lacerte, Steven Rona and Jeno Solymar. Constant Intraesophageal Antacid Drip as a Method of Treatment of Reflux Esophagitis. Canad. M. A. J. 90:570, Feb. 29, 1964.

REGIONAL ENTERITIS

"Is there a place in the treatment of regional enteritis for such drugs as propantheline bromide (Pro-Banthine) and the preparation trade-named Donnatal?"

Reply: In Pro-Banthine you have pure anticholinergic action and in Donnatal there is this action plus the sedative effect of the contained phenobarbital. Since both anticholinergic and/or sedative actions often appear to be indicated in this malady, the use of the drugs you mentioned is rational. One may use almost any anticholinergic agent, however, and perhaps in some instances replace the Donnatal with a plain anticholinergic agent or such an agent together with a tranquilizer—meprobamate (Miltown, Equanil), or chlordiazepoxide (Librium), or diazepam (Valium)—in place of the phenobarbital. But be careful—it is not difficult to precipitate a state of ileus in this bowel that may be partially obstructed.

"Does the antibiotic, chemotherapeutic and corticosteroid therapy of regional enteritis differ essentially from that of ulcerative colitis?"

Reply: No, but the results have not been as good.

REITER'S DISEASE

"Since Reiter's disease is rare in females, might it be advisable to use an estrogen in the treatment of the male patient?"

Reply: In Manchester, England, S. M. Laird and associates found that the mean duration of attack of cases followed to recovery in patients treated with stilbestrol was shorter than that for cases not so treated, but the series was a very small one. If you wish to undertake such therapy it is well to remember that your patient cannot be truly diagnosed as having Reiter's disease unless he satisfies all three of the criteria: nongonococcic urethritis, conjunctivitis and subacute or chronic polyarthritis.

S. M. Laird, A. J. Gill and D. A. Pitkeathly. Treatment of Reiter's Disease with Stilbestrol. Brit. M. J. 1:970, Apr. 10, 1965.

RELAPSING FEVER

"With our military involvement in the Far East are we not likely to have some cases of relapsing fever appearing in returning soldiers? In any case, what is the preferred drug therapy?"

Reply: The arsenical therapy of former times, which was never very satisfactory, has been completely replaced by the antibiotics. It now appears that penicillin is the preferred agent in louse-borne cases and the tetracyclines in tick-borne cases. Chloramphenicol (Chloromycetin) may be resorted to in either type of the disease if the less toxic agents are not effective.

RENAL TUBULAR ACIDOSIS

"In a case of renal tubular acidosis the result of vitamin D and calcium therapy has been very pleasing, and the occasional episodes of paralysis resulting from potassium depletion have responded nicely to administration of potassium salts. Is there any other drug therapy to be recommended?"

Reply: Nothing that I know of.

RHEUMATIC FEVER

"I have heard that a swing away from penicillin in the prophylaxis of recurrent rheumatic fever is pending. Can you enlighten?"

Reply: Some time ago the American Heart Association suggested that 200,000 units of penicillin twice daily was the preferred regimen, but recently in New York, Alvan Feinstein and associates have expressed the opinion that this suggestion was an arbitrary one that was made without clinical trial to test its value. They therefore undertook a comparative study of sulfadiazine vs. a double daily dose of penicillin in a group of 153 children under the age of 14 years, who unquestionably qualified for such a trial. Randomly allocating these subjects to the receipt of 1 Gm. of sulfadiazine daily or 200,000 units of penicillin G twice daily, they found the annual attack rates of streptococcic infection fluctuating over each of the 3 calendar years of the study, but that the total results showed almost identical rates for the two regimens of prophylaxis: when "carrier states" were eliminated, the attack rate was 19% in each group. Therefore, since sulfadiazine costs less and carries less risk of sensitization than penicillin, one must feel that this study was an important one and that schedule changes throughout the country are quite likely to reflect its findings.

Alvan R. Feinstein, Harrison F. Wood, Mario Spagnuolo, Angelo Taranta, Esther Tursky and Edith Kleinberg. Oral Prophylaxis of Recurrent Rheumatic Fever: Sulfadiazine vs. Double Daily Dose of Penicillin. J.A.M.A. 188:489, May 11, 1964.

"In a patient with rheumatic fever who is being treated with corticosteroids, what is the best protective measure against a post-therapeutic rebound when the drugs are withdrawn?"

Reply: In studying the 100 clinical rebounds, manifested by clinical and laboratory abnormalities, that occurred in 64 of 415 children and adolescents with acute rheumatic fever, Spagnuolo and Feinstein, at Irvington House, Irvington-on-Hudson, New York, determined that it is possible to reduce the incidence of subsequent clinical rebound by adding salicylates if not initially at least when reduction of the corticosteroids begins, and maintaining them for several weeks after the other drugs have been stopped.

Mario Spagnuolo and Alvan R. Feinstein. Rebound Phenomenon in Acute Rheumatic Fever: II. Treatment and Prevention. Yale J. Biol. & Med. 33:279, 1961.

"What about treating the rheumatic fever patient, if the attack is mild and the initial one, on bed rest alone without the use of drugs; would that be malpractice?"

Reply: I am going to dodge the *malpractice* aspect of the question because you know there are lawyers in each of our 50 sovereign states; but as for the efficacy of bed rest itself, I can cite the report of E. G. L. Bywaters and G. T. Thomas, in Taplow, England, whose evidence may be summarized about as follows: (a) if the attack is mild the patient will do pretty well on bed rest alone; (b) salicylates will not alter the course of the disease or the cardiac status but they may help relieve the symptoms; (c) in mild cases the corticosteroids may shorten the course but will not alter the cardiac prognosis; (d) there is definite indication for use of corticosteroids in a severe case with serious cardiac involvement.

E. G. L. Bywaters and G. T. Thomas. Bed Rest, Salicylates and Steroids in Rheumatic Fever. Brit. M. J. 1:1628, June 10, 1961.

"Rheumatic fever is occurring in a fairly mild form in our area nowadays, especially in adolescents and adults, but there is nevertheless a high incidence of cardiac involvement which demands utmost care in treatment. How well is a combination of aspirin and penicillin succeeding without the use of corticosteroids?"

Reply: I shall cite the experience of Thomas Begg and associates, at the Western Infirmary in Glasgow, who reviewed the records of 139 patients in whom routine treatment was in most instances complete bed rest and salicylate sufficient to maintain the serum level at about 35 mg./100 ml.; 115 of the patients also received penicillin orally or intramuscularly, usually phenoxymethylpenicillin (Pen-Vee, V-Cillin, etc.) orally, 250 mg. four times daily. In 116 of these patients there was abatement of fever and joint pains within a week, within 48 hours in 20 instances. The erythrocyte sedimentation rate dropped to normal within 4 weeks in 92, within 8 weeks in 32, and was elevated for more than 12 weeks in only 8. Electrocardiographic abnormalities compatible with rheumatic carditis occurred in 53% of the patients, well-substantiated clinical signs of carditis in only 18%. The abnormalities subsided within 4 weeks in 66% of the patients with ECG changes, but persisted for more than 12 weeks in 11%. Reduction or discontinuance of salicylate dosage provoked symptoms and signs of relapse in 17% of the patients, but in all but two instances these subsided spontaneously or with further salicylate therapy in a few days. There were no fatalities in the series and there was a prolonged severe illness that required corticosteroid therapy in only 2 patients. Several authoritative studies, both in Great Britain and the United States, have shown that prognosis regarding the cardiac outcome in rheumatic fever is excellent if there is no carditis when the disease is first recognized.

Thomas B. Begg, J. W. Kerr and B. R. Knowles. Rheumatic Fever in Adolescents and Adults. Brit. M. J. 2:223, July 28, 1962.

"In acute arthritic states we are accustomed in our hospital to attempt to reach and maintain for as long as necessary a salicylate level of 30–35 mg./100 ml. serum. But many patients are made uncomfortable by the dosage necessary to maintain such a level and we are required to back off from it. Just what is the dangerously toxic serum titer?"

Reply: In discussing their experience in acute salicylate poisoning in 208 cases, G. W. Beveridge and associates (Royal Infirmary, Edinburgh) said that patients with serum salicylate levels of over 70 mg./100 ml. are unlikely to survive either deterioration in the level of consciousness or circulatory collapse unless they are immediately hemodialyzed. This figure is only about twice that mentioned by you as an ideal therapeutic level. I had not realized myself that the drug's margin of safety is so narrow as that, but I think that we must accept this statement as authoritative.

G. W. Beveridge, W. Forshall, J. F. Munro, J. A. Owen and I. A. G. Weston. Acute Salicylate Poisoning in Adults. Lancet 1:406, June 27, 1964.

"I have a patient in whom it appears that aspirin provokes a state of hypoglycemia. Has such a thing been recorded?"

Reply: Yes, there are a few such instances on record. Actually, it is not unlikely that the occurrence is more frequent than is noted because it has been established both experimentally and clinically that the drug causes metabolic derangements. Very likely there is an interference with key enzyme systems. In one of their cases, George Limbeck's group, in Seattle, demonstrated that an increase in blood insulin concentration was not involved.

George A. Limbeck, Rogelio H. A. Ruvalcaba, Ellis Samols and Vincent C. Kelley. Salicylates and Hypoglycemia. Am. J. Dis. Child. 109:165, 1965.

"I have tried choline salicylate (Arthropan) as well as the soluble aspirin preparation, Calurin, and have not found them superior to aspirin itself for analgesic and antiphlogistic effects in the arthritides. What of Pabalate, which contains para-aminobenzoic acid as alleged synergist of the salicylate; is it really a superior preparation?"

Reply: Some years ago para-aminobenzoic acid (PABA), which is a constituent of the vitamin B complex, was administered empirically with sodium salicylate and sodium bicarbonate at the Mayo Clinic to a rheumatic fever patient in whom the plasma salicylate titer could not be pushed above 15 mg. per 100 ml. even with high salicylate dosage. In several trials PABA consistently raised the level to 37.5 mg. per 100 ml., and the desired clinical response was obtained. These findings have since been amply confirmed. It appears that 3 Gm. (45 grains) of PABA, every 3–4 hours by mouth, is satisfactory dosage. But the hitch with regard to Pabalate is that in the recommended average dosage of 2 tablets four times daily there would not be provided nearly this much PABA, and therefore I think it likely that your patient would obtain no more relief than from a comparable amount of aspirin alone. Of course the Pabalate tablets are enteric-coated and this allegedly protects the gastric mucosa, but you do know I am sure that sometimes enteric-coated tablets come on through the entire tract without having undergone complete disintegration and liberation of their contents.

R. M. Salassa, J. L. Bollman and T. J. Dry. Effect of PABA on Metabolism and Excretion of Salicylate. J. Lab. & Clin. Med. 33:1393, 1948.

"Is the use of a corticosteroid together with aspirin more effective than aspirin alone in treatment of acute rheumatic fever?"

Reply: The Combined Rheumatic Carditis Study Group, drawn from eight hospitals in New York City, Baltimore, Boston and Cleveland, concluded that when corticosteroids in high dosage are given during the first attack complicated by carditis in a child under 12 years of age, with a first manifestation of the disease within 28 days of beginning therapy, there is accomplished a reduction in the incidence of residual heart disease that is too insignificant to justify the risks inherent in the therapy. In London, J. D. H. Slater concluded from his study in 28 young men treated with salicylate alone or combined with a corticosteroid, that the addition of corticosteroids to salicylate therapy in the acute attack hastens its defervescence but does not lower the incidence of chronic rheumatic heart disease; at least that seems to me to be the gist of his report. Then, in Taplow, England, G. T. Thomas, reviewing the cases of 198 patients with rheumatic fever treated with and without salicylates and corticosteroids, found that treatment with neither corticosteroids nor salicylates during the acute attack affects the cardiac status, on 5 year follow-up, but that the reduction of recurrences through prophylactic use of sulfonamides is definitely beneficial from the cardiac standpoint. And I would draw to your attention the report of the Rheumatic Fever Working Party of the Medical Research Council of Great Britain and the Subcommittee of Principal Investigators of the American Council on Rheumatic Fever and Congenital Heart Disease, American Heart Association, which was remarkable for two things: one, for having offered a 5 year

follow-up report on 445 of the 497 patients initially involved in the studies; and two, for making the fact quite clear that the status of the heart when rheumatic fever is first manifested is the determinant factor in cardiac outcome. However, the matter is really not yet settled, for the very next year after the appearance of the above report a group at the House of the Good Samaritan, and also Dorfman and associates, using as criteria the same that had been employed by the other investigators, namely, the disappearance of murmurs, reported that they found evidence of greater effectiveness in steroid-treated than in aspirin-treated patients. And more recently, a group from the House of the Good Samaritan, Gabor Czoniczer and associates, have reported corticosteroids to be especially striking in cases of severe rheumatic carditis with congestive heart failure. A lengthy and unsatisfactory answer, I am afraid.

J. D. H. Slater. Combined Aspirin and Cortisone Treatment of Acute Rheumatic Fever: Controlled Trial in Young Men. Ann. Rheumat. Dis. 20:173, 1961. Combined Rheumatic Carditis Study Group. Comparison of Effect of Prednisone and Acetylsalicylic Acid on Incidence of Residual Rheumatic Heart Disease. New England J. Med. 262:895, May 5, 1960. G. T. Thomas. Five-Year Follow-up on Patients with Rheumatic Fever Treated by Bed Rest, Steroids or Salicylate. Brit. M. J. 1:1635, June 10, 1961. Rheumatic Fever Working Party of the Medical Research Council of Great Britain and the Subcommittee of Principal Investigators of the American Council on Rheumatic Fever and Congenital Heart Disease, American Heart Association. Evolution of Rheumatic Heart Disease in Children: Five-Year Report of Co-operative Clinical Trial of ACTH, Cortisone and Aspirin. Brit. M. J. 2:1033, Oct. 8, 1960. Gabor Czoniczer, Francisco Amezcua, Salvatore Pelargonio and Benedict F. Massell. Therapy of Severe Rheumatic Carditis: Comparison of Adrenocortical Steroids and Aspirin. Circulation 29:813, 1964.

"I have heard it rumored that intermittent penicillin therapy is fully as effective in the prophylaxis of streptococcic infections in rheumatic fever patients as continuous therapy. Is this correct?"

Reply: This matter was studied by Alvan Feinstein's group, at Yale, who concluded that a continuous prophylactic program is the most effective method of prevention of recurrent rheumatic fever. Some of their patients received 1,200,000 units of benzathine penicillin G and others 400,000 units of oral potassium penicillin G one-half hour before breakfast, one-half hour before the evening meal and at bedtime for 10 consecutive days each month. There were 118 patients in the oral group and 119 in the injection group, but 17 of the latter were later transferred to the oral group. The attack rate of streptococcic infection was 7.7/100 patient years in the injection group and 43.2 in the oral group; for rheumatic recurrences, the attack rates were 0.9/100 patient-years for the injection group and 10.7 for the oral group.

Alvan R. Feinstein, Mario Spagnuolo, Saran Jonas, Esther Tursky, Edith K. Stern and Muriel Levitt. Prophylaxis of Recurrent Rheumatic Fever: Ineffectiveness of Intermittent "Therapeutic" Oral Penicillin. J.A.M.A. 191:451, Feb. 8, 1965.

"I understand that phenylbutazone (Butazolidin) has been shown in England to be better than aspirin in controlling the symptoms in acute rheumatic fever. What inference do you draw from this?"

Reply: The inference of course—if it is as much better as it was shown to be by Will and Murdoch in a very careful study—is that it should be used in preference to the classical drug. But I think you should be informed that in a broad experience with phenylbutazone in other disorders the occurrence of side actions has required discontinuance of therapy in about 15% of instances, most frequently occurring reactions being nausea, edema from sodium chloride retention, rash, epigastric pain, vertigo and stomatitis. And there have been such serious reactions as peptic ulcer reactivation, agranulocytosis, purpura, exfoliative dermatitis, psychoses, hypertension and toxic hepatitis. Add these things to a good many other side effects of relatively low incidence, and I think you must admit that in phenylbutazone we have a drug that is much more potentially toxic than aspirin. Under ordinary circumstances I would give it with considerable trepidation.

G. Will and W. R. Murdoch. Treatment of Rheumatic Fever: Comparison of Effects of Aspirin and Phenylbutazone. Brit. M. J. 2:281, Aug. 1, 1964.

"Are all the streptococci associated with rheumatic fever still susceptible to the action of penicillin?"

Reply: Yes, all strains of group A streptococci concerned in the events leading to rheumatic fever still show in vitro susceptibility to penicillin, but it is undeniable that some treatment failures with this drug are occurring. Perhaps a partial explanation for this state of affairs is supplied by the study of Ruth Kundsin and Joseph Miller, at Harvard, who found that individuals carrying a strain of penicillin-resistant *Staphylococcus aureus* in the nasopharynx interfered with streptococcus eradication in a community survey of disease due to group A streptococci.

Ruth B. Kundsin and Joseph M. Miller. Significance of Staphylococcus Aureus Carrier State in Treatment of Disease Due to Group A. Streptococci. New England J. Med. 271:1395, Dec. 31, 1964.

"Our pathologist claims that aspirin invariably causes an increase in the urine cell count, and he can actually demonstrate what appear to

be renal tubular cells. Is this a fact or is our leg being pulled; and if there is truth in the allegation, what is its significance?"

Reply: If your fellow is like some I know, he probably enjoys seeing internists squirm, but there is truth in what he says and demonstrates, all the same. But I shouldn't worry, for J. T. Scott and associates, who I believe were the first to demonstrate these evidences of renal irritation at the Postgraduate Medical School in London, expressed themselves as doubtful that any serious damage is done to the kidney by salicylates in therapeutic dosage even after long periods.

J. T. Scott, A. M. Denman and J. Dorling. Renal Irritation Caused by Salicylates. Lancet 1:344, Feb. 16, 1963.

"Would there be any advantage in using the new drug indomethacin (Indocin) in place of aspirin in the treatment of rheumatic fever?"

Reply: I have seen only one report, that of Alberto Vignau I. and associates, in Chile, who found no significant differences between the two drugs either in effects on acute manifestations or the incidence of valvular heart disease after one year. As of the present moment therefore, since indomethacin administration is associated with some very objectionable side effects, I should say that it is not to be preferred to aspirin in the treatment of rheumatic fever.

Alberto Vignau I., Enrique Correa T., Julio Guasch L., Augusto Schuster C., Alfredo Patri M., Samuel Vaisman B. and Edward A. Mortimer, Jr. The Effects of Indomethacin on Rheumatic Fever. Arthritis & Rheum. 8:501, 1965.

"Controlled studies of the therapy for streptococcal pharyngitis have shown convincingly that the administration of penicillin in adequate dosage for 10 days prevents the obvious clinical manifestations of acute rheumatic fever. But what of the use of penicillin during an acute attack of rheumatic fever; does the drug really exert any effect on the development of valvular heart disease?"

Reply: The thorough study of a group of investigators at the University of Chile, comprised of both Chilian and American personnel, failed to demonstrate that it does. Indeed, such therapy appeared actually to exert an unfavorable effect. The conclusion drawn from this study by the observers themselves was that by the time symptoms of rheumatic fever have appeared, persistence of the *Streptococcus* does not seem to be necessary for the further evolution of valvular heart disease; i.e., although the presence of the organism is essential for some days or weeks subsequent to the onset of the inciting streptococcal infection, the role of the bacterium appears to be completed by the time rheumatic manifestations occur. Furthermore, eradication of the group-A streptococcus from the rheumatic fever patient fails to alter either the acute phase or the ultimate outcome of the disease; hence it appears inescapable that penicillin is of no therapeutic benefit at this time. This does not mean that its use may not be justified for the protection of other susceptibles who may be exposed to the patient, and therefore despite the findings that have been cited the antibiotic should be used in all cases.

Samuel Vaisman B, Julio Guash L., Alberto Vignau I., Enrique Correa T., Augusto Schuster C., Edward A. Mortimer, Jr., and Charles H. Rammelkamp, Jr. Failure of Penicillin to Alter Acute Rheumatic Valvulitis. J.A.M.A. 194:1284, Dec. 20, 1965.

RHEUMATOID ARTHRITIS

"Has anything new been proposed in the therapy of that old devil, rheumatoid arthritis?"

Reply: In Gloucester, England, G. R. Fearnley and associates, reasoning from the fact that blood fibrinolytic activity tends to be lower in patients with rheumatoid arthritis and other inflammatory conditions than in healthy individuals, used the antidiabetic drug, phenformin (DBI)—known to increase the blood fibrinolytic activity—in 16 patients with the malady. Twelve patients responded to the treatment, as judged by change in fibrinolytic activity, clinical improvement and reduction of the erythrocyte sedimentation rate and plasma fibrinogen levels; and in 5 of these interruption with a placebo confirmed that the effects observed were due to phenformin. Of course nothing whatsoever may come of this.

G. R. Fearnley, R. Chakrabarti and Elizabeth D. Hocking. Phenformin in Rheumatoid Arthritis. Lancet 1:9, Jan. 2, 1965.

"Is anything ever gained by determining the salicylate blood levels in a rheumatoid arthritic who is being treated with aspirin?"

Reply: Indeed one may occasionally gain a great deal because individuals vary widely in their handling of aspirin. Your patient who is not doing as well as you think he should may simply not be absorbing the drug as fully as most other individuals. The salicylate determination is a very simple laboratory procedure.

"When it is necessary to administer fairly high dosage of aspirin in rheumatoid arthritis are there any other maladies which the patient might have concomitantly that could effect an increase in

the toxicity of the drug through hindering its elimination?"*

Reply: Salicylate elimination is impaired in kidney disease, chronic alcoholism, morphinism and hyperthyroidism. Hepatic disease does not seem to affect the elimination.

"Is there any danger of damaging the parenchymatous organs when giving high dosage of salicylates in rheumatoid arthritis?"

Reply: High therapeutic dosage of salicylates increases the flow of bile, and when the really toxic dosage range is reached it appears that some liver damage is caused. Aspirin has no effect upon the kidneys in low dosage such as is used for ordinary analgesic effects, but both aspirin and sodium salicylate may temporarily impair renal function to some extent in very high therapeutic dosage. The effect is completely reversible. Because of the possible effects upon carbohydrate metabolism, which somewhat resemble those of insulin, one should be cautious in using high salicylate dosage in diabetics.

"I have a patient with rheumatoid arthritis whom I can keep reasonably comfortable only with slightly subtoxic dosage of aspirin. She is in fact able to titrate dosage by the degree of tinnitus and deafness experienced; fortunately, she does not experience vertigo, though she is ambulatory. Sometimes the deafness progresses pretty far before she reduces dosage. Am I in danger of causing progressive and permanent deafness with this therapy?"

Reply: No you are not. At Harvard Medical School, Eugene Myers and associates studied this matter in a group of 25 patients with rheumatoid arthritis and other connective tissue diseases and found that each time they withdrew the salicylate the effect on hearing loss was completely reversible within 2 or 3 days. They believe that salicylate intoxication merely produces an inhibition of oxidative enzymes in the cochlea, thus depressing the bioelectric and biochemical properties of this organ so that hearing is temporarily reduced.

Eugene N. Myers, Joel M. Bernstein and George Fostiropolous. Salicylate Ototoxity. New England J. Med. 273: 587, Sept. 9, 1965.

"I have recently had a patient whose hallucinations seemed definitely to be associated with the high dosage of aspirin she was taking for rheumatoid arthritis. Is this a well recognized occurrence?"

Reply: Yes, though the incidence is not high. However, in addition to the familiar gastrointestinal disturbances, dermatitis, alteration in blood coagulation mechanisms, tinnitus, deafness, vertigo, etc., the drug can cause confusion, bizarre behavior, hallucinations, stupor, movement disorders and even papilledema. The patients are frequently individuals who have been taking aspirin in excessive dosage for prolonged periods and have "written off" the hearing and mild gastrointestinal disturbances and are brought to the office or hospital with an acute episode of mental derangement. Usually it will be found in these cases that the serum salicylate level is above 35 mg./100 ml., and this, coupled with the presence of hyperventilation, will point to the diagnosis.

Hugh D. Greer, III, Harry P. Ward and Kendall B. Corbin. Chronic Salicylate Intoxication in Adults. J.A.M.A. 193: 555, Aug. 16, 1965.

"I have recently had a patient with rheumatoid arthritis who developed severe salicylate intoxication when I tapered off the corticosteroids that he had been receiving simultaneously with aspirin. Has anything of this sort been recorded?"

Reply: Yes, Klinenberg and Miller have reported 4 cases of this sort in which toxic levels of salicylate were reached and mentioned several other instances in which it was difficult to achieve therapeutic serum salicylate concentrations despite oral administration of high dosage if corticosteroids were being given concomitantly. These workers speculated that long-term corticosteroid therapy may augment the renal clearance of salicylate. There is some work, however, which makes this explanation not easily acceptable.

James R. Klinenberg and Frederick Miller. Effect of Corticosteroids on Blood Salicylate Concentration. J.A.M.A. 194:601, Nov. 8, 1965.

"I have a patient with rheumatoid arthritis who has been on phenylbutazone (Butazolidin) for more than 2 years, which seems to me a rather long time. What has been the usual experience?"

Reply: R. M. Mason and V. L. Steinberg (London Hospital) studied 315 patients with rheumatoid arthritis to determine the length of time they had taken the drug and the reasons for stopping. Discontinuance within 3 months, 37.1%; within 6 months, 53.6%; within 1 year, 67.6%; within 2 years, 80%; within 4 years, 87.9%. Fifty of the 117 withdrawing at 3 months did so because of intolerance; as the duration of administration continued, intolerance played a progressively decreasing part in causing withdrawals, which is strikingly in contrast to the situation with corticosteroid therapy.

R. M. Mason and V. L. Steinberg. Long-Term Use of Phenylbutazone (Butazolidin) in Rheumatoid Arthritis. Brit. M. J. 2:828, Sept. 17, 1960.

"I have a patient with rheumatoid arthritis who, in his acute exacerbations, responds to nothing so well as to oxyphenbutazone (Tandearil), but the erythrocyte sedimentation rate remains stationary despite the clinical improvement. Can you explain this?"

Reply: No I cannot, but the phenomenon has been observed by others. For example, Neil Cardoe, in England, remarked upon this and also said he had the impression that his patients become anemic under the drug, though his hemoglobin studies did not substantiate this. By and large, this is an agent whose use should not be too lightly entered upon. If the patient is receiving other potent drugs, such as the oral antidiabetic compounds, insulin or the anticoagulants, you must be very careful or you may have toxic reactions of very great severity on your hands. A number of things contraindicate the use of the drug: history of a blood dyscrasia (agranulocytosis, leukopenia, thrombocytopenia have been recorded), peptic ulcer or history of the same, hepatic, renal and heart disease. Discontinue administration at once if a skin rash appears, because there have been some instances of exfoliative dermatitis.

Neil Cardoe. The Place of Oxyphenbutazone in the Treatment of Rheumatoid Arthritis and Allied Conditions. M. J. Australia 2:986, Dec. 19, 1964.

"I have a patient with long-standing rheumatoid arthritis of moderate degree who maintains himself in an ambulatory state through regular use of pheylbutazone (Butazolidin) in moderate dosage. But I am puzzled by the fact that upon several occasions blood specimens taken in the late afternoon have revealed an abnormal amount of uric acid which is never present in a specimen drawn in the morning. The patient does not have clinical gout. What is going on?"

Reply: I think it not unlikely that your patient, like so many other victims of rheumatoid arthritis, takes considerable amounts of aspirin throughout the day in addition to the drug that you prescribe for him. At Northwestern University, John Oyer's group have shown that the combination of a salicylate and phenylbutazone will decrease uricosuria. Phenylbutazone is a long-acting drug but aspirin is eliminated much more rapidly; thus the salicylate titer in your patient's blood in the morning could be quite low whereas it might rise sufficiently during the day as a result of the aspirin ingestion to bring about the urico-suria-suppressing effect by afternoon.

John H. Oyer, Sheldon L. Wagner and Frank Schmid. Suppression of Salicylate-Induced Uricosuria by Phenylbutazone. Am. J. M. Sc. 251:1, 1966.

"Are all of the antimalarial compounds equally effective in the treatment of rheumatoid arthritis, and what is the explanation for their action?"

Reply: I have answered this question elsewhere as follows: "It is an interesting and as yet unexplained fact that efficacy of the antimalarial compounds in the collagen disorders resides only in quinacrine (Atabrine), chloroquine (Aralen), hydroxychloroquine (Plaquenil) and amodiaquin (Camoquin), i.e., only those compounds that are built on either the acridine or the 4-amino quinoline nucleus. Little is known regarding the anticollagen action and, in fact, not much more regarding the action in malaria. However, a high concentration of the drugs occurs in the parenchymatous organs—the liver, spleen, lungs and kidneys—and the leukocytes contain several times as much as the plasma; and since sequestration in tissues indicates nucleoprotein binding, one may speculate that if there is faulty nucleoprotein metabolism in the collagen disorders these drugs may act by inactivating some of this structure through attachment to it."

Harry Beckman. 1961–62 Year Book of Drug Therapy, p. 531.

"A patient of mine, who had been on chloroquine (Aralen) for a prolonged period in treatment of rheumatoid arthritis, developed a syndrome that closely resembled progressive muscular dystrophy of the limb-girdle type, which gradually but completely cleared when I took her off the chloroquine. Could it actually be that the drug had caused this thing?"

Reply: Yes it could. A small number of such cases has been reported, the patients usually having been on chloroquine in daily dosage of 250–500 mg. for from 6 months to a year. It appears characteristic of the picture that the symptoms continue to progress for several weeks after withdrawal of the drug, improvement then setting in slowly and sometimes not reaching completion until the lapse of a full year.

S. Blom and P. O. Lundberg. Reversible Myopathy in Chloroquine Treatment. Acta med. scandinav. 177:685, 1965.

"In the treatment of rheumatoid arthritis and other connective tissue disorders the two antimalarial compounds, chloroquine phosphate (Aralen) and hydroxychloroquine sulfate (Plaquenil) have proved to be of some value, but some of us hesitate to use them because of reports of the ocular damage they may cause. Could you provide a statement of the extent and seriousness of such damage?"

Reply: The ocular lesions are of two types: reversible corneal changes, and a retinopathy that has usually been found irreversible; regarding this universal irreversibility, however, there is now some question since a few reports have appeared in which complete recovery was described after discontinuance of the therapy. The most complete study of the matter that has come to my attention was that of Arthur Scherbel and associates at the Cleveland Clinic. The chloroquine-treated group of these investigators comprised 408 patients who had received the drug for 1–9 years, the mean duration of their illness being 8.6 years; the 333 patients who had never received a chloroquine compound were of comparable sex distribution but their mean age was 12.6 years greater and mean duration of illness 1.4 years longer than the treated group. Corneal deposits typical of chloroquine keratopathy were observed in 10% of the treated group and were reversible; chloroquine had been used in 83% of these cases, hydroxychloroquine in 8.5% and both drugs at different times in 8.5%. None of the patients with corneal lesions had retinopathy. Although various posterior ocular lesions were observed in 7.4% of patients receiving a chloroquine derivative, there were only 2 cases of bilateral macular pigmentation in which these changes might, though questionably, have been related to the drug. Neither resembled the "doughnut" or "bull's-eye" macula supposedly diagnostic of chloroquine retinopathy. Vision remained normal and there were no changes in the visual fields. Three patients who had never received the chloroquine drug exhibited similar bilateral macular changes. In both groups retinal changes of all types were found exclusively in patients over 40 years of age.

A noteworthy feature of this Cleveland Clinic study is that none of the treated patients received dosage of chloroquine greater than 250 mg. once daily, or of hydroxychloroquine 200 mg. twice daily, older children receiving half these amounts and those weighing less than 50 pounds, one-fourth the adult dose. In practically all the other reports of severe retinal damage from these drugs the dosages have been much higher than these. Certainly it would appear the part of wisdom not to increase chloroquine dosage if moderate amounts of the drug do not appear to be effective.

Arthur L. Scherbel, Allen H. Mackenzie, James E. Nousek.

Ocular Lesions in Rheumatoid Arthritis and Related Disorders with Particular Reference to Retinopathy. New England J. Med. 273:360, Aug. 12, 1965.

"One of the bright young interns in our hospital has become quite enthusiastic about the use of antimalarial compounds and wants to try them in almost every recalcitrant malady. Would you kindly supply a list of the principal entities in which they have been used with some satisfaction and also a list of the serious toxic reactions to them that I may bring to this young man's attention?"

Reply: The disorders in which these drugs — principally chloroquine (Aralen), amodiaquin (Camoquin) and hydroxychloroquine (Plaquenil) — have been rather widely used are discoid and systemic lupus erythematosus, pemphigus, scleroderma, lichen planus, photosensitivity reaction, sarcoidosis, rheumatoid arthritis and probably numerous other unrecorded maladies. When these drugs are used in antimalarial dosage in the treatment or prophylaxis of that specific infection they have very low toxicity, but serious toxic reactions have often occurred in connection with their use in high dosage in these other diseases. Aralen: skin reactions that have sometimes gone on to exfoliative dermatitis, increased pigmentation, worsening of pre-existent psoriasis, alopecia, graying or bleaching of the hair, visual disturbances and usually irreversible retinopathy, usually reversible corneal changes, severe gastrointestinal disturbances, widespread but reversible muscular weakness, toxic psychosis. Camoquin: pigmentation, melanosis, corneal edema, lethargy, weakness, fever, headache, severe gastrointestinal distress, liver damage, bladder incontinence, tremors, tinnitus, arrhythmias, muscular degeneration, agranulocytosis. Plaquenil: toxicity is lower than with the other two, but it is advisable to consider that all of the reactions characteristic of Aralen may eventually be seen with this drug also.

"What is the position of indomethacin (Indocin) vis-à-vis corticosteroids in the therapy of rheumatoid arthritis?"

Reply: It is really difficult to answer this question because, although a number of studies have been made and reported, the disease itself is so unpredictable in its course that an assessment of the benefit truly derived from use of any agent is difficult to make. Long-term double-blind studies in the disease can hardly be counted upon to produce anything of value, since practically all patients will take aspirin or some other analgesic regularly during any trials that are being made

with other drugs and thus vitiate interpretation of subjective responses to the trial agent. However, it does appear that indomethacin is probably a valuable addition to our armamentarium, and in specific reply to your question I can cite the report of Charley Smyth, at the University of Colorado, who made a comparative objective evaluation of the new drug with the standard corticosteroids. Using the most reliable techniques of drug testing, and disregarding entirely the subjective responses of the patients to the drugs, Smyth found that in 16 of 30 patients receiving corticosteroids when they entered the study it was possible to withdraw these agents completely and in 4 additional patients to reduce the total corticosteroid dosage by 50% or more. In four (inflammatory index, shoe-tie time, grip strength and walking time) of the six most reliable tests of inflammation and function, he found the anti-inflammatory effect of the two agents to be about parallel, though as I read his charts it seemed that the advantage was with the corticosteroids. Significant changes were obtained with the sedimentation rate and ring-size tests with corticosteroids but not with indomethacin. The majority of the patients in the study were maintained on 100–200 mg. of indomethacin daily. It was necessary to stop the drug in 37 of the 97 cases in the series of Albert Katz and associates, in Los Angeles: the principal reactions were gastrointestinal, light-headedness, giddiness, headache and psychic changes. Ulcers developed in 6 patients, in 4 of them very rapidly after onset of treatment. In the 234 patient-trials of Norman Rothermich, in Columbus, Ohio, reversible central nervous system side effects required discontinuance of the drug in 20%, and gastrointestinal symptoms in 12.5%, but the dosage was high. In Australia, Michael Kelly has found the drug cumulative in its effects; in 2 years nearly half of his patients had to stop taking it.

Charley J. Smyth. Indomethacin in Rheumatoid Arthritis. A Comparative Objective Evaluation with Adrenocorticosteroids. Arthritis and Rheum. 8:921, 1965. Albert M. Katz, Carl M. Pearson and Joseph M. Kennedy. Clinical Trial of Indomethacin in Rheumatoid Arthritis. Clin. Pharmacol. & Therap. 6:25, 1965. Norman O. Rothermich. An Extended Study of Indomethacin. J.A.M.A. 195:531, Feb. 14, 1966. Michael Kelly. Treatment of 193 Rheumatic Patients with Indomethacin, A New Anti-Rheumatic Drug. J. Am. Geriatrics Soc. 14:48, 1966.

"I have a patient with active rheumatoid arthritis who is doing fairly well on phenylbutazone (Butazolidin). Would anything be gained by switching her to the newer drug, indomethacin (Indocin)?"

Reply: As in the case of most new drugs that are enthusiastically promoted, increasing experience indicates that it is perhaps not as good as it was earlier thought to be. However, experience with it is still insufficient to provide adequate answer to your question. The study of Hart and Boardman, in London, was designed to effect comparison between phenylbutazone and indomethacin. This was a double-blind crossover trial using 75 mg. of indomethacin daily and 300 mg. of phenylbutazone, each being given for a period of 28 days to 26 patients. There were no significant differences between the two groups in relief of symptoms afforded by the two drugs, but there seemed to be greater reduction of early morning stiffness on phenylbutazone and of joint swelling on indomethacin. When the patients expressed their personal preference at the end of the trial it was in favor of phenylbutazone. In a mixed group of patients treated by these observers over 2½ years it was found that indomethacin effectively improved the symptoms in 50.5% of instances. Side effects occurred in 36.6% of the patients, most commonly headache, giddiness, "muzziness," nausea and vomiting.

F. Dudley Hart and P. L. Boardman. Indomethacin and Phenylbutazone: A Comparison. Brit. M. J. 2:1281, 1965.

"If a patient reacts adversely to a corticosteroid in the treatment of rheumatoid arthritis, is anything to be gained by switching him to another compound of the same series?"

Reply: Quite often this is the case in a long-term therapeutic regimen. For example, cortisone, hydrocortisone (Cortef, etc.) or prednisone (Meticorten, etc.) may cause fluid retention and edema in a patient who will do very well on prednisolone (Meticortelone, etc.) or dexamethasone (Decadron, etc.) or perhaps best of all on triamcinolone (Aristocort, Kenacort). Or triamcinolone may suppress the appetite in a patient who eats too much and gains excessive weight under dexamethasone. There are also instances in which a patient will not respond fully to a corticosteroid but will progress favorably on corticotropin (ACTH), which must of course be injected.

"How does the toxicity of corticosteroid therapy in rheumatoid arthritis compare with that in gold and phenylbutazone therapies?"

Reply: In the study reported by Norman Rothermich, at Ohio State University, he found an incidence of 10% of serious corticosteroid toxicity comparing favorably with the 35% incidence in gold therapy and the 44% incidence in phenylbutazone therapy. It should be noted, however, that this investigator considers a large initial corticosteroid dosage as hazardous

and that he therefore starts with the smallest dose possible to enable the patient to be up and about and not disabled but not entirely free from symptoms. And he only institutes corticosteroid therapy if the patient's condition is not controllable by a basic program of increased rest, salicylate therapy, appropriate physical therapy and general health measures. He also feels it important to incorporate in his program an "anticatabolic" feature, which includes a diet high in protein and calcium, anabolic gonadal hormones or their analogues, supplemental vitamins (especially B_{12}) and active exercise and massage. His data definitely offer confirmatory evidence that the harmful effects of corticosteroids are dose-related, for only 4% of those who received 5 mg. of prednisone or its equivalent daily had serious effects, while at the 10 mg. daily dose there was a 10% incidence and at the 15 mg. level a 25% incidence.

Norman O. Rothermich. Corticosteroid Therapy in Rheumatoid Arthritis: Criteria and Results. Postgrad. Med. 36:117, 1964.

"Which are the more dangerous of the two types of drugs in the collagen disorders, corticosteroids or antimalarials?"

Reply: The antimalarials are potentially the more toxic of the two groups because they are entirely foreign compounds to the body economy, whereas the "toxic" reactions to the corticosteroids are really not toxic reactions at all but only evidences of the excessive physiologic actions of these compounds, which in their simplest forms are normal body constituents. In true antimalarial dosage, the antimalarial compounds do not cause the types of toxic reaction that are seen when they are used in the high dosage employed in the collagen disorders.

"Is it true that the antidepressant drugs will enable one to lower the dosage of corticosteroids in rheumatoid arthritis through some potentiating action on these agents?"

Reply: It has been alleged by several investigators that the monoamine oxidase inhibitors do have a "steroid-sparing" effect, but in a recent study in the General Infirmary, Leeds, England, V. Wright's group, who used the antidepressant drug, nialamide (Niamid), in 50 mg. dosage three times daily in patients who had been on constant corticosteroid therapy for at least 6 months, felt that any steroid-sparing action of the drug was not by means of a direct biochemical mechanism or other direct influence on corticosteroids, but rather by an elevation of mood and an increase in the patient's tolerance of pain.

V. Wright, W. C. Walker and E. A. M. Wood. Nialamide (Niamid) as "Steroid Sparing" Agent in Treatment of Rheumatoid Arthritis. Ann. Rheumat. Dis. 22:348, 1963.

"A number of comparative studies were made in England a few years ago of the corticosteroids and aspirin in the treatment of rheumatoid arthritis. What was the upshot of this?"

Reply: The report of the early trials conducted by the Joint Committee of Medical Research Council and Nuffield Foundation on Clinical Trials of Cortisone, ACTH and Other Therapeutic Measures in Chronic Rheumatic Diseases produced little evidence that there is much on which to base a choice between cortisone and aspirin in long-term management of the disease, and a similar result came out of a trial conducted by the Empire Rheumatism Council Research Subcommittee, in 1955–57. Then, in 1959, the Joint Committee reversed itself, reporting favorably on the use of a corticosteroid vs. aspirin. Professor Kellgren, of the Rheumatism Research Center, Manchester, who spoke for the Joint Committee, when asked why the new trial had shown such a different result from the earlier ones, said that it was due to the fact that a different corticosteroid had been used, i.e., prednisolone instead of cortisone. It seemed to me, however, at that time that the fact was being very lightly overlooked that more than half of the patients on prednisolone were also receiving aspirin or other analgesics during the trial. Furthermore, adverse effects of the steroid were also not lacking—moonface, rise in blood pressure, etc.—but this was not much emphasized in the report. Then, in a further extension of the trials in 1960, it appeared that the advantages earlier claimed for prednisolone were not perhaps being fully sustained and that the side effects of the drug might in the long run considerably detract from its value. One of those whose group had been fully involvéd in these therapeutic trials, H. F. West, of the Sheffield Center for the Investigation and Treatment of Rheumatic Diseases, expressed the view that *was* and *is* that of many observers in this field, namely that corticosteroid therapy should be used in the severely affected patient only, which meant in West's opinion about 1 in 20.

Comparison of Prednisolone with Aspirin or Other Analgesics in Treatment of Rheumatoid Arthritis: Second Report by Joint Committee of Medical Research Council and Nuffield Foundation on Clinical Trials of Cortisone, ACTH and Other Therapeutic Measures in Chronic Rheumatic Diseases. Ann. Rheumat. Dis. 19:331, 1960. Comparison of Cortisone and Aspirin in Treatment of Early Cases of Rheumatoid Arthritis: Report by Joint Committee of Medical Research Council and Nuffield Foundation on Clinical Trials of Cortisone, ACTH and Other Therapeutic Measures in Chronic Rheumatic Diseases. Brit. M. J. 1:1223, May 29, 1954. Empire Rheumatism

Council. Multicenter Controlled Trial Comparing Cortison Acetate and Acetylsalicylic Acid in Long Term Treatment of Rheumatoid Arthritis: Results up to One Year. Ann. Rheumat. Dis. 14:353, 1955. Empire Rheumatism Council Multicenter Controlled Trial Comparing Cortisone Acetate and Acetylsalicylic Acid in Long-Term Treatment of Rheumatoid Arthritis: Results of Three Years' Treatment. Ann. Rheumat. Dis. 16:277, 1957. Comparison of Prednisolone (Meticortelone, Etc.) with Aspirin or Other Analgesics in Treatment of Rheumatoid Arthritis. Ann. Rheumat. Dis. 18:173, 1959.

"When contemplating the beginning of corticosteroid therapy in rheumatoid arthritis, what are the main drawbacks to be thought of?"

Reply: Increased susceptibility to infection, provocation of peptic ulceration, development of osteoporosis, induced adrenal insufficiency, the psychic shock to the patient when he is forced to discontinue use of the agents and then experiences reversion to his former state.

"Can you give me guidance in the choice of corticosteroid for use in treatment of rheumatoid arthritis?"

Reply: At the University of Southern California, Edward Boland studied several compounds on a long-term basis and found little to choose between prednisone (Meticorten, etc.), prednisolone (Meticortelone, etc.), methylprednisolone (Medrol, Wyacort), fluprednisolone (Alphadrol) and paramethasone (Haldrone) for the ordinary patient requiring therapy of this nature. He did, however, find dexamethasone (Decadron, etc.), betamethasone (Celestone) and triamcinolone (Aristocort) less desirable for routine use because they are more prone to cause certain troublesome side effects.

Edward W. Boland. Clinical Comparison of Newer Antiinflammatory Corticosteroids. Ann. Rheumat. Dis. 21:176, 1962.

"When may help be obtained through the intra-articular injections of corticosteroids?"

Reply: The chances of effecting relief are very good, provided infection does not exist or is not suspected, when there is active inflammation of one or a few joints, bursae or tendon sheaths. If the condition is self-limited, such as a subdeltoid bursitis or traumatic arthritis, it may require only a few or perhaps only one injection to effect suppression of the inflammatory process. But in such chronic conditions as rheumatoid arthritis and osteoarthritis, one must expect no more than an ameliorating effect from the individual injection, and that even though such effect is obtainable through reinjections, the indicated systemic therapy must also be employed.

"The intra-articular administration of cortico-steroids in cases of rheumatoid arthritis is rather popular in our area, and does not appear to be associated with many complications, but I am never quite at ease with it. Have there been serious results?"

Reply: You should be aware of the possibility of producing a Charcot arthropathy. The incidence of this complication is unknown, but the British literature a few years ago suggested that it is more frequent than is generally realized. In the case of Charles Steinberg and associates, in Rochester, New York, the patient had received 22 injections of hydrocortisone acetate into the right knee during 27 months. When operated upon, on suspicion of a Charcot joint, the knee revealed marked destruction of the articular cartilage of both tibial and femoral condyles, with multiple osteophytes and general fragmentation and fibrillation of the cartilage. Both menisci seemed to have been dissolved completely, and the synovia was brownish, villous and nodular. There was about 15 ml. of clear yellow, thick fluid in the joint. Microscopic study revealed changes more typical of a Charcot joint than of progressive rheumatoid disease. The Rochester investigators felt that a course of intra-articular corticosteroid injections should be limited to three to four during a few weeks, followed by a period of more conservative management; and such joints, particularly if weight-bearing, should be carefully examined for excessive effusion formation, ligamentous instability and the like.

Charles Le Roy Steinberg, Robert B. Duthie and Agustin E. Piva. Charcot-Like Arthropathy Following Intra-articular Hydrocortisone. J.A.M.A. 181:851, Sept. 8, 1962.

"In recent years I have been preferring hydro-cortisone for the corticosteroid injection of the knee joint, but I now have a patient in whom the joint involvement appears to be worsening after repeated injections. What is present opinion regarding the preparation to be preferred?"

Reply: A good many men have turned to hydrocortisone in preference to prednisolone because it has seemed that systemic effect could thus be minimized, but opinion has been mounting latterly that methylprednisolone acetate (Medrol), or a similar long-acting steroid, should be used instead of hydrocortisone precisely because of such experiences as you are now having, i.e., progressive joint deterioration in a patient repeatedly injected with hydrocortisone. Some men are now using betamethasone (Celestone) with satisfaction. I think that in using corticosteroids by direct injection into the joint, one should always be guided by the same principles that apply to the systemic use of the drugs, namely, that as the duration of therapy increases the risk of complications increases, that the dose should be reduced as quickly as possible, and that attempt should not be made to achieve absolute elimination of all symptoms.

Martti Oka and Kaija Lähdesmäi (Central Hospital, Kuopio, Finland). Systemic Effects of Large Doses of Hydrocortisone Acetate (Hydrocortone Acetate, etc.) and Prednisolone Acetate Administered Intra-articularly to Patients with Rheumatoid Arthritis. Acta rheumat. scandinav. 8:192, 1962. W. R. Murdoch and G. Will. Methylprednisolone Acetate in Intra-articular Therapy: Clinical, Biochemical and Chromatographic Studies. Brit. M. J. 1: 604, Mar. 3, 1962. Abraham Cohen and Joel Goldman. Intra-articular Injection of Betamethasone (Celestone) in Treatment of Osteoarthritis and Rheumatoid Arthritis. Pennsylvania M. J. 68:47, 1965.

"Would there be any advantage to be expected from using an anabolic steroid together with anti-inflammatory agents in treating the rheumatic disorders?"

Reply: As a matter of fact, a very interesting report on therapy of this sort appeared several years ago from the clinic of William Kuzell and associates, in San Francisco. They sought to determine whether they could favorably alter the asthenia, anorexia, physical status, number and severity of rheumatic symptoms and requirement for anti-inflammatory drugs in 320 patients of both sexes with primary diagnoses of one or more of the following: rheumatoid arthritis, ankylosing spondylitis, osteoarthritis, gout and symptomatic osteoporosis. Some of the patients were given 5 mg. of methandrostenolone (Dianabol) daily for a mean period of 14 months, and others, 2.5 mg. for 12 months. The drug had to be discontinued in 6 women because of acne or symptoms of virilism. Improvement did indeed appear to be associated with use of the anabolic agent in 134 (82.7%) of 162 patients. When corticosteroid requirement was reduced in this combined therapy it occurred most often in patients with rheumatoid arthritis, whereas reduction in salicylates, antimalarials or phenylbutazone occurred most often in osteoarthritic patients.

William C. Kuzell, Richard P. Glover, David L. Bruns and John O. Gibbs. Methandrostenolone (Dianabol) in Rheumatic Diseases and Osteoporosis. Geriatrics 17:428, 1962.

"I have heard that Canadian investigators have shown that corticosteroids and nitrogen mustard are capable of reducing the amount of recoverable rheumatoid factor in rheumatoid arthritis. Is this true, and what is the significance of the finding?"

Reply: Yes, at Queen's University, Kingston, Ontario, H. G. Kelly and N. A. Hinton did report such a finding, but it does not seem to me that its significance is clear. There have been several suggestions in recorded investigations of the rheumatoid factor that it may be quantitatively related to the course of rheumatoid arthritis. But numerous observers doubt that the production of these macroglobulins that are designated "rheumatoid factor" are primarily related etiologically to the disease. Actually these bodies may be recovered from the blood of normal persons, may be transfused without provoking the disease, and may be absent in the presence of the disease.

H. Garfield Kelly and Norman A. Hinton. Effect of Dexamethasone and Nitrogen Mustard on Production of Rheumatoid Factor in Rheumatoid Arthritis. Canad. M. A. J. 91:57, July 11, 1964.

"I have heard that methotrexate (Amethopterin) has been employed effectively in the treatment of that type of arthritis that is nowadays known as psoriatic arthritis, but is this not a very toxic agent to use in such a malady?"

Reply: Indeed it is, and such treatment should certainly be reserved for patients with severe disabling disease who have failed to respond to more conservative measures. At the National Institutes of Health, Roger Black and associates compared the response of 21 patients with psoriatic arthritis to a series of three parenteral injections (intravenous when possible, otherwise intramuscular) of methotrexate in progressively increasing doses of 1–3 mg./kg. at intervals of 10 days. In comparison with placebo, the drug was found to be effective in suppressing skin manifestations, decrease in joint tenderness and swelling, improving joint range of motion, and decreasing the erythrocyte sedimentation rate. But among the 21 methotrexate-treated patients there were the following side effects: anorexia or nausea in 13, burning sensation in the skin in 10, depression of the white blood cell count below 4000/cu. mm. in 7, oral ulcerations in 2, and mild hair loss in 1.

Roger L. Black, William M. O'Brien, Eugene J. Van Scott, Robert Auerbach, Arthur Z. Eisen and Joseph J. Bunim. Methotrexate Therapy in Psoriatic Arthritis. J.A.M.A. 189:743, Sept. 7, 1964.

"I concluded some time ago that since gold is a very toxic agent whose worth has never been really proved, I would stop using it, which I did. But now I have heard that it is being effectively used in combination with chloroquine (Aralen). Can you tell me anything of this?"

Reply: I have seen only one report of a study of these two agents used in combination, that of Sievers and Hurri, at the Rheumatism Foundation Hospital, Heinola, Finland. They were unable to show a statistically significant difference in favor of the combined therapy, and they felt that a long-term fully controlled study would be needed to make a final assessment of the method.

K. Sievers and L. Hurri. Combined Therapy of Rheumatoid Arthritis with Gold and Chloroquine (Aralen): I. Evaluation of Therapeutic Effect. Acta rheumat. scandinav. 9:48, 1963.

"For reasons that are far from clear to me some men in our area are again showing interest in the use of gold in the treatment of rheumatoid arthritis. What are the untoward reactions to be expected and the contraindications to the use of gold?"

Reply: This is a toxic drug. The organs especially affected are those through which gold is excreted, the kidneys, stomach and intestine. The following reactions occur: temporary increase in pain, skin eruptions (some of these are possibly due to the sesame oil in which the salts are suspended), exfoliative dermatitis, edema, stomatitis, conjunctivitis, ocular chrysiasis (gold impregnation of the ocular tissues, a rare occurrence), "gold bronchitis," gastroenteritis, hepatitis with jaundice, albuminuria, acute nephritis, nephrotic syndrome (rare), hematopoietic damage (agranulocytosis, leukopenia, platelet reduction, purpura, aplastic anemia) and neurologic and psychic manifestations.

There is no way of anticipating or preventing the reactions. In various published series of cases in the period some years ago when this therapy was much in vogue and high dosage was used, the incidence of significant toxicity ran as high as 40–80%; it may be lower nowadays.

The principal contraindications to gold seem to be the following: pregnancy, severe anemia, history of purpura or agranulocytosis, ulcerative colitis, diabetes, hepatic disease, congestive heart failure, chronic skin affections such as eczema (but not psoriasis, though it is said that patients with complicating psoriasis respond less favorably), active pulmonary tuberculosis and hypertension. Old age and arteriosclerosis do not in themselves constitute contraindications, in the opinion of some observers. It seems advisable to withhold the drug in patients with an allergic history. Eosinophilia has long been recognized as an accompaniment of chrysotherapy, but its occurrence does not appear to be an absolute contraindication to the continued use of the agent.

"Although gold salts have some bactericidal action against streptococci and some other organisms in vitro, they are less effective in this regard than either sulfonamides or antibiotics; and since neither of the latter types of compound is effective in the treatment of rheumatoid arthritis, what can be the rationale of using gold salts in this malady?"

Reply: Since we are really ignorant of the fundamental cause of rheumatoid arthritis, I wonder whether one can legitimately speak of any therapy as being rational? Stimulation of the reticuloendothelial system to effect immune body response is generally conceded to be the nature of gold's action. The true value of gold therapy in rheumatoid arthritis remains uncertain after 20 years' use of the compounds, but it is undeniable that a few men who have persisted in use of the element still believe that any patient should be given the benefit of a trial of gold therapy who has not improved under other types of treatment.

"I have heard that a mixture of proteolytic enzymes derived from the pineapple plant, known as Ananase, is sometimes helpful in resolving the fibrin deposits and reducing the inflammatory process in rheumatoid arthritis. But I know nothing about this product and am fearful of employing it because of possible toxicity. Can you enlighten me?"

Reply: The agent has not been used a great deal, I believe, though I have seen the report of Abraham Cohen and Joel Goldman who recorded that in most of their 29 patients on maintenance corticosteroid dosage there was a reduction of residual joint swelling and a corresponding gain in joint mobility soon after the start of Ananase therapy. I believe that there has been no report of untoward effects from the use of this agent.

Abraham Cohen and Joel Goldman. Bromelains (Ananase) Therapy in Rheumatoid Arthritis. Pennsylvania M. J. 67:27, 1964.

"Is the colchicine test for differentiation of rheumatoid arthritis and gout a reliable one?"

Reply: I think the answer must be no. At least Jack Zuckner (St. Louis University) found it not to be reliable in his 30 patients with rheumatoid arthritis who were given 0.6 mg. colchicine orally every hour for a maximum of 12 hours, being instructed to stop medication upon improvement or appearance of toxicity. Ten patients had satisfactory subjective relief, and 4 also had good objective evidence of improvement 18-24 hours later. Of 14 who received the drug intravenously in 2 or 3 mg. doses, there was satisfactory objective response and objective signs of improvement in 7. There was some favorable response

to placebos also in the small number of patients put to the test. Thus, despite the placebo responses, it appeared that a significant number of the patients improved because of the colchicine itself; and since these were fully established rheumatoid arthritis cases, the evidence is clear that gout cannot be reliably differentiated from rheumatoid arthritis by the colchicine test. It is a fact, however, that a gouty patient who responds to colchicine remains free of symptoms until another exacerbation or acute attack of gout occurs, whereas the rheumatoid arthritis patient who responds satisfactorily does not maintain the improvement for as long as a week. Therefore, extension of the period of observation after giving the colchicine will strengthen the value of the test.

Jack Zuckner. Responses to Colchicine Therapeutic Trial in Rheumatoid Arthritis. New England J. Med. 267:682, Oct. 4, 1962.

"There was a time when Nature helped us mightily with our rheumatoid arthritis patients if we just gave them some aspirin and put them to bed, i.e., enforced a period of bed rest even upon those who were not already more or less incapacitated. Then came the great corticosteroid breakthrough and the prospect of accomplishing with the new drug, in an ambulatory patient and very quickly, what it took us a long time to do with the older regime. But now that we have become pretty much disillusioned with the corticosteroids, I find some of my younger colleagues unable to believe that anything can be accomplished, or indeed was ever accomplished, by the measures employed before the advent of corticosteroid therapy. Can you cite any recent article extolling bed rest as a therapeutic measure in rheumatoid arthritis that I may spread out before these young fellows?"

Reply: Why not show them the report of J. W. Zeller and associates (Boston), whose 200 patients were subjected to "sanatorium management?" Arthritis had been present for more than a year before entry in 87% of these patients and for 6 years or more in 54%; nearly all had active inflammatory involvement, and the sedimentation rate was in the normal range in only 13 of them. About 45% of the group had hemoglobin levels of 12 Gm. or below. Treatment: general rest and splinting of acutely inflamed joints; active exercises after subsidence of the acute involvement; hot packs, hot soaks, hot baths, Hubbard tub; orthopedic care and appliances; adequate amount of salicylate; reduction of corticosteroid dosage as rapidly as possible consistently with safety. When discharged, 74 patients had major improvement or complete remission, and 50 had advanced to minor incapacity or full functional ability after severe or complete functional incapacity. Steroid toxicity contributed significantly to the number of patients responding unsatisfactorily to the "sanatorium" regime, and there was no evidence that these drugs had an extended beneficial effect in the disease.

J. Wallace Zeller, Hans Waine and Kurt Jellinek. Sanatorium Management of Rheumatoid Arthritis. J.A.M.A. 186:1143, Dec. 28, 1963.

"I have a patient with destructive and deforming rheumatoid arthritis complicated by chronic leg ulcers due to coexistent arteritis. L. E. cell tests have been repeatedly positive and rheumatoid factor is present in high titer. Can you suggest any therapy to effect improvement in the ulcers?"

Reply: In a similar case R. Z. Jaffe, in New York, used penicillamine, 2 Gm. daily, for about a year and achieved healing of the ulcers with significant fall in the level of rheumatoid factor. The drug was given in divided dosage of 0.5 Gm. four times daily after meals and at bedtime. Other drugs for which some successes have been claimed have been corticosteroids in high dosage, anticoagulants and 6-mercaptopurine (Purinethol).

Israeli A. Jaffe. Rheumatoid Arthritis with Arteritis: Report of a Case Treated with Penicillamine. Ann. Int. Med. 61:556, 1964.

"In the case of any one of the variants of rheumatoid arthritis—ankylosing spondylitis, Sjögren's syndrome, palindromic rheumatism, Felty's syndrome, Still's disease, Caplan's syndrome, intermittent hydrarthrosis, the arthritis accompanying psoriasis or ulcerative colitis—is there any reason to depart essentially from one's usual therapeutic approach to rheumatoid arthritis itself?"

Reply: I take it you mean to inquire whether there are drugs that approach any of these variants more specifically than those we use in the classical disorder. The answer is no.

"Practically always when I find it necessary to put a rheumatoid arthritis patient on corticosteroids I continue the use of aspirin. Has there ever been published a well-controlled evaluation of the combination of these two agents?"

Reply: Yes, at the Lemuel Shattuck Hospital, in Boston, Hershel Jick and associates performed two sequential crossover controlled double-blind trials, in the first of which 1.5 mg. of dexamethasone (Decadron, etc.) was found to be superior to 0.75 mg. for symptomatic relief; in the second trial the addition of 1.5 Gm./day of aspirin to the lower dose of dexa-

methasone increased the therapeutic efficacy to the level of the higher dose of the corticosteroid.

Hershel Jick, Robert S. Pinals, Robert Ullian, Dennis Slone and Hugo Muench. Dexamethasone and Dexamethasone-Aspirin in the Treatment of Chronic Rheumatoid Arthritis: A Controlled Trial. Lancet 2:1203, Dec. 11, 1965.

"I have a patient with rheumatoid arthritis in whom posterior subcapsular cataracts are developing. Are there confirmed findings that such cataracts may be associated with protracted systemic corticosteroid therapy?"

Reply: Yes, there are.

Robert W. Spencer and S. Yale Andelman. Steroid Cataracts: Posterior Subcapsular Cataract Formations in Rheumatoid Arthritis Patients on Long-Term Steroid Therapy. Arch. Ophth. 74:38, 1965.

RICKETTSIAL DISEASES

"I understand that all of the rickettsial diseases respond favorably to antibiotics, but which of them is the drug of choice?"

Reply: You are quite correct in saying that they all respond to antibiotics but one exception must be made, since we do not have adequate information regarding trench fever in the period in which these drugs have been available. As to choice, the tetracyclines and chloramphenicol seem to be equally effective.

SALMONELLOSES

"In the salmonelloses other than typhoid fever what is the antibiotic of choice?"

Reply: These organisms actually often show as much in vitro susceptibility to the action of chlortetracycline (Aureomycin) and streptomycin as to chloramphenicol (Chloromycetin), but chloramphenicol is by far the most effective agent clinically.

SANDFLY FEVER

"Since we are becoming more deeply involved day by day in the Far East, some of our soldiers are going to be acquiring sandfly fever. Is there any specific drug therapy available?"

Reply: No.

SARCOIDOSIS

"I have had a patient with sarcoidosis on chloroquine (Aralen) therapy with good effect, but the malady relapsed when I discontinued the drug. How am I to know whether I am to resume this therapy; in other words, did the drug bring about the remission or was this simply a spontaneous resolution?"

Reply: In reporting the largest series of chloroquine-treated sarcoidosis cases that has come to my attention, Louis E. Siltzbach and Alvin S. Teirstein, at the Mount Sinai Hospital in New York, made the point that spontaneous resolution is a commonplace event in this disease but that relapse after spontaneous resolution is quite uncommon. They therefore felt that frequent "rebound" relapse after discontinuing chloroquine is a more reliable measure of the drug's suppressive action than is the patient's improvement under the therapy. When chloroquine was stopped in the 7 cases reported by Stephen Morse's group, at the Rockefeller Institute, there were clinical relapses in 4 patients within 3 months; the lesions again receded in 2 of them under a second course of the drug. In Toronto, Barbara Hunt and Edmund Yendt reported a single case in which the accompanying hypercalcemia, and the consequent nausea and vomiting, frequency and nocturia, irritability and muscular weakness, was remarkably well combated through use of antimalarials. Discontinued after 17 months, the drugs had to be resumed when the serum calcium began to rise again after 7 weeks.

Stephen I. Morse, Zanvil A. Cohn, John G. Hirsch and Russell W. Schaedler. Treatment of Sarcoidosis with Chloroquine. Am. J. Med. 30:779, 1961. Louis E. Siltzback and Alvin S. Teirstein. Chloroquine Therapy in 43 Patients with Intrathoracic and Cutaneous Sarcoidosis. Acta med. scandinav. (Supp. 425) 176:302, 1964. Barbara Hunt and Edward Yendt. Response of Hypercalcemia in Sarcoidosis to Chloroquine. Ann. Int. Med. 59:554, 1963.

"I have started a patient with advanced pulmonary sarcoidosis on corticosteroids; what may I expect?"

Reply: In Göteborg, Sweden, Lars Andér and associates employed such therapy in 12 cases with the progressive type of the disease, using the drugs for at least 1 year. In 7 cases there was a significant improvement, usually evident within 1 month from the onset of therapy, optimal improvement occurring between 1 and 24 months. In 1 case with initial improvement the patient stopped the medication and experienced a temporary marked relapse. In 5 of the cases the progressiveness of the disease appeared to be totally unaffected by the therapy.

Lars Andér, Erik Berglund and Rolf Malmberg. Long-Term Steroid Medication in Advanced Pulmonary Sarcoidosis. Acta med. scand. (Supp. 425) 176:299, 1964.

"I heard several years ago of the successful use of colchicine in treating sarcoid arthritis. Has this been followed up?"

Reply: Yes, Herbert Kaplan, who initially described the dramatic response to colchicine therapy in 2 patients, has since reported 3 additional cases. The drug was used about as in the treatment of an acute episode of gout: 1 mg. initially followed by 0.5 mg. hourly until diarrhea appears.

Herbert Kaplan (MC, USAR). Further Experience with Colchicine in Treatment of Sarcoid Arthritis. New England J. Med. 268:761, Apr. 4, 1963.

SCABIES AND LOUSE INFESTATION

"Is there some one combination of drugs that can be easily used in an individual who is infested with both lice and the scabies mite?"

Reply: A much used preparation is an emulsion (Enbin) containing 1% of chlorophenothane (DDT), which destroys lice; 2% of ethyl aminobenzoate (Benzocaine, Anesthesin), which destroys the eggs (nits) as chlorophenothane does not; and 10% of benzyl benzoate, which destroys the scabies mites. Thus the preparation is useful in both scabies and pediculosis and is indeed employed in both infestations. For treatment of pediculosis it is customary to anoint the affected area thoroughly and leave the application in place for 24–48 hours, after which it is washed out with soap and water; clothing must be thoroughly laundered and the treatment repeated in a week if necessary. In scabies, a hot bath is taken, with thorough rinsing away of the soap afterward, before applying the lotion or ointment over the entire body below the neck, with special care to the elective sites; a bath after 24 hours, and repeating in a week if necessary.

SCIATICA

"I have a patient with severe diabetic sciatica. Would treatment with epidural injections of procaine and hydrocortisone likely be beneficial?"

Reply: According to Goebert's group, at the Cleveland Clinic, sciatica due to carcinoma with bone metastasis, intradural or extradural tumor, arachnoiditis or postherpetic or diabetic neuralgia is not benefited. They felt that the main indication of this type of treatment is sciatica of the type indicating pathologic involvement of the spinal nerve roots that contribute to the sciatic nerve. The clinical picture here may suggest protruded or degenerated disk, radiculopathy, adhesions after laminectomy, arthritis, trauma or sciatica without demonstrable cause. They felt that an additional indication may be nocturnal gastrocnemius cramps following an otherwise successful operation for protruded disk.

H. William Goebert, Jr., Stanley J. Jallo, W. James Gardner, Carl E. Wasmuth and Elmars M. Bitte. Sciatica: Treatment with Epidural Injections of Procaine and Hydrocortisone. Cleveland Clin. Quart. 27:191, 1960.

SCLERODERMA

"I have heard that chelating agents have been used with some effect in scleroderma and related maladies but can find no reference to this therapy in the literature available to me. Could you cite the work?"

Reply: The study to which you doubtless refer was reported by Sture Johnson (University of Wisconsin) several years ago in the Wisconsin Medical Journal, which you are unlikely to have seen. He observed that treatment with ethylenediamine-tetra-acetic acid (EDTA, Endrate Disodium) effected improvement in patients with sarcoidosis, arsenical keratoses, generalized scleroderma, and stasis ulcers occurring in sclerodermatous skin of the legs. There was no improvement in patients with atopic eczema, psoriasis, dermatitis herpetiformis, extracellular calcinosis and blastomycosis. Patients were almost routinely given 3 Gm. diluted with 500 ml. of 5% dextrose, intravenously during 4 hours for 5 consecutive days, followed by 2 days of rest, and repeated twice. There was also a daily dose of 75 mg. pyridoxine. Greater dilution, or slower infusion, or the use of a larger vein usually obviated the burning sensation and pain. (See also the immediately following Reply.)

Sture A. M. Johnson. Use of Chelating Agent Edathamil Disodium in Acrosclerosis, Sarcoidosis and Other Skin Conditions with Comments on Tryptophan Metabolism in Sarcoidosis. Wisconsin M. J. 59:651, 1960.

"I have heard that in scleroderma the drug disodium edetate (Endrate) has some value, but since I understand that to embark upon therapy with this chelating agent is quite a project, I would want to know whether the thing would be worthwhile. What has careful study revealed?"

Reply: At the Mayo Clinic, Neldner's group did study the matter very carefully and concluded that the small chance for improvement did not seem to warrant routine use of the agent. That is to say, in a review of 727 cases seen at the Clinic it was found that there was an overall 5 year survival rate of 70.3%. Therefore, any type of therapy to be effective in this disease must demonstrate definite improvement in more than 70% of unselected patients over 5 years. This the chelating agent did not do.

Kenneth H. Neldner, R. K. Winkelmann and Harold O. Perry. Scleroderma: Evaluation of Treatment with Disodium Edetate (Versenate, Endrate). Arch. Dermat. 86: 305, 1962.

"I have heard that spectacular results have been achieved by the use of potassium para-amino-benzoate (Potaba) in scleroderma and dermatomyositis. Since it seemed that the agent should be safe to use, I have begun its employment in a patient with scleroderma. What is the mechanism of the action?"

Reply: It is postulated that the fibrotic changes in these maladies are the result of the depression of monoamine oxidase activity through tissue anoxia. Potassium para-aminobenzoate increases tissue oxygenation. Some years ago, J. A. Evans' group used PABA instead of KPAB with disappointing results, but half of their patients could not tolerate the therapy for a period that might have been long enough. Chris Zarafonetis initiated the KPAB therapy in localized forms of scleroderma several years ago, and more recently Grace and associates, New York, have effected dramatic improvement with it in 2 generalized cases of scleroderma and 2 of dermatomyositis. Dosage 20 Gm. daily, later reduced to 15 Gm.

J. A. Evans et al. J.A.M.A. 151:891, 1953. William J. Grace, Richard J. Kennedy and Anthony Formato. New York J. Med. 63:140, Jan. 1, 1963. Chris J. D. Zarafonetis. Treatment of Localized Forms of Scleroderma. Am. J. M. Sc. 243:147, 1962. W. Silver and N. Gitlin. Progressive Systemic Sclerosis (Diffuse Scleroderma): Treatment with Potaba: Preliminary Report. South African M. J. 39: 453, May 29, 1965.

SCURVY

"An elderly patient, who has been subsisting for several years on nothing more than coffee, doughnuts and hamburger, has just come into my practice. The clinical diagnosis of scurvy is very evident. May I hope to correct the associated megaloblastic anemia as well as the vitamin C deficiency by the administration of ascorbic acid alone?"

Reply: No, you had better give him folic acid in addition.

SHEEHAN'S SYNDROME

"I have a patient with Sheehan's syndrome who is extremely anxious to bear a child. Do women with this malady ever become pregnant?"

Reply: It has been accomplished a few times. In a case reported by Polishuk and associates, in Israel, the medication employed was human menopausal gonadotropin for its FSH activity and human pregnancy urine gonadotropins (Pregnyl, etc.) for their LH-like activity. Dosage was 300 mg. of the menopausal gonadotropin daily for 12 days and a total of 25,000 units of the pregnancy urine in 3 days. On the presumed day of ovulation and subsequent 2 days the patient was inseminated by donor semen (because her husband happened to be sterile) and became pregnant.

W. Z. Polishuk, Z. Palti, E. Rabau, B. Lunenfeld and A. David. Pregnancy in a Case of Sheehan's Syndrome Following Treatment with Human Gonadotrophins. J. Obst. & Gynaec. Brit. Common. 72:778, 1965.

SHIGELLOSIS

"A case of bacillary dysentery, which does not often appear in my practice, is being treated cautiously, and I must admit unsuccessfully, with low dosage of sulfonamides. I should like to terminate the infection sharply now, and have heard that this is being done with single, very high antibiotic dosage. Can you particularize?"

Reply: This sort of thing, which is referred to as "Stosstherapy," has been reported by Stoker at the RAF Hospital in Cyprus. He gave 2.5 Gm. of tetracycline (Achromycin) in a single dose to 91 patients and declared that his results were as good or better than with the more orthodox dosage. In 1 patient, who vomited the tablets immediately after ingestion, the pattern was set for spreading the medication out during an hour when the patient had nausea. The mean hospital stay of patients receiving a streptomycin/sulfonamide mixture was 13 days, and of those on the tetracycline Stosstherapy 9 days. In more "orthodox" therapy, tetracycline is used in 500 mg. dosage every 8 hours for the first 24 hours and then in half dosage at the same intervals until a normal temperature and negative fecal culture is achieved for at least 3 consecutive days.

D. J. Stoker. Treatment of Bacillary Dysentery, with Special Reference to Stosstherapy with Tetracycline. Brit. M. J. 1:1179, Apr. 28, 1962.

"May one use tetracycline to clear up a bout of shigellosis without provoking superinfection?"

Reply: Yes, this is possible with care. At the U.S. Naval Hospital in Philadelphia, H. Leonard Jones and Orville Nielsen advocate the use of oxytetracycline (Terramycin) or tetracycline (Achromycin, etc.) in oral dosage of 500 mg. every 6 hours for 5–7 days, and

advise that one should obtain at least one negative stool culture.

H. Leonard Jones, Jr., and Orville F. Nielsen. Colitis: Management Based on Pathogenic Mechanisms. M. Clin. North America 49:1271, 1965.

SHOCK

"When a patient who has sustained some type of physical trauma enters the emergency receiving service in a state of impending or actual clinical shock, what guideposts are there to rational therapy? Our residents almost invariably administer metaraminol (Aramine) and start blood transfusion as soon as possible, but the results do not seem to me to support this routine procedure."

Reply: Here we have one of the most vexing problems in medicine, and yet the *principles* of shock therapy (not, mark you, the *etiology* of shock) are really quite forthright and simple. The cerebrovascular failure reflects an imbalance between vascular tone, cardiac output, blood volume and oxygenation of the blood; and you must determine which one or more of these elements is altered pathologically. Do not overlook the possibility that deficient ventilation, due to decreased chest excursion because of pain, airway obstruction, pulmonary compression, abdominal distention or brain injury, may be producing hypoxia and respiratory acidosis, which will be directly myocardial depressant. So the shock may be due to deficient cardiac output and call for correction of the respiratory deficiency through mechanical respiratory support, administration of oxygen and nonopiate analgesic and sedative drugs, and possibly surgical measures. Of course in rare instances there may be obstruction in venous return as a result of mediastinal compression or pericardial tamponade, which would require thoracotomy or aspiration. If the major fault lies in hypovolemia, there will be quick improvement in arterial pressure upon rapid administration of 500–750 ml. of blood, or a blood volume expander such as a 250 ml. unit of plasma protein fraction (Plasmanate). But if the fault should lie in myocardial depression rather than in loss of blood volume, the introduction of these fluids may easily worsen the situation, which can only mean that some means of determining blood volume must be resorted to in order to learn whether volume expanders are indicated or not. The most feasible method of accomplishing this quickly and accurately is by monitoring the central venous pressure through cannulation of the superior vena cava by percutaneous puncture of the subclavian vein (a simple technique, but the pleura or lung may be easily punctured – Residents beware!). If the central venous pressure is low there will not be danger in administering fluids, and a good response can be expected; and here, too, a vasopressor drug may be used rationally because there is probably a state of peripheral vasodilatation to be combated. In any case, if a vasopressor is used it should be one, such as metaraminol (Aramine), which stimulates the heart as well as constricting the vessels. But if the pressure is high it indicates a failing myocardium and reflex constriction of peripheral vasculature; and persistence in fluid administration, or the injection of a vasopressor drug, could be disastrous. If you have established adequate ventilation, and restored blood volume if study of the central venous pressure has indicated the necessity for this, and the cardiovascular failure continues, you must look to the state of the heart. There may be arrhythmias to be corrected by quinidine or procainamide (Pronestyl), or digitalis may be indicated to increase myocardial performance and correct arrhythmias in its own peculiar way. Acidosis from respiratory embarrassment or hypoxic metabolic disorientation will be revealed by pH and CO_2 studies, and indicate the use of sodium bicarbonate. Electrocardiographic studies will reveal hyperkalemia before it is otherwise clinically apparent; this electrolyte derangement is particularly to be anticipated if much blood is being given and will of course be aggravated by a decrease in urine output. A cation-exchange resin, such as Kayexalate, may be used to reduce the potassium, but this can be hazardous unless the serum electrolyte pattern can be closely followed; glucose and insulin may also be useful. Oliguria should be looked upon as merely reflecting the circulatory embarrassment, correctable through one or the other of the measures already discussed, but if there is increased central venous pressure the use of a diuretic drug may offer additional support to the handicapped heart through reducing the hypervolemic load. The matters dealt with in this reply are fully discussed by J. N. Wilson and associates, of Denver. Elsewhere in these Replies I have considered the matter of using vasodilators rather than vasoconstrictors in shock.

John N. Wilson. The Management of Acute Circulatory Failure. S. Clin. North America 43:469, April, 1963.
John N. Wilson, J. B. Grow, C. V. Demong, A. E. Prevedel and J. C. Owens. Central Venous Pressure in Optimal Blood Volume Maintenance. Arch. Surg. 85:563, 1962.
Robert Matz. Complications of Determining the Central Venous Pressure. New England J. Med. 273:703, Sept. 23, 1965.

"As in many other entities nowadays, the therapy of shock has become confused by a plethora of new drugs. What, precisely, is the comparative status of the three vasopressor agents, levarterenol (Levophed), metaraminol (Aramine) and angiotensin (Hypertensin)?"

Reply: Of the numerous studies that have been performed with these drugs in the treatment of shock, I know of only one in which the pharmacodynamic properties of the three were assessed simultaneously. The 12 patients employed in the study of Vasant Udhoji and and Max Weil at the Los Angeles County General Hospital were in a state of shock from bacterial infection (4 patients), myocardial infarction (3), hypovolemia (2), and neurogenic hypotension (3), barbiturate intoxication in 2 and insulin shock in 1. In 6 patients, studies with Hypertensin preceded observations of the effects of Levophed or Aramine. In an additional 6, the response to Levophed or Aramine was studied first, the action of Hypertensin next, and studies with one of the other two agents were then repeated. Infusion of the drugs was regulated to achieve equal pressor response with all. No definitive advantages of Hypertensin over Levophed or Aramine in the treatment of shock emerged from this investigation. In fact, Hypertensin affected cardiac output less favorably than did the other two drugs, and when it was given peripheral vascular resistance was disproportionately higher. There was also a significant reduction in urine flow in 10 of 12 patients during Hypertensin infusion. These investigators concluded that the rationale for the use of Hypertensin in the treatment of shock may be questioned, especially its use in preference to Levophed and Aramine.

Vasant N. Udhoji and Max H. Weil. Circulatory Effects of Angiotensin (Hypertensin), Levarterenol (Levophed) and Metaraminol (Aramine) in Treatment of Shock. New England J. Med. 270:501, Mar. 5, 1964.

"Is it admissible to use morphine to allay the apprehension and pain of a patient in shock?"

Reply: Unless severe pain makes its use mandatory, which will be in the exceptional case, the patient in secondary shock either of traumatic or hemorrhagic origin should probably not be given morphine. It may add to the circulatory and respiratory embarrassment by: (a) slowing the pulse through vagus stimulation, (b) diminishing oxygen consumption and carbon dioxide output through respiratory slowing, (c) lessening the response of the respiratory center to carbon dioxide and to asphyxia. These things will aggravate the condition of the patient already suffering from reduced circulating blood volume, reduced peripheral circulation, depression of blood pressure and poor cardiac output. Furthermore, morphine may dilate the cutaneous vessels and further decrease circulatory efficiency. The cerebral hypoxia of a patient in shock makes him restless and apprehensive, but a small subcutaneous dose of a barbiturate will soothe him sufficiently and is unlikely to have so much respiratory and circulatory depressant action. Blood transfusion can then be given to supply oxygen. The patient will usually complain of pain only when the blood pressure begins to recover. Morphine may then be given with greater safety, preferably in low dosage intravenously. In any case, one should not give an injection and then, after a while, another and another while waiting to have the patient transfused. These "shots" will lie where placed until the circulation improves, and then the patient, who may be weathering the shock, will die of morphine poisoning. It happened often in World War II.

"If a patient in shock does not respond to phenylephrine (Neo-Synephrine) or metaraminol (Aramine) as well as it appears he should, other things being equal, what might be at fault?"

Reply: The necessity to have a satisfactory blood stream titer of thyroidal hormone for best action of the vasopressor agents is pretty well established in animal experimentation, and therefore, if one may safely extrapolate into human affairs, your patient may be in a borderline myxedematous state, in which the shock, from whatever cause, is operating only as a complication. There is some reason to believe, too, that corticosteroids are essential to the proper action of the sympathomimetic vasopressors. So your patient may need corticosteroids as well as liothyronine (Cytomel) before you can pull him out of shock with the vasopressor agents. Or the vasopressor approach may be altogether wrong and a vasodilator agent, such as phenoxybenzamine (Dibenzyline), may be what is really indicated.

Boris Catz and Stephen Russell. Myxedema, Shock and Coma: Seven Survival Cases. Arch. Int. Med. 108:407, 1961.

"In our area it has become popular to supplant levarterenol (Levophed), as a potent vasopressor substance for the treatment of shock, by metaraminol (Aramine) because the newer drug does not produce skin necrosis. Recently I have had the experience of a patient going into deep shock after a brief period in which I was supporting her blood pressure by continuous intravenous infusion of Aramine. I stopped the drug, and by good fortune she survived, but I am left with a puzzle. Has this sort of thing been observed often?"

Reply: It is certainly being seen increasingly, not only with Aramine but with Levophed also. W. E. Spoerel and associates (University of Western Ontario, London, Ontario) have reported 4 cases of what they call "shock caused by continuous infusion of Aramine."

The 4 patients suffered from entirely different diseases, Aramine treatment being undertaken because of hypotension in 3, and the desire to maintain an elevated blood pressure in the fourth. All had a satisfactory initial response to the vasopressor agent, but then it became increasingly difficult to maintain the pressure within a normal range and the dosage had to be progressively increased. It was with this increasing dosage that the picture of profound shock developed. Clinically the picture was that of extreme vasoconstriction with a markedly elevated hematocrit due to reduced plasma volume. The investigators felt that because of the intense vasoconstriction and stagnation of the peripheral circulation induced by the drug, the accompanying tissue hypoxia caused the loss of plasma; compensation for the resulting hypovolemia and hypotension was accomplished by greater vasoconstriction, which in turn led to further deterioration of the peripheral circulation and loss of plasma. "Thus the patient entered a vicious circle, and further treatment with metaraminol (Aramine) only contributed to the progression of the already existing state of shock." In combating this form of iatrogenic collapse, the logical approach is toward restoration of the plasma volume and of course discontinuing the drug. One must be careful, however, in using blood and dextran not to provoke pulmonary edema in the presence of this intense vasoconstriction.

W. E. Spoerel, F. L. Seleny and R. D. Williamson. Shock Caused by Continuous Infusion of Metaraminol Bitartrate (Aramine). Canad. M. A. J. 90:349, Feb. 1, 1964.

"What a time this is to live in! In our hospital we are actually considering the use of a vasodilator agent in the treatment of shock, but intend proceeding slowly and cautiously. Is the matter rational and practical?"

Reply: The answer is "yes" to both portions of your question, but I should certainly not as yet consider the adoption of any sort of "policy" in this regard. In the state of shock there is a reflex sympathetic vasoconstriction that effects a redistribution of the circulating blood in such a way as to maintain a preferential flow to the heart and brain. This is a wonderfully effective survival measure, but the blood deprivation in other vital organs, if too prolonged, can have dire consequences. The rationale, then, of employing a vasodilating agent is to overcome this vasoconstriction and relieve the situation before the shock becomes "irreversible." The drug phenoxybenzamine (Dibenzyline), which abolishes the arteriolar and venous constrictor effects of l-norepinephrine, is the one that has been widely studied experimentally and is now beginning to be used clinically. The most satisfactory report of hemodynamic studies made with this drug in patients in clinical shock that I have seen is that of Robert Wilson and associates at Wayne State University, Detroit. These investigators made hemodynamic measurements in 19 patients before and after intravenous administration of Dibenzyline in treatment of shock that had been refractory to conventional methods. Dosage was 0.2–0.5 mg./kg. in 2 cases; 1 mg./kg. in 10 cases and 1.5–2 mg./kg. in 7 cases. The drug was given in a small intravenous drip over a period of 60 minutes unless the patient was deteriorating rapidly, in which cases the full dose was given in 5 minutes. All other measures were not discontinued when the Dibenzyline treatment began, since it was necessary in many instances to provide large additional volumes of fluid in order to maintain cardiac output and blood pressure, and attempts were also made to correct acid-base aberrations when they were present. It should be remarked, however, that similiar measures had failed to prevent deterioration in the patients before institution of the vasodilator approach. The drug frequently produced an improved clinical picture, the patient becoming quieter, the extremities dry, pink and warm, respirations less labored, urine output increased, fluid administration much better tolerated. The blood pressure fell in 16 of the 19 patients, the decrease in systolic (21%) and diastolic (25%) being greater than in pulse pressure (14%). Pulse pressure rose after the first hour, and the central venous pressure decreased in 13 of the 18 patients in whom it was measured, average net change being a decrease of 28%. The pulse rate rose in 9 of 17 patients studied and dropped in 8. Cardiac output increased in 8 of 9 patients in whom it was studied, and was accounted for chiefly by an increase in stroke volume. Urine output rose in 7 of the 19 patients, three of whom had previously been anuric. Six patients remained anuric, urine output remaining unchanged in 2 and decreasing in 4. Thus it can be seen that in this study the overall clinical effects of Dibenzyline were beneficial; even in patients considered moribund on admission to the study there was transient and sometimes prolonged improvement. However, in closing the discussion that followed presentation of their paper, the authors emphasized that the drug should be used very discretely since there were sometimes precipitous falls in pressure. Bear in mind that the pressure-sustaining reflexes, mediated through the carotid sinus, are eliminated by Dibenzyline; however, the cardiac inotropic (force of contraction) and chronotropic (rate) actions are not blocked, and there is no direct effect on coronary circulation.

Robert F. Wilson, Donald V. Jablonski and Alan P. Thal. Usage of Dibenzyline in Clinical Shock. Surgery 56: 172, 1964.

"What are the advantages of dextran (Dextran, Gentran) that justify its apparently increasing employment as a plasma volume expander?"

Reply: The theoretical advantages of dextran as a plasma volume expander over other nonprotein colloids are said to be: (1) that it is free from acidic radicals and therefore not likely to form storage complexes; (2) that it can be hydrolyzed into glucose by acids and certain living organisms, which suggests that the human body may also be able to metabolize it slowly. Jaenike and Waterhouse gave large amounts to normal human subjects and observed striking salt and water retention and rapid plasma volume expansion. Although serum protein left the circulation during rapid plasma volume expansion, in some subjects total circulating protein, later reached supernormal levels, indicating that plasma volume remains expanded or continues to expand when serum dextran concentration is falling. The cardiac output, stroke volume, right atrial pressure and venous pressure increases noted by Witham's group are adjusted by homeostatic mechanisms before the dextran effect is over.

Dextran has been found to be unquestionably useful in expanding plasma volume and maintaining blood pressure for a period of 12 hours or more following a single injection in the emergency therapy of hemorrhagic and traumatic shock and extensive burns. For example, Amspacher and Curreri concluded from their Korean experience that battle casualties who have mild to moderate blood loss can frequently be satisfactorily treated with dextran alone and that many of the severely wounded who require whole blood and extensive surgical treatment can be maintained by its use during first aid and transportation. Køster and associates found that 1 gram of dextran retains about 18 ml. of fluid. One must remember, however, that this agent only temporarily restores volume and nothing else; nutritive and hematologic losses are not combated.

An anomalous situation exists with regard to dextran, for although Kabat and Berg, independently confirmed by Maurer, found it definitely antigenic in man, allergic reactions to it under clinical conditions are very unusual when the most refined American product is used. Since injection of the large amount usually employed does not provoke reactions except in infrequent instances, it is possible that such reactions are to be expected only in individuals who may have been sensitized by ingestion over a prolonged period of commercial sugar, which contains some dextran, or by dextran-producing organisms in the intestine.

The parenchymatous organs do not appear usually to be injured by the compound, although Vickery reported the finding of nephrosis-like tubular changes in the kidneys of Korean battle casualties, which he thought would have been transient and reversible. Roche and associates observed no interferences with the typing or cross matching of bloods or with Rh determinations. Jaenike and Waterhouse observed nitrogen and phosphorous sparing, indicative of retarded tissue protein catabolism, and an antiketogenic effect, but these things were transient and subsided soon after discontinuance of the injections. They also found that bleeding time might be prolonged, but clotting time and platelet counts were not affected. However, the increase in bleeding time has been found subsequently to be of some practical significance: Langdell and associates gave 1000 ml. of solutions of various concentrations to 257 volunteer personnel and found a bleeding time in excess of 30 minutes in 8% of instances; maximum incidence occurred 3–9 hours after termination of the infusion. It was felt that the phenomenon may be due to interference with platelet activity.

It is probable that dextran infusion should be considered contraindicated in patients with a known bleeding tendency or to whom blood was been transfused in considerable amount.

Dextran does not deteriorate at room temperature and hence may be stockpiled and used without warming or any other preparatory procedures.

J. R. Jaenike and C. Waterhouse. Metabolic and Hemodynamic Changes Induced by Prolonged Administration of Dextran. Circulation 11:1, 1955. A. C. Witham, J. W. Fleming and W. L. Bloom. The Effect of the Intravenous Administration of Dextran on Cardiac Output and Other Circulatory Dynamics. J. Clin. Invest. 30:897, 1951. W. H. Amspacher and A. R. Curreri. Use of Dextran and Control of Shock Resulting from War Wounds. Arch. Surg. 66:730, 1953. K. H. Køster, V. Sele, M. Schwartz and E. Sindrup. Blood Volume Changes After Infusion of Dextran Solutions. Lancet 2:262, 1957. E. A. Kabat and D. Berg. Dextran, as Antigen in Man. J. Immunol. 70:514, 1953. P. H. Maurer. Dextran, as Antigen in Man. Proc. Soc. Exper. Biol. & Med. 83:879, 1953. A. L. Vickery. The Fate of Dextran in Tissues of the Acutely Wounded: A Study of the Histologic Localization of Dextran in Tissues of Korean Battle Casualties. Am. J. Path. 32:161, 1956. P. Roche, Jr., R. A. Dodelin and W. L. Bloom. Effect of Dextran on Blood Typing and Cross-matching. Blood 7:373, 1952. R. D. Langdell, E. Adelson, F. W. Furth and W. H. Crosby. Dextran and Prolonged Bleeding Time. J.A.M.A. 166:346, 1958.

"The new attitude toward shock, which would have us consider the use in some cases of a vasodilating agent rather than a vasoconstrictor, has directed attention to phenoxybenzamine (Dibenzyline), an agent that appears actually to have been around for some time. But I must confess to practically complete ignorance of the drug beyond the fact that it is alleged to effect the dilatation of peripheral vessels through adrenergic blocking. Has it had any useful clinical employment prior to the present time?"

Reply: Phenoxybenzamine is used with some success in dilating the uninvolved vessels in arteriosclerotic peripheral vascular disease. The progress of the lesion is not arrested, but symptomatic relief is afforded, since promotion of collateral circulation lessens the localized hypoxia that has caused the pain and tissue necrosis. A satisfactory result is also sometimes achieved in cases of peripheral arterial embolism, but infrequently in thromboangiitis obliterans (Buerger's disease). In Raynaud's disease in its early stages, in which the episodes are patently due to arterial and possibly venous spasm and there are not yet any residual trophic changes, it might be expected that best success would be attained, and this seems actually to be the case. Usefulness has also been reported in acrocyanosis, causalgia, the "post-frostbite syndrome" and in the treatment of chilblains. It has also been used effectively in high dosage to maintain pressure reduction in a period of emergency preceding the surgical removal of a malignant pheochromocytoma, and on a rather tentative basis it has been given intravenously in severe asthma to permit exceptionally high dosage of epinephrine. In addition it has some importance as a prognostic agent when used in cases of chronic peripheral vascular disease in which sympathectomy is contemplated; if a dose of the drug, with its unalloyed adrenergic blocking action, affords definite improvement in the peripheral circulation (as measured in terms of maximal digital blood flow and temperature changes) it is likely that the operation will be rewarded with an appreciable measure of success.

"What is the best drug with which to combat the necrosis due to levarterenol (Levophed) extravasation?"

Reply: Probably phentolamine (Regitine). In such an emergency, Gary Zucker, at Beth Israel Hospital, New York, milked out as much of the levarterenol solution as possible through several puncture holes and then infiltrated the involved area with 5 mg. of phentolamine dissolved in 20 ml. of water.

G. Zucker. Use of Phentolamine to Prevent Necrosis Due to Levarterenol. J.A.M.A. 163:1477, 1957.

"I understand it has been found in animal experimentation that the circulatory effects of mephentermine (Wyamine) are not entirely like those of metaraminol (Aramine) and levarterenol (Levophed). Are there any clinical implications of this?"

Reply: It does indeed appear that in the experimental animal mephentermine does not act as a vasoconstrictor drug but rather improves circulation by increasing myocardial contractility, reducing the volume of blood stored in the venous circuit, and increasing venous return. The same action has been shown by Udhoji and Weil, at the University of Southern California, in 11 patients with circulatory shock. In these patients the drug consistently increased cardiac output without increasing arterial pressure; indeed peripheral arterial resistance was usually reduced, indicating that mephentermine more often acted as a vasodilator drug. However, in so doing it does not restore the arterial pressure to a level that might maintain optimal perfusion of the coronary, cerebral and renal circuits. Therefore it might be that eventually we will develop some combination of mephentermine with metaraminol or levarterenol that would have the desired effect of increasing blood flow and at the same time maintaining sufficient arterial pressure to perfuse the vital organs effectively. Another drug that should be mentioned here is isoproterenol (Isuprel, etc.), which you did not include in your list because you probably thought of it only as a bronchodilator. It does have cardiovascular actions much like those of mephentermine, however, and has been shown by Gary Kardos, in San Francisco, to be very useful in states of endotoxin (bacteremic) shock where cardiac output often appears to be low and peripheral vascular resistance elevated.

Vasant N. Udhoji and Max Harry Weil. Vasodilator Action of a "Pressor Amine," Mephentermine (Wyamine) in Circulatory Shock. Am. J. Cardiol. 16:841, 1965. Gary G. Kardos. Isoproterenol in Treatment of Shock Due to Bacteremia with Gram-Negative Pathogens. New England J. Med. 274:868, Apr. 21, 1966.

SHOULDER-HAND SYNDROME

"What does one do for this awful thing, the shoulder-hand syndrome, known also as causalgia and under numerous other names?"

Reply: The vicious circle of pain, sympathetic nervous system dysfunction and central nervous system aggravation that characterizes this malady, can be interrupted early by stellate ganglion block or procaine injected locally into a trigger area. But it appears that equally good results may be obtained by physical treatment alone, irrespective of the duration of the disease. In England a number of years ago, Plewes obtained good results with physical treatment that included prolonged periods of exposure to hot air (105° F.) with the extremity elevated; he also recommended paraffin baths and exercise twice daily. Much more recently, in Columbus, Ohio, Ernest Johnson and Anthony Pannozzo have employed this approach very effectively. The program consists of paraffin baths for up

to 8 hours each day, with at least three sessions of vigorous active and passive exercise interposed. The paraffin-dip wrap is changed every hour for six times. Cold packs are used if the patient's pain is aggravated by heat. The active-exercise program consists of pendular shoulder swings with a 5 pound weight strapped at the wrist, wall climbing with shoulder flexed forward and abducted, and the wheel for rotation. All the exercises are performed with 10 repetitions. Stretching the shoulder is done by forward flexion, abduction, and rotation of the shoulder slowly 10 times, with the patient in supine position. Active finger and wrist exercises include individual finger flexion, extension and opposition to the thumb. There are also passive finger exercises.

L. W. Plewes. Sudeck's Atrophy in the Hand. J. Bone & Joint Surg. 38 B:195, 1956. Ernest W. Johnson and Anthony N. Pannozzo. Management of Shoulder-Hand Syndrome. J.A.M.A. 195:108, Jan. 10, 1966.

SILICOSIS

"Is there any drug of specific value in the treatment of silicosis?"

Reply: No, the disablement in symptomatic cases simply reflects ventilatory obstruction, and one is thus ultimately confronted with such complications as bronchitis and emphysema, tuberculosis and cor pulmonale. The dilemmas encountered in the drug therapy of these maladies are considered elsewhere in these Replies.

SJÖGREN'S SYNDROME

"Since Sjögren's syndrome is closely related to rheumatoid arthritis and systemic lupus erythematosus, might one expect it to respond to antimalarial therapy similarly to these maladies?"

Reply: In London, J. M. Heaton has put the matter to the test, using 800 mg. daily of hydroxychloroquine (Plaquenil) in a double-blind test lasting a year in 15 patients who had had ocular symptoms for 2–30 years. Twelve patients improved on the drug and 6 on the placebo; no patient became worse. The erythrocyte sedimentation rate, which had been raised in 9 patients before the trial, was reverted to normal in 7 on the drug and in none on the placebo. It is to be noted that this was a very small series of cases; conclusions as to the efficacy of the therapy cannot really be drawn from the study. Furthermore, one must always be alert to the possibility of damage to the fundus when using an antimalarial compound in high dosage.

J. M. Heaton. Treatment of Sjögren's Syndrome with Hydroxychloroquine (Plaquenil). Am. J. Ophth. 55:983, 1963.

SPRUE

"We have a case of imported tropical sprue in our practice that we seem unable to influence by use of folic acid and vitamin B_{12}. What else may be done?"

Reply: In Puerto Rico, Ricardo Guerra and associates have described their experience in 9 patients who had persistent symptoms and malabsorption despite prolonged treatment with folic acid and vitamin B_{12}. All of these patients responded with clinical and laboratory improvement to a 6 month course of therapy with tetracycline (Achromycin, etc.) or oxytetracycline (Terramycin). There was an average weight gain of 16 pounds, return of serum carotene to normal in all, return of xylose test to normal in 8 of the 9, and decrease in fecal fat excretion from an average of 25 grams/day/patient to 5.8 grams, becoming normal in 5 of the 9 individuals. See also the following Reply.

Ricardo Guerra, Munsey S. Wheby and Theodore M. Bayless. Long-Term Antibiotic Therapy in Tropical Sprue. Ann. Int. Med. 63:619, 1965.

"A patient has just entered my practice with a diagnosis of tropical sprue. He requests antibiotic therapy because he says that such is the general practice in his native Puerto Rico. Is this the case?"

Reply: It is certainly not routinely the therapy of choice but has met with some successes. Sheehy and Perez-Santiago, at the University of Puerto Rico, treated 12 patients who had classic manifestations of the disease with tetracycline, 1 Gm. daily for 7 days followed by chloramphenicol, 1 Gm. daily for 7 days. Observations were repeated during the next 2 weeks. Four patients obtained hematologic remission and excellent clinical improvement; 1 week after beginning of the antibiotic therapy they felt better, appetite increased and diarrhea decreased. In the other patients there was only partial clinical improvement. In a thorough study of a case of this sort in New York, Frederick Klipstein postulated an improved absorptive capacity consequent upon antibiotic administration, but I do not believe that this has been demonstrated experimentally. The "explanation" that antibiotics in the intestinal tract change the flora into one productive of increased amounts of folic acid, has not been disproved. It seems to be established fact that megaloblastic anemia in these cases is secondary to a combined deficiency of folic acid and vitamin B_{12}.

T. W. Sheehy and E. Perez-Santiago. Antibiotic Therapy in Tropical Sprue. Gastroenterology 4:208, 1961. Frederick A. Klipstein. Antibiotic Therapy in Tropical Sprue: Role of Dietary Folic Acid in Hematologic Remission Associated with Antibiotic Therapy. Ann. Int. Med. 61:721, 1964.

"I have recently seen a few cases of tropical sprue in immigrants from the West Indies. Folic acid therapy has produced rapid clinical improvement but x-ray studies have not supported this. Is this the usual experience?"

Reply: Despite the fact that it is fairly well established that tropical sprue is a chronic disease ascribable to vitamin deficiency and malabsorption, the whole of the etiology does not seem to be explained in this way. Indeed, transients are sometimes afflicted with the disease shortly after reaching the tropics. And such experiences as yours are frequent. In Puerto Rico, Sheehy's group attained rapid clinical improvement with folic acid therapy in their patients, but the x-ray pattern showed reversion to normal in only 7 of the 20 individuals after 2–3 years of treatment.

Thomas W. Sheehy, Barbara Baggs, Enrique Perez-Santiago and Martin H. Floch. Prognosis of Tropical Sprue: Study of Effect of Folic Acid on Intestinal Aspects of Acute and Chronic Sprue. Ann. Int. Med. 57:892, 1962.

STAPHYLOCOCCIC INFECTION

"Has the newest of the semisynthetic, penicillinase-resistant penicillins, nafcillin (Unipen), been well studied for effectiveness in comparison with the others?"

Reply: Finland's group at the Boston City Hospital reported on the use of the drug during a 15 month period in the treatment of 86 patients with serious staphylococcal infections. They found it an effective and well tolerated agent giving results entirely comparable to those previously observed with the other penicillinase-resistant penicillins and cephalothin (Keflin). Of the three agents—methicillin (Dimocillin-RT, Staphcillin), oxacillin (Prostaphlin, Resistopen) and nafcillin (Unipen)—the two latter may be given both orally and parenterally but the former can be given only parenterally.

Theodore C. Eickhoff, Jay Ward Kislak and Maxwell Finland. Clinical Evaluation of Nafcillin in Patients with Severe Staphylococcal Disease. New England J. Med. 272:699, Apr. 8, 1965.

"It seems to me that an acute staphylococcal enterocolitis is a prime type of infection with a resistant staphylococcus upon which to base a typical therapy with the newer agents that are effective against resistant staphylococci. Would you therefore make a statement of the method of using such drugs in this infection?"

Reply: The situation has altered quite radically from that of just a relatively few years ago and we now find ourselves in possession of a large number of effective agents. The following may be given in dosage of 1 Gm. every 4 hours until diarrhea ceases and persisting until staphylococci can no longer be recovered from the stool: oxacillin (Prostaphlin, Resistopen), methicillin (Dimocillin-RT, Staphcillin), nafcillin (Unipen). Methicillin is given intramuscularly, the other two either by that route or orally. Then there are three equally effective slightly older agents: kanamycin (Kantrex), vancomycin (Vancocin) and ristocetin (Spontin); each of these may be given orally in dosage of 1 Gm. hourly for 4 hours and then every 4 hours until the situation clears as with the other drugs.

"The influx of new semisynthetic penicillins on the market, each with high claims for superiority in staphyloccic infections, has become somewhat confusing. Could you cite an authoritative study in which the next to the newest of these compounds, oxacillin (Prostaphlin, Resistopen) has really been shown to be as good as or better than methicillin (Dimocillin-RT, Staphcillin)?"

Reply: Yes, in a careful study at the Boston City Hospital, Klein and associates of Maxwell Finland's group, established a fine record for the drug, which was particularly impressive since the great majority of the patients had hospital-acquired staphylococcic infections and serious underlying diseases and had previously failed to respond to other antibiotics. Also, in the same city, Rutenburg and Greenberg obtained a good response to therapy in 79% of 302 patients with staphylococcic infections, the failures being accountable for as follows: gram-negative bacteria resistant to oxacillin in 11 patients, discontinuance after discovery that the infection was due to *Streptococcus faecalis* in 5, indwelling foreign bodies or inadequate drainage of an abscess in 18, therapy too late in the course of illness in 8, and side effects requiring withdrawal of the drug before control of the infection in 4. It would therefore seem that at present oxacillin appears to be one of the best antibiotics in serious systemic staphylococcic infections. But it does not seem of outstanding value in the pyodermas, as evidenced in the double-blind controlled study of Cotts and Sellers (Emory University). Actually, I wish that word of this failure in the pyodermas would get around rapidly so that the drug would not be used indiscriminately for every little pimple that comes into the office.

Jerome O. Klein, Leon D. Sabeth, Bruce W. Steinhauer and Maxwell Finland (Harvard Med. School). Oxacillin (Prostaphlin, Resistopen) Treatment of Severe Staphylococcic Infections. New England J. Med. 269:1215, Dec. 5, 1963. Alexander M. Rutenburg and Harold L. Greenberg (Harvard Med. School). Oxacillin (Prostaphlin, Resistopen) in Staphylococcic Infections: Clinical Evaluation of Oral and Parenteral Administration. J.A.M.A. 187:281, Jan. 25, 1964.

"Since it has been well documented that the newborn nursery can be a critical determinant in the community spread of staphylococcal disease, might it be of protective value to the community to prevent the colonization of hospital strains of staphylococci in neonates through prophylactic use of penicillin?"

Reply: At the University of Oklahoma, Russell Shaw's group addressed themselves to this question. Methicillin (Dimocillin-RT, Staphcillin) and oxacillin (Prostaphlin, Resistopen) were given prophylactically to 81 newborns with a control group of the same size. It was found that this measure significantly reduced the nasal staphylococcal colonization rates of the infants but did not eradicate the carrier state once it was established. Nor did the treatment have any long-term effect on subsequent colonization rates or on incidence of infection when the infant left the hospital nursery and was exposed to the home environment.

Russell F. Shaw, Harris D. Riley, Jr., and E. C. Bracken. The Influence of Prophylactic Methicillin and Oxacillin in the Prevention of Staphylococcal Colonization and Subsequent Clinical Infection in Newborn Infants. Clin. Pharmacol. & Therap. 6:492, 1965.

"What is the best drug to use in combating a severe staphylococcic enterocolitis following broad-spectrum antibiotic therapy?"

Reply: Not all of the cases of this severe malady have followed the use of broad-spectrum antibiotics, as was shown in the analysis of the 155 cases seen in the Surgical Services of the University of Cincinnati, by William Altemeier's group. The drugs involved were as follows: 5 patients received penicillin alone, 80 penicillin in combination with a broad-spectrum antibiotic, 79 tetracycline, 44 neomycin alone or with sulfasuxidine, chloromycetin 36, terramycin 12 and erythromycin 4. It is also true that in occasional instances a patient enters the hospital with staphylococcal enterocolitis rather than developing it while hospitalized on antibiotics. However, the treatment comprises discontinuance of whatever antibiotic is being used and the institution of supportive therapy: hydration, replacement of electrolyte losses, transfusion, vasopressor and other symptomatic therapy. The antibiotics with which staphylococcic infections of this sort are currently being most effectively combated are methicillin (Dimocillin-RT, Staphcillin), in dosage of 1–2 Gm. intramuscularly or intravenously at 4–6 hour intervals; nafcillin (Unipen), in dosage of 500 mg. intramuscularly or intravenously at 4–6 hour intervals or 250 mg.–1 Gm. orally every 4–6 hours, preferably 1–2 hours before meals; oxacillin (Prostaphlin, Resistopen), in dosage of 500 mg.–1 Gm. orally at 4–6 hour intervals, preferably 1–2 hours before meals, or the same dosage intramuscularly or slowly intravenously well diluted.

William A. Altemeier, Robert P. Hummel and Edward O. Hill. Staphylococcal Enterocolitis Following Antibiotic Therapy. Ann. Surg. 157:847, 1963.

"In our hospital we have been unable to rid a number of the personnel of their status as nasal carriers of coagulase-positive Staphylococcus aureus. Has anyone solved this problem?"

Reply: At the VA Hospital in Montrose, New York, Hussar enthusiastically reported a simple and effective measure for terminating this carrier state, but I do not know how widely it has been adopted. After the third of three positive nasal swab cultures taken several days apart, he liberally sprayed the nares and deeper nasal cavities with a solution of 5 mg. neomycin sulfate per ml. normal saline. Thereafter, daily cultures were taken and followed by an additional spraying. Treatment was discontinued when there had been two negative cultures, and repeated if the culture became positive again after 1–3 weeks. In 32 of the 44 courses of treatment in 28 nurses the culture became negative after the first spray, after the second in seven instances, and after the third in four instances. The only failure was one that remained positive after the fifth spray.

Allen E. Hussar. Neomycin Spray in Treatment of Nasal Carriers of Staphylococcus. Clin. Pharmacol. & Therap. 3:441, 1962.

"In a case of staphylococcic enterocolitis I have run the gamut of the well established antibiotics without success. What next?"

Reply: Have you tried the newer drug, vancomycin (Vancocin)? In treating 7 cases, all resistant to all of the other antibiotics that were tried, James Wallace and associates at the University of Washington, obtained very prompt results with the administration of this drug in doses of 0.5 Gm. orally every 6 hours. Unfortunately the drug is expensive, but apparently a relatively short course of therapy with it suffices. So far as I am aware, vanco-

mycin-resistant staphylococci have not yet appeared.

James F. Wallace, Ronald H. Smith and Robert G. Petersdorf. Oral Administration of Vancomycin (Vancocin) in Treatment of Staphylococcic Enterocolitis. New England J. Med. 272:1014, May 13, 1965.

"The prevalent opinion in our area is that treatment of nasopharyngeal carriers in an attempt to eliminate staphylococci has practically no value. Is this a justified position?"

Reply: Yes, that is practically the unanimous opinion (but see nevertheless one of the immediately preceding Replies). Here in Milwaukee, Meyer Fox and Lois Almon recently put the thing to the test again, using methicillin (Dimocillin, Staphcillin) topically and concluding that what was gained by reducing the numbers of the total carrier reservoir did not outbalance the hazards of developing strains of staphylococci resistant to methicillin.

Meyer S. Fox and Lois Almon. Topical Treatment of Nose and Throat Carriers of Staphylococcus Aureus with Methicillin (Dimocillin; Staphcillin). Wisconsin M. J. 64:147, 1965.

STEVENS-JOHNSON SYNDROME

"I have a patient with the Stevens-Johnson syndrome. Have drugs been implicated in the causal role of this malady?"

Reply: In reporting the apparent association of the long-acting sulfonamides, sulfamethoxypyridazine (Kynex, Midicel) and sulfadimethoxine (Madribon, and also contained in the mixture Madricidin), with the Stevens-Johnson syndrome, Carroll's group at the Food and Drug Administration listed the following drugs as having been implicated: penicillin, sulfonamides, antipyrine, belladonna, quinine, mercury preparations, aspirin, phenylbutazone (Butazolidin), chlorpropamide (Diabinese) and several anticonvulsants. Some of the vaccines and antitoxins, and deep x-ray therapy, have been associated with the syndrome, as well as malignancies and viral, fungal and parasitic infections. And in addition, no causal agent or condition can be identified in many cases.

Oree M. Carroll, Paul A. Bryan and Robert J. Robinson. Stevens-Johnson Syndrome Associated with Long-Acting Sulfonamides. J.A.M.A. 195:691, Feb. 21, 1966.

STONE

"I have a patient from whom a large cystine stone was recently removed elsewhere. Is there any effective treatment for cystinuria?"

Reply: Cystinuria results in stone formation because of the relative insolubility of cystine. Treatment through increased fluid intake, alkalinization of the urine and dietary restriction of methionine has had only limited success. The use of penicillamine to form the more soluble penicillamine cysteine appears to be of better promise. At the Seton Hall College of Medicine, McDonald and Henneman had 3 patients on penicillamine for periods of 20, 12 and 8 months respectively at the time of their report, all patients having maintained a low urinary cystine value. In 1 patient an elevated sedimentation rate developed after 6 months of therapy, and 2 patients showed an elevated alkaline phosphatase after 1 year and 6 months of penicillamine, respectively. In the 1 patient with cystine stones there was definite reduction in the size of the stones and complete dissolution after 1 year of therapy.

Joseph E. McDonald and Philip H. Henneman. Stone Dissolution in Vivo and Control of Cystinuria with D-Penicillamine. New England J. Med. 273:578, Sept. 9, 1965.

"In a patient with recurrent renal uric acid calculi and hyperuricemia without symptomatic gout would it be advantageous to use probenecid (Benemid)?"

Reply: A. Bernstein and associates reported the case of a patient who had been in this sort of situation for 18 years in whom probenecid therapy promptly reduced the number and frequency of calculus formation and stopped it altogether after 29 months.

A. Bernstein, D. Bronsky and A. Dubin. Successful Treatment of Recurrent Uric Acid Renal Calculi with Probenecid (Benemid). Ann. Int. Med. 49:203, 1958.

"A new patient of mine, who has gout and frequent renal colic, has been placed on the uricosuric agent, probenecid (Benemid). What may I expect the effect to be on the renal calculi?"

Reply: None of the 39 patients of Elmer Bartels and Lester Corn, at the Lahey Clinic, became worse. One patient, who had had 12–17 calculi a year before treatment, passed 2 calculi in the first year of therapy, 1 in the second year and none in the third. In the fourth year, he passed 3 within 8 days. His gout had been under complete control throughout. In 1 case, although the gout was brought under control, five operations were necessary for calculi that presumably had been present before treatment was begun.

Elmer C. Bartels and Lester R. Corn. Renal Calculi and Hyperuricemia: Preliminary Report. Postgrad. Med. 33:7, 1963.

"Is there any drug that will reduce calcium

absorption? I am wanting to protect a patient against hypercalciuria and the threat of a stone."

Reply: Sodium phytate (Rencal), in dosage of 3–4.5 Gm. three times daily, has been reported to have some value in cases of idiopathic hypercalciuria. Encouraging results have also been achieved with thiazide diuretics.

P. F. Maurice and P. H. Henneman. Medical Aspects of Renal Stones. Medicine 40:315, 1961. Edmund R. Yendt, Raymond J. A. Gagné and Moussa Cobanim. The Effects of Thiazides in Idiopathic Hypercalciuria. Am. J. Med. Sc. 251:449, 1966.

"I have heard that pyridoxine may have some value in reducing the formation of calcium oxalate stones. Is this true?"

Reply: No, unfortunately, I do not believe that it is. In fact many attempts to reduce oxalate formation—such as the low protein diet to reduce the glycine intake, the use of sodium benzoate to trap precursor glycine as hippurate, or the use of pyridoxine because pyridoxine deficiency is productive of hyperoxaluria in experimental animals—have been made and none has been successful. Since calcium oxalate stones may be secondary to hypercalciuria, as well as occurring without apparent cause, it is probably advisable in some instances to attempt the reduction of calcium absorption as one might in hypercalcuria per se; and fluids should be forced.

T. D. R. Hockaday and Lloyd H. Smith, Jr. Renal Calculi. Disease-A-Month, Nov. 1963.

"Is alkalinization of the urine an effective treatment for the patient with a tendency to form uric acid stones?"

Reply: Yes, it is, but it is not sufficient merely to prescribe alkali since it is necessary to maintain the urine pH at 6.5 or above; the patient must keep an actual urine pH chart.

T. D. R. Hockaday and Lloyd H. Smith, Jr. Renal Calculi. Disease-A-Month, Nov. 1963.

"Why is it that atropine, with its ability to relax spasmodic smooth muscle structure, is of so little help in the treatment of renal colic?"

Reply: At the University of Michigan, Jack Lapides has demonstrated that the human ureter is an autonomous organ highly specialized for the propulsion of urine from the kidneys to the bladder but apparently devoid of parasympathetic or sympathetic stimulating or relaxing influences. He found the sole stimulus for its contractions and peristalsis to be the volume of urine and that no drug affected it. This probably accounts for the fact that atropine, though routinely employed, is not often effective in relieving renal colic. In anesthetized dogs with recording balloons in the ureters, we can demonstrate a relaxing effect of atropine, but it is likely that the presence of the immovable obstruction, coupled with the heroic dosage employed, accounts for the difference. Of course in renal colic the presence of a stone in the ureteral tract would also constitute an obstruction.

J. Lapides. The Physiology of the Intact Human Ureter. J. Urol. 59:501, 1948.

STREPTOCOCCIC INFECTION

"Word is going around that the new agent, lincomycin (Lincocin), is superior to penicillin in the treatment of β-hemolytic streptococcal pharyngitis. Is it?"

Reply: I am unaware of the evidence. To be sure, Jackson's group, at Fort Morgan, Colorado, found it just as good in a fairly large number of patients with adequate controls, but they themselves made the point that their evidence was not sufficient to challenge the status of penicillin and erythromycin as the drugs of choice in this disease.

Ham Jackson, Jack Cooper, W. J. Mellinger and A. R. Olsen. Group A β-Hemolytic Streptococcal Pharyngitis—Results of Treatment with Lincomycin. J.A.M.A. 194:1189, Dec. 13, 1965.

"In an individual with β-hemolytic streptococcal infection, who is sensitized to penicillin, what drug should one turn to when the upper respiratory tract is particularly involved?"

Reply: The broad-spectrum antibiotics have not been uniformly effective in these infections and should furthermore be reserved if possible for other uses. The sulfonamides generally have also failed to be fully satisfactory in treatment, though they have a better record in prophylaxis despite the emergence of resistant strains during their massive prophylactic use in the Armed Forces. Nevertheless, each of the new sulfonamides has been hopefully studied, and we now have the record of quite good results achieved by Jan Alban, in San Francisco, with the use of sulfamethoxazole (Gantanol) in a pediatric population. The drug was used in treatment of 229 patients, in all but 13 of whom the upper respiratory tract was involved; the presence of β-hemolytic streptococci was demonstrated culturally in all cases. Initial dosage varied from 1 to 2 Gm. at once and daily maintenance dosage of 0.5–2 Gm., except in a small number of instances in which lower or higher dosages were used. Duration of treatment varied from 2 to 33 days with the majority of patients being treated for 10–14 days. A bacteriologic conversion rate and a clinical cure rate of 96% was obtained. The bacteriologic conversion was considered to be comparable with that generally seen with penicillin, apparently superior to that obtained with erythromycin, and definitely superior to that observed with broad-spectrum antibiotics.

Jan Alban. Treatment of β-Hemolytic Streptococcal Infection. Am. J. Dis. Child. 109:304, 1965.

"Is the recommendation of the American Heart Association, that 125 mg. (200,000 units) of phenoxymethyl penicillin (Pen-Vee, V-Cillin) be given three times daily for 10 days in treatment of streptococcic pharyngitis, still authoritative?"

Reply: This is the rule that is being almost universally followed, but Stillerman and Bernstein (Long Island Jewish Hospital, New Hyde Park, N. Y.) have recently shown that double that dosage is more effective. Their study seems to have been well planned and executed and one wonders whether practice is going to change.

Maxwell Stillerman and Stanley H. Bernstein. Streptococcic Pharyngitis Therapy. Am. J. Dis. Child 107:35, 1964.

"In treating streptococcal infections in children, in which it is essential that a therapeutic titer of penicillin be maintained in the blood stream for at least 10 days, is it safe to prescribe a penicillin preparation for oral administration?"

Reply: This simply means of course, can parents be trusted to administer the drug as directed to their children for a period as long as 10 days, considering the fact that after the first few days there will usually be no evidence of illness in the child. The answer must surely depend on the type of family with which one is dealing. In a *private* pediatric practice in Oneida, N.Y., Joseph Leistyna and John Macaulay treated β-hemolytic streptococcic infections in 162 children whose families saw the same physician at each visit, paid for his services, and bought the prescribed medication. Through personal, instructive communication with the family physician and the utilization of precise, mimeographed instruction sheets, parents successfully treated 144 children (89%) for the prescribed 10 day period. But another type of study may also be cited. At the State University of New York, Syracuse, Abraham Bergman and Richard Werner prescribed a 10 day course of oral penicillin (tablets or liquid) for 59 children with suspected streptococcic infection seen in the *clinic* and then visited at home 3, 6 or 9 days later. The families were told that medication was free of charge, a known amount was dispensed, and the instruction was that the drug was to be taken three times daily for the full 10 days. Despite protestations on the part of the parents that they knew what the medication was and understood the directions for its use, counts of the remaining tablets or measurement of remaining liquid revealed that administration of the drug had been stopped by the third day in 56% of the cases, by the sixth day in 71%, and by the ninth day in 82%. Study of urine specimens substantiated these findings.

Putting this all together, it seems to me that a simple reply to your question would be: inject a long-acting-penicillin preparation at the time of diagnosis.

Joseph A. Leistyna and John C. Macaulay. Therapy of Streptococcal Infections. Am. J. Dis. Child. 111:22, 1966. Abraham B. Bergman and Richard J. Werner. Failure of Children to Receive Penicillin by Mouth. New England J. Med. 268:1334, June 13, 1963.

SUICIDE

"A young college student in my practice has recently committed suicide without anything to warn us that such an event was pending. Had we considered suicide as a possibility in this case, are there any drugs that might have been helpful in avoiding the culmination?"

Reply: I think not in the case of the college student. These college student suicides are in the main the result of an immature individual's sudden and complete inability to deal with an emotional situation, and they almost invariably occur without any warning indications to friends and associates that the precipitating cause was of such completely overwhelming importance to the individual. Excluding accidents, suicide is now the leading cause of death among college students, accounting for more deaths than all diseases taken together. In the mature person suffering from depression it is probable that alcohol should be prohibited, even though the case against alcohol in a causative role is not clear-cut. The well known fact, however, that in some persons alcohol intensifies depression, whereas in others it increases aggressiveness (which in some instances may be turned against themselves), makes it a matter of mere good sense to attempt at least the denial of alcohol to individuals in whom there exists the likelihood of resort to extreme measures. The record of the antidepressant drugs in preventing suicide of depressed patients appears to be pretty good, and conversely the record of a large supply of barbiturates in the hands of an individual with suicidal tendencies is very bad. It is also highly advisable to refrain from using rauwolfia drugs in patients under suspicion because this group of agents has long been suspected of inducing depression of suicidal depth. It is quite evident that the action of a tranquilizing drug in persons of a certain type may well prevent their anxiety and agitation from reaching the point of aggression against themselves, but whether the patient attains relief from a tranquilizer or an antidepressant, it is of utmost importance not to cease use of the drug suddenly; such deprivation may precipitate an overwhelming return to the previous state and a plunge into self-destruction.

F. M. Berger. The Role of Drugs in Suicide. Symposium on Suicide, George Washington University School of Medicine, Oct. 14, 1965. E. D. Freis. Mental Depression in Hypertensive Patients Treated for Long Periods with Large Doses of Reserpine. New England J. Med. 251: 1006, Dec. 16, 1954. H. Jacobziner. Attempted Suicides in Adolescence. J.A.M.A. 191:7, Jan. 4, 1965. E. M. Litin, R. L. Faucett, R. W. P. Anchor. Depression in Hypertensive Patients Treated with Rauwolfia Serpentina. Mayo Clin. Proc. 31:233, Apr. 18, 1956.

SUNBURN

"I have heard it rumored that an experimenter in England has found the antihistaminic, triprolidine (Actidil) protective against sunburn. Has this been verified?"

Reply: In England, Lloyd and Johnson, and in Denmark, Osmundsen and Brodthagen, have failed to confirm the claim that this drug will abolish the abnormal responses to sunlight in photosensitive patients and reduce significantly the sunburn reaction in normal individuals.

P. E. Osmundsen and H. Brodthagen. Triprolidine and Light Protection. Brit. J. Dermat. 77:249, 1965. Jennifer Lloyd and B. E. Johnson. Triprolidine and the Response of Skin to Ultra-Violet Radiation. Brit. J. Dermat. 77:244, 1965.

"Some of my patients, who are hell-bent on acquiring the tanned look, will simply not believe that the 'quickie' preparations they smear over themselves will not protect them against sunlight exposure even though it turns them brown. Can you support me with reference to a study of the matter?"

Reply: Yes, Shaffer and his associates, at the University of Pennsylvania, studied the compound dihydroxyacetone, at that time available in Man Tan, and found that it neither enhanced nor diminished either the erythema reaction or melanogenesis resulting from ultraviolet light exposure. In short, it was *not* protective against sunlight exposure. A fellow I know once expostulated as follows on this subject: "I must confess that the craze for sun-tanning mystifies and disgusts me. To be sure, the end result in the ladies is fetching, for their brown pins are mighty pretty when later revealed below the skirt line; but the men! Why should any full-grown man be concerned about his color in the altogether? And the time they waste, lying brainlessly on their blankets, one ear cocked for the maudlin radio and the other full of dirty sand. Ugh!"

Bertram Shaffer, Milton M. Cahn and Edwin J. Levy. Use of Dihydroxyacetone (Man Tan) for Skin Tanning. Arch. Dermat. 83:437, 1961. Harry Beckman. Editorial comment *in* Year Book of Drug Therapy 1961–1962, p. 165.

SUPPURATIVE ARTHRITIS

"I have in my practice a case of suppurative arthritis in which the response to systemic antibiotic therapy, combined with repeated aspiration of the joint, has provided only moderately satisfactory results. Should I proceed to intraarticular antibiotic therapy?"

Reply: In reviewing the features of pyogenic arthritis in 42 patients seen in a period of 4½ years, Ralph Argen and associates, in Buffalo, concluded that such therapy is best avoided because it appears to be associated with the development of postinfectious synovitis.

Ralph J. Argen, C. H. Wilson, Jr., and Philip Wood. Suppurative Arthritis: Clinical Features of 42 Cases. Arch. Int. Med. 117:661, 1966.

SYDENHAM'S CHOREA

"I have a 5 year old child with Sydenham's chorea but no sign of joint involvement or heart disease. Is it still considered unnecessary in such a case to institute the prophylactic therapy of rheumatic fever?"

Reply: This has certainly been the impression as the result of a report made about 25 years ago, but the recent study of Alan Aron and associates, at Columbia University, has challenged the concept that chorea is a benign manifestation of rheumatic fever. In one third of their patients, followed for many years, heart disease subsequently developed in the absence of any additional recognizable manifestations of rheumatic fever. These observers quite understandably felt that all patients with Sydenham's chorea should be given continuous antibiotic prophylaxis such as would be carried out if they had acute rheumatic fever.

Alan M. Aron, John M. Freeman and Sidney Carter. Natural History of Sydenham's Chorea: Review of the Literature and Long-Term Evaluation with Emphasis on Cardiac Sequelae. Am. J. Med. 38:83, 1965.

SYRINGOMYELIA

"Are there drugs that will slow the progress of syringomyelia?"

Reply: No, nor even be of much alleviating effect; the most potent analgesics may ultimately fail to obtund this pain.

TEMPORAL ARTERITIS

"I have a patient with temporal arteritis who is suffering considerable pain but is not much relieved by the usual nonopiate analgesics, and I do not want to use corticosteroids in her. What would you suggest?"

Reply: Try phenylbutazone (Butazolidin) in dosage of 0.2 Gm. three times daily. S. E. Björkman (University of Lund) reported very favorably on this therapy some time ago. He felt that the thrombophlebitis, which was indicated by the swelling and reddening of the skin in the temporal region, was probably responsible for the clinical symptoms in temporal arteritis, and that this accounted for the relief effected by the antiphlogistic drug.

S. E. Björkman. Phenylbutazone (Butazolidin) in Treatment of Temporal Arteritis. Lancet 2:935, Nov. 1, 1958.

TETANUS

"Has penicillin really proved to be highly valuable in the treatment of tetanus?"

Reply: Oh yes, and tetracycline also. But of course there is very much more to the effective handling of a case of severe tetanus than the giving of an antibiotic: the use of antitoxin, of sedative measures, the maintenance of the airway, débridement, the use of skeletal muscle–relaxant drugs, etc.

"Can you cite the experience of some one observer who has not bounced around among all the proposed therapies but consistently used one type of treatment of tetanus in a sufficient number of cases to give his results true significance?"

Reply: Yes I can. At the University of Texas, Quellin Box reviewed all the cases that were treated in his hospital during the period of 1956–62 in which he treated as follows. A well lighted, air conditioned, special area separate from other patients; nurse in attendance at all times and physician essentially so; sodium phenobarbital the only antispasmodic, given subcutaneously or intramuscularly but only on an individual dose order, seeking a level of sedation that permits as much activity as is consistent with prevention of prolonged or apneic seizures or a potentially exhausting level of seizure activity (in most infants and children this is a dosage of 50–200 mg./2–6 hours, in newborns 8–32 mg./2–6 hours); except in mild cases, nothing by mouth or gastric tube for 5–10 days; penicillin in large dosage, intravenously initially; tetanus antitoxin, 40,000 units for newborns and 60,000 units for infants and children, in a single dose, half intravenously and half intramuscularly (recent newborns have received 5000 units infiltrated about the umbilicus); antitoxin is given in 5% glucose in ½ and 2 hours, usually without preliminary skin tests; tracheostomy not routine; pharyngeal suction transorally; postural tracheobronchial drainage in patients requiring heavy sedation; periodic surveillance of the bacterial flora of the respiratory tract, with vigorous antimicrobial therapy as indicated; urethral catheterization discouraged; initial injection of gamma globulin, 4 ml. for newborns and 10 ml. for others; wound care deferred until the seizure status is carefully appraised, adequate sedation is accomplished and antitoxin has been given.

Quellin T. Box. Treatment of Tetanus. Pediatrics 33:872, 1964.

THROMBOSIS AND THROMBOPHLEBITIS

"Is it true that the taking of phenobarbital lessens the efficacy of the oral anticoagulants?"

Reply: At least in the case of bishydroxycoumarin (Dicumarol), Goss and Dickhaus, in Denver, showed this to be the case in 8 patients receiving long-term anticoagulant therapy.

J. E. Goss and Donald W. Dickhaus. Increased Bishydroxycoumarin Requirements in Patients Receiving Phenobarbital. New. England J. Med. 273:1094, Nov. 11, 1965.

"We have recently had a case of adrenal hemorrhage associated with anticoagulant therapy, which was not diagnosed during life. What symptoms might have aided us in recognizing the situation in time to institute corticosteroid therapy?"

Reply: At the Peter Bent Brigham Hospital, Elias Amador searched the 4325 adult necropsy records since the adoption of anticoagulant therapy in the hospital in 1949, and found 9 cases of adrenal hemorrhage, none of which

had been diagnosed clinically. Five of the patients had received heparin and 5 (including 1 personal case) had received heparin plus dicumarol, adrenal hemorrhage occurring after 2–10 days of therapy. The records showed that localizing manifestations were steady pain of sudden onset, located to the upper abdomen or flanks, accompanied by tenderness and guarding. There was also anorexia, nausea and vomiting, listlessness and weakness progressing to lethargy. Late signs were tachycardia, hypotension, fever and cyanosis, with death in 2–8 days. It was felt that a direct eosinophil count above 50 cells/mm.^{3} might be the most helpful laboratory test for detecting an adrenal crisis.

Elias Amador. Adrenal Hemorrhage During Anticoagulant Therapy. Ann. Int. Med. 63:559, 1965.

"Since one's intricate medical or surgical management of a case can often be defeated by fatal pulmonary embolism, might it not be justifiable practice to anticoagulate any seriously ill medical patient or preoperative surgical patient who has a history of an episode of thrombophlebitis at any preceding time?"

Reply: Your question presupposes, I presume, that the patient is not presenting evidences of venous thrombosis at the time of his present confinement to bed, but has only revealed that he has had such an episode in the past. Could one not question how reliable such a history would be? I mean to say, if you are going to anticoagulate only those individuals who have definite recollection of a thrombophlebitis at some preceding time, would you not always be wondering whether you were not failing to use the measure in individuals who simply did not remember or were uncooperative or too unintelligent to supply reliable information. Furthermore, you are assuming, I take it, that the occurrence of a thrombotic episode in the past predisposes to recurrence and thus to embolism, but actually I do not know that this is the case. If we did know this to be the fact, it would seem to me that, other things being equal, one should anticoagulate the patient with such a history provided it has been shown that anticoagulation will reliably prevent the occurrence of thrombosis in a patient confined to bed under circumstances generally believed to predispose to the malady. I do not know that this has been proven to be the case. In fairness, I will cite the most recent favorable controlled clinical trial that has come to my attention, that of S. Borgström and associates, in Sweden, but there have also been a number of contradictory reports. Indeed, it seems to me that the evidence regarding the efficacy of anticoagulation when thrombosis has been diagnosed is not entirely satisfactory. A continuous study of the prevention of pulmonary emboli in clinically manifest phlebitis has been in progress at the Boston City Hospital since 1943, and in the 1963 report of John Byrne of that hospital it was shown that among patients who had no treatment there was a mortality of 41.6% whereas among those who were anticoagulated the mortality was only 16.5%. However, the number of untreated patients was 408 while the number of treated patients was only 176, and I think one can question the validity of direct comparison here. Furthermore, there is always the question of the underlying condition predisposing to the phlebitis in the individual patient and, still more importantly, the age of the patients in the treated and untreated groups. In Byrne's report, tabular evidence is offered of the striking increase in mortality with increase in age, but the ages of the patients in the untreated and treated groups are not specifically given. The matter is not a simple one therefore, and I at least am unable to supply a categorical reply to your question.

John J. Byrne. Phlebitis and Pulmonary Embolism. S. Clin. North America 43:827, 1963. S. Borgström, T. Greitz, W. Van Der Linden, J. Molin and I. Rudics. Anticoagulant Therapy of Venous Thrombosis in Patients with Fractured Neck of Femur. Acta chir. scandinav. 129:500, 1965.

"I have a patient with thrombophlebitis in whom sudden, localized, hemorrhagic skin lesions, culminating in hemorrhagic infarcts and even small areas of gangrenous necrosis, occurred on the third day after she was placed on warfarin (Coumadin, etc.). Has such a thing been heard of before?"

Reply: It has been very little known in the United States but somewhat better known in Europe, though it is certainly one of the rarer complications associated with the use of the coumarin group of anticoagulants. One can merely describe this as an idiopathic hemorrhagic infarct of the skin and subcutaneous tissues, since allergy to the drugs, the Arthus and the Schwartzman phenomena, has apparently been ruled out by several investigators.

Robert M. Nalbandian, Ivan J. Mader, John L. Barrett, James F. Pearce and Edson C. Rupp (Royal Oak, Michigan). Petechiae, Ecchymoses and Necrosis of Skin Induced by Coumarin Congeners: Rare, Occasionally Lethal Complication of Anticoagulant Therapy. J.A.M.A. 192:603, May 17, 1965.

"I have a case in my practice that causes me to wonder whether there may be any relationship between prolonged use of heparin and the development of osteoporosis?"

Reply: A relationship between heparin administration and osteoporosis has been demonstrated in the experimental animal, and George Griffith's group at Harvard Medical School has reported a small series of cases demonstrating such association in man. But it appears that dosage level rather than duration of treatment with heparin is the determining factor in developing the osteoporosis.

George C. Griffith, George Nichols, Jr., John D. Asher and Barry Flanagan. Heparin Osteoporosis. J.A.M.A. 193:91, July 12, 1965.

"In using the Quick one stage prothrombin time in the routine management of patients on oral anticoagulants, what should be one's aim?"

Reply: It is usually considered satisfactory to maintain the patient's prothrombin time at two to two and one-half times control values, reckoning such control at 11–12 seconds.

"Would you consider that the morbidity from hemorrhage as a complication of anticoagulant therapy is negligible?"

Reply: This is a matter of definition, is it not? In studying prophylactic anticoagulant therapy on an orthopedic service in Springfield, Missouri, Leo Neu and associates felt that the incidence of hemorrhage that was more than twice as great in the treated as in the untreated group, and the necessity to transfuse the treated three times as often as the untreated, was negligible morbidity. Your opinion on this?

Leo T. Neu, Jr., Jim R. Waterfield and Charles J. Ash. Prophylactic Anticoagulant Therapy in the Orthopedic Patient. Ann. Int. Med. 62:463, 1965.

"I have a patient on long-term anticoagulant therapy after myocardial infarction who has become quadriplegic in a matter of 18 hours after first noting a feeling of unusual fatigue. Could this be attributable to the anticoagulant therapy?"

Reply: Yes it could. In reviewing the subject, I. Jacobson's group in England found that nearly 20% of the instances of spontaneous spinal epidural hemorrhage have been associated with anticoagulant therapy.

I. Jacobson, J. J. Maccabe, P. Harris and N. M. Dott. Spontaneous Spinal Epidural Hemorrhage During Anticoagulant Therapy. Brit. M. J. 1:522, Feb. 26, 1966.

"How nearly perfect should our control of anticoagulant therapy be in a community hospital with a satisfactory laboratory and resident staff?"

Reply: At St. Joseph Mercy Hospital, in Pontiac, Michigan, Paul Sullivan and Michael Kozonis, defining an "escaped" patient as one having less than one and one-half times or greater than two and one-half times the normal Quick control value, found that 8 of 100 patients were in the therapeutic range at least 70% of the time. It would have been of great interest if careful record had been kept of the drugs other than anticoagulants that were being used in these patients during the period of study, since the number of drugs that may decrease prothrombin concentration (elsewhere listed in this present volume) is quite large.

At the Kingston, Ontario General Hospital, George Mayer found that errors made by the house staff produced inadequate anticoagulant therapy in 30% of the patients, and he therefore concluded that hospitals should not administer anticoagulant drugs unless this can be done by especially trained and experienced full-time staff. This hardly sounds feasible for most community hospitals, but I certainly think that the control of this therapy should not be in the hands of interns.

Paul M. Sullivan and Michael C. Kozonis. How Effective is Clinical Control of Anticoagulant Therapy? Postgrad. Med. 38:49, 1965. George A. Mayer. Efficiency of the House Staff in Management of Anticoagulant Therapy. Vasc. Dis. 2:30, 1965.

"Is it true that fresh thrombotic attacks are more likely to occur shortly after anticoagulant treatment is stopped?"

Reply: I believe that this clinical impression has been to some extent substantiated. Gradual withdrawal of the drugs—halving the dosage for the first 2 weeks and then halving that dosage again for 2 weeks more—has been shown to eliminate rebound hypercoagulability.

L. Poller and Jean M. Thompson (Manchester, England). Reduction of "Rebound" Hypercoagulability by Gradual Withdrawal ("Tailing Off") of Oral Anticoagulants. Brit. M. J. 1:1475, June 5, 1965. John Marshall and E. H. Reynolds (London). Withdrawal of Anticoagulants From Patients with Transient Ischemic Cerebrovascular Attacks. Lancet 1:5, Jan. 2, 1965.

"I had a patient who died while on anticoagulants and was found at necropsy to have extensive hemorrhages in both adrenal glands. Has there been a record of such an occurrence?"

Reply: Two such cases have been reported in Germany and 1 here in the United States.

F.-J. Krause. Fatal Adrenal Hemorrhage with Heparin Administration. Deutsche med. Wchnschr. 90:955, May 21, 1965. Robert E. Miller and Ricardo Ceballos. Anticoagulant Therapy as Cause of Bilateral Adrenal Necrosis. Alabama J. M. Sc. 1:404, 1964.

"Would you kindly supply a list of the contraindications to the use of the oral anticoagulant drugs?"

Reply: Anticoagulants are definitely contraindicated in the following instances: blood dyscrasias with bleeding tendency, purpura, surgical and traumatic wounds with open raw surfaces, ulcer and cancer of the gastrointestinal or genitourinary tract, severe hypertension, after surgery on the brain or spinal cord or when sympathectomy or regional blocking injections are contemplated, liver disease, jaundice, marked renal failure, in vitamin K or vitamin C deficiency, subacute bacterial endocarditis. Many observers feel that pregnancy should be added to this list, both because of danger to the fetus and of severe hemorrhage in approaching term or in threatened or incomplete abortion. And one should add that any patient who is to be anticoagulated should be sufficiently intelligent and cooperative to follow instructions meticulously and sufficiently stable not to alter or discontinue therapy upon a whim.

"Is there any significant difference in the adequacy of prothrombin levels that can be maintained with the various anticoagulants?"

Reply: Donald Mosley's group, at the Henry Ford Hospital in Detroit, found no such difference when they aimed to maintain prothrombin time between one and one-half and two times the control value in their 970 outpatient cases. Phenprocoumon (Liquamar) was used in 42% of the cases, warfarin (Coumadin) in 30%, phenindione (Danilone) in 16% and bishydroxycoumarin (Dicumarol) in 12%. Of 2668 determinations in 300 patients selected randomly, 65% were within the desired range, 8% above and 27% below control values.

Donald H. Mosley, Irwin J. Schantz, Gerald M. Breneman and John W. Keyes. Long-Term Anticoagulant Therapy: Complications and Control in Review of 978 Cases. J.A.M.A. 186:914, Dec. 7, 1963.

"Is the erythrocyte sedimentation rate or the hematocrit determination altered in the heparinized patient?"

Reply: No.

"Will you please supply a list of the various uses for the anticoagulant agents?"

Reply: The following maladies are ones in which anticoagulants are frequently employed, either upon an acute therapeutic or prophylactic basis or in the form of long-term prophylaxis: (1) extensive surgical intervention, especially for carcinoma, when prolonged immobilization will be required; (2) situations in which vessels must be kept open, as when vascular sutures, anastomoses or transplants are involved; (3) frostbite, to prevent thrombosis in the injured vessels; (4) acute deep thrombophlebitis, to prevent phlebothrombosis; (5) in women about to undergo pelvic or abdominal surgery of a sort normally associated with a relatively high incidence of thrombosis and fatal embolism; (6) peripheral arterial embolism; (7) acute basilar artery insufficiency; (8) internal carotid insufficiency, while awaiting surgical procedures; (9) arteriosclerosis obliterans with recurring arterial occlusions; (10) cerebrovascular accident when it can be reasonably established that the episode is one of thrombosis and not hemorrhage; (11) intractable cardiac decompensation with complicating atrial fibrillation; (12) myocardial infarction. (13) pulmonary embolism (heparin).

"Is there any means of predicting which of 2 patients placed on anticoagulants is the more likely to have a bleeding episode?"

Reply: Unfortunately it appears that there is not. At least, when Charles Baugh (University of Saskatoon) performed coagulation studies on 10 patients who bled during anticoagulant therapy (there being no other demonstrable underlying cause for the bleeding) and 10 patients with similar degrees of hypoprothrombinemia who were not bleeding (the average age and sex distribution of the two groups being similar), no association was found between the occurrence of hemorrhage and the type of anticoagulant used, the duration of treatment or the nature of the underlying disease. No differences were found in the levels of Factors II, VII, IX and X or in the glass and silicone clotting time, the thromboplastin generation test and thrombotest. One must simply agree with Baugh that all patients on anticoagulant drugs, whose prothrombin time is in the therapeutic range or longer, are potential bleeders.

Charles W. Baugh. An Investigation of the Hemorrhagic Diathesis in Patients Receiving Coumarin and Indanedione Anticoagulants. Canad. M. A. J. 92:116, Jan. 16, 1965.

"An acid-citrate-dextrose (A-C-D solution) is now generally used in preparing bank blood. Since it is the citrate in this blood that maintains it in the incoagulable state, and we subsequently transfuse this drug with impunity, why can we not use a simple citrate such as the sodium salt for ordinary anticoagulant therapy instead of the more expensive and potentially toxic agents that are now in use?"

Reply: Simply because the amount of cit-rate that would be necessary to maintain all of the blood in the body in an incoagulable state would be fatally depressant to the myocardium.

"How can one best abolish the anticoagulant effects of heparin?"

Reply: Whole blood transfusion will suspend heparin action, but the blood must be relatively fresh. Another means of instantly abolishing all heparin effects is through intravenous administration of protamine sulfate, which neutralizes the negative charge of heparin with its own electric charge. It appears that 1.5 mg. of protamine is required fully to neutralize 1 mg. of heparin, but it is customary not to give more than 50 mg. of protamine, in sterile 1% solution, at one time. The neutralizing effect on heparin wears off in about 2 hours. In high dosage, protamine may actually have an anticoagulant effect itself, but this is unlikely to be a matter of clinical importance. The substance is a complex, noncrystalline, nonhomogeneous protein-like material obtained from fish sperm; sensitization to it is occasionally seen, and prolonged hypotension and bradycardia not infrequently accompany its use. The compound is not useful in idiopathic or congenital hyperheparinemia.

"Why is it that we can get an anticoagulant action with heparin so much more rapidly than with the coumarin compounds that are given orally? Is this simply because the latter require more time to be absorbed or is there a radical difference in the nature of the action of the two types of agents?"

Reply: The quicker action obtained with heparin is due to the fact that it operates quite differently in affecting the coagulation process. To understand this difference you must keep before you the following simple statement of the steps in blood coagulation: thromboplastin complex plus prothrombin complex plus calcium equals thrombin; then thrombin plus fibrinogen equals fibrin. Heparin affects the constituents of this process in four different ways: (1) it has a nondestructive reaction with prothrombin (with the aid of a plasma cofactor) to prevent its conversion into thrombin; (2) it inactivates thrombin nondestructively (again with the aid of a plasma cofactor); (3) it has an antithromboplastin action of unknown nature; and (4) it prevents the disintegration of platelets (and it is this disintegration of platelets, liberating thromboplastinogenase, that is important in the formation of thromboplastin). Thus the drug prevents coagulation by the exertion of inhibiting actions upon all the main factors concerned in the coagulation process except calcium and fibrinogen. And since the action is exerted directly in the blood stream it is a very quick one. Coumadin (Warfarin), on the other hand (using it as representative of the orally administered coumarin compounds), does not directly affect any of the blood stream constituents of the coagulation process but only acts indirectly to bring about a hypo-prothrombinemia. The action consists not in the destruction of prothrombin in the blood stream but in the prevention of its formation in the liver. And the reason for the delay in the evidence of its action is merely that it takes a while for the preformed prothrombin to be used up. The intimate nature of the coumarin action is not fully known, but the similarity and chemical structure of vitamin K and the compounds of this group supports the idea that the latter compete with the former in the formation of an enzyme essential to prothrombin synthesis in the liver.

"As a clinician I am faced with the decision, when I have diagnosed venous thrombosis in a peripheral vessel, to anticoagulate or not anticoagulate the patient, and in doing so I must of course take into account such bedside matters as the local symptoms, the temperature, the erythrocyte sedimentation rate and the thrombotic history of the patient. But in any case, I can only affect the process of blood coagulation. What of the other factors in this situation; indeed, what are these other factors?"

Reply: One of the most interesting of the "other factors" is the question of hypercoagulability; i.e., may it be that a state of hypercoagulability of the blood precedes the formation of the thrombus rather than following upon the state of blood stasis that is usually associated with the initiating damage to a blood vessel? Then we know that when a vessel is injured a platelet clump develops at the site and appears to release there a clot-promoting factor. Under the electron microscope evidence is developing that some granular material disappears from the clumped platelets. Attention has also been drawn by investigators to the fact that undamaged vascular intima, which is electrically negatively charged, repels platelets that are also negatively charged, and that injury to a vessel, which dispels its electronegativity, would cause it to attract platelets. And then there are factors which through diminishing the diameter of a vessel decrease the rate of flow of blood through it, and thus decrease the negative charge of the intima which appears to be bolstered by the negative "streaming" poten-

tial of the fluid moving through the tube. This is certainly not a very satisfactory answer to your question, but it is all that I know about the subject.

Charles A. Owen, Jr. (Mayo Clinic). Hypercoagulability and Thrombosis. Mayo Clin. Proc. 40:830, 1965.

"The properties of dextran suggest that it might be capable of decreasing the propagation of the clot in thrombophlebitis and lessen the incidence of pulmonary embolism. Do you know of a study in which the drug has been carefully tried?"

Reply: Yes, at Brooke Army Medical Center, Robert Sawyer and associates, after studies in the experimental animal, used dextran with considerable success in 39 patients with acute thrombophlebitis. Following initial evaluation, the patients were given 6% clinical dextran, 600 mg./kg. intravenously, following this by daily infusion of half this dosage as long as signs and symptoms persisted. Ninety per cent of the patients experienced dramatic subjective relief in the first 24 hours, and complete resolution of signs and symptoms occurred in the average time of 4.14 days with superficial thrombophlebitis and 4.22 days with deep thrombophlebitis. Other patients, treated by conventional methods, remained symptomatic for an average of 11–15 days. There were also 3 patients who had failed to respond to anticoagulant therapy who improved rapidly under dextran. In Baltimore, Villasanta has reported satisfactory use of dextran in antepartum thrombophlebitis.

Robert B. Sawyer, John A. Moncrief and Peter C. Canizaro. Dextran Therapy in Thrombophlebitis. J.A.M.A. 191: 740, Mar. 1, 1965. Umberto Villasanta. Therapy of Antepartum Thrombophlebitis. Obst. & Gynec. 26:534, 1965.

"The most important objective of fibrinolytic therapy in thrombophlebitis is the prevention of pulmonary embolism. Do we have evidence that this is being accomplished?"

Reply: No, I do not think that we have. It is simply that not enough careful clinical studies of the matter have been done or at least reported. Of course, the end point in the study of embolism, i.e., whether or not such an episode develops, is easy enough to determine in the individual case, but to accumulate a sufficient number of observations to be of statistical significance would be a protracted affair that has not yet attracted a team of investigators, to my knowledge. It is actually difficult, as a matter of fact, to determine whether thrombolytic measures have succeeded unless one has definite knowledge of the presence of a clot before therapy and demonstration of its absence after therapy. In Hecker's (Stanford University) study, suggestive evidence was provided by venograms that thrombolysis of varying degree occurred in 8 of 23 patients with comparable pre- and post-treatment venograms. Flow through a major venous channel was restored in only 2 of these patients.

Sydney P. Hecker. Fibrinolytic Therapy of Thrombophlebitis: Twenty-five Cases Studied with Serial Venograms. California Med. 101:23, 1964.

"I have just had the frightening experience of a patient on anticoagulants who developed generalized hemorrhagic manifestations when I administered a drug for the relief of skeletal-muscle spasm. Has this sort of thing been noted by others?"

Reply: You do not name the drug used, but I can tell you that there is on record precisely such an occurrence when phenyramidol (Analexin) was the relaxant drug used. You should probably be reminded at this time also that anyone on anticoagulant drugs should avoid exposure to all potentially hepatotoxic and nephrotoxic agents. Edgar Luton has reported the case of a patient on a long-term anticoagulant regimen who experienced a striking hypoprothrombinemia upon accidentally ingesting a very small amount of the hepatotoxic carbon tetrachloride.

Stefan A. Carter (St. Boniface, Manitoba, Canada). Potentiation of the Effect of Orally Administered Anticoagulants by Phenyramidol Hydrochloride. New England J. Med. 273:423, Aug. 19, 1965. Edgar F. Luton. Carbon Tetrachloride Exposure During Anticoagulant Therapy. J.A.M.A. 194:1386, Dec. 27, 1965.

"When patients who are being maintained on anticoagulants are admitted for necessary surgery, it seems to be increasing experience that closely controlled prothrombin levels are desirable during and after the operation, with gradual resumption of full therapeutic levels on the third or fourth day. Just how reliable is the Quick method of prothrombin estimation in this situation?"

Reply: This is being squabbled over, as you know. Armand Quick has been one of my close associates through many years, and it therefore may be assumed that I am prejudiced in my opinion that his method is very reliable when performed by meticulously careful people who know their way about in techniques of this sort. But others, with no axe of friendship to grind at all, have also concluded that this is the case; one such report is that of Alexander Bradford at the University of Colorado, who said that experience with his entire group of patients treated over the past 16 years by the same individuals using a single laboratory, assured him that there is only occasionally a need to reassess therapy with the thrombotest, especially if bleeding of any kind is observed. And at the Michael Reese Hospital, Chicago, S. F. Rabiner has, more recently, concluded that "the Quick one-stage prothrombin time alone is adequate for daily management of patients receiving oral anticoagulants."

In the section on Coronary Disease in this book there is discussion of drugs that may affect the prothrombin time.

Alexander Bradford. Anticoagulants in Management of Various Thromboembolic Diseases. Angiology 15:35, 1964. S. Frederick Rabiner. The Relationship of Coagulation Defects to Hemorrhage in Patients Receiving Oral Anticoagulants. Am. J. M. Sc. 249:404, 1965.

"We have just had a patient in whom laparotomy was performed for small bowel obstruction. A 25 cm. thickened, violacious and hemorrhagic segment of proximal jejunum was resected and a jejunojejunostomy performed. There were about 500 ml. of unclotted blood in the peritoneal cavity. The patient had been on bishydroxycoumarin (Dicumarol) for several months preceding the episode of cramping, midabdominal pains, nausea and vomiting that brought him in. Have instances of anticoagulant-induced intestinal obstruction been previously observed?"

Reply: Yes, they have. Indeed, Walter Goldfarb at Barnes Hospital, St. Louis, reported 11 cases of intestinal obstruction in 9 patients, secondary to hypoprothrombinemia associated with coumarin therapy. Intramural intestinal hematomas form the basis of the obstruction, and Goldfarb has made the point that with appropriate supportive measures (intestinal intubation and small amounts of vitamin K) this process is readily reversible and operative measures unnecessary.

Walter B. Goldfarb. Coumarin-Induced Intestinal Obstruction. Ann. Surg. 161:27, 1965.

"When Thrombolysin is being used in the treatment of thrombophlebitis, should anticoagulant therapy be employed also?"

Reply: Hecker (Stanford University) concluded that this is the case; in fact, he found no evidence in most instances that administration of Thrombolysin added significantly to the results of heparin therapy.

Sydney P. Hecker. Fibrinolytic Therapy of Thrombophlebitis. Twenty-five Cases Studied with Serial Venograms. California Med. 101:23, 1964. A. Amery, J. Vermylen, H. Maes and M. Verstraete (Univ. of Louvain). Pitfalls in Thrombolytic Treatment of Venous Occlusion. Vasc. Dis. 1:89, 1964.

"I am puzzled to understand why the fibrinolysin therapy of thrombophlebitis and pulmonary embolism has not been more effective; theoretically the thing is sound?"

Reply: Sandy and Perrett (University of British Columbia) concluded from their studies that the possible reasons for the apparent failure of this type of therapy are that the series of cases studied by them was too small to bring out possible advantages; that the ideal method of extraction, purification and activation of fibrinolysin has probably not been achieved; that there may be inhibitor substances in the blood stream preventing an effective amount of fibrinolysin from reaching the thrombus; and that dosages are still empirical and may be inadequate in individual cases. To this I think that one may add as a possible additional reason for failure, the beginning of the administration too late. It has been shown in animal experimentation that a clot more than 3 days old has increased considerably in resistance.

J. T. Sandy and T. S. Perrett. Fibrinolysin (Actase) Therapy of Thrombophlebitis and Pulmonary Embolism: Double-Blind Study. Canad. M. A. J. 88:1139, June 8, 1963.

"There is some agitation among our surgical residents for the introduction of intermittent intravenous injection of heparin in the treatment of acute venous thrombosis. How has this method been employed?"

Reply: At the University of Pittsburgh, Leslie Morris and Philip Balk inject intravenously a dilute aqueous heparin (1000 U.S.P. units/ml.) every 4 or 6 hours, so as to maintain the Lee-White coagulation time at two and one-half to three times the control 30 minutes before the next dose of heparin is due. Some of their patients have required as much as 9000 units/4 hours. A small polyethylene catheter is introduced into a forearm vein and secured with adhesive tape; a sterile rubber cap is attached to the catheter and all doses of heparin are injected through it. Elastic bandages and/or stockings are applied to the affected extremity and changed frequently to avoid "binding." When feasible, ambulation is commenced on the second day of therapy, always immediately after an injection of heparin.

Leslie E. Morris and Philip Balk. The Management and Mismanagement of Acute Venous Thrombosis (Thrombophlebitis) of the Extremities. Angiology 16:339, 1965.

"Has heparin ever been used as an aerosol?"

Reply: Yes, Stuart Rosner, in Washington, had 1 or 2 ml. of a solution containing 10,000

to 40,000 units of heparin as an aerosol delivered through a positive pressure respirator during 10–20 minutes in 9 patients. A clotting time twice the control value was achieved in only 2 patients, but further study of this method appears warranted.

Stuart W. Rosner. Heparin Administered as an Aerosol. Vasc. Dis. 2:131, 1965.

THYROIDITIS

"I have an 11-year-old girl in my practice with lymphocytic thyroiditis. Shall I treat her with desiccated thyroid substance?"

Reply: There is certainly a good deal we do not know about this malady and the use of thyroid substance in it, but the consensus is that use of the drug is the safest and indeed the only indicated form of therapy. Usually recommended dosage is 120 mg./sq. meter/day; in the experience of Leboeuf and Ducharme, who have studied the matter intensively at the University of Montreal, whenever lower dosage than this was used or the drug was taken in a sporadic fashion, the effect was disappointing and the natural course of the disease unaltered.

Gilles Leboeuf, Jacques R. Ducharme. Thyroiditis in Children. Pediat. Clin. North America 13:19, 1966.

"In our area roentgen therapy is often used for subacute thyroiditis, but there is frequently a 1 or 2 week delay before symptoms begin to be relieved, there is a relatively high relapse rate, and the treatment is expensive. What success has been had with corticosteroids?"

Reply: At the Cleveland Clinic, Penn Skillern controlled the signs and symptoms of this malady quite well in 32 patients, using dosage of 10 mg. three times daily for the more acutely ill individuals and 5 mg. four times daily for those less acutely ill. Dosage was then reduced after 3 days to 5 mg. three times daily for 4 days and finally to 5 mg. twice daily for 3 weeks. If symptoms returned, a maintenance dose of 5 mg. twice daily was used. Within 1 or 2 days no analgesic drugs were needed, though in some patients fatigue persisted for varying periods; goiter disappeared in all the patients.

Penn G. Skillern. Prednisone for Treatment of Subacute Thyroiditis: Study of 32 Patients. Postgrad. Med. 28: 232, 1960.

"I have a patient with a painful, nonsuppurative swelling of the thyroid not associated with hemorrhage into an adenoma, that I have diagnosed as subacute thyroiditis. Since she is diabetic and also has a history of peptic ulcer, I am unwilling to use corticosteroids. Would it be rational to treat her with l-triiodothyronine (Cytomel)?"

Reply: I suppose your assumption would be that suppression of TSH might prove beneficial. Actually the trial has been made with some success by H. P. Higgins and associates, in Toronto. They gave 100 μg. of Cytomel daily to 32 patients, and if there was a definite response continued at this dosage level for 1–2 weeks, then reducing dosage and discontinuing after another 2–4 weeks. Twenty of the patients responded completely to this therapy, and the 12 non- or incomplete responders were treated satisfactorily in most instances with prednisone (Meticorten, etc.), starting with 5 mg. four times daily. Four of the patients successfully treated with Cytomel had exacerbations when the dose was reduced or the drug discontinued, followed by suppression of the disease again when therapy was reinstituted.

H. Patrick Higgins, T. Arnold Bayley and Andrew Diosy. Suppression of Endogenous TSH: New Treatment of Subacute Thyroiditis. J. Clin. Endocrinol. 23:235, 1963.

"Are the corticosteroids of any value in the treatment of Hashimoto's thyroiditis?"

Reply: I have only seen one report of their use, but it is favorable. R. M. Blizzard and associates treated three adolescent hypothyroid girls who had this disorder, and in 20–40 days all three became euthyroid and the glands were no longer palpable. When the corticosteroid dosage was reduced, the goiters reappeared and so did clinical signs of hypothyroidism. Nevertheless, these observers felt that desiccated thyroid remains the hormone of choice in the treatment of Hashimoto's thyroiditis, though the gland does not decrease in size as rapidly as it does under the corticosteroids.

R. M. Blizzard, W. Hung, R. W. Chandler, T. Aceto, Jr., M. Kyle and T. Winship. Hashimoto's Thyroiditis: Clinical and Laboratory Response to Prolonged Cortisone Therapy. New England J. Med. 267:1015, Nov. 15, 1962.

THYROTOXICOSIS

"If a patient with thyrotoxicosis develops hypersensitivity to propylthiouracil is it safe to try methimazole (Tapazole)?"

Reply: At the University of Louisville, Maurice Best and Charles Duncan recorded an instance in which such a switch was made without disturbance; but of course a transfer to radioiodine could also be made.

Maurice M. Best and Charles H. Duncan. Lupus-Like Syndrome Following Propylthiouracil Administration. J. Kentucky M. A. 62:47, 1964.

"A pregnant patient has just entered my practice whose thyrotoxicosis has been inadequately treated, but it nevertheless appears that she is going to carry to term. What drug shall I use to give me the best chance of delivering a nontoxic infant?"

Reply: I would be inclined simply to advise you to use the iodides for their rapid onset of action rather than the thiouracils, since the pregnancy will probably terminate before these drugs have outlived their usefulness. Nevertheless, I must add that there is considerable diversity of opinion in this matter. At the Peter Bent Brigham Hospital in Boston, Herbst and Selenkow are of the opinion that, except for preoperative preparation, iodides alone should not be used in the treatment of hyperthyroidism during pregnancy, saying that they are neither reliable nor effective for long-term management, that they obscure interpretation of the protein-bound iodine or butanol-extractable iodine, and that such fetal complications as cretinism and obstructive goiter could result from prolonged use of iodides during pregnancy. This statement has not gone unchallenged, however, and several observers have cited their experience of bringing both mothers and infants safely through the pregnancy with iodide dosage of 3–5 drops daily of Lugol's solution. Some men, eschewing iodine, would have the patient treated solely with low dosage of antithyroid drugs. For example, at Western Reserve University, Richard Levy and associates report satisfactory results with 200 mg. of propylthiouracil or its equivalent dose of methimazole (Tapazole) daily, the object of such therapy being to use the minimal dose of the drug to bring the patient close to the normal state. But Selenkow and Herbst will have none of this and insist upon using the antithyroid drug *plus* thyroid hormone. They use an amount of propylthiouracil daily to achieve the desired control of the thyrotoxicosis, and then when there is amelioration of the signs and symptoms of the malady they add U.S.P. thyroid, 120–180 mg. daily. They do admit that the rate of transplacental passage of thyroid hormone is uncertain but feel nevertheless that their type of therapy is superior, and they certainly show no worse results than those who treat with either propylthiouracil alone or Lugol's solution. So you see there *is* a difference of opinion

"You alone shall be the judge
Of what to condemn and what
to agree to.

Damned you be if you falter
Damned again if you be
    too firm.
You should follow a method
Modeled on Janus—
    and me too!"

—and I plump for iodine.

Arthur L. Herbst and Herbert A. Selenkow. Hyperthyroidism During Pregnancy. New England J. Med. 273:627, Sept. 16, 1965. In discussion of the preceding, William S. Reveno and Herbert Rosenbaum, New England J. Med. 274:164, Jan. 20, 1966; Joel I. Hamberger, ibid. 274:165, 1966; Richard P. Levy, Marvin Kopelson and Kenneth J. Ryan, ibid. 274:165, 1966; Herbert A. Selenkow and and Arthur L. Herbst, ibid. 274:165, 1966.

"I have a patient who has been on propylthiouracil for about a month in treatment of her thyrotoxicosis, and now she has developed ecchymotic areas over the arms, chest and legs and purpuric areas in the mouth. Her prothrombin time is prolonged to 33.6 seconds (our control here is 14 seconds). Could this situation be attributable to the drug?"

Reply: Yes, a few instances of hypoprothrombinemia and a severe bleeding tendency were reported a few years ago by D'Angelo and Le Gresley, and Kolars and Gonyea, the former in Canada and the latter at the University of Minnesota.

G. D'Angelo, L. P. Le Gresley. Severe Hypoprothrombinaemia After Propylthiouracil Therapy. Canad. M. A. J. 81: 479, 1959. Charles P. Kolars and Lorraine M. Gonyea. Deficiency of Prothrombin and Proconvertin After Therapy with Propylthiouracil. J.A.M.A. 171:2315, Dec. 26, 1959.

"What are the evidences of excessive or toxic action of the thioamide goitrogens (i.e., drugs of the propylthiouracil type) and the contraindications to the use of these agents?"

Reply: If fever, sore throat, skin rash, lymphadenopathy or malaise develops under thioamide therapy, the drug should be stopped at once. When the white blood cell count is below 2500 with a normal differential count, or below 3000 with diminished granulocyte percentage, penicillin should be given to prevent or control the full picture of agranulocytic angina. It has become rather clear from statistical studies that leukocyte counts at weekly intervals will often, but not infallibly, warn of developing agranulocytosis. Shall we say that in about half the cases the first indication of impending disaster is a fall in the leukocyte count? Unfortunately, leukopenia is common in untreated thyrotoxicosis, and therefore a study of the blood should be made before therapy is begun, to serve as a reference base line.

Vomiting and febrile reactions occurring early in the treatment are probably of allergic origin and may be rapidly self-terminating. Very occasionally, however, these drugs cause an exacerbation of all the symptoms of hyperthyroidism when their use is begun. Febrile reactions, accompanied by muscle and joint pain and multiform skin lesions are not easily attributable to them because such symptoms may occur in hyperthyroid patients who are not receiving this type of therapy. A few instances of hypoprothrombinemia and a severe bleeding tendency have been reported.

Serum precipitable iodine (protein-bound iodine) reflects altered thyroid secretion more rapidly than does the basal metabolic rate. Therefore, a subnormal finding in this item always indicates overdosage even though symptoms of clinical myxedema may not have appeared—or would if it were not that in a few instances this index becomes inexplicably elevated during prolonged therapy, without correlation with either the basal metabolic rate or the patient's clinical condition.

The consensus is that these drugs may be safely used in pregnancy, but hypothyroidism must of course be avoided; the infant should not be allowed to suckle. The advisability of using them in the presence of liver disease is still a moot point; there is animal work showing liver damage from high dosage.

"In a patient with thyrotoxicosis in whom it is contemplated to use radioiodine, is it advisable to use the antithyroid drugs while waiting for radioiodine to take effect?"

Reply: Not unless it is urgently necessary to obtain early control of the situation. If the patient has been on antithyroid drugs and it is decided to switch to radioiodine, it is advisable to stop the use of the drugs at least 2 weeks before beginning the radioiodine therapy. In a study of this matter at the Karolinska Hospital, Stockholm, Einhorn and Säterborg found that only 39% of 208 doses of I^{131} given led to euthyroidism and only 2% resulted in hypothyroidism within 1 year after the therapy. Further I^{131} treatment was required by 59% of the patients. Patients receiving I^{131} therapy during antithyroid drug medication showed a significantly lower incidence of remissions than those in whom antithyroid drugs had been omitted for 15–30 days before beginning I^{131} therapy. It is probable that premedication with antithyroid drugs causes the gland to become radioresistant by reason of the sulfhydryl group contained in thiouracil. It would be interesting to learn whether carbimazole (Neo-Mercazole) reduces thyroid uptake of I^{131} less than the other antithyroid preparations since it contains no sulfhydryl group.

J. Einhorn and N. -E. Säterborg. Antithyroid Drugs in Iodine-131 Therapy of Hyperthyroidism. Acta radiol. 58:161, 1962.

"What drug therapy, if any, is effective in infiltrative ophthalmopathy of Graves' disease?"

Reply: In Los Angeles, the study of Josiah Brown and associates in 19 patients with this severe form of infiltrative eye disease left little doubt in their minds that high dosage corticosteroid therapy was beneficial. They felt that inflammatory changes alone did not of themselves warrant such therapy, but that rapid progression of proptosis or ophthalmoplegia often did so, and that an absolute indication for the use of these compounds was a development of visual field defects or decreased visual acuity.

Josiah Brown, Jack W. Coburn, Richard A. Wigod, John M. Hiss, Jr., and J. Thomas Dowling. Adrenal Steroid Therapy of Severe Infiltrative Ophthalmopathy of Graves' Disease. Am. J. Med. 34:786, 1963.

"In our area there has been a definite swing toward radioactive iodine rather than the antithyroid drugs in the treatment of thyrotoxicosis, but I am still using the drugs myself. Can you cite the recorded experience of any group which has been using these drugs over a long period of years?"

Reply: At Harper Hospital, Detroit, W. S. Reveno and H. Rosenbaum reviewed the effectiveness of this form of therapy during an experience of 20 years. Of their 167 patients, 96 had been in permanent remission for 4 years or more at the time of their review. They found that patients with toxic nodular goiters who responded favorably had relatively small goiters; in successfully managed patients with toxic diffuse goiter, the symptoms had preexisted for an average of 15 months, the goiters were not large, and it took 5 months for remission to occur. There was favorable response in patients with postoperative hyperthyroidism, but 20 months was required to achieve euthyroidism. Remission of hyperthyroidism improved diabetic control in patients with toxic nodular goiters only if the diabetes was stable or mild. While unfavorable reactions in this series rarely exceeded 3% overall, there was an incidence of agranulocytosis of 1%, which was certainly astonishingly high and would be prohibitive in general experience.

W. S. Reveno and H. Rosenbaum. Observations on Use of Antithyroid Drugs. Ann. Int. Med. 60:982, 1964.

"Since it is pretty well agreed that the treatment of thyrotoxicosis with drugs tends to increase the degree of exophthalmos, I am wondering whether the rate at which the control of the malady is obtained is a factor in this result?"

Reply: At the University of Aberdeen, W. R. Greig and associates measured the degree of exophthalmos before and after control of the hyperthyroidism in 72 patients, 30 treated with methylthiouracil and 42 with I^{131}. Exophthalmos was found to increase equally in both groups irrespective of the rate of control or type of treatment used.

W. R. Greig, S. A. Aboul-Khair, S. D. Mohamed and J. Crooks. Effect of Treatment of Thyrotoxicosis on Exophthalmos. Brit. M. J. 2:509, 1965.

"How is thyroxine best used to reduce exophthalmos in thyrotoxicosis?"

Reply: In a study of this matter, in Glasgow, D. A. Koutras and associates divided a series of 68 thyrotoxic patients into four groups: one treated with antithyroid drugs alone, one with antithyroid drugs plus thyroxine, one with radioiodine alone, and one with radioiodine plus thyroxine. Exophthalmos was measured before treatment began, when the patient became euthyroid, and 3 months later. An increase in the exophthalmos was recorded in the first three groups, but in the fourth group, treated with radioiodine plus thyroxine, no significant change occurred.

D. A. Koutras, W. D. Alexander, W. W. Buchanan, R. McG. Harden and R. D. Hunter. Effect of Thyroxine on Exophthalmos in Thyrotoxicosis. Brit. M. J. 1:493, Feb. 20, 1965.

"I have a patient with suspected thyrotoxicosis in whom it appears that the administration of androgens has lowered the PBI level. What other agents may do this?"

Reply: The following have been listed by Aron Fisher and associates (Cleveland): androgens, triiodothyronine (Cytomel), diphenylhydantoin (Dilantin), salicylates, mercury and gold.

Aron B. Fisher, Richard P. Levy and Waide Price. Gold—An Occult Cause of Low Serum Protein-Bound Iodine. New England J. Med. 273:812, Oct. 7, 1965.

"A few years ago several clinical studies were reported in which a beneficial effect of reserpine on the symptoms of thyrotoxicosis was claimed. To my knowledge no one in our area has tried this therapy, but I now have an unusually severe case of this malady in my practice and am wondering whether I should make a trial of reserpine in this patient?"

Reply: I think that most of the more recent studies have seriously questioned the usefulness of this measure. For example, in Minneapolis, Malcolm Blumenthal and associates used 2.5 mg. of reserpine intramuscularly every 6 hours in 7 hyperthyroid and 4 control subjects and observed that not only were none of the hyperthyroid patients improved, but their clinical state was actually aggravated through development of a carcinoid syndrome characterized by an erythematous flush of the face and trunk, diarrhea, increased tremor, nausea, fatigue, nervousness and in one instance bronchial asthma. Three of the 4 control patients noted similar but less severe symptoms.

Malcolm Blumenthal, Richard Davis and Richard P. Doe. Carcinoid Syndrome Following Reserpine Therapy in Thyrotoxicosis. Arch. Int. Med. 116:819, 1965.

"I have heard that guanethidine (Ismelin) is being used in the treatment of thyrotoxicosis but do not understand this; can you enlighten?"

Reply: This drug has a very potent and unique sympatholytic effect through which it may promptly and effectively ameliorate those signs and symptoms of thyrotoxicosis that are due to sympathetic hyperactivity, and will do so without affecting the function of the thyroid gland. This latter point is an important one in the case in which it seems imperative to institute immediate treatment with antithyroid drugs without waiting for diagnostic tests. At the Cook County Hospital, Sheldon Waldstein's group reported on the use of guanethidine in 90 patients between the ages of 3 and 79 years. They used initial dosage of 50–100 mg. for adults in a single oral dose daily, usually in the morning. Three children, aged 3, 11 and 12 years, tolerated well a starting dose of 1 mg./kg. The response to guanethidine was evaluated daily and the dose increased by 25 mg. increments every third day until therapeutic end point was achieved: i.e., complete control of symptoms and signs of the disease; the appearance of distinct eyelid ptosis; or the development of distinct orthostatic hypotension. When end point dosage was achieved it was continued as the maintenance dosage. The drug was found to be a very potent one for adjunctive therapy of thyrotoxicosis before or concomitantly with specific antithyroid treatment, but it should not be used unless the patient is distinctly thyrotoxic because those with mild or doubtful symptoms of hyperthyroidism tolerate it badly. Furthermore the drug should not be used for 1–2 weeks prior to general anesthesia because sympatholytic agents enhance the risk of anesthetic complications, such as shock and ventricular fibrillation.

Sheldon S. Waldstein, George H. West, Jr., Winfred Y. Lee and David Bronsky. Guanethidine in Hyperthyroidism. J.A.M.A. 189:609, Aug. 24, 1964.

"Although there can be no doubt of the efficacy of the antithyroid drugs in the treatment of thyrotoxicosis, it is certainly difficult to persuade a patient to adhere rigidly to the taking of the drugs at 8 hour intervals for a long period of time. Has any other dosage scheme been investigated?"

Reply: Yes, at the University of Oregon, Monte Greer and associates studied the use of a single daily dose of propylthiouracil, and the data collected over a 4 year period on 31 patients convinced them that a single daily dose of this drug is as effective in inducing or maintaining a remission as the same total daily dose divided into equal fractions given every 8 hours. The dosage used was 300 mg., and severe forms of the disease with marked agitation, tremor and weight loss appeared to respond as well as milder forms, though the number of the former was really not sufficient to establish this fact with certainty.

Monte A. Greer, Walter C. Meinhoff and Hugo Studer. Treatment of Hyperthyroidism with a Single Daily Dose of Propylthiouracil. New England J. Med. 272:888, April 29, 1965.

"What result might be expected from the mistaken administration of an antithyroid drug for a prolonged period to a euthyroid patient?"

Reply: In San Francisco, Louis Levy and John Vogel studied the effects of administering methimazole (Tapazole) to 24 euthyroid patients for 6–12 months. Clinically apparent hypothyroidism, most frequently evidenced by constipation, decreased activity, hoarseness and infraorbital edema, occurred in 14 patients after an average duration of treatment of 30 weeks; there was palpable enlargement of the thyroid gland in 12 after about the same length of time. The response of the 24 hour thyroidal uptake of radioactive iodine was variable, but the serum protein-bound iodine decreased markedly in 17 individuals and the red-blood-cell radiotriiodothyronine uptake decreased below the normal range in 13.

Louis Levy and John M. Vogel. The Effect of Methimazole on the Thyroid Function of Euthyroid Patients. Am. J. M. Sc. 250:199, 1965.

"The postoperative thyroid crisis, which was formerly seen so often, has practically disappeared in most hospitals because of the preoperative use of thyroid-suppressive medication. So one is out of touch with latest developments in the therapy of this emergency. Have the corticosteroids or other newer agents been effectively employed in the occasional case that undoubtedly still occurs?"

Reply: This is certainly a true emergency in which the patient may easily be lost unless steps are quickly taken to counteract the effects of the severe hypermetabolism. Anoxia must be prevented and replacement must quickly be made of the fluid, electrolyte and caloric losses. And sedation is mandatory. In reporting the 2 cases seen by them in the last 10 years, Norman Thompson and William Fry, at the University of Michigan, found hydrocortisone (Cortef, etc.) effective in dosage of 100 mg. intravenously or intramuscularly daily. They also said that a rapid and occasionally dramatic response to reserpine has been seen; intramuscular or intravenous dosage of 2.5–10 mg. is recommended.

Norman W. Thompson and William J. Fry. Thyroid Crisis. Arch. Surg. 89:512, 1964.

"What is the ideal treatment for thyrotoxicosis in children?"

Reply: I do not think that the "ideal" treatment has been developed as yet or will ever be, because it must always depend to some extent upon the calibre of the surgery available in the area. Hayles and Chaves-Carballo, at the Mayo Clinic, reported on a group of 16 children under 15 years of age treated within a 9 year period; 7 had relapses and 2 had recurrences at least 2 years after completion of therapy. Only 4 patients had a remission, and these observers felt, on the basis of previous surgical experience and the results of this trial with drugs, that subtotal thyroidectomy is the most satisfactory treatment in these young people. Upon the other hand, at Johns Hopkins Hospital, Wellington Hung and associates concluded that surgical therapy should be resorted to only in patients who do not cooperate in medical therapy or relapse after such therapy has been used for a prolonged period. Their experience in a series of 34 patients, with age of onset of symptoms between 1 and 5 years in 9, between 6 and 10 in 14, and between 11 and 15 in 11, was that propylthiouracil is the drug of choice, with low incidence of toxicity. Initial daily dosage used was 300 mg., which was progressively reduced after 3–4 weeks to maintenance dosage of 100–150 mg. If the thyroid gland enlarged during therapy, 2–3 grains of desiccated thyroid was added and the propylthiouracil dosage was increased to the initial amount. I shall cite also the therapy used by Kogut's group at the Children's Hospital of Los Angeles, in 10 males and 35 females aged 2–16 years. Treatment was with I^{131} in 23 cases and with antithyroid medication in 15; surgery in 12 cases (1 patient given I^{131} and 4 given antithyroid medication included).

Total I^{131} dosage varied from 0.7 to 4.3 μc. The drug of choice in the medically treated patients was propylthiouracil, with methimazole (Tapazole) or potassium perchlorate used only if the response was poor or if there were untoward reactions. Usual initial propylthiouracil dosage was 300 mg. daily; perchlorate, 2 Gm. daily; methimazole, 30 mg. daily. The patients coming to surgery were given 300–900 mg. propylthiouracil daily until the day of surgery and 5–10 drops of Lugol's solution three times daily for 10–14 days before operation.

Alvin B. Hayles and Enrique Chaves-Carballo. Exophthalmic Goiter in Children: A Therapeutic Trial with Antithyroid Drugs. Mayo Clin. Proc. 40:889, 1965. M. D. Kogut, S. A. Kaplan, P. J. Collipp, T. Tiamsic and D. Boyle. Treatment of Hyperthyroidism in Children: Analysis of 45 Patients. New England J. Med. 272:217, Feb. 4, 1965. Wellington Hung, Ross N. Wilkins and Robert Blizzard. Medical Therapy of Thyrotoxicosis in Children. Pediatrics 30:17, 1962.

"If a woman with thyrotoxicosis has been treated throughout her pregnancy with antithyroid drugs should the infant be allowed to nurse?"

Reply: No.

TRICHOMONIASIS

"Since about 20% of women manifest vaginal moniliasis after successful treatment of trichomonal vaginitis with metronidazole (Flagyl), has anyone tried the local application of gentian violet or some other fungicide at the initiation of the metronidazole therapy?"

Reply: Yes, at the Royal Hospital in Sheffield, England, Mary Beveridge determined that the effect of concurrent administration of the local fungicide, nystatin (Mycostatin), with Flagyl in a study group of 100 consecutive patients did not decrease the incidence of moniliasis very much. Perhaps you should try gentian violet on your own? At Baylor University, Herman Gardner and Dean Dukes observed that Flagyl appears neither to encourage nor to suppress growth of candida.

M. Mary Beveridge. Local Fungicide Used Concomitantly with Flagyl in Trichomonal Infection. Brit. J. Ven. Dis. 40:198, 1964. Herman L. Gardner and C. Dean Dukes. Clinical and Laboratory Effects of Metronidazole (Flagyl). Am. J. Obst. & Gynec. 89:995, 1964.

"May I feel perfectly at ease in using metronidazole (Flagyl) in the treatment of trichomoniasis in the pregnant patient?"

Reply: Yes. At Mount Sinai Hospital, in New York, Gisella Perl has made an intensive study of this matter. A total of 151 women were followed through delivery and the post-partum period, each having an unquestionable diagnosis of trichomonal infection. Treatment was initiated in the first trimester in 2.71%, in the second trimester in 51% and in the third trimester in 46.3%. In 43% of the women, both moniliasis and trichomoniasis were present. Dosage of Flagyl was 1 tablet of 250 mg. three times daily for 10 days. The infant was checked in the neonatal period and the mothers were recalled 6–10 weeks after the baby was discharged and again at 3–6 months after delivery. All 151 of the patients were cured: 142 after one treatment, 8 after two treatments and 1 after three treatments. There were 148 live babies and 3 stillborns, metronidazole not having been shown to be a contributing factor in the intrauterine deaths. When seen 3–6 months after delivery, all 148 babies showed normal development and, though there was the usual number of serious and minor congenital defects, it could not be shown that metronidazole was in the causative role of any of them. Similar findings have been reported by Robinson and Mirchandani, in Halifax, and Peterson's group in Washington.

Gisella Perl. Metronidazole (Flagyl) Treatment of Tri-chomoniasis in Pregnancy. Obst. & Gynec. 25:273, 1965. S. C. Robinson and G. Mirchandani. Trichomonas Vagi-nalis: Further Observations on Metronidazole (Including Infant Follow-up). Am. J. Obst. & Gynec. 93:502, 1965. William F. Peterson, John E. Stauch and Constance D. Ryder. Metronidazole in Pregnancy. Am. J. Obst. & Gynec. 94:343, 1966.

"In our practice we have been using metronida-zole (Flagyl) quite freely in the treatment of trichomoniasis with results that have been upon the whole quite gratifying. The only side effects have been mild, transient vaginal inflammation, un-pleasant taste, dry mouth and coated tongue, nausea, cramps, weakness and dizziness — until recently, when one patient experienced a tem-porary fall in polymorphonuclear neutrophils from 6000/cu. mm. to 1500/cu. mm. Do we really know how toxic this drug is?"

Reply: Not yet, I believe, though to be sure nothing very frightening has been experienced apparently in use of the drug in most private practices. Even in the larger experi-mental series, such as that of Forster and associates (University of Puerto Rico), the drug has not been reported to have consistent adverse effects on the hematopoietic system or to decrease the incidence of abnormal Papanicolaou smears. Should one neverthe-less keep an eye on the blood count of individ-uals taking this drug? The study of Kotcher's group (University of Louisville) appears to answer this question in the negative, but still we do not have the total picture. For example,

there is not considerable enlightenment in the fact that in Forster's study, 7 of the 150 placebo treated patients experienced side effects warranting discontinuance of the drug while 20 of the 300 Flagyl treated patients fell into the same class. Again, in Porapakkham's study, in Bangkok, only 1 of 122 women was unable to tolerate the drug — but there were an additional 39 women who started the treat-ment and failed to return for follow-up, and we do not know that some of them may not have dropped out because of very disagreeable side effects. As drugs go, one can certainly look upon this one as having quite low toxicity, but the specific answer to your question is that we do not know as yet what its full toxic proclivities are. M. Scott-Gray has found Flagyl secreted in the breast milk.

Stanley A. Forster, Oscar Garcia Ramirez and Alan H. Rapoport. Metronidazole (Flagyl) and Trichomonal Vagi-nitis: Report of Double-Blind Clinical Investigation of 450 Women. Am. J. Obst. & Gynec. 87:1013, 1963. Saroj Porapakkham. Metronidazole (Flagyl) Treatment of Vaginal Trichomoniasis. Obst. & Gynec. 22:516, 1963. Emil Kotcher, Carolyn A. Frick and L. O. Giesel. Effect of Metronidazole (Flagyl) on Vaginal Microbiology and Maternal and Neonatal Hematology. Am. J. Obst. & Gynec. 88:184, 1964. M. Scott-Gray. Metronidazole in Obstetric Practice. J. Obst. & Gynaec. Brit. Common. 71:82, 1964.

"With the advent of a therapeutic agent, metronidazole (Flagyl), that is effective in eradica-tion of the *Trichomonas* parasite from the vagina, urinary tract and adjacent glands in the female, as well as from the genitourinary system of the male, it becomes important to know precisely what is the best treatment regimen to employ. What is the most careful study that has been made to date?"

Reply: It seems to me that the study made by Armand Pereyra and J. Dee Lansing, in California, is the most satisfactory, since it was performed in a women's prison where conditions provided an ideal environment for a valid therapeutic evaluation because the schedules of medication could be maintained, long-term observation was possible, examina-tions following treatment could be completed on practically all patients, and the findings were not vitiated by sexual contacts. A total of 2002 women inmates at the institution studied were found infested with *T. vaginalis* during a period of 36 months and treated with metronidazole. A 3 day course of the drug proved inadequate, but statistical analysis showed 5, 7, and 10 day treatment schedules essentially equally effective. The best treat-ment comprised 250 mg. given three times daily orally, plus 250 mg. administered once daily vaginally, concurrently for 5 days. There was a transient drop in white blood cell count in less than one fourth of 200 women in whom this parameter was investigated. Except for discoloration, no urinary changes were produced, and the compound was equally well tolerated in patients with various chronic disease states. A few women were treated during the second and third trimesters of pregnancy, without the appearance of abnormalities in the infants; but conclusions on this point cannot be drawn from this small number of cases.

Armand J. Pereyra and J. Dee Lansing. Urogenital Trichomoniasis. Obst. & Gynec. 24:499, 1964.

TRIGEMINAL NEURALGIA

"In a trigeminal neuralgia patient who refuses alcohol injections or surgery, have any of the newer non-narcotic analgesics been found effective?"

Reply: I think one must say that the strictly analgesic drugs do not have a very good record in this malady, but the antiepileptic agent, diphenylhydantoin (Dilantin) has been used with some effect. Indeed, the paroxysmal quality of the pain attracted Braham and Saia to a trial of the drug. Of their 20 patients, 14 received some benefit, 8 being completely relieved. Improvement began within 24–48 hours of the initiation of therapy.

J. Braham and Alma Saia. Phenytoin (Dilantin) in Treatment of Trigeminal and Other Neuralgias. Lancet 2: 892, Oct. 22, 1960.

"I have a trigeminal neuralgia patient in whom the good effects obtained with diphenylhydantoin (Dilantin) are rapidly decreasing. Could you suggest any other drug that I might resort to?"

Reply: B. L. Crue's group has found King's use of mephenesin carbamate (Tolseram) useful in a number of cases. The usual starting dosage was 1 teaspoonful of the commercially available suspension every 3 or 4 hours as needed to control the pain, but some patients increased the dosage to 2 or 3 teaspoonfuls every 2 or 3 hours, and there were others who did not tolerate even 1 teaspoonful. Best effects were obtained in patients who had not had the syndrome very long, were not extremely aged, and had not had too many previous alcohol blocks or surgical procedures. Another drug, carbamazepine (Tegretol) has been reported upon favorably in England, but I do not believe that it is available here in the United States. Dosage of this agent is 100–200 mg. four times daily.

B. L. Crue, E. M. Todd and A. G. Loew. Clinical Use of Mephenesin Carbamate (Tolseram) in Trigeminal Neuralgia. Bull. Los Angeles Neurol. Soc. 30:212, 1965. B. R. King. The Medical Control of Tic Douloureux: Preliminary Report of the Effect of Mephenesin on Facial Pain. J. Neurosurg. 15:250, 1958. J. G. Graham and K. J. Zilkha. Treatment of Trigeminal Neuralgia with Carbamazepine: A Follow-Up Study. Brit. M. J. 1:210, Jan 22, 1966.

TROPICAL PULMONARY EOSINOPHILIA

"All sorts of exotic tropical diseases are turning up in the temperate zones in this era of rapid transportation. We have recently had in our practice a case of tropical pulmonary eosinophilia in which we gained a rapid relief of symptoms through the use of intravenous arsenicals. But we do not know that we have really effected a cure by this therapy; is there anything new?"

Reply: The cause of this malady is not yet absolutely determined, but there has recently been a swing back toward the earlier contention that filariasis is to be considered in an etiologic role. Microfilaria have been reported in the lymph nodes of some patients presenting with lymphadenopathy even though they have not been found in the blood upon repeated examinations. Whatever may be the truth, Robert Peter and Milton Campbell (Duke University) reported a very successful use of diethylcarbamazine (Hetrazan), an antifilarial compound, in their single case, and in India, Kedar Nath and S. N. Pandeya considered that 91% of their 44 patients, though not definitely established as having worm infestations, were cured, the criteria being disappearance of symptoms and an absolute eosinophil count of 1000/cu. mm. or less.

Robert H. Peter and Milton F. Campbell. Tropical Pulmonary Eosinophilia, Cause Unknown, Treatment Dramatically Effective. Ann. Int. Med. 59:231, 1963. Kedar Nath and S. N. Pandeya. Diethylcarbamazine (Hetrazan) Therapy in Tropical Eosinophilia. Brit. M. J. 1:104, Jan. 9, 1960.

TRYPANOSOMIASIS

"What therapy is most effective in trypanosomiasis?"

Reply: Unfortunately, in the American type of case (Chagas' disease) there is usually no response to any of the drugs with the very rare exceptions that perhaps just prove the rule. In the African cases, however, the effective drugs are suramin (Antrypol, Bayer 205), Melarsen and Mel B and tryparsamide. All of these drugs have curative value in the early, or fever and lymphadenopathy, stage of the disease, but in the late stage, when the central nervous system has been invaded, suramin is not effective.

TUBERCULOSIS

"Upon the basis of long-term follow-up of proved cases of previously untreated, far-advanced, cavitary tuberculosis, what drug combinations have been found to be most effective?"

Reply: At the Battey State Hospital, in Georgia, 151 patients were employed in a study designed to settle this point through employment of two United States Public Health Service regimens. Regimen Number 1 comprised streptomycin (1 Gm.) daily plus pyrazinamide (40 mg./kg.) daily for 12 weeks, followed by isoniazid (300 mg.) daily in two or three equal doses plus PAS (12. Gm.) daily for 20 weeks. Regimen Number 2 comprised alternating 4 week courses of streptomycin (1 Gm.) daily plus pyrazinamide (40 mg./kg.) daily, and isoniazid (300 mg.) daily and PAS (12 Gm.) daily for a period of 32 weeks, starting treatment with streptomycin and pyrazinamide. Clinical, roentgenologic and sputum studies were made every 4 weeks through 40 weeks, and isoniazid and streptomycin susceptibilities were determined for all positive cultures. In essence the study showed that alternating courses of streptomycin-pyrazinamide and isoniazid-PAS are very effective in treating advanced pulmonary tuberculosis, and it is concluded that strong consideration should be given to these regimens in selecting initial therapy for advanced pulmonary tuberculosis. No patient died from the progressive disease in this series, and whereas 7% of the patients had toxic reactions necessitating drug discontinuance, no patient had an irreversible reaction. No patient died from a drug reaction. Cavity obliteration was obtained in 77% of the patients and reversal of infectiousness in 97%. The relapse rate was less than 1% with a follow-up period of 30–40 months.

United States Public Health Service Cooperative Study Group. Alternating Regimens of Streptomycin-Pyrazinamide, Isoniazid-Para-Aminosalicylic Acid at Battey State Hospital. Am. Rev. Resp. Dis. 90:262, 1964.

"I know that it is currently the accepted thing to recommend pulmonary resection for tuberculosis when there is persistence of cavitary disease after sputum cultures have become negative for the organism; i.e., in the type of case that is usually called the 'open negative case.' Has this position ever been soundly challenged?"

Reply: Yes, at the University of Kentucky, Don Pearl told of 12 patients with tuberculosis of this sort who refused recommended resection during a 2 year period. They were followed for 4–6 years and tuberculosis remained inactive in all of them.

Don C. Pearl. Treatment of Open Negative Tuberculosis without Resection: Review of 13 Cases. Am. Surgeon 31: 370, 1965.

"In a rather limited experience of the treatment of tuberculosis I am surprised at the high incidence of drug intolerance that I am encountering. Is this general experience and is it related directly to dosage?"

Reply: In an analysis of this matter on 1744 patients at Valley Forge General Hospital, Stephen Berté's group found the following overall drug intolerance rates: all drugs, 12.2%; streptomycin, 10.3%; PAS, 8.8%; and isoniazid, 1.3%. Reactions occurred more frequently when the dose of isoniazid or streptomycin was increased and when the latter was added to an isoniazid-PAS treatment regimen. It appeared that the incidence of multiple-drug reactions was related more to the number of drugs administered than to the dosage of each drug.

Stephen J. Berté, Joseph D. DiMase and Charles S. Christianson. Isoniazid, Para-Aminosalicylic Acid, and Streptomycin Intolerance in 1,744 Patients. Am. Rev. Resp. Dis. 90:598, 1964.

"Is primary drug resistance of tubercle bacilli increasing in the United States?"

Reply: In the Veterans Administration, Gladys Hobby and associates are making a continuing study of this matter. In their 1965 report they compared the data from a group of hospitals which had previously been studied between the period of 1960 and 1962 and concluded that no significant increase in primary drug resistance has occurred in geographic areas under study in the survey.

Gladys L. Hobby, Tulita F. Lenert, Joyce Maier and Patricia O'Malley. Primary Drug Resistance. Am. Rev. Resp. Dis. 91:30, 1965.

"Will the use of isoniazid in a prophylactic program prevent reactivation of inactive tuberculosis?"

Reply: The New York State Departments of Health and Mental Hygiene studied this matter in the period of 1958–1965, and in the final report Julius Katz and associates stated that the administration of isoniazid for 2 years to patients with inactive tuberculosis is effective in reducing the frequency of reactivation not only during the period of drug administration but also for a 2 year period after it is discontinued. These observers did not, however, believe it to be a practicable matter to launch a large scale program to find and treat patients with inactive tuberculosis in the general population.

Julius Katz, Solomon Kunofsky, Vytautas Damijonaitis, Albert Lafleur and Theresa Caron. Effect of Isoniazid Upon the Reactivation of Inactive Tuberculosis. Am. Rev. Resp. Dis. 91:345, 1965.

"Rapid reversal of infectiousness in pulmonary tuberculosis can now be achieved with use of the new drugs in effective combinations, but there is not always a comparable advance in the speed with which improvement can be detected in the roentgenogram. Has the possibility been investigated of using corticosteroids to hasten resolution of the pulmonary process?"

Reply: Yes, the United States Public Health Service has made extensive trial of this among 1674 patients with newly diagnosed pulmonary tuberculosis in 25 hospitals. A daily maintenance dose of 10 mg. of prednisolone (Meticortelone, etc.) was given for 5 weeks to one group of patients and for 9 weeks to another, placebo being given to a third group. Half the patients in each group received isoniazid plus PAS for 32 weeks, the other half receiving streptomycin plus pyrazinamide (Aldinamide, PZA) daily for 12 weeks followed by isoniazid plus PAS for 20 weeks. Infectiousness was reversed to the same extent in the corticosteroid and placebo groups, and there was little effect on cavity closure. The drug did, however, effect more frequent and more rapid clearing of the infiltrate in Negroes than in whites.

A United States Public Health Service Tuberculosis Therapy Trial. Prednisolone in the Treatment of Pulmonary Tuberculosis. Am. Rev. Resp. Dis. 91:329, 1965.

"We have recently had rheumatic symptoms appearing in one of our patients during tuberculosis therapy, with strong suspicion of isoniazid as the causative agent. Has such a thing been recorded?"

Reply: Yes, a rheumatic syndrome has been associated with tuberculosis therapy, most often appearing in the fourth week of drug treatment. Armin Good and associates at the University of Michigan have reported 7 cases in their hospital, but they emphasized that the incidence of the syndrome is low, that liver disease and malnutrition may be important cofactors, and that the association with isoniazid must remain tentative in the absence of definitive studies.

Armin E. Good, Robert A. Green and Chris J. D. Zarafonetis. Rheumatic Symptoms During Tuberculosis Therapy. A Manifestation of Isoniazid Toxicity? Ann. Int. Med. 63:800, 1965.

"Does isoniazid ever cause actual damage to the central nervous system?"

Reply: The neurotoxic effects of this drug are rather well known. Peripheral neuropathy is the commonest, but there have also been instances of optic atrophy, convulsions, major psychoses, Korsakoff's psychosis, neuromyelitis optica, myelopathy and toxic encephalopathy. Fortunately these occurrences are quite rare.

Peter Adams and Chester White. Isoniazid-Induced Encephalopathy. Lancet 1:680, Mar. 27, 1965.

"I have heard that the administration of streptomycin during pregnancy may cause defective hearing in the infant. Is this true?"

Reply: In a study of the etiology of hearing loss in 200 preschool children in Vancouver, Geoffrey Robinson and Kenneth Cambon did not find that the prenatal administration of streptomycin or dihydrostreptomycin for treatment of tuberculosis in pregnant women was involved, but in the subsequent 100 cases, 2 children with congenital hearing loss were found whose mothers had received the drug for treatment of tuberculosis during their pregnancies. These observers stated that similar cases had been reported in the literature by six other investigators.

Geoffrey C. Robinson and Kenneth G. Cambon. Hearing Loss in Infants of Tuberculous Mothers Treated with Streptomycin During Pregnancy. New England J. Med. 271:949, Oct. 29, 1964.

"Like everyone else dealing with tuberculosis, we have found the isoniazid-PAS combination to be the backbone of effective therapy, but we believe it advisable to include a third drug not so much because we are convinced of the superiority of a triple drug regimen as because we feel safer in the knowledge that when a patient feels that one of the drugs is excessively upsetting his stomach and he arbitrarily discontinues its use he will still be under the influence of a two drug regimen. As a third drug we have habitually used streptomycin, but understandably many of our patients grow very tired of the protracted series of intramuscular injections necessary with this drug. What is being done in this situation in specialized groups?"

Reply: At the Presbyterian and Kingsbridge VA Hospitals, in New York City, John Lattimer's group has found in recent years that they can get on well without the streptomycin injections even in the treatment of renal tuberculosis. The regimen they like best is isoniazid 100 mg. three times daily, sodium

PAS 5 Gm. three times daily, and cycloserine (Seromycin) 250 mg. twice daily. In addition they give 50 mg. of pyridoxine twice daily as a precautionary measure against peripheral neuritis from the isoniazid. This regimen is maintained for at least 2 years, and if intolerance to any one of the drugs develops they substitute ethionamide (Trecator) for the offender in dosage of 250 mg. three times daily by mouth. When they have to resort to ethionamide they feel it advisable to perform liver function studies monthly, but they say that only in case of urgent need would they resume streptomycin at the rate of 0.5 Gm. twice daily or 1 Gm. twice weekly, intramuscularly, or viomycin (Viocin, Vinactane) at dosage of 2 Gm. twice weekly, intramuscularly, or kanamycin (Kantrex), 1 Gm. twice weekly intramuscularly for only a very limited time (possibility of deafness). I think that in the experience of most men it is the PAS, even though used in the sodium form, that is most likely to be omitted from any regimen — you doubtless know the old story that there is a patch under every sanatorium window in which grass will not grow because of the PAS tablets that have been thrown out.

John K. Lattimer. Renal Tuberculosis. New England J. Med. 273:208, July 22, 1965. John K. Lattimer, Robert J. Reilly, Akio Segawa, Herman Wechsler, Jerald Siegel, Amir Girgis and Donald Gleason. Injections Are No Longer Necessary in the Treatment of Renal Tuberculosis. J. Urol. 93:735, 1965.

"I have an epileptic patient on phenobarbital and diphenylhydantoin (Dilantin) to whom I have given isoniazid in attempting to control the complicating tuberculosis. She has become much more stuporous than expected from the dosage of the antiepileptic drugs; could this be due to the isoniazid?"

Reply: Yes, it very definitely could be, according to the experience of Francis Murray in an epileptic institution in which even a very small dose of isoniazid in a prophylactic attempt against tuberculosis had the effect, in a number of instances, that you described. However, the drug may also *provoke* seizures, in individuals with a history of epilepsy or childhood convulsions, if there is not antiepileptic drug protection.

Francis J. Murray. Outbreak of Unexpected Reactions Among Epileptics Taking Isoniazid. Am. Rev. Resp. Dis. 86:729, 1962.

"A patient has just appeared in my practice whose pulmonary tuberculosis is complicated with pneumoconiosis. This is a new combination in my experience; may I expect a poorer response to chemotherapeutic agents?"

Reply: On the basis of a British Medical Research Council report, the answer is yes.

British Medical Research Council. Chemotherapy of Pulmonary Tuberculosis with Pneumoconiosis: First Report to Medical Research Council From Joint Investigators. Tubercle 44:47, 1963.

"A good many people are spontaneously tuberculin positive without demonstrable tuberculous foci. Suppose one of these persons should require long-term corticosteroid medication, what should be done?"

Reply: Follow him with regular chest x-rays. If he is one who has an active or an inactive tuberculous lesion in the lungs, he should be treated prophylactically with the antituberculosis chemotherapeutic agents while he is receiving the corticosteroids.

Einar Espersen. Corticosteroids and Pulmonary Tuberculosis: Activation of Four Cases. Acta tuberc. scandinav. 43:1, 1963.

"Those of us who practice in rather remote areas cannot always easily refer our recalcitrant tuberculosis cases to, or consult with, specialists and are sometimes tempted to abandon chemotherapy rather than subject our patient to the toxic potentialities of 'second-line' drugs about which we know very little. What, specifically, is current opinion regarding ethionamide (Trecator)?"

Reply: I think that the following statements may be made with confidence: First, that it may be considered a valuable addition to the armamentarium if one keeps in mind certain reservations; second, that it may be usefully combined with streptomycin or isoniazid, but that when doing so fully effective dosage may be prohibitively high for prolonged use; third, that its toxicity may be augmented by the concomitant administration of isoniazid; and fourth, that primary resistance to it has occurred. Among the reported reactions have been severe gastrointestinal disturbances, peripheral neuritis, liver function abnormalities, headache, acne, drug rash that may eventuate in exfoliative dermitis, and mental depression.

Marian Zierski (Warsaw, Poland). Value of Ethionamide (Trecator) in Retreatment of Pulmonary Tuberculosis. Acta tuberc. scandinav. 43:48, 1963. A. W. Lees (Ruchill Hosp., Glasgow). Ethionamide (Trecator) and Streptomycin Therapy in Previously Untreated Cases of Pulmonary Tuberculosis. Am. Rev. Resp. Dis. 88:399, 1963. A. W. Lees. Ethionamide (Trecator) and Isoniazid in Previously Untreated Cases of Pulmonary Tuberculosis. Dis. Chest 45:247, 1964. A. W. Lees. Toxicity in Newly Diagnosed Cases of Pulmonary Tuberculosis Treated with Ethionamide. Am. Rev. Resp. Dis. 88:347, 1963. J. Pernod. Hepatic Tolerance of Ethionamide. Am. Rev. Resp. Dis. 92:39, 1965.

"In the long-haul treatment of tuberculosis, daily drug taking becomes such a burden that undoubtedly this alone accounts for some of our failures since it is really an exceptional sort of individual who will strictly adhere to the regimen throughout a long period of time. What experimentation has been done with wider spacing of dosage?"

Reply: In Finland, Lennart Brander gave one daily dose of isoniazid, varying between 3.5 and 13.3 mg./kg. body weight, to 195 patients whom he observed from 30 to 480 days. All patients wese also treated simultaneously with PAS and streptomycin, and 127 of them were given 300 mg. of pyridoxine daily. He found that 169 of the patients were able to take the whole daily amount of isoniazid in a single dose, and since side effects were rare and usually mild at 3.5–6 mg./kg. body weight, he naturally concluded that it is rational to give the whole daily amount of isoniazid in a single dose. In Denver, Joseph Hawkins' group actually found conversion earlier and cavity closure more frequent on a single dose regimen of all standard drugs than on a twice daily dose. Also, but this time at the Tuberculosis Chemotherapy Center, Madras, India, a study was performed in which it appeared that twice weekly isoniazid plus streptomycin was as effective as a standard regimen of daily isoniazid plus PAS. And at the Hammersmith Chest Clinic, in London, after an initial 3 month period of daily streptomycin 0.75 Gm., isoniazid 300 mg. and PAS 12 Gm., patients were placed for a subsequent 15 month period on streptomycin 1.0 Gm. plus isoniazid 600 mg. on 3 alternate days each week. So the reply to your question is that the matter is being looked into very definitely. It seems to me that while once daily dosage might prove to be quite feasible, and indeed might be expected to guarantee greater faithfulness in dosing on the part of the discharged patient than the three times daily dosing, the twice or thrice weekly regimens could hope to be effective only if they could be carried out under the closest supervision. However, Graham Poole and Peter Stradling, at the Hammersmith, were able to keep 97% of their patients on the regimen for 6 months, 84% for 15 months and 77% for the planned 18 months. The subject certainly will have to be exhaustively investigated before reliable and authoritative pronouncement can be made by any of the specialist groups in this field.

Lennart Brander (Mjölbolsta Hosp., Finland). Tolerance of Isoniazid in One Daily Dose. Acta tuberc. scandinav. 43:299, 1963. Tuberculosis Chemotherapy Center, Madras, India. Intermittent Treatment of Pulmonary Tuberculosis: Concurrent Comparison of Twice-Weekly Isoniazid Plus Streptomycin and Daily Isoniazid Plus PAS in Domiciliary Treatment. Lancet. 1:1078, May 18, 1963. Graham Poole and Peter Stradling. Long-Term Use of Intermittent Streptomycin Plus Isoniazid in Treatment of Tuberculosis. Tubercle 46:290, 1965. Joseph A. Hawkins, Clifton W. Arrington, Warren C. Morse and James E. Hansen. Once Versus Twice Daily Administration of Antituberculosis Drugs. Dis. Chest 48:573, 1965.

"The results I am getting from the use of the antituberculosis drugs are making me suspect that some of my patients are simply not taking them with regularity despite their assertions that they are. What has been the experience of others in this field, and is there any way of determining accurately whether a patient is faithfully taking his drug?"

Reply: In a study of this matter at Tripler General Hospital, Honolulu, David Preston and Frank Miller compared a physician's opinion and his patient's opinion as to the drug-taking reliability of the latter. The accuracy of these estimates was determined by chemical analysis of the patient's urine. Of 25 patients, 24 stated that they were faithfully taking the prescribed medication, and it was the judgment of the physician that 20 of them were actually doing so. However, analysis for PAS and metabolites of isoniazid on the day of the clinic visit indicated that only 18 had taken the drugs as prescribed. And amazingly, 7 patients had erred in the evaluation of their own drug-taking reliability. In a comprehensive treatise dealing with this subject, W. Fox concluded that in patients who are expected to continue with therapy for many months after they feel perfectly fit, it is a combination of forgetfulness and indifference that causes them to default in the self-administration. There is a type of patient also, of course, who will blame every little symptom he feels on the drug and, therefore, stop taking it. So far as testing to determine faithfulness is concerned, random urinalysis for metabolites of the drugs under the guise of routine urinalysis, is the only way to accomplish this. But here, too, one can be deceived because some patients will hurriedly take a dose of their medication before coming to the clinic even if they have not taken it at any other time.

David F. Preston and Frank L. Miller. Tuberculosis Outpatient's Defection From Therapy. Am. J. M. Sc. 247:55, 1964. Wallace Fox. Chemotherapy and Epidemiology of Tuberculosis: Some Findings of General Applicability From Tuberculosis Chemotherapy Center, Madras. Lancet. 2:413, Sept. 1; 473, Sept. 8, 1962.

"I have a tuberculosis patient on isoniazid-PAS who has become pronouncedly hypothyroid. Could this be attributable to the use of these drugs?"

Reply: Could be, but this would certainly be a rare occurrence. However, the study of Seinfeld and Starr (University of California) showed that patients who have been on prolonged therapy with these drugs, say for 6 months or more, may experience a depression of thyroxine production without any overt signs of goiter or hypothyroidism; i.e., a subclinical hypothyroidism.

Edward Seinfeld and Paul Starr. Studies of Thyroid Function in Patients Treated with Para-aminosalicylic Acid and Isoniazid. Am. Rev. Resp. Dis. 80:845, 1959.

"In cases of tuberculous meningitis treated with the standard chemotherapeutic agents, what factors are of prognostic importance?"

Reply: The review of the records of 73 patients at the Philadelphia General Hospital, by Weiss and Flippin, revealed that 76% of children, 56% of young adults and only 17% of patients over age 40 survived. Of the deaths, 97% were in nonwhites. Sex seemed unrelated to outcome and so also was the duration of symptoms before admission or the presence of coma. Miliary tuberculosis was as common in those who survived as in those who died, but pulmonary and other extrameningeal tuberculosis was more frequent in those who died. Significant cerebrospinal fluid findings: survivors seldom had a protein concentration above 300 mg./100 ml. or a chloride concentration below 585 mg./100 ml. High protein measurements were recorded in 25% of patients who died and low chloride levels in 39%.

William Weiss and Harrison F. Flippin. Prognosis of Tuberculous Meningitis in the Isoniazid Era. Am. J. M. Sc. 242:423, 1961.

"In household contacts of an active case of tuberculosis what are the factors of prognostic import?"

Reply: In a study of 25,512 contacts in 6219 households, Ferebee and Mount (USPHS) found the three factors of prognostic import to be age, weight and initial status of tuberculosis infection. Prognosis was good for children under 5, poor for those 5–9, fair for those 10–14, and then good again for those 15–30. Initially underweight patients were more susceptible, and the risk was proportional to the size of the initial tuberculin reaction, being lowest for those with reactions of less than 5 mm. of induration.

Shirley H. Ferebee and Frank W. Mount. Tuberculosis Morbidity in Controlled Trial of Prophylactic Use of Isoniazid Among Household Contacts. Am. Rev. Resp. Dis. 85:490, 1962.

"Can it be stated with assurance that isoniazid prophylaxis should be given to all contacts of persons with known tuberculosis?"

Reply: It appears that definitive answer cannot be given, although I believe it is the consensus that such prophylaxis is desirable. In a large scale study in Japan, performed in cooperation with the USPHS, a difference in the results in the treated and untreated groups was doubtfully significant, whereas in a much larger study under the USPHS in the United States, there was a significantly greater development of tuberculosis in the untreated than in the treated group. In the Japanese report, the more recent of the two, further study of the matter is recommended, but the investigators nevertheless felt that prophylaxis should be administered to contacts pending final decision in the matter.

S. H. Ferebee and F. W. Mount. Tuberculosis Morbidity in a Controlled Trial of the Prophylactic Use of Isoniazid Among Household Contacts. Am. Rev. Resp. Dis. 85: 490, 1962; ibid (reversed authors) 85:821, 1962. Ovid B. Bush, Jr., Masamitsu Sugimoto, Yoshihiko Fujii and Frank A. Brown, Jr. Isoniazid Prophylaxis in Contacts of Persons with Known Tuberculosis. Am. Rev. Resp. Dis. 92:732, 1965.

"Could you tersely list the categories of patients in whom tuberculosis chemotherapy is indicated?"

Reply: Of course nothing is static in this field any more than in any other, and I am sure that increasing experience will foster new authoritative pronouncements from time to time. But I do not believe that major alterations in viewpoint have yet come about since the report of the members of the Committee on Therapy of the American Thoracic Society appeared in late 1961. According to this group chemotherapy is mandatory in: (1) patients discharged without completion of a full course of therapy; and (2) the exceptional patient with clinically active disease in whom hospitalization is not feasible. It is strongly indicated in: (1) tuberculin-positive children under 3 years of age, who must be presumed to have active disease in the absence of clinical evidence; (2) patients with previously diagnosed tuberculosis in whom activity is uncertain or shown only by minor roentgen changes, even in the absence of symptoms or bacteriologic evidence; (3) tuberculin-positive persons receiving corticosteroid therapy for other reasons; (4) tuberculin-positive persons with an inactive pulmonary lesion who are to undergo or have had gastric resection; (5) persons with unstable or severe diabetes who are tuberculin positive; and (6) patients with nodular silicosis who are tuberculin positive. It is discretionary in: (1) household contacts of patients with positive sputum regardless of age; (2) children under 14 years who are tuberculin positive; (3) tuberculin-positive persons with indeterminate pulmonary lesions; (4) tuberculin-positive children with severe viral infection, especially measles; (5) a pregnant woman with inactive tuberculosis; (6) the case of a definite conversion from a negative to a positive reaction to 5 T.U. tuberculin (intermediate PPD) in an adult. Since pleural effusion in a young adult with a positive tuberculin skin test should be considered tuberculous until proved otherwise, such a patient should probably be added to the mandatory list.

Committee on Therapy, American Thoracic Society: Thomas B. Barnett, Benjamin Burrows, Kurt Deuschle, William Lester, Frank M. MacDonald, Donald E. Olson, Robert R. Shaw and William W. Stead. Use of Chemotherapy as Public Health Measure in Tuberculosis. Arch. Environ. Health 3:441, 1961. Abraham Falk. Tuberculous Pleurisy with Effusion: Diagnosis and Results of Chemotherapy. Postgrad. Med. 38:631, 1965.

"I have a patient with tubal occlusion caused by healed genital tuberculosis. What might I do to promote the possibility of pregnancy?"

Reply: Isaac Halbrecht, in Israel, gave combined cortisone and antituberculosis drugs to 42 such patients: 50 mg. cortisone or 5 mg. Meticorten daily plus 250 mg. isoniazid, 12 Gm. PAS and 1 Gm. streptomycin three times weekly for 4 months. There was complete restitution of tubal patency in 7 individuals, and 2 of the 3 who became pregnant immediately after treatment had an intrauterine pregnancy. In 12 other patients, antituberculosis drugs were begun immediately after tuboplasty, cortisone was added 4–5 days later, and the combination of drugs was continued for 6–8 weeks. Patency was restored in 2 of these 12 persons.

Isaac Halbrecht. Cortisone in Treatment of Tubal Occlusion Caused by Healed Genital Tuberculosis. Fertil. & Steril. 13:371, 1962.

"In my practice in one of the less developed countries, where facilities for chest surgery are poor, do you think that I am placing my patients under added risk of developing empyema when I treat their acute pulmonary tuberculosis with corticosteroids in addition to the antituberculosis agents?"

Reply: Probably not sufficiently so to overcome the advantage you probably gain through concomitant use of both types of drugs under your working conditions. However, Simmonds reported a case of spontaneous pneumothorax and tuberculous empyema occurring in a patient with such combined therapy.

F. A. H. Simmonds. Tubercle 43:448, 1962.

"I have a child with tuberculous pleural effusion whom I am treating with chemotherapeutic agents but without corticosteroids. In average cases, what would be the outcome of such a regimen?"

Reply: Filler and Porter found that the various indexes of pulmonary function in 40 children with healed tuberculous pleural effusion were the same as those in normal children and that the addition of corticosteroids had not altered the end result.

J. Filler and M. Porter. Am. Rev. Resp. Dis. 88:181, 1963.

"When treating tuberculous pleurisy with chemotherapeutic agents it is often 5 or 6 months before one can see clinical and laboratory improvement. Why this prolonged period of subclinical response?"

Reply: I do not know precisely, but Sohn's group (Capital Army Hospital, Seoul, Korea) studied the effect of chemotherapy on morphologic changes in such patients and found that the healing process of pleural granulomatous lesions began immediately after institution of the therapy and reached a peak within 3 months.

Esuk Sohn, Bin Hwang and Taik Koo Yun. Effect of Chemotherapy on Tuberculous Pleurisy: Serial Study of 191 Needle Biopsy Specimens in 41 Patients. Am. Rev. Resp. Dis. 86:197, 1962.

"I am going for medical missionary service into a remote region in one of the primitive countries in which much tuberculosis will be encountered. In fact, I am informed that because of the malnourished, poverty-stricken overcrowded city in which I shall work, and the fear that patients treated at home might become chronic excretors of drug-resistant organisms, most of my patients will be in a far advanced cavitary stage of the disease in a mass domiciliary situation in which they have been brought together. Can you give me any guidance from the experience of others who have faced a problem of this sort?"

Reply: To this extent only, that under quite similar circumstances in Madras, India, Wallace Fox found that those who were treated under domiciliary conditions such as you will encounter were at a disadvantage in comparison with those who were treated in their own homes. In the sanatorium there was a decidedly superior diet and the treatment was carried out in airy, well ventilated wards, and none of the patients was allowed up for over 4 hours a day, whereas most of the home-treated patients were on partial or full activity at the end of 12 months. But there was very little nursing care available for the sanatorium patients, and there was some irregularity in the taking of their drugs. Actually, however, the home-treated patients had more severe disease. At the end of the first year the disease was quiescent in 92% of the sanatorium cases and 86% of the home cases. Nothing therefore was gained by the resort to domiciliary care, which had a very important effect of disrupting family life and presenting major social problems. Bacteriologic relapse occurred in 9% of those whose disease had become quiescent in the sanatorium and in 5% of those at home during a 2 year follow up. Fox also observed that exposure to the active case under treatment did not increase the risk of home contacts. It is certainly not surprising that he concluded that there is no special reason for not treating the patient at home. One of the greatest problems presenting in this study was the difficulty in getting patients to take their drugs, either in the sanatorium or at home, with necessary regularity.

Wallace Fox. Chemotherapy and Epidemiology of Tuberculosis: Some Findings of General Applicability From Tuberculosis Chemotherapy Center, Madras. Lancet 2:413, Sept 1; 473, Sept. 8, 1962.

"We are using the antituberculosis drugs with great confidence, which is certainly justified; however, we are also just as certainly getting relapses. Just what is the incidence of these relapses in general experience?"

Reply: I do not think any one knows precisely what the incidence is in private practice among a class of people in whom faithfulness in taking the drugs might be expected to be (whether justifiably or not!) somewhat greater than in a group of clinic patients. So I shall recite to you the relapse incidence as reported by Samuel Phillips from the VA Hospital in Memphis, based on follow-up information on 109 of 115 patients with bacteriologically proved and previously untreated pulmonary tuberculosis, in almost all of whom the disease was considered "inactive" at the time of discharge. Of these patients, 68% were white, 32% Negro, and all but 1 were males. Of the whole group, 54% had moderately advanced disease, 27% far advanced disease, and 19% minimal disease. At the beginning of treatment, 48% were under age 40, 33% were 40–60 and 19% over 60. Of streptomycin-treated patients, the relapse incidence was 13%; of isoniazid treated, 7%; of isoniazid and pyrazinamide treated, 0%. The rate was 16% for those treated up to 2 years but only 4% for those treated for 2 years or more. The rate among those having such procedures as pneumoperitoneum, extraperiosteal plombage, thoracoplasty or some form of pulmonary resection, the rate was 5% as compared with

10% of those whose treatment did not include any of these procedures, but the disparity in numbers between these two groups of patients was rather large. The rate was twice as high in Negroes as in whites and considerably higher in those over 50 than in those who were under that age.

Samuel Phillips. Relapse in Treated Cases of Pulmonary Tuberculosis. Am. Rev. Resp. Dis. 89:61, 1964.

"Has the value of continuous chemotherapy in pulmonary tuberculosis for a long period after hospitalization been fully established?"

Reply: Indeed, yes. In fact, since relapses usually occur within 2–5 years after discontinuance of treatment, most men arbitrarily attempt to continue the use of the drugs for 5 years at least. Using the three standard drugs, streptomycin, PAS and isoniazid, Morris Dressler (VA Hospital, Coral Gables, Florida) compared two groups. In the long-treated group of 202 patients, 39% had far advanced disease, 49% moderately advanced and 12% minimal; operation had been performed in 19%. In this group, 93% received chemotherapy for 19–60 months or longer. In the control group of 105 patients, all of whom received chemotherapy for less than 19 months, disease was far advanced in 40%, moderately advanced in 46% and minimal in 14%; there had been operation in 18%. In this control group relapse occurred in 30% and in the treated group only 1%, and actually the 2 patients who constituted this 1% had been transferred to another area where their drugs had been discontinued.

Morris Dressler. Posthospital Outpatient Treatment of Pulmonary Tuberculosis by Prolonged Chemotherapy: Study of Relapse Rate. Dis. Chest 41:425, 1962.

"All of us who are treating tuberculosis are wondering to what extent we are piling up a backlog of drug-resistant organisms in our communities. Can you enlighten?"

Reply: Not with the clarity that could be wished. In two studies from authoritative sources (one of them being that of Gerszten and associates in a sanatorium population of American Negroes of the lower socioeconomic class, and the other that of the Research Committee of the British Tuberculosis Association in random sampling of 38 chest clinics in Britain) there has been provided dramatic and somewhat frightening evidence of the high incidence of drug-resistant tuberculosis in these two situations. However, in an authoritative review of this subject, Gladys L. Hobby of the VA Special Research Laboratory, concluded that the true prevalence of resistant strains cannot be satisfactorily estimated until more refined laboratory methods have been devised. She did warn, though, of the advisability of proceeding on the assumption that such strains may not be rare and could become an important public health problem.

Enrique Gerszten, Donald L. Brummer, Marvin J. Allison and Miles E. Hench (Med. College of Virginia). Increased Resistance of Mycobacterium Tuberculosis to Drug Therapy: Study of Frequency of Drug-Resistant Tubercle Bacilli Among 482 Patients and Its Effect on Recovery. J.A.M.A. 185:6, July 6, 1963. Gladys L. Hobby. Am. Rev. Resp. Dis. 86:839, 1962; ibid, 91:30, 1965. The Research Committee of the British Tuberculosis Association. Acquired Drug Resistance in Patients with Pulmonary Tuberculosis in Great Britain—National Survey, 1960–61. Tubercle 44:1, 1963.

"I have heard that the long-term administration of para-amino salicylic acid (PAS) is capable of causing a decrease in absorption of vitamin B_{12}. Is this the result of a general malabsorption induced by the drug?"

Reply: According to the observations of O. Heinivaara and associates, in Helsinki, the malabsorption concerns specifically or at any rate chiefly, vitamin B_{12}. But I do not understand why, if this is the case, megaloblastic anemia is not known to be a complication of PAS therapy. Hemolytic anemia, purpura, leukopenia and neutropenia have been reported, but not megaloblastic anemia.

O. Heinivaara and I. P. Palva. Malabsorption and Deficiency of Vitamin B_{12} Caused by Treatment with Para-Aminosalicylic Acid. Acta med. scandinav. 177:337, 1965. O. Heinivaara, I. P. Palva, M. Siurala and R. Pelkonen. Selectivity of the PAS-Induced Malabsorption of Vitamin B_{12}. Ann. med. int. Fenniae 53:75, 1964.

"What effect do the corticosteroids have on the exudate and cavity closure in pulmonary tuberculosis?"

Reply: In the USPHS Tuberculosis Therapy Trial involving 1674 patients with newly diagnosed pulmonary tuberculosis in 25 hospitals, it was found that low dosage of prednisolone (Meticortelone, etc.) had little effect on cavity closure, but it produced more frequent and more rapid clearing of the infiltrate in Negro than in white patients. As little as 5 weeks of therapy, of course in combination with antituberculosis agents, seems to have accelerated the clearing process by at least a month in Negroes.

U.S.P.H.S. Tuberculosis Therapy Trial. Am. Rev. Resp. Dis. 91:329, 1965.

"Could you cite the results of a careful study of local instillation of a corticosteroid in the treatment of tuberculous pleural effusion?"

Reply: In India, Mathur and associates used intrapleural hydrocortisone acetate (Cortef Acetate) emulsion in dosage of 125 mg., repeating at 2 week intervals up to a maximum of four instillations. Of the 77 patients, 60 obtained fluid absorption completely after the first instillation, and this occurred after two administrations in 10 others. In 25 controls, the effusion cleared up in 8% within a month and in 36% within 6 weeks.

Krishna S. Mathur, Jyoti S. Mathur and Rajendra P. Sapru. Treatment of Tuberculous Pleural Effusion with Local Instillation of Hydrocortisone. Dis. Chest 47:83, 1965.

"Would it be of advantage to continue chemotherapy in a patient with inactive tuberculosis for several years after one would normally discontinue it?"

Reply: In Albany, New York, Julius Katz and associates put this matter to the test and determined that such a procedure would be of definite value. Two hundred and forty-seven of their 513 patients with inactive tuberculosis received 300 mg. of isoniazid daily for 2 years, the observation period being almost 6 years, of which almost 4 were post-treatment. The reactivation rate in the first year of treatment was 2.5 per 100 person-years among treated patients and 3.9 among controls, the respective rates in the second year being 1.4 and 4.3. But thereafter the difference in the rates decreased, and they were essentially the same in the third and fourth post-treatment years. Of course a large scale program to find and treat such patients in the general population must be considered completely impractical; but it should be completely feasible in infants and children in contact with active cases.

Julius Katz, Solomon Kunofsky, Vytuatas Damijonaitis, Albert Lafleur and Theresa Caron. Effect of Isoniazid on Reactivation of Inactive Tuberculosis: Final Report. Am. Rev. Resp. Dis. 91:345, 1965.

"What standardized treatment of acute pulmonary tuberculosis has been settled upon in large institutions where the thing has been expertly studied?"

Reply: At the well known Battey State Hospital, in Rome, Georgia, patients with proved cases of previously untreated, far advanced, cavitary tuberculosis were treated by one or two regimens of a USPH Service protocol. No. 1: 1 Gm. streptomycin daily plus pyrazinamide, 40 mg./kg., daily for 12 weeks, followed by 300 mg. of isoniazid daily in two or three equal doses plus 12 Gm. PAS daily for 20 weeks. No. 2: alternating 4 week courses of 1 Gm. streptomycin daily plus pyrazinamide, 40 mg./kg. daily, and 300 mg. isoniazid daily plus 12 Gm. PAS daily for 32 weeks, starting treatment with streptomycin and pyrazinamide. Both regimens were entirely successful in preventing deaths from progressive tuberculosis. Of the patients on regimen No. 1, 9.3% were removed because of drug toxicity, and 5% of those on regimen No. 2. The reactions were due to PAS, none to isoniazid and a few to pyrazinamide and streptomycin. Of the patients on regimen No. 1, 74% had no visible cavities by the end of the study, 9% having their cavities excised. In 77% of patients on regimen No. 2, the cavities had closed or had been excised. Both regimens were effective in sputum "conversion" and both reached peak conversion at the end of 7 months. After 5 months of therapy with either of the regimens, 85% of the patients with far advanced cavities had noninfectious sputum; after 6 months the sputum of 92% was noninfectious; and after 7 months 97% had noninfectious sputum. No patient died of progressive tuberculosis during the follow-up period (30–40 months) and of those who had eliminated tubercle bacilli from their sputum at the end of the study, 0.8% had a bacteriologic relapse.

Raymond F. Corpe and Frank A. Blalock. Alternating Regimens of Streptomycin-Pyrazinamide, Isoniazid-Para-Aminosalicylic Acid at Battey State Hospital. Am. Rev. Resp. Dis. 90:262, 1964.

"In the chemotherapy of miliary tuberculosis is race a significant factor in affecting survival?"

Reply: It certainly appeared to be in a Veterans Administration–Armed Forces Cooperative Study reported by Abraham Falk. Although the number of white and Negro patients was about equal, only 39% of the Negroes died of tuberculosis whereas 69% of the white patients died. This was a series, however, in which many of the individuals had meningeal as well as miliary involvement.

Abraham Falk, U.S. Veterans Administration–Armed Forces Cooperative Study on Chemotherapy of Tuberculosis. Am. Rev. Resp. Dis. 91:6, 1965.

"How often does one find an individual with tuberculosis who is resistant to more than one of the chemotherapeutic agents?"

Reply: At Battey State Hospital, Rome, Georgia, Raymond Corpe's group reported 16 patients who were resistant to two of the three major drugs (isoniazid, streptomycin and PAS) plus one of the secondary drugs (pyrazinamide, viomycin and cycloserine); 21 who were resistant to two of the three major drugs plus two secondary drugs; and 41 who were resistant to all three of the major drugs plus two of the secondary drugs.

Raymond F. Corpe, Frank A. Blalock, John H. Gross and Egon J. Goldhammer. Retreatment of Drug-Resistant Pulmonary Tuberculosis at Battey State Hospital. Am. Rev. Resp. Dis. 90:957, 1964.

"In the retreatment of drug-resistant pulmonary tuberculosis, what has been attained?"

Reply: At Battey State Hospital, Rome, Georgia, Raymond Corpe's group, using a therapy schedule designed to obtain peak serum concentrations of their drugs, with a regimen consisting of ethambutol, ethionamide and isoniazid, obtained 76% reversal of infections in the 92 patients in the series, as indicated by sputum culture. Of the 24% that were treatment failures, 13 were white males, 2 were white females, 5 were Negro males and 2 were Negro females. None of the patients under age 20 failed to respond to the treatment, which was unsuccessful in 3 of 12 aged 20–39, 11 of the 52 aged 40–59, and 8 of the 25 aged 60–79.

Raymond F. Corpe, Frank A. Blalock, John H. Gross and Egon J. Goldhammer. Retreatment of Drug-Resistant Pulmonary Tuberculosis at Battey State Hospital. Am. Rev. Resp. Dis. 90:957, 1964.

"Among those of us in general practice who often handle our own cases of tuberculosis now that the chemotherapeutic agents are available, the winds blow hot and cold regarding the matter of accompanying the use of these drugs with corticosteroids. What is the authoritative position in this matter nowadays?"

Reply: I shall cite the report of the Research Committee of the British Tuberculosis Association. The 346 patients with acute pulmonary tuberculosis in this study were allocated randomly to treatment with chemotherapy alone: 1 Gm. streptomycin, 16 Gm. PAS and 300 mg. isoniazid daily (as control group); the same chemotherapy with 30 IU of corticotropin daily for 3 months; or the same chemotherapy with 30 mg. prednisone (Meticorten, etc.) daily for 3 months. The antituberculosis chemotherapy was continued for an overall period of 12 months, with the patients in hospital and in bed during much of this time. The conclusion reached was that the antituberculosis drugs, as used, provided an effective means of recovery for patients with pulmonary tuberculosis, and that the addition of prednisone in the early months of therapy not only hastened clinical improvement initially, but produced significantly greater radiographic progress by 12 months. I would emphasize to you, however, that before concluding that these findings have significance for routine practice, you bear carefully in mind that this study was carried out under close supervision in a specialized hospital. In a similar study in the United States, at the Madison and Minneapolis Veterans Administration Hospitals, results favorable to the use of corticosteroids were also obtained, and these observers reported that "Results from this study and seven other controlled studies indicate that corticosteroids are a worthwhile adjunct to the chemotherapy of seriously ill patients with extensive pulmonary tuberculosis."

Research Committee of the British Tuberculosis Association. Trial of Corticotropin and Prednisone with Chemotherapy in Pulmonary Tuberculosis: Two-Year Radiographic Follow-Up. Tubercle 44:484, 1963. J. R. Johnson, B. C. Taylor, J. F. Morrissey, J. W. Jenne and F. M. MacDonald. Corticosteroids in Pulmonary Tuberculosis. Am. Rev. Resp. Dis. 92:376, 1965.

"What has been the incidence of intolerance to the three principal antituberculosis agents: isoniazid, PAS and streptomycin?"

Reply: The most thorough study I have seen of this matter was that of Stephen J. Berté's group at Valley Forge General Hospital. The overall incidence of drug intolerance in their 1744 patients was 12.2%. Of the 400 patients given streptomycin, 10.3% showed intolerance, about twice as many reactions occurring when the drug was given daily as when it was given twice weekly. Of the 1698 receiving PAS, 8.8% showed intolerance, and among 1724 receiving isoniazid, 1.3% showed intolerance, with the greatest incidence in patients who received more than 100 mg. three times daily.

Stephen J. Berté, Joseph D. DiMase and Charles S. Christianson. Isoniazid, Para-Aminosalicylic Acid and Streptomycin Intolerance in 1,744 Patients: Analysis of Reactions to Single Drugs and Drug Groups Plus Data on Multiple Reactions, Type and Time of Reactions and Desensitization. Am. Rev. Resp. Dis. 90:598, 1964.

TULAREMIA

"What is the antibiotic of choice in tularemia?"

Reply: This infection usually yields quickly to streptomycin, with chlortetracycline (Aureomycin) probably the second most effective agent.

TYPHOID FEVER

"Unlike in my younger days when typhoid fever was rampant, we now rarely see a case in our hospital and when we have done so recently have been wondering whether it would be advantage-

ous to use corticosteroids together with the specific chloramphenicol (Chloromycetin)?"

Reply: In Haiti, where the disease still prevails in high incidence, Philip Eskes recently made a limited study of this matter in 99 infants and children with initially uncomplicated disease, i.e., those with such other prevailing diseases as malaria and tuberculosis were excluded from the observation. There were both inpatient and outpatient groups; corticosteroid was given either as prednisone (Meticorten, etc.) or prednisolone (Meticortelone, etc.) 1 mg./kg./day in divided doses for 3 consecutive days, starting at the moment the diagnosis was made; chloramphenicol dosage was 50–75 mg./kg./day in divided doses for a minimum of 2 weeks. There was a sufficiently striking reduction in mortality and morbidity in the corticosteroid treated patients to warrant further investigation, but Eskes warned against use of these drugs in patients with a history of fever for 2 weeks or more, as most typhoid perforations occur in the third week. It should also be noted that a rebound phenomenon after cessation of steroid therapy (return of fever without toxicity for 24–36 hours) as previously described by other observers, was seen in 9 of the patients.

Philip W. H. Eskes. The Effects of Steroids in the Treatment of Typhoid Fever. Pediatrics 36:142, 1965.

"The word is going around that *somebody somewhere* has found *some* drug to be better than chloramphenicol (Chloromycetin) in the treatment of typhoid fever. It seems too bad for such a rumor to get started unless it has good basis in fact because chloramphenicol has truly been an effective drug in this disease. Has something startling really been achieved?"

Reply: Hardly startling, but it is true that in Beirut, Lebanon, Uwaydah and Shamma'a have found that ampicillin (Penbritin) is an effective drug when chloramphenicol cannot be used. This is surely reassuring news. *Dosage*: 1 Gm. orally every 6 hours until fever subsides, followed by 0.5–0.75 Gm. every 6 hours for 7–10 days or longer. In Durban, Natal, South Africa, Whitby obtained a good response in 5 of 6 typhoid carriers given 1 Gm. of the drug every 6 hours for 21–28 days.

Marwan Uwaydah and Munir Shamma'a. Treatment of Typhoid Fever with Ampicillin (Penbritin). Lancet 1:1242, June 6, 1964. J. M. F. Whitby. Ampicillin in Treatment of Salmonella Typhi Carriers. Lancet 2:71, July 11, 1964.

"It has developed that a middle-aged patient of mine who has gallstones is also a typhoid carrier. Can I hope to rid her of the carrier state without getting rid of the gallstones?"

Reply: Tynes and Utz, at the National Institutes of Health, have findings suggesting that antibiotics cannot sterilize the center of an infected stone and that infection of bile occurs as soon as antibiotic concentrations fall below the inhibiting level for the organism. Thus it seems that a salmonella carrier with gallstones should have cholecystectomy combined with pre- and postoperative antibiotic therapy. However, Simon and Miller, in California, have reported the ampicillin (Penbritin, Polycillin) treatment of 15 chronic carriers, 5 of whom had gallstones, and all of whom achieved negative stool cultures during therapy, 13 of them remaining negative after 7–54 months of observation at time of publication. Dosage was high: 75–100 mg./kg./day for 3 weeks in most cases, with 1 week of rest and then another week of dosing.

Bayard S. Tynes and John P. Utz. Factors Influencing Cure of Salmonella Carriers. Ann. Int. Med. 57:871, 1962.
Harold J. Simon and Raymond C. Miller. Ampicillin in Treatment of Chronic Typhoid Carriers. New England J. Med. 274:807, Apr. 14, 1966.

UREA DECOMPRESSION

"Has a large-scale experience with urea decompression in neurosurgery been recorded?"

Reply: The study most likely to meet your requirement was that of Stig Jeppsson and associates, at the University of Lund, who reported the use of intravenous hypertonic urea in 174 craniotomies in which there were signs of increased intracranial pressure in all but 7 instances. A 30% solution of urea crystals in 10% invertose was given as intravenous drip at a usual rate of 60 drops/minute, the total dose being kept at 1.5 Gm./kg. with a tendency to reduce this to 1 Gm./kg. Two thirds of the amount was given while elevating the bone flap, and the remainder, at a rate of about 18–20 drops/minute, during the course of the operation. Good results were received in 93.1% of the cases, "good" meaning a completely slack dura with considerable free space between the skull bone–dura and the brain surface; in 4.6% of additional cases there was a slightly tense dura which could be opened without any prolapse of the brain. In 16 of the cases urea was given postoperatively because of symptoms presumably due to brain swelling. During the first postoperative day there was a rise in nonprotein nitrogen level to 60.8 mg./100 ml., but the level was normal again within 3 days. There was no undue fluctuation of serum electrolytes; a slight tendency toward hemoconcentration during

the first day; potassium deficiency in several cases but without untoward effect; 7 cases of postoperative clotting, but a decreasing incidence of this in recent experience; frequent superficial phlebitis and in 1 case localized necrosis with complete healing; no toxic cortical effects revealed in electrocorticograms; no rebound phenomena. It was found possible with the urea to reverse fulminant tentorial herniation with respiratory arrest and fixed-dilated pupils.

Stig Jeppsson, Sven E. Järpe and Lennart Rabow. Treatment of Increased Intracranial Pressure in Neurosurgery: Clinical Report on Use of Intravenous Hypertonic Urea in 174 Craniotomies with Evaluation of This and Other Decompressive Methods, Alone and in Combination. Acta chir. scandinav. supp. 312, 1963.

URETHRAL STRICTURE

"The results of corticosteroid therapy following dilatation for urethral stricture have been favorably reported in the literature but I do not know anyone who has used or is using this method. What is its present status?"

Reply: The effects of both systemic and local administration of corticosteroids have been regarded as good in the main, but the method has not come into wide use nevertheless. The systemic treatment is of the usual sort and local treatment is usually followed one or a few times after dilatation. In employing the local therapy in Stockholm, Ekström and Hultengren used prednisolone tertiary butyl acetate (Hydeltra-T.B.A., Hydeltrasol), injecting from 20 to 60 mg. at several sites beneath the mucous membrane after dilatation. After the treatment, a Foley 20 catheter was inserted and left in position for 24 hours. The conclusion of these observers was that the long-term results of injection treatment were favorable in patients with a single short stricture of fairly short standing and poorer in cases of long and of multiple strictures previously treated with dilatation for a lengthy period.

Tore Ekström and Nils Hultengren. Effect of Local Corticosteroid Therapy for Urethral Stricture. Acta chir. scandinav. 130:379, 1965.

URINARY TRACT INFECTION

"I have a pregnant patient with a clinical urinary tract infection and a urine culture positive for *Aerobacter aerogenes*. Would there be any risk involved in treating her with tetracycline?"

Reply: I should not do it. Both Schultz and associates and Whalley and associates have reported severe liver and pancreatic dysfunction in obstetrical patients who were treated with one of the tetracyclines. To be sure, the drug was given in high dosage intravenously in all of the cases, but still I would not risk it even orally. An interesting corollary question would be how long after her delivery it might be safe to begin the use of a tetracycline compound, but I cannot find the answer to this in any literature available to me, although in the 1966 edition of the A.M.A. "New Drugs" the statement is made that this serious reaction has occurred "most often in pregnant or postpartum patients."

J. C. Schultz, J. S. Adamson, W. W. Workman and T. M. Norman. Fatal Liver Disease After Intravenous Administration of Tetracycline in High Dosage. New England J. Med. 269:999, 1963. P. J. Whalley, R. H. Adams and B. Combes. Tetracycline Toxicity in Pregnancy. J.A.M.A. 189:357, 1964.

"In a patient with urinary tract infection who has not responded to other drugs, would I be justified in trying cycloserine (Seromycin)?"

Reply: J. McC. Murdoch's group (Edinburgh) used it in 5 female patients in dosage of 250 mg. every 8 hours for 14 days. All responded dramatically, being afebrile and free of urinary tract symptoms within 3 days. The urine became sterile and follow-up during several months revealed no evidence of clinical or bacteriologic relapse. But 1 patient with impaired renal function developed a mild personality change during treatment, but this was reversible. Be careful, however, if there is disturbed renal function, and do not give this drug to an epileptic. In Houston, Arnold and Fahlberg found 500 mg. of the drug daily for 7–14 days effective in about 50% of the ordinary pyogenic infections.

J. McC. Murdoch, J. D. Sleigh and S. C. Frazer. Cycloserine in Treatment of Infection of Urinary Tract. Brit. M. J. 2:1055, Nov. 21, 1959. Jasper H. Arnold and Willson H. Fahlberg. Evaluation of Seromycin in Pyogenic Infection of the Urinary Tract. J. Urol. 94:462, 1965.

"Why is it that one cannot always sterilize a urinary tract infection when using the proper antibiotic or chemotherapeutic agents as revealed by sensitivity studies?"

Reply: In many instances the failure is due to replacement of the original infecting organism upon which the therapy was based by a new organism making its presence known after elimination of the other one; in these instances both organisms were probably present together originally but the overgrowth of the one toward which therapy was directed masked the presence of the other in the beginning. In some instances the necessary level of the therapeutic agent is not effectively delivered to the infecting organism because its concentration is diluted by residual urine, or there is a complicating hydronephrosis or severe azotemia. In some instances the presence of a stone or other morphological alteration will prevent complete eradication of the organisms so that, although they will apparently disappear during the period of active treatment, they return very quickly when treatment is interrupted. And then there is the very small group of cases in which the organisms truly develop resistance to the drugs. A further matter to be taken into account of course is the apparent persistence of infection in the bladder or above when the organisms demonstrated are really only urethral contaminants.

Thomas A. Stamey, Duncan E. Govan and John M. Palmer. The Localization and Treatment of Urinary Tract Infections: The Role of Bactericidal Urine Levels as Opposed to Serum Levels. Medicine 44:1, 1965.

"When an elderly individual (it will usually be a woman) presents with asymptomatic bacteriuria of unknown duration, how shall I treat?"

Reply: One must bear in mind that in most such cases the bacteriuria will have been present for many years and that it is unlikely to cause significant morbidity from either hypertension or uremia. In studying this matter at the University of Washington, Petersdorf and Plorde have made the important point that very often all that is accomplished by antimicrobial therapy in such cases is an alteration of the urinary flora and replacement of a sensitive microorganism by a more resistant one. They favored a conservative therapeutic approach as the most rational one considering the relative resistance of the pathogens usually encountered and the potential toxicity of most of the antimicrobial agents that are effective against them. However, in a patient with an elevated BUN who is unable to elaborate a concentrated urine or who has symptoms suggesting vesical outlet obstruction or stone they definitely advocate further evaluation for two reasons: first, to determine the extent of renal parenchymal involvement, and second, to detect surgically correctable lesions. They generally recommend surgery in elderly men with vesical outlet obstruction because of the likelihood that acute urinary retention, with or without symptomatic cystitis, pyelonephritis or bacteremia, may occur at some time in the future. But they feel that in the case of the cystoceles, urethroceles, urethral caruncles and other lesions of women, that are often associated with bacteriuria, the situation is best left alone since correction of these things may have little effect on the urinary infection. When there is no correctable lesion or when surgery is contraindicated they feel that antibiotics may be used though not with the certainty that they are going to deter or prevent further renal parenchymal damage in this way. Here in Milwaukee, Paul Kimmelstiel has made the following authoritative statement: "If we could show that bacteriuria precedes or causes pyelonephritis, treatment would be justified. Presently available evidence, however, merely proves that this sequence of events is possible, for factual data in the human are still controversial. Statistics proving the causative role of bacteriuria are no better than the information fed into the calculation. Indeed, such information, establishing the diagnosis of pyelonephritis following bacteriuria, is shockingly scant. The relationship of bacteriuria to chronic pyelonephritis is not established beyond the occasional association." However, I think that I should bring to your attention the position stated by the Seattle group (Turck et al.) that intensive treatment is indicated in young patients with urinary sepsis in whom deterioration in renal function may be anticipated if infection is permitted to persist. These observers feel that in such cases the use of bactericidal drugs capable of achieving antibacterial levels in both urine and tissues may be warranted.

Robert G. Petersdorf and James J. Plorde. Management of Urinary Tract Infection in the Elderly. Geriatrics 20:613, 1965. Paul Kimmelstiel. In Controversy in Internal Medicine (F. J. Ingelfinger, A. S. Relman and M. Finland, eds.). Phila. W. B. Saunders Co., 1966, p. 313. Marvin Turck, Ann A. Browder, Robert I. Lindemeyer, Norman K. Brown, Kenneth N. Anderson and Robert G. Petersdorf. Failure of Prolonged Treatment of Chronic Urinary Tract Infections with Antibiotics. New England J. Med. 267: 999, Nov. 15, 1962.

"The patient has an indwelling catheter. Should one try to prevent urinary infection through the systemic use of antibiotics?"

Reply: I believe it is the consensus that this is the wrong thing to do and that indeed it may actually worsen the situation. In most practices the drugs are not used so long as the patient is free of symptoms, but the urine is regularly cultured and sensitivity tests performed on the pathogens. If, then, fever, chills or flank pain develop you will be ready to attack the organism with the suitable antibiotic, using it only long enough to control the symptoms. It has been amply shown that the infections cannot be cleared so long as the catheter is in place; once it is removed, then one can attack the thing with full vigor.

Robert G. Petersdorf and James J. Plorde. Management of Urinary Tract Infection in the Elderly. Geriatrics 20: 613, 1965.

"In 2 of the 6 cases in which I have used colistin (Coly-Mycin) in treatment of urinary tract infections there has occurred a reversible circumoral paresthesia, which bothers me somewhat. Have instances of more severe central nervous system involvement been reported?"

Reply: No, not to my knowledge, but the reaction you describe is seen rather frequently. When the injectable form of this drug, sodium colistimethate (Coly-Mycin Injectable), is used there appears a myasthenic type of reaction (apnea, muscle weakness, ptosis) fairly often it seems, particularly in patients with impaired renal function.

"Is ampicillin (Polycillin, Penbritin) suitable for use in urinary tract infections?"

Reply: The experience of Kennedy and associates (City Hospital, Edinburgh) indicated to them that its use should be limited to the initial and long-term treatment of sensitive proteus infections. They found it not as effective as cycloserine (Seromycin) and at the time of their writing more expensive.

W. P. U. Kennedy, A. T. Wallace and J. McC. Murdoch. Ampicillin in Treatment of Certain Gram-Negative Bacterial Infections. Brit. M. J. 2:962, Oct. 19, 1963.

"I have been using Mesulfin, which contains equal amounts of sulfamethizole and methenamine mandelate, with good effect in a few urinary tract infections, but in some instances the urine becomes quite turbid. Is there any danger attached to this?"

Reply: I believe the manufacturers maintain that the turbidity is due to inorganic salts, mostly amorphous urates, but Joseph Lipton (Lynn, Massachusetts, Hospital) found 69% of the material causing the turbidity to be a sulfonamide derivative. I do not believe that this has been reported as yet to be of practical importance, but if the finding is a true one it would certainly at least theoretically increase the risk of renal blockage or urinary calculus.

Joseph H. Lipton. Incompatibility Between Sulfamethizole and Methenamine Mandelate. New England J. Med. 268:92, Jan. 10, 1963.

"One of my associates has been using ascorbic acid with indifferent success in combating urinary tract infections. Has this matter been studied?"

Reply: Yes, at the VA Hospital in Topeka, Kansas, Francis Murphy and associates found the agent palatable, harmless and effective as a urinary acidifying agent in patients with uninfected urine, but in those with a chronic urinary infection its effect was vitiated by bacterial ureases. However, when combined with antibacterial therapy, the urinary acidity was effectively maintained as well as, or better than, by antibacterial therapy alone. The lowest urinary pH obtained clinically in infected patients in their series was achieved by a combination of ascorbic acid with nitrofurantoin (Furadantin). Ascorbic acid was given orally as tablets or solution every 4 hours in dosage varying from 3 to 6 Gm. daily. Down in Texas, Luther Travis's group found it an effective acidifying agent with methenamine mandelate (Mandelamine).

Francis J. Murphy, Samuel Zelman and Walter Mau. Ascorbic Acid as a Urinary Acidifying Agent: Its Adjunctive Role in Chronic Urinary Infection. J. Urol. 94:300, 1965. Luther B. Travis, Warren F. Dodge, Aaron A. Mintz and Manuchelar Assemi. Urinary Acidification with Ascorbic Acid. J. Pediat. 67:1176, 1965.

"One of my associates has just told me of an elderly woman under treatment with nitrofurantoin (Furadantin) for a urinary tract infection in which he strongly suspects that the sudden onset of dyspnea at rest, orthopnea and vomiting is due to the drug. Is this possible?"

Reply: Instances of this general sort have been very rarely reported and have most probably been upon an allergic basis. In 2 of Murray and Kronenberg's cases, in Minneapolis, there was a picture resembling acute pulmonary edema and these patients were treated for pulmonary edema of cardiac origin. In Robinson's case, in Woodland, California, in which there was pulmonary infiltration and pleural effusion, the symptoms returned when medication was resumed after a period without the drug.

M. J. Murray and Richard Kronenberg. Pulmonary Reactions Simulating Cardiac Pulmonary Edema Caused by Nitrofurantoin. New England J. Med. 273:1185, Nov. 25, 1965. Benjamin R. Robinson. Pleuropulmonary Reaction to Nitrofurantoin. J.A.M.A. 189:239, July 20, 1964.

"Can you provide a brief statement of the present status of the new urinary tract antiseptic, nalidixic acid (NegGram)?"

Reply: Yes, but only with the understanding that any present statement must be entirely tentative since adequate comparison of this agent with the other urinary tract antiseptics has not yet been made. It appears that the most important indications for use of nalidixic acid are *Escherichia coli* and proteus infections, but an important limitation to the usefulness of the drug is the tendency of organisms to develop resistance to it. And it appears likely that it is not ideal as an initial drug in an acute infection because

of its limited gram-negative spectrum. I have not seen firm evidence that the drug causes disturbances of liver or kidney function. Among the 100 patients treated by Akbari's group, at Cornell University, there were skin rashes severe enough in 2 to warrant discontinuance of the drug. In Lionel Reese's 70 patients, the drug had to be discontinued in 6: nausea and vomiting in 3, diarrhea in 1 and urticaria in 2.

Ahmad Akbari, Joseph N. Ward, Morris M. Hilf, Russell W. Lavengood and John W. Draper. NegGram (Nalidixic Acid) in Treatment of Urinary Infections. J. Urol. 92: 552, 1964. Lionel Reese. Nalidixic Acid (NegGram) in Treatment of Urinary Infections. Canad. M. A. J. 92:394, Feb. 20, 1965. R. A. Sleet, W. Gray, M. Calder and J. McC. Murdoch. Treatment of Urinary Tract Infections with Nalidixic Acid: Clinical Trial. Chemotherapia 8:137, 1964.

"Has nalidixic acid (NegGram) been found effective in cases of nongonococcic urethritis?"

Reply: At St. Mary's Hospital, in London, Willcox used the drug in a small number of patients and concluded that it is unlikely to be effective in such cases.

R. R. Willcox. Treatment of Nongonococcic Urethritis with Nalidixic Acid (NegGram). Brit. J. Ven. Dis. 40:196, 1964.

"Is it true that nalidixic acid (NegGram) is dangerous to use because it is likely to cause convulsions?"

Reply: Unfortunately there have been several reports of convulsions in association with the use of this drug, but in all instances that have come to my attention the dosage used has either been excessive or the patient had a history of convulsive seizures or was a person with advanced cerebral arteriosclerosis or parkinsonism. It is unfortunate that these occurrences should have engendered the rumor that the drug is prone to cause convulsions, because it is apparently a valuable addition to our armamentarium in the treatment of urinary tract infections since it will sometimes handle a *Proteus* infection when other drugs have failed.

"Methenamine mandelate (Mandelamine) was formerly much used in our hospital in the treatment of urinary tract infections but has latterly given way before the newer drugs. Is this not nevertheless still a very good agent?"

Reply: Thorough study has established Mandelamine as effective in controlling about 75% of the common urinary tract infections in 3–14 days, perhaps usually in 6–7 days. The sulfonamides will not ordinarily do much better than this and organisms originally susceptible to them may become insusceptible though susceptibility to Mandelamine is not lost; this advantage is possessed in comparison with the antibiotics also. *Escherichia coli* is particularly well attacked by the drug and so also is *Streptococcus faecalis*, but *Aerobacter aerogenes, Pseudomonas aeruginosa* and *Proteus vulgaris* are often resistant. In neurogenic bladder cases the most usually found organisms are *Escherichia coli, Staphylococcus albus* and *Proteus vulgaris*. Unless there is a retention catheter, which makes sterilization of the urine impossible with any drug, Mandelamine will cure about a third of these cases in 30–90 days. It is certainly the safest of all drugs for such prolonged use. However, the consensus is that its use had as well be abandoned if bacteria are still present after 6 months of therapy. When a patient is to be operated upon many men feel it advisable to use Mandelamine in preparation, then give sulfonamides or antibiotics maximally for a few days before and after operation, and return to Mandelamine. In this way maximal efficacy can be expected with minimal toxicity.

The adult dosage is 3 of the 250 mg. tablets taken orally after meals and also on retiring, without any restrictions regarding diet or liquids ingested. Infants may be given 250 mg. twice daily in the form of the suspension, children over 5 years of age, three times daily. The urine must be acid to obtain the sterilizing action residing in both fractions of this compound. Mandelic acid acts bactericidally as such in acid urine; the active antiseptic property of methenamine is the formaldehyde which will split off from it only in an acid medium. Mandelamine tends to acidify the urine, but if there is a urinary pH of 7.0 or more this should be reduced to 6.0 or less (Nitrazine Paper changes color at pH 5.5). Advisable practice when the pH is too high in the beginning is to give ammonium chloride in 3 or 4 day courses of 1–2 Gm. at 4–6 hour intervals around the clock; resting a few days between courses is sufficient. The commercially available enteric-coated tablets are designed to lessen gastric irritation, which they undoubtedly do, but it is not unlikely that some of them also traverse the entire tract undissolved. The drug may also be acceptably given in the form of a flavored prescription containing 1 Gm. (15 gr.) per teaspoonful.

Since ammonium chloride cannot be used continuously without losing its acidifying properties, and during the rest period between courses the Mandelamine is not effectively chemotherapeutic, some men prefer to use methionine (Meonine) as an acidifying agent. Initial daily dosage is 8–18 Gm. in adults and 2–6 Gm. in children. But this medication is rather expensive.

D. P. Zangwill, P. J. Porter, A. L. Kaitz, R. S. Cortran, P. T. Bodel and E. H. Kass (Boston). Antibacterial Organic Acids in Chronic Urinary Tract Infection: Use in Long-Term Management. Arch. Int. Med. 110:801, 1962.

"When acidifying the urine in connection with the use of Mandelamine in the treatment of a urinary tract infection, is there any danger of going too far in the process?"

Reply: You should not raise the urinary acidity too much in elderly individuals and not forget either that the susceptibility of the kidney to infection could be increased by acidification unless, of course, the acidification is completely suppressing the bacteriuria.

"One of my urologist associates is using cephalothin (Keflin) in bladder irrigation during cystoscopy. What is the record of this agent?"

Reply: At the New York Presbyterian Hospital, Seneca and associates found the drug to be an excellent antibacterial agent for incorporation into bladder and kidney irrigating solutions. They made careful comparison of 106 patients cystoscoped with use of cephalothin instillation, with a similar number in which only saline solution was used, and not only found a larger number of cases negative at the end of the procedures using cephalothin but that a statistically significantly smaller number became positive after instrumentation in the treated group. The spectrum of the drug was found sufficiently broad to cover most contaminants, there was no toxicity locally, and the drug was felt to have the advantage over neomycin and bacitracin of not being nephrotoxic.

Harry Seneca, John K. Lattimer, Margaret Reilly and Patricia Peer. Cephalothin in Cystoscopy and Retrograde Pyelography. J. Urol. 94:489, 1965.

"I have a young patient with urinary tract infection that has not responded to any of the drugs in current use. Could I hope for anything from kanamycin (Kantrex)?"

Reply: Yes. Yahiro and Rosenthal (University of Illinois) studied the use of this antibiotic in children with urinary tract infections, since it is related to neomycin and streptomycin and has an antibacterial spectrum in both gram-positive and gram-negative organisms. The results were very good in acute cases, not quite so good in the chronic ones. But you must remember that the drug has considerable aural and renal toxicity, and that it must be given intramuscularly. *Dosage*: 20 mg./kg./day, in divided doses every 6 or 12 hours for 7 days.

Ernest I. Yahiro and Ira M. Rosenthal. Kanamycin (Kantrex) in Urinary Tract Infections in Childhood. J. Pediat. 55:744, 1959.

"In our hospital we have been studying first acute urinary tract infections in infants and children, finding as others have done a predilection for females. *Escherichia coli* and *Paracolobactrum* have been the predominating organisms, and the patients have received either a triple sulfonamide (Sulfose, including sulfadiazine, sulfamerazine and sulfamethazine) in dosage of 100–150 mg./kg. daily or nitrofurantoin (Furadantin) in dosage of 5.7 mg./kg daily. Both drugs are given orally in three or four divided doses per day. We have achieved eradication of bacteria from the urine in all instances, but recurrence has taken place in 24% of the patients, equally divided between the two drug-treated groups. Now what has caused these relapses?"

Reply: At Boston University, Charles Pryles and associates studied this matter very closely and concluded that a relapse must be regarded as evidence of a complication until the possibility is ruled out. In their series pyelography revealed an abnormality in one fourth of the cases, but these were mild abnormalities and not helpful in uncovering patients most likely to have a recurrence. Measurement of residual urine by catheter was also not helpful. BUN was somewhat elevated in a few patients but returned to normal in all, and serum creatinine was normal in every instance.

Charles V. Pryles, Brian A. Wherrett and Joan M. McCarthy. Urinary Tract Infections in Infants and Children: Long-Term Prospective Study; Interim Report on Results of Six Weeks' Chemotherapy. Am. J. Dis. Child. 108:1, 1964.

"Of course it is axiomatic that the treatment of urinary infections in children include an attempt to prevent persistence or recurrence because the end result of recurrent urinary infection may frequently be progressive renal damage. But how often is it successful?"

Reply: Oh, prolonged maintenance chemotherapy has been encouragingly reported upon a number of times. A recent favorable study was that of Normand and Smellie at the University College Hospital, London, who treated 29 boys and 87 girls with continuous maintenance dosage for at least 6 months after control of the presenting infection. Ages of these children at onset ranged from 3 weeks to 12 years, the mean age at onset being 1.9 years in the 46 children with single attacks and 6.1 years in the 70 with recurrent attacks. The 31 patients with normal radiologic findings and no history of previous urinary infection received chemotherapy for a total of 38 patient-years. One child had a recurrence during treatment, and another had one after treat-

ment. Three of the 19 children with normal radiologic findings and a history of recurrent infection and recurrences during treatment, and 5 of the 8 who completed treatment, had recurrences after treatment. Only 2 of the 15 children with x-ray changes and no history of previous infection had relapses during treatment. In the 38 patients with x-ray changes and a history of recurrent infection who were treated by chemotherapy alone, the average frequency of attacks was reduced from about 2.6 to about 0.3 per year, and 25 patients had no recurrence. The 26 patients treated surgically after recurrent infection had 117 attacks in 56 patient-years before treatment and 25 attacks in 45 patient-years after discharge from the hospital.

I. C. S. Normand and Jean M. Smellie. Prolonged Maintenance Chemotherapy in Management of Urinary Infection in Childhood. Brit. M. J. 1:1023, Apr. 17, 1965.

VAGINITIS

"In the treatment of nonspecific vaginitis with its multiplicity of causes, I try to keep medication as simple as possible and have relied principally upon simple vinegar douches. The patients frequently feel that I should know some trick better than that. What are some of the useful agents?"

Reply: Well, of course what you are trying to accomplish with your vinegar douche is to provide a vaginal acid pH to encourage regrowth of normal vaginal flora through elimination of pathogens, and it is doubtful if the commercial preparations will do it any more satisfactorily than the household agent you have been using. However, the ones that have considerable vogue are Domogyn douche powder, Massengill Powder and Aci-Jel. Unless you feel that there is special indication, I should hesitate to use antibacterial agents topically in this situation—such for example as Sultrin Triple Sulfa Cream, Ortho-Creme, Gantrisin Cream, or the nitrofurazone preparations, Furacin Insert and Furacin Vaginal Suppositories—for fear of inducing a local or systemic allergic reaction.

"I have used gentian violet with fair satisfaction through the years in the treatment of *Candida albicans* vaginitis, but latterly there has been increasing complaint of irritation following painting of the vaginal walls with the solution, and I have not found suppositories effective. Can you suggest anything?"

Reply: Perhaps you have been using the agent in too great concentration? The 0.5% aqueous solution is much less irritating than the stronger solutions and usually found to be just as effective. Or you might switch to an iodine compound, though with these you may have some irritation also: Betadine Vaginal Gel or Betadine Douche. The hydroxyquinoline preparations (Floraquin, Vioform) are sometimes useful, but of course they also contain some iodine. Then there are the preparations containing propionic, ricinoleic and caprylic acids, of which Caprylium Vaginal Creme and Propion Gel are examples.

"In a menopausal woman in whom estrogens do not seem indicated for systemic effect, has success usually been achieved with their local use for atrophic (senile) vaginitis?"

Reply: They are certainly so used frequently, usually in combination with a chemotherapeutic agent. For example, at Baylor University, James Friedman and Norman Olsen reported satisfactory clinical improvement in 84% of a group of 50 patients in this category and corresponding changes in vaginal cytology in 86%. Of the 5 patients requiring retreatment, 4 obtained satisfactory results. The preparation used was Furestrol Vaginal Suppository, which contains 0.006 grams of nitrofurazone and 0.00025 grams of diethylstilbestrol. The course of treatment comprised the insertion of a suppository into the vagina nightly for 12 nights.

James A. Friedman and Norman Olsen. Nitrofurazone-Estrogen Vaginal Suppositories in Treatment of Atrophic Vaginitis. J. Am. Geriatrics Soc. 13:828, 1965.

VARICOSE VEINS

"What are the contraindications to injection treatment of varicose veins?"

Reply: E. J. Orbach offered the following list: (1) huge superficial veins with wide open communications to deeper veins; (2) allergic conditions and acute infections; (3) acute superficial phlebitis; (4) underlying arterial disease; (5) varicosities caused by abdominal and pelvic tumors; (6) uncontrolled diabetes mellitus, thyrotoxicosis, tuberculosis, neoplasms, asthma, sepsis, blood dyscrasias, acute respiratory or skin diseases; (7) last trimester of pregnancy; (8) uncooperative and undependable patient.

One should perhaps add to this that any condition causing the patient to be bedridden is a contraindication; further, neurotic individuals stand these treatments, like everything else, very poorly.

E. J. Orbach. Has Injection Treatment of Varicose Veins Become Obsolete? J.A.M.A. 166:1964, 1958.

VENEREAL DISEASES

"Now that the incidence of syphilis and gonorrhea is increasing throughout the world it would be interesting to know to what extent the concomitant increase in penicillin allergic sensitivity will force us to the use of the less satisfactory alternative orally administered tetracyclines. Has this matter been studied?"

Reply: Yes, in data collected from the large material available to him at St. Mary's Hospital in London, R. R. Willcox has determined that prescribed penicillin schedules can be followed in 94–96% of cases. He believes that, since the degree of "penicillinization" of the population has become stabilized and is no longer increasing, and provided the drug is withheld from suspected allergic subjects, his evidence suggests that the problem of allergic reactions in venereal disease patients is not one that continues to increase in magnitude.

R. R. Willcox. Influence of Penicillin Allergic Reactions on Venereal Disease Control Programs. Brit. J. Ven. Dis. 40: 200, 1964.

"The two principal venereal diseases, gonorrhea and syphilis, resemble each other closely nowadays in that they are both increasing considerably in incidence. Are there still the marked therapeutic similarities also?"

Reply: If by "therapeutic similarity" you mean in their striking and absolute response to penicillin in the acute stages, the answer must be no, for the gonococcus is becoming resistant to the classic drug and the necessity for devising new ways of combating it is upon us, whereas syphilis has not in the least diminished in its responsiveness. The latter point is made very clearly in the study of Jefferiss and Willcox, using the vast material at St. Mary's Hospital, London. In their series of 547 males and 89 females there were 211 with seronegative primary syphilis, 179 with seropositive primary syphilis, 196 with secondary syphilis, and 50 with early latent syphilis in the first year of infection. The patients were instructed to return for examination monthly for 6 months, every 3 months for a year and every 6 months for a second year. Follow-up of 11–15 months or more was achieved in 57.9% and for 2–2½ years or more in 37.4%. Results were excellent. Ignoring 1 woman treated for secondary syphilis and retreated 7 months later while completely seronegative (because she was pregnant), retreatment was necessary within 2½ years for 17 patients, or 3.1% of those followed. The serologic findings were also impressive. By 22 months or more after treatment, the Wassermann test was negative in 98.6% of the patients and the VDRL test in 95%. The results of cerebrospinal fluid examinations when indicated were all normal except that 1 patient who had seronegative primary syphilis had a protein content of 40 mg./100 ml. with a colloidal gold reaction of 11111000. Actually it was felt that most, possibly all, of the cases in which retreatment was required were due to reinfection, an opinion which was supported by the high proportion showing chancres at new sites; another supporting fact was the high proportion of extremely promiscuous homosexuals among those requiring retreatment. Certainly, then, it appears that the treatment of early syphilis with penicillin is yielding as good effects now as formerly and that it is still unnecessary to supplement the drug with the use of other agents.

F. J. G. Jefferiss and R. R. Willcox. Treatment of Early Syphilis with Penicillin Alone. Brit. J. Ven. Dis. 39:143, 1963.

"How frequent are penicillin reactions in patients with venereal disease? How often are they serious or fatal? To what extent do they interfere with the treatment of the patient or with venereal disease control as a whole? Is the problem increasing?"

Reply: In London, R. R. Willcox has answered these questions from the immense material at St. Mary's Hospital. Data on over 74,500 cases of venereal disease showed a reported incidence of under 1% of penicillin reactions when only one injection of the drug was made, but with multiple injection techniques the reaction rate was 6.6–10.2%. From a survey of 858,024 patients it was estimated that there was one death per 78,002 treated. Willcox feels that once the degree of "penicillinization" of the population has become stabilized and is no longer increasing, and provided that the drug is withheld from suspected allergic patients, the evidence suggests that the problem of allergic reactions is not one that continues to increase in magnitude. A previous history of allergy contraindicated the use of penicillin in 1.75–3.58% of the cases in and around London. He makes the additional point that though some reactions occur if multiple injections are given, the late occurrence of many of them will insure that all but a few patients will have already received a curative dose of the antibiotic.

R. R. Willcox. Influence of Penicillin Allergic Reactions on Venereal Disease Control Programs. Brit. J. Ven. Dis. 40:200, 1964.

"Recent experience with a case of gonorrhea

causes me to wonder whether the asymptomatic male carrier of living gonococci exists as a companion to the well known asymptomatic female carrier?"*

Reply: Suggestive evidence that this may be the case was offered by John Lentz and associates (Philadelphia) several years ago; 2 patients were found to be asymptomatic carriers of gonococci after apparent cure of their acute gonorrheal urethritis. Organisms isolated from the urine fulfilled all cultural criteria for gonococci, but whether these organisms were present as a result of the original treated infection or a subsequent asymptomatic reinfection could not be determined; it seemed to the observers, however, that the former possibility was more likely. But certainly neither the prevalence of asymptomatic male carriers nor their importance in control of gonorrhea has been established; much study needs still to be done.

John W. Lentz, Donald N. MacVicar and Henry R. Beilstein. Use of Tetracycline with Amphotericin B for Gonorrhea in Males. Pub. Health Rep. 77:653, 1962.

"What are the other drugs that have been shown to be effective in the treatment of acute gonorrhea when penicillin fails?"

Reply: The following is probably a full list of the drugs shown to date to be effective in gonorrhea: penicillin, the newer penicillins, tetracyclines, spiramycin, erythromycin, chloramphenicol, actinospectacin, streptomycin with a sulfonamide.

R. R. Willcox (St. Mary's Hospital, London). Review of Treatment of Gonorrhea with Drugs Other Than Penicillin. Acta dermat.-venereol. 42:484, 1962.

"Gonorrhea is increasing sufficiently in our area so that we must all become conversant again with the treatment methods. Has the controversy been resolved regarding the existence nowadays of penicillin-resistant strains of the organism?"

Reply: Oh, I think so. There is an immense literature, but I believe that the study of Kjellander and Finland (Harvard Medical School) adequately answered the investigators who have doubted that increasing resistance of the gonococcus adequately explains the failure of some cases to respond to penicillin dosage that had been previously effective. They found that one can still expect 100% of success with penicillin in usual dosage if the organism is sensitive to in vitro tests and if there are no other penicillinase-producing organisms present. In 1960, Gentele and associates first drew attention to the concomitant presence of penicillinase-producing organisms in the urethra; and Finland's study supplied at least suggestive support for this.

Jan Olof Kjellander and Maxwell Finland. Penicillin Treatment of Gonorrheal Urethritis: Effects of Penicillin Susceptibility of Causative Organism and Concomitant Presence of Penicillinase-Producing Bacteria on Results. New England J. Med. 269:834, Oct. 17, 1963. B. Gentele and A. Lagerholm. Penicillinase-Producing Concomitant Organisms in the Male Urethra in Gonorrhea. Acta dermat.-venereol. 40:256, 1960.

"Is there any reason to believe that one should treat a male gonorrheal patient whose infection has been of rather long standing more intensively than one would treat a fresher infection?"

Reply: The answer to this question has been difficult to determine, but on the basis of relatively limited experience, by which I mean a relatively small number of cases, Pamela Wray, at the Royal Hospital in Sheffield, found that relapses are commoner in individuals with prolonged duration of infection than in more acute cases, and she therefore felt it possibly true that treatment for acute gonorrhea of comparatively long standing in the male should be more intensive than for that of short duration.

Pamela M. Wray. Clinical Aspects of Penicillin Failure in Gonorrhoea. Brit. J. Ven. Dis. 41:117, 1965.

"In a patient with acute gonorrhea, who was sensitive to penicillin, I recently tried nalidixic acid (NegGram) in dosage of 2 Gm. twice daily for 2 days and could not observe that it had much effect. Has the matter been studied?"

Reply: Yes it has, but by only one observer so far as I am aware. In Bradford, England, Leonard Oller gave the drug to 74 male patients, with results indicating definitely limited antigonorrheal action. He advised that the drug be taken at intervals of not less than 6 hours over at least 30 hours, and that individual doses should not be less than 2 grams with an initial loading dose of 4 grams. Even with this regimen some patients could not reach what he considered to be the adequate plasma level, 25 μg./ml., probably because of either poor absorption or rapid elimination. Of course the necessity to give the drug in multiple doses is a disadvantage, but the fact that it has no effect on *Treponema pallidum* makes it a probable drug of choice in cases of gonorrhea in which concomitant early syphilis is suspected.

Leonard Z. Oller. Treatment of Gonorrhoea with Nalidixic Acid. Brit. J. Ven. Dis. 40:256, 1964.

"What is the efficacy of ampicillin (Penbritin, Polycillin) in acute gonorrhea in men?"

Reply: At St. Mary's Hospital, London, R. R. Willcox determined in an adequate number of cases that 1,200,000 units of aqueous procaine penicillin gives the best results in acute gonorrhea; that indifferent results may be obtained with single injections of 250–500 mg. of ampicillin, and that the failure rates obtained with this method of using ampicillin can be halved by giving 500–1000 mg. in a single oral dose.

R. R. Willcox. Ampicillin by Injection and by Mouth in the Treatment of Acute Gonorrhoea. Brit. J. Ven. Dis. 40:261, 1964.

"What dosage of penicillin appears nowadays to be required in the treatment of acute gonorrhea in the male?"

Reply: The 600,000 unit daily dosage for 4 consecutive days, formerly recommended, has now been found relatively ineffective. The Venereal Disease Branch of the USPHS recommends a total dosage of 1,200,000–2,400,000 units and maintenance of blood levels for at least 48 hours. Actually, numerous observers have found that the administration of a single dose of 2,400,000 units (concurrent injections of 1,200,000 units in each hip) is the treatment to be preferred.

H. C. Gjessing (Dept. of Health, Oslo) and K. Ödegaard (State Inst. of Public Health, Oslo). Sensitivity of Gonococcus to Antibiotics and Treatment of Gonorrhea. Acta dermat.-venereol. 44:132, 1964. Lynn T. Staheli. Duration of Therapy in Management of Gonorrhea. J.A.M.A. 190:854, Nov. 30, 1964.

"How do the several penicillins fit into the therapeutic picture in gonorrhea nowadays when there is such an upsurge in the prevalence of the disease?"

Reply: In a considerable experience at Saint Mary's Hospital, London, in which 1,200,000 units of aqueous procaine penicillin was used as standard therapy, R. R. Willcox obtained better results with 0.5 Gm. ampicillin (Polycillin, Penbritin) and observed that the same drug produced substantially better results than obtained with double the dose of phenethicillin (Syncillin, etc.) and phenoxymethyl penicillin (V-Cillin, etc.). Benzathine penicillin (Bicillin, etc.) proved entirely unsatisfactory in his hands. Ampicillin, the successful competitor with aqueous penicillin, in the dosage used was more effective than four times the dosage of oxytetracycline (Terramycin).

R. R. Willcox. Ampicillin (Penbritin) in Treatment of Gonorrhea. Brit. J. Ven Dis. 39:164, 1963.

"In view of the current rising incidence of gonorrhea, how shall one approach the prophylaxis of

gonorrheal ophthalmia neonatorum: silver nitrate or penicillin?"

Reply: In reviewing this subject, Paul Barsam, at the Massachusetts Department of Public Health, concluded that the continued routine use of 1% silver nitrate appears to be still the necessary prophylactic measure.

Paul C. Barsam. Specific Prophylaxis of Gonorrheal Ophthalmia Neonatorum: A Review. New England J. Med. 274:731, Mar. 31, 1966.

"What is the law regarding the prophylaxis of gonorrheal ophthalmia neonatorum in the several states?"

Reply: The following recapitulation was prepared by the National Society for the Prevention of Blindness, as of October, 1965, according to Paul Barsam: Twenty-two states now require the use of silver nitrate as the sole prophylactic agent specified by law or regulation. Eight states permit the substitution of other substances for investigation purposes only. Alaska, California, Iowa, Maryland, Mississippi and Missouri specifically allow for the administration of penicillin. Idaho discontinued the use of penicillin, February, 1964. Five states allow for the alternative use of silver nitrate or "an equally effective agent." In four states substances other than silver nitrate may be given only by physicians in hospitals. Montana, Nevada and Ohio make no stipulation about the substance that may be administered. Wyoming requires the use of erythromycin ophthalmic ointment, but an attending physician can prescribe any additional medication. Alabama, Delaware and New Mexico allow for the use of silver nitrate, Argyrol, Protargol or acceptable equivalents as specified by the state board of health. Seven states permit the administration of antibiotics in addition to silver nitrate. Finally, the health departments of 33 states furnish silver nitrate for use as prophylaxis. No other prophylactic agent is similarly supplied by any state.

Paul C. Barsam. Specific Prophylaxis of Gonorrheal Ophthalmia Neonatorum: A Review. New England J. Med. 274:731, Mar. 31, 1966.

"With the upswing in the incidence of gonorrhea one may expect at almost any time to see again a case of acute purulent gonorrheal conjunctivitis as in earlier times. How should one treat such a case?"

Reply: In Portland, Oregon, Terry Hansen and associates have reported 4 such cases, 2 in adults and 2 in newborns, the 2 latter occurring despite the fact that the hospital records showed that 1% silver nitrate drops

had been placed in the eyes at birth. The patients were isolated and examined for gonorrheal infection in other parts of the body, and treatment was started before cultural confirmation was obtained. All 4 patients responded rapidly to topical eyedrops containing penicillin G, 10,000 units/ml., instilled initially every 15 minutes. Additional penicillin was given intramuscularly in appropriate dosage and sterile sodium chloride solution was used to wash out the purulent discharge which collected in the conjunctival sac.

Terry Hansen, Robert P. Burns and Aurelia Allen. Gonorrheal Conjunctivitis: An Old Disease Returned. J.A.M.A. 195:1156, Mar. 28, 1966.

"In a practice in which the patient with acute gonorrhea will be seen only a single time, what would seem to be the best treatment in view of the fact that some strains of the gonococcus are partially resistant to penicillin?"

Reply: In Oslo, Gjessing and Ödegaard give an injection of 600,000 units of procaine penicillin G combined with a single dose of 1 Gm. ampicillin (Penbritin, Polycillin), the latter taken as 4 tablets of 0.25 Gm. each, swallowed under supervision. In their series of 500 males there was a 3% failure rate. I would like to add, however, that in several very active venereal disease clinics it has been found that a single intramuscular injection of 2,400,000 units of procaine penicillin G effects a very high cure rate; 97.9% in the experience of Gamil Ashamalla's group in a California jail population.

H. C. Gjessing and K. Ödegaard. Intramuscular Injection of Procaine Penicillin Combined with Oral Administration of Ampicillin in the Treatment of Gonorrhoea. Brit. J. Ven. Dis. 41:48, 1965. Gamil Ashamalla, Ronald Walters and Marcus Crahan. Recent Clinicolaboratory Observations in the Treatment of Acute Gonococcal Urethritis in Men. J.A.M.A. 195:1115, Mar. 28, 1966.

"I have not had much experience with syphilis because during my time in training, and since in practice, the disease has been very little in evidence, but in the last couple of years I have had a number of fresh infectious cases—and what is worrying me particularly is that I have recently had what appears to be a recrudescence of the disease in a patient whom I felt certain I had cured. Is penicillin losing its grip? What is going on?"

Reply: What is going on is that the times have changed so that numerous factors are now conspiring to produce the increase in the incidence of syphilis that is occurring throughout the world. Penicillin is to a considerable extent both directly and indirectly responsible for this. During the early penicillin years, when the drug was widely prescribed for all sorts of ailments, it is very likely that a good many cases of syphilis were inadvertently cured during the incubation period without coming to the knowledge of either the patient or his physician. But then penicillin reactions came to the fore, the scare set in, and the promiscuous use of penicillin decreased very much. One result of this has been the appearance of more fresh cases of syphilis than were being seen in the early days of penicillin. Another reason for the disease's reappearance is the fact that when penicillin is used in treatment of an early case the cure is so rapid that the patient has little or no time to develop an appreciable immunity, and as a result he may be quickly reinfected. This is almost certainly what has happened to your patient if you were sure that your treatment of his initial infection was effectively curative. Penicillin has definitely not lost its antitreponemal power; indeed you can see from what I have just said how the retention of its power contributes to the present upsurge in the number of acute cases. Another factor in this situation having directly to do with drugs is that gonorrhea, having become to some extent resistant to penicillin, is now often treated with antibiotics other than penicillin, and these drugs are much less likely to suppress incubating syphilis in the patient. Another contributing factor is the fact that young people who were formerly to a considerable extent protected through the widespread use of penicillin for other maladies now tend quite often to have broad-spectrum antibiotics used for these maladies rather than penicillin. Then, too, the widespread knowledge that penicillin is a fully effective agent in the cure of syphilis has engendered a feeling of security in the general population, who no longer feel syphilis to be the serious matter that it was formerly held to be. And then there is that great congeries of things that has altered life so much in the industrialized nations in recent decades: the surge of country folk into the cities and the congested living conditions in many of the latter; the alteration in transportation facilities which will now take almost anyone from anywhere to somewhere else in a matter of hours or of days at most, and much syphilis is "foreign" contracted; the good wages being earned by young people, the increase in consumption of alcohol by them, the increased freedom with which the sexes intermingle, the lowering of moral standards (or should one say the recession of fear?), the rise in homosexuality. No, very definitely, penicillin is not failing us but other things are.

Brit. M. J. (Leading Article) 1:433, Aug. 21, 1965. W. H. O. Chronicle 18:451, 1964. A. C. Curtis. J.A.M.A. 186:46, 1963. I. L. Schamberg. Brit. J. Ven. Dis. 39:87, 1963.

"Is there any evidence that *Treponema pallidum* survives in humans after adequate antisyphilitic penicillin therapy?"

Reply: There is not.

"Now that syphilis has 'returned' and we are all acquainting or reacquainting ourselves with its penicillin treatment, I should like very much to know what happens to the untreated syphilitic."

Reply: Several thorough investigations of this matter have been made, notably the Tuskegee study in male Negroes in the South, the Rosahn study at Yale and the Oslo study in Norway. The latter, being probably the most informative, has been succinctly reviewed by Clark and Danbolt at Columbia University and the University of Oslo. This study stemmed from the deep conviction of Professor Boeck of Oslo that the specific treatment of his time was completely inadequate, which led him to hospitalize 1978 patients with primary and secondary syphilis for periods of from 1 to 12 months until all traces of the disease had disappeared. His study covered a 20 year period, 1891–1910. In 1929, E. Bruugaard, Boeck's successor, reported on a follow-up study of 473 of these patients, and then from 1928 to 1951, Gjestland made an epidemiologic restudy of this entire unique clinical material. From Clark and Danbolt's 1964 review of this important contribution to the syphilologic literature, the following items may be gleaned to satisfy your wish.

Clinical secondary relapse was shown not to be related only to inadequate treatment of early syphilis, since it developed in 23.6% of this untreated group within 5 years of discharge from the hospital, approximately one fourth of the patients having multiple episodes. Benign late syphilis occurred in 14.4% of males and 16.7% of females as early as the first and as late as the forty-sixth year, developing in most instances by the fifteenth year. Cardiovascular syphilis developed in 13.6% of males and 7.6% of females, but it did not develop in either sex if the individual had been infected before the age of 15. There were twice as many males as females who developed neurosyphilis, and this complication did occur in those infected before the age of 15 but not in males infected after the age of 40. Of those with neurosyphilis who died, the death was attributed to this complication in two thirds of the instances. Syphilis was the primary cause of death in 15.1% of the males and 8.3% of the females; among males the disease ranked second and among females fifth as a cause of death; I think, however, that one must interpolate here the statement that much of this information was gathered in a period when tuberculosis still was a leading cause of death. While it could be estimated from the study that between 60 and 70 out of every 100 of the patients went through life with a minimum of inconvenience despite no treatment for early syphilis, this can be restated to mean that syphilis can cause serious difficulties among 30–40% of all those who remain untreated; and finally, if an additional reason for treatment is needed, it must be pointed out that untreated syphilis is a transmissible disease.

E. Gurney Clark and Niels Danbolt. The Oslo Study of the Natural Course of Untreated Syphilis. M. Clin. North America 48:613, 1964. Donald H. Rockwell, Anne Roof Yobs and M. Brittain Moore, Jr. The Tuskegee Study of Untreated Syphilis. Arch. Int. Med. 114:792, 1964. P. D. Rosahn. Autopsy Studies in Syphilis, J. Vener. Dis. Inform. (Suppl. 21) 24:684, 1940.

"Has acquired resistance to penicillin in syphilis ever been recorded?"

Reply: In the resurgence of syphilis that is now occurring throughout the world there has been no evidence of initial or acquired resistance to the drug in acute cases. However, in Poland, Dowzenko and Krysztofiak have shown that in some rare cases of meningo-vascular syphilis the disease process may relapse even after several years of improvement in the cerebrospinal fluid findings and after the disappearance of a positive Wassermann reaction in the fluid. They reported 2 cases of this sort in which the syphilitic process was at first penicillin-sensitive and then became resistant not only to penicillin but to Aureomycin, Chloromycetin and Signemycin and also to malaria therapy.

A. Dowzenko and B. Krysztofiak. Relapses in the Cerebrospinal Fluid and Acquired Resistance to Penicillin in Cases of Neurosyphilis. J. Neurol. Sci. 2:197, 1965.

"What is the most frequently employed antibiotic for the treatment of syphilis in a patient with known penicillin allergy, and has it been successfully used in the pregnant woman?"

Reply: To the first part of your question I would reply that probably erythromycin estolate (Ilosone) is most frequently employed in dosage of 500 mg. four times daily for 10 days, although 15 instead of the 20 Gm. spread out through this 10 day period has also been shown to be effective. Regarding your second question, I can only answer that Mary Ann South and associates, in Houston, successfully treated a young woman with secondary syphilis 2 months before her delivery with 500 mg. of erythromycin estolate three times daily for 10 days (thus totalling 15 Gm.), but

that the infant developed signs of congenital syphilis and died during the third day of life. There have been reports that a total dose of 30 Gm. is satisfactory during pregnancy, but the fact has not been fully established.

Mary Ann South, David H. Short and John M. Knox. Failure of Erythromycin Estolate Therapy in In Utero Syphilis. J.A.M.A. 190:182, Oct. 5, 1964.

"I have a patient in my practice who is experiencing the severe lightning pains of tabes dorsalis. Was any non-narcotic analgesic measure of worth developed during the days before the 'disappearance' of syphilis?"

Reply: No, I am afraid not, though I will bring to your attention Joseph Green's successful treatment of 2 patients with diphenyl-hydantoin (Dilantin). The relief accomplished was said not only to have been remarkable while use of the drug was persisted in, but it could also be obtained recurrently when the pain came back after use of the drug had been stopped.

Joseph B. Green. Dilantin in Treatment of Lightning Pains. Neurology 11:257, 1961.

"Which of the antibiotics is used most successfully in treating granuloma inguinale?"

Reply: The tetracyclines, streptomycin and chloramphenicol appear to be equally effective.

"Shall I use an antibiotic or a sulfonamide in treating lymphogranuloma venereum?"

Reply: Here is one of the maladies that is still more susceptible to sulfonamides than to the antibiotics, among which latter, however, the tetracyclines may sometimes be equally useful particularly in the early stages of the disease. It is doubtful if either sulfonamides or antibiotics truly eradicate this infection.

"With the resurgence of acute syphilis we are planning for a broad-scale therapeutic attack upon the disease in our area. Included in the plan is an examination of the cerebrospinal fluid as a test of cure not less than 2 years after adequate treatment of early syphilis. We recognize of course that such testing will be difficult of accomplishment, and some of us are wondering whether it is really necessary. Has the matter been studied?"

Reply: At a large venereal disease clinic in Ceylon the test of cure that you propose was applied to a group of 151 patients at least 2 (average 3.05) years after their adequate treatment with penicillin in the acute stage of the disease. Of these cases, 25 had been seronegative primary, 90 seropositive primary, and 36 in the secondary stage. The VDRL was positive at the time of the lumbar puncture in 10 cases, of which 2 were possibly serorelapses (there was no history of reinfection), 4 had had one or more attacks of gonorrhea during the follow-up period, and 2 were reinfected with syphilis. None of these 10 patients had any abnormality in the cerebrospinal fluid. The remaining 141 (93%) of the 151 patients were seronegative at the time of lumbar puncture. Reporting these findings, W. L. Fernando felt that the matter of abandoning the cerebrospinal fluid examination as a routine test of cure needs reconsideration.

W. L. Fernando. Cerebrospinal Fluid Findings After Treatment of Early Syphilis with Penicillin. Brit. J. Ven. Dis. 41:168, 1965.

"How is it most advisable to treat chancroid?"

Reply: Of the several antibiotics to which the Ducrey bacillus is sensitive, streptomycin seems to be the most effective in daily dosage of 1.0 gram intramuscularly for 7–10 days. However, since this antibiotic also has some activity against the treponema of syphilis, it is considered preferable by most observers to begin the treatment of chancroid with one of the sulfonamides in dosage of 1.0 gram four times daily for the 7–10 days.

VINCENT'S ANGINA

"While it is true that penicillin effects a fairly rapid cure in most cases of Vincent's angina there are nevertheless a few that are stoutly resistant. Has anything new been suggested?"

Reply: Yes, in England, D. L. S. Shinn found to his surprise that a patient suffering from trichomonal vaginitis and Vincent's angina was cured of both diseases when treated with metronidazole (Flagyl) prescribed for the trichomoniasis. With associates he then treated 20 cases of the Vincent disorder alone and obtained an excellent response in all. Pain had in most instances disappeared by 24 hours and halitosis by 48 hours; ulceration and hemorrhage were resolving at 48 hours, and at 96 hours had cleared completely except in 3 patients who had some slight ulceration. All the patients seen at 14 days showed complete resolution and no recurrence of the disease.

D. L. S. Shinn. The Treatment of Vincent's Disease with Metronidazole. Dent. Practit. 15:275, 1965.

VITILIGO

"I have a case of vitiligo in my practice. What does one do for this thing?"

Reply: Perhaps the most effective treatment employed in recent decades is that with 8-methoxypsoralen (Meloxine, Oxsoralen). Lanceley's group (Kampala, Uganda) reported encouraging results in 41 Asians and 4 Africans. Dosage varied from 2.5 mg. in infants to 5 or 10 mg. in older children, with daily maintenance never exceeding 30 mg. Patients took the drug 2 hours before exposure to sunshine or ultraviolet light and began exposure to sunshine with 5 minutes daily followed by an increase of 1 minute daily. These investigators took care to select only otherwise healthy individuals for their study and excluded those with impaired hepatic or renal function. The trial included only a small number of individuals, and some of them had not been long under treatment, but it was said that in many of the patients repigmentation began in about 3 weeks; older children with extensive lesions of long duration responded slowly. You may expect that the regimen will be long, tedious, and time-consuming even in the most favorable cases. In reviewing the subject in 1958, Sulzberger and Lerner said that a satisfactory response is achieved in only about 1 out of every 7 patients treated. The most frequently seen toxic effects are headache, giddiness, anorexia, nausea, vomiting, epigastric pain, retrosternal discomfort, excessive sweating, jitteriness and failure to gain weight comparable to growth. The fact that derivatives of the plant *Ammi majus Linn* could restore pigment in vitiliginous lesions was known to the ancient Egyptians, but the active principals, the psoralens, were not extracted from the plants until 1947.

J. L. Lanceley, E. S. Lanceley and D. B. Jelliffe. Treatment of Vitiligo with 8-Methoxypsoralen in Uganda Children. J. Pediat. 60:572, 1962. Marion B. Sulzberger Aaron B. Lerner (Yale Univ.). Sun Tanning—Potentiation with Oral Medication. J.A.M.A. 167:2077, Aug. 23, 1958.

WARTS

"In my area in one of the effete Eastern states the natives practice all sorts of hocus-pocus in the treatment of warts. And it seems to work. What about this?"

Reply: I permit myself the most reprehensible of practices, quotation of self: "In Kentucky, in my childhood, the method was to rub the cut side of a potato on the wart, bury the potato and wait: I do not recall the results. A bit further west, in the land of Tom Sawyer, there was something about a bloody bean and a cat in the graveyard at midnight, if memory serves me correctly. The practice in Timbuctoo is not known to me. In Zurich some years ago, Bloch risked his reputation by asserting his belief that warts could be cured by suggestion; Sulzberger, who studied under Bloch, has stated that he also uses hocus-pocus effectively at times, and others have reported in the same vein. I wonder if this advances us very much?"

Harry Beckman. Treatment in General Practice. 6th Ed. Phila. W. B. Saunders Co., 1948, p. 916.

"What is being done with the topical injection of warts?"

Reply: At the University of Helsinki, M. H. Frick and associates injected 238 warts in 81 school children with 2% procaine hydrochloride solution or some modification of this. The injections were intracutaneously beneath the wart, blanching the skin and elevating the wart from its bed. Dosage was 0.4–0.8 ml./wart/injection. Two injections were made at an interval of 2 weeks except when cure was obtained after the first injection. They ascribed the results, which were said to be good, to the local pressure effect of the injected fluid causing a disturbance in the nutrition of the wart; nothing was said about a possible psychologic effect. The trouble was, which they admitted, that the business was very painful; the children probably had to be dragged in bodily for that second injection. In Tampa, Florida, Wesley Wilson reported the intralesional injection of hydroxychloroquine (Plaquenil) in a total of 637 warts; best response was had in plantar warts; injections of 0.1–0.5 ml./sq. cm. of a 40 mg./ml. preparation were said to result in no discomfort; treatments were given every 2–3 weeks.

M. H. Frick, L. Kantele and T. Putkonen. Treatment of Warts by Procaine Injections. Acta dermat.-venereol. 38:394, 1958. Wesley W. Wilson. Clinical Evaluation of Intralesional Administration of Hydroxychloroquine Sulfate (Plaquenil) in Several Diseases. South. M. J. 56:794, 1963.

"I have a patient with several small but unsightly warts on one eyelid, and I am fearful of attempting cauterization or other physical methods of removal at that site. Is there any drug that has been effective in such a situation?"

Reply: Rudolph Bock, in Palo Alto, has reported the successful use of a cantharides preparation in 22 of 27 cases. The drug was used as Cantharone, which is a 0.7% solution in equal parts of acetone and collodion. He recommends that the solution be kept stoppered to minimize evaporation and that it be handled very carefully because it is potentially dangerous to individuals hypersensitive to it. He applies a small drop to the surface of the wart, being careful to avoid touching the surrounding normal skin; a thin gray film of dry collodion forms in a few seconds, and no dressing is applied. On the second to fourth day the patient may experience some pain and a blister may form, lifting the wart. The application may be repeated two or three times at 8–10 day intervals if the wart has not disappeared after the first treatment. Thirteen of Bock's 27 patients had their warts removed with one application, 9 required repeated applications, and 5 did not respond at all.

Rudolph H. Bock. Treatment of Palpebral Warts with Cantharone. Am. J. Ophth. 60:529, 1965.

WEGENER'S GRANULOMATOSIS

"I have a patient with Wegener's granulomatosis, who has of course been everywhere and had all drugs poured into her. Is there anything _new_ that is worth trying?"

Reply: I really know of nothing.

WHIPPLE'S DISEASE

"I have a patient with Whipple's disease who has not done well on the corticosteroids but has been improving steadily for a short period of time on tetracycline. Since this disease is characterized pathologically by infiltration of the intestinal wall and lymphatics by macrophages filled with glycoprotein, how is it that an antibiotic can be helpful?"

Reply: In reporting their cases of the disease studied by electron microscopy, C. T. Ashworth's group, in Dallas, found large number of extracellular and intracellular bacilliform bodies in lesions, which disappeared completely from the intestinal mucosa concomitantly with clinical remission after tetracycline therapy. They presented reasons for the belief that these bodies are bacteria of a specific type which may possibly play a primary etiologic role in the disease, and that the characteristic foamy periodic acid–Schiff-positive macrophages of the disease result from persistence of the cell walls of the phagocytozed bodies.

C. T. Ashworth, F. C. Douglas, R. C. Reynolds and P. J. Thomas. Bacillus-Like Bodies in Whipple's Disease; Disappearance with Clinical Remission After Antibiotic Therapy. Am. J. Med. 37:481, 1964.

"I have recently had what appeared to be at

least limited success in a case of Whipple's disease through the use of antibiotics alone. What has been the general experience?"

Reply: In their carefully studied 10 patients at Duke University Medical Center, Ruffin's group tested the value of this therapy. Without going into a detailed discussion of their findings, I can say that the experience was sufficiently satisfactory so that patients at the Center were thereafter to be hospitalized and given 1,200,000 units of penicillin and 1 Gm. of streptomycin daily for 10–14 days, and then followed by 1 Gm. of tetracycline by mouth daily for 3–6 months. Nevertheless, one should remember that strong doubts regarding the efficacy of antibiotics versus the corticosteroids have been expressed by Gross et al., England et al. and Holt et al.

J. B. Gross et al. Gastroenterol. 36:65, 1959; M. T. England et al. ibid. 39:219, 1960; and P. R. Holt et al. New England J. Med. 264:1335, 1961. Julian M. Ruffin, Stanley M. Kurtz and Walter M. Ronfail. Intestinal Lipodystrophy (Whipple's Disease) J.A.M.A. 195:476, Feb. 7, 1966.

WHOOPING COUGH

"When one sees a case of whooping cough in this country nowadays, which is fortunately not often, it is in a quite young child and the situation is likely to be a serious one. Are any of the antibiotics really helpful?"

Reply: Hattie Alexander, who participated in a very thorough study of this matter at The Willard Parker Hospital, New York, in which streptomycin and chloramphenicol were compared with rabbit and human antibodies, says that while no definitive answers regarding efficacy of therapy were provided, it seemed to her that, if one is to use an antibiotic, chloramphenicol is the one of choice. She recommended dosage of 100 mg./kg. daily in three divided portions (not exceeding 2 Gm. daily) for 7 days.

Hattie E. Alexander. *In* Beeson and McDermott: Textbook of Medicine. Phila. W. B. Saunders Co., 1963, p. 215.

WILSON'S DISEASE

"I have a patient with hepatolenticular degeneration (Wilson's Disease) who has improved somewhat under penicillamine (Cuprimine) but has now developed the nephrotic syndrome. Is this a manifestation of the disease or due to the drug?"

Reply: It appears that the fatalities in this malady are the result of irreversible damage to the central nervous system or the liver, and the nephrotic syndrome is not a part of the picture. Some of the toxic effects of penicillamine can be very severe but are reversible if the drug is discontinued; such things as erythematous rashes, fever, leukopenia and pronounced thrombocytopenia. The nephrotic syndrome as part of the reaction to the drug, first reported in 1959, has been seen in at least 6 patients to my knowledge. In the patient of Hirschman and Isselbacher, at Massachusetts General Hospital, described in 1965, the manifestation gradually disappeared after discontinuance of the penicillamine and the administration of moderate doses of corticosteroids. The possibility of optic neuritis in association with the use of penicillamine has been brought to attention recently.

Shalmom Z. Hirschman and Kurt J. Isselbacher. The Nephrotic Syndrome as a Complication of Penicillamine Therapy for Hepatolenticular Degeneration (Wilson's Disease). Ann. Int. Med. 62:1297, 1965. Irmin Sternlieb and I. Herbert Scheinberg (New York). Penicillamine Therapy for Hepatolenticular Degeneration. J.A.M.A. 189:748, Sept. 7, 1964. Norman P. Goldstein, Robert W. Hollenhorst, Raymond V. Randall and John B. Gross. Possible Relationship of Optic Neuritis, Wilson's Disease and DL-Penicillamine Therapy. J.A.M.A. 196:734, May 23, 1966.

"Which of the symptoms of Wilson's disease can one hope most to influence through the use of penicillamine (Cuprimine)?"

Reply: Since penicillamine is a "decoppering agent" it may be presumed capable of abstracting the copper accumulated in all of the tissues. Deposition of copper in individuals with this disease leads to the tremor-rigidity syndrome as a result of effects upon the basal ganglions; in the liver it causes cirrhosis; in the kidneys, disturbances in renal tubular function with resultant glycosuria, aminoaciduria, phosphaturia and uricosuria of the low threshold type. There is also corneal deposition of copper. This is a rare disease and few individuals have seen many cases. The largest reported series that has come to my attention was that of J. M. Walshe, University of Cambridge, who reported on the use of penicillamine in 22 patients collected from 16 hospitals. Dosage in these patients varied from 500 mg. to 3 Gm. daily, 1 Gm. being given in most instances. Duration of therapy was from 4 weeks to 3 years, with an average of 1 year. Two of these patients, given the drug prophylactically before there was clinical evidence of neurologic involvement, did not present evidence of central nervous system involvement and neither of them deteriorated on maintenance therapy. Three patients did not improve or actually deteriorated under treatment, and in 17 there was a degree of benefit varying from slight to complete recovery.

One patient developed a serious erythematous rash and jacksonian convulsions, ascribable to the drug.

J. M. Walshe. Treatment of Wilson's Disease with Penicillamine. Lancet 1:188, Jan. 23, 1960.

"In my practice I have a 10-year-old boy with Wilson's hepatolenticular degeneration. With the aid of dedicated personnel I was able to maintain him for some time on a 75 Gm. protein diet with 24 hour copper intake limited to 1 mg.; potassium sulfide, 20 mg. three times daily with meals, with the intent of limiting copper absorption from the gut; and d-penicillamine, 1 Gm. daily in four divided doses. He was also given water-soluble vitamins and the diet was supplemented with 4 Gm. calcium lactate daily; ascites and peripheral edema were combated with monthly infusions of salt-poor albumin. But then an intensely pruritic maculopapular rash appeared over the trunk and extremities, accompanied by eosinophilia, and I was obliged to discontinue the penicillamine. When these disorders had disappeared, and penicillamine was resumed, we proceeded for some months without incident and with some evidences of improvement in the patient's clinical state; but recent studies are revealing diminution in the cupriuretic effect of the penicillamine and I am having to increase the dosage. What reasons for hopefulness may I present to the patient's family?"

Reply: Since you were only able to speak of "some evidences of improvement" when the patient was already on high penicillamine dosage and you are now having to give increased amounts of the drug, I am afraid that you have about reached the limit of what can be accomplished. However, dimercaprol (BAL) has been used with good effect. J. M. Walshe (University of Cambridge) gave this drug in short courses of 5–7 days, alone or combined with penicillamine, to 16 patients. There was notable improvement in 1, limited improvement in 3, and only temporary improvement in 1; but he felt that 5 of the patients had probably received inadequate amounts of the drug. As a guide to BAL dosage one may probably best follow the plan used in mild cases of arsenic or gold poisoning: four intramuscular injections daily (6 hour intervals) with 3 mg./kg. body weight on the first and second days, two injections on the third day, and one injection daily thereafter for 10 days or until recovery. At the University of Virginia, Fritz Dreifuss and William McKinney described a patient who had two successful pregnancies while under continuous therapy with BAL for 6 years. Dosage was 175 mg. twice daily for 10 days in each month with continuous administration of potassium sulfide capsules, 20 mg.

three times a day. A great handicap in approaching Wilson's disease therapeutically is that it is a congenital disorder in which there is a defective synthesis of ceruloplasmin, a protein that combines with and holds copper in the plasma; in the absence of sufficient amount of this protein, copper is free to escape into the tissues, which it does to a disastrous extent in the liver, kidneys and brain especially. Until we can develop more effective chelators of copper, or actually learn to overcome the ceruloplasmin deficiency, the situation seems pretty hopeless.

Victor G. Herring, III, Gerald Klatskin and Ira K. Brandt (New Haven, Connecticut). Hepatolenticular Degeneration: Observations on a Case Treated with d-Penicillamine. J. Pediat. 63 (Part 1):550, 1963. J. M. Walshe. Treatment of Wilson's Disease with Penicillamine. Lancet 1:188, Jan. 23, 1960. Fritz E. Dreifuss and William M. McKinney. Wilson's Disease and Pregnancy. J.A.M.A. 195:960, Mar. 14, 1966.

WORM AND FLUKE INFESTATIONS

"With the recent increase in the influx of persons from foreign lands we are seeing more worm infestations on the East Coast than formerly and are not entirely at ease in our handling of the anthelmintics. Would you kindly supply a statement of what may be achieved with the respective drugs, their dosage and their toxicities and contraindications?"

Reply: PIPERAZINE CITRATE (ANTEPAR, ETC.). With this drug successful riddance may be expected in well over three fourths of the cases of *pinworm infestation* (actually in 93.2% of the cases reviewed by Bumbalo and Plummer in 1957), though of course reinfestation is a notoriously frequent occurrence in this malady no matter what drug is used. The combination of piperazine and senna (Pripsen) is palatable and easy to take. Recent studies also indicate high efficacy of piperazine in *roundworm infestation*, a 4–7 day course of treatments sufficing again in over three fourths of the cases; Brown (1960) says, in fact, that therapy on 2 consecutive days will eliminate approximately 95% of the worms. A great advantage from the standpoint of use in *Ascaris* infestations is that the worms are not stimulated into primary activity as is the case with some of the previously used drugs, and therefore it may be expected that rupture of the bowel or occlusion of the common bile duct by large and muscular worms attempting to escape from a violently antagonistic agent will not occur with this drug. Recommended dosage of the syrup in *Enterobius* (pinworm) cases is ½ teaspoonful daily during each day of treatment (7 days of therapy, 7 days of rest and another 7 of therapy) for children up to 15 pounds body weight; ½ teaspoonful twice daily for children up to 30 pounds; 1 teaspoonful twice daily for those up to 60 pounds; 2 teaspoonfuls twice daily for those over 60 pounds. In *Ascaris* (roundworm) cases, the same dosage is used but only for a 4–7 day course.

Therapeutic dosage appears to be associated with no toxicity except very rare gastrointestinal disturbances and urticaria. Accidental ingestion of excessively large amounts has caused muscular weakness, blurred vision and other evidences of reversible effects upon the central nervous system. Combes and associates suggested that piperazine should be given very cautiously to individuals with impaired renal function.

DIETHYLCARBAMAZINE (HETRAZAN). This drug has a good record in roundworm infestation. Since pronounced and sustained reductions in microfilariae occur with the drug in practically every patient with *bancroftian filariasis*, and since there appear to be no recurrences without reinfestation, it is highly regarded in this disease. The disappearance of inflammatory and allergic reactions seems to reflect the death of adult worms in filariasis; when symptoms persist despite disappearance of microfilariae from the blood stream it is tentatively assumed that some of the adults have not been killed. Of course well advanced elephantiasis is not affected by the agent more than through relief from recurrent lymphangitis, though some softening of indurated tissue apparently may take place. The drug is used with as much success in *loiasis* as in bancroftian filariasis, but in *onchocerciasis* the action appears to be less rapid and permanent. Shanker and associates used diethylcarbamazine with excellent results in a large series of cases of *tropical pulmonary eosinophilia* in India.

Usual dosage in filariasis is 2 mg./kg. orally, three times daily for several weeks. In the beginning of the treatment period there is an acute exacerbation of symptoms, thought to reflect release of filarial protein by dead worms. In patients who have had unusually severe attacks and are presumably hypersensitized to such protein it appears advisable to begin treatment with dosage of only 0.2–0.5 mg./kg. Treatment should continue for 3 weeks after the protein reactions are no longer obtained. In patients who do not have such reactions, either because they are not sensitized or because the drug is not killing the worms, treatment should persist for 4–6 weeks. Under conditions in which it has not been possible to treat native populations for several weeks, one dose daily for 7 days has been used satisfactorily. In such instances the giving of 12 mg./kg. about 8:30 p.m., when the microfilarial tide is rising, causes disappearance of 60–80% of the microfilariae within 30 minutes. Intravenous injection of 50 mg. of the citrate salt has caused disappearance of 60% of the organisms in 4 minutes.

In ascariasis (roundworm) it appears that 15 mg./kg. in a single dose daily for 4 consecutive days suffices. Neither pretreatment dietary alteration nor post-treatment purging is necessary when this drug is used.

When the higher dosage is used, nausea and vomiting and epigastric pain sometimes occur, especially if the drug is taken on an empty stomach. But the lower doses cause, if anything, only headache, nausea, sedation and malaise that are both mild and brief. It has been reported that diethylcarbamazine is well tolerated by patients with hepatic and renal insufficiency, hypertension and coronary disease. The drug causes no changes in blood urea or cholesterol. It should be noted, however, that in onchocerciasis the allergic reactions due to larval destruction are likely to be prohibitively severe.

HEXYLRESORCINOL. This is an excellent all-round anthelmintic, being very effective in *roundworm, hookworm, pinworm, whipworm* and *dwarf tapeworm* cases. It has the disadvantage, though, of requiring preliminary starvation and post-treatment purgation. It is given orally in the same dosage for all infestations in which it is useful. After a saline purge the night before, it is administered on an empty stomach in the morning. When the specially coated Crystoids capsules in 0.1 or 0.2 Gm. size are used, a child under 6 years is given 0.4 Gm.; 6–10 years, 0.8 Gm.; older children and adults, 1.0 Gm. No food is allowed for 4 hours and a saline purge (not magnesium sulfate) is given 24 hours later. The treatment may be repeated after 3 days. Successful use of hexylresorcinol enemas in whipworm cases has been reported, repeating at 3–7 day intervals until parasites and eggs no longer appear in the feces. If fluoroscopic control is to be employed, the formula used contains 1 Gm. of hexylresorcinol, 30 Gm. of barium sulfate and 300 ml. of lukewarm water; otherwise, 30 Gm. of acacia is given to replace the barium sulfate. The patient is given only liquids for supper, a cleansing enema at 9 p.m. and another at 6 the next morning, and then the anthelmintic enema at 8 a.m. in dosage of 20 ml. of the formula per pound body weight up to 60 pounds. The anal region and adjacent areas must have petrolatum liberally applied to them for protection against the irritating suspension, a no. 22 French catheter is introduced as far as possible before the enema tube is connected, and effort should be made—through massaging the abdomen while the patient lies on his right side with the catheter in place—to have the fluid carried up to the cecum. Retention should be for about 10 minutes.

Systemic toxicity is practically unknown, but if the capsule is chewed it may burn the mouth and cause some local gastrointestinal discomfort. Hexylresorcinol is contraindicated in gastroenteritis and in peptic ulcer.

TETRACHLOROETHYLENE. The superiority of tetrachloroethylene to all other anthelmintics in *hookworm infestation* is well established because of the ease of administration, relatively low cost, low toxicity and relatively high efficacy in a single treatment. However, efficacy is very much greater in *N. americanus* than in *A. duodenale* cases. Effectiveness in *pinworm* cases is only fair, and the drug is practically useless in all the other infestations except that its trial may be worthwhile in a patient with *intestinal flukes*.

Tetrachloroethylene is given in the morning on an empty stomach and nowadays not followed by a cathartic of any sort because recent studies indicate that to do this both increases toxicity and lessens efficacy. Dosage for children is 0.2 ml. per year of age up to 15 years; adult dose 3–4 ml. Treatment may be repeated at 4 or 5 day intervals if eggs continue to be found in the stool.

DITHIAZANINE IODIDE (DELVEX). This drug, which is a fairly new one, is probably the most effective agent we have against *whipworm* and *strongyloides infestations* and it also has some efficacy against *pinworm* and *roundworm* infestations. But the reactions to it are both so frequent and often severe that its employment is doubtfully advisable unless the strongyloides and whipworm cases are associated with definitely disturbing symptomatology, and it appears to be the consensus that it should not be used in roundworm infestations for the reason that we have a more effective and much less toxic drug in piperazine.

The drug is given two or three times daily for a 5–10 day course in the whipworm cases and for 7–21 days in strongyloidiasis. Brown's total daily dosage for children was: 20–30 pounds, 200 mg.; 30–40 pounds, 300 mg.; 40–50 pounds, 400 mg.; 50–60 pounds, 500 mg.; over 60 pounds, 600 mg.

The drug frequently causes severe gastrointestinal irritation—anorexia, nausea, vomiting, abdominal cramps, diarrhea. Other reactions occurring less frequently have been transient albuminuria, edema, urticaria and fever; and there have been some instances of hypotension, acidosis, coma and death. The drug should certainly not be used in individuals with renal insufficiency or in those with electrolyte imbalance or dehydration. The drug stains the stools blue.

PYRVINIUM PAMOATE (POVAN). This new drug is highly effective in *pinworm infestations*. In the experience of J. W. Beck and associates a single-dose treatment eliminated the worm in 96 of 100 children without evidence of toxicity. However, it may be necessary to give one or more subsequent treatments at intervals of 2 or 3 weeks in order fully to clear the situation. There is also some efficacy in *Strongyloides infestations*. Usual dosage for children and adults as well is 5 mg./kg. as a single dose. There has been a low incidence of nausea, vomiting and abdominal cramping, and photosensitivity has been reported but in only one instance so far as I am aware.

QUINACRINE (ATABRINE) is used quite effectively in the treatment of *tapeworm infestations* (T. saginata, T. solium, D. latum). On the day preceding treatment the patient eats a light supper and then takes no breakfast on the treatment morning. Adult dosage is 0.2 Gm. quinacrine and 0.6 Gm. of sodium bicarbonate by mouth every 10 minutes for four doses; 2 hours after the last dose a saline cathartic is given. Dosage should probably be cut in half for children 3 years of age and under.

METHYLROSANILINE CHLORIDE (GENTIAN VIOLET) is useful in *Strongyloides* infestation and also in *pinworm* cases. For children with pinworm infestation, dosage is 10 mg. daily with meals for 8 days for each year of apparent age, then a rest of 1 week and the course is repeated; adult dosage, 65 mg. three times daily. In *Strongyloides* cases the administration is usually continued for twice as long.

Nausea, vomiting, abdominal pain, diarrhea, headache and dizziness sometimes accompany gentian violet medication but subside quickly when dosage is reduced or the drug is omitted for a day or two. It has been felt that contraindications to this therapy are concomitant infestation with roundworms, gastrointestinal, cardiac, hepatic or renal disease, and pregnancy, but Brown gave full dosage for 10 consecutive days to 20 children infested with *Ascaris lumbricoides* and did not observe indications of migration or of intestinal or pharyngeal obstruction. He also stated that in regions of heavy *Ascaris* infestation he had found local physicians routinely employing gentian violet against pinworms without noting any untoward reactions resulting from the presence of *Ascaris*. Alcohol should not be ingested during the period of treatment.

THE ANTIMONIALS. The symptoms in *schistosomiasis* are due to the local processes in the bladder and intestine resulting from the lodgment of the paired male and female flukes in the submucosal veins in the two sites. Obviously, anthelmintic agents that are given by mouth and are not absorbed would not be effective in the treatment of this condition. We were helpless in the disease until tartar emetic was introduced for intravenous use in the early part of this century. It is remarkably effective, not only in killing the flukes but, at least in the opinion of some experienced observers, in killing the ova as well, though Maegraith has trenchantly remarked that no entirely satisfactory agent has yet been discovered. At any rate it is unquestionably more effective than either of the other two trivalent compounds, antimony thioglycollamide and stibophen, though the latter are considerably less toxic.

Tartar emetic is nowadays given intravenously in schistosomiasis in a 0.5% solution in glucose-saline, injecting at a maximum rate of 8 ml./minute. Injections are given every other day, being increased from the initial 8 ml. injection by 4 ml. each dose until a 28 ml. dose is reached. Thereafter 28 ml. is given at each injection (or 14 ml. at each of two injections) on alternate days until 444 ml. have been given.

Stibophen (Fuadin) is given to adults with schistosomiasis in a 34 ml. course of the commercially available 6.3% solution. On the first day, three intramuscular injections of 2.4 and 4.0 ml. are given at 4 hour intervals; on each of the 2 subsequent days, three injections of 4 ml. each at 3 hour intervals. Children are given 17 ml. during the 3 days: a first dose of 1 ml., followed by two doses of 2 ml. each at 3 hour intervals and then three doses of 2 ml. each at 3 hour intervals on each of the 2 succeeding days.

Antimony thioglycollamide dosage, intramuscularly or intravenously, is a course of 15–25 injections of 0.08 Gm. each on alternate days, at least 12 additional injections being given later to prevent relapse. This drug is not presently commercially available in the United States and indeed is used very little anywhere, I believe.

A systemic antimony reaction has the following features: dizziness, coughing, vomiting, diarrhea, muscle and joint pains, hepatitis (necessitating immediate cessation of the treatment), severe headache and rigor, electrocardiographic changes, striking bradycardia and frightening respiratory standstill. The considerable likelihood of these things occurring during a tartar emetic course has made this drug very unpopular with the patients, but I believe that governmental agencies charged with the treatment of large native populations still feel that the old drug is the best despite the drawbacks of toxicity and the necessity for intravenous administration. The general systemic toxicity of the other antimony preparations is certainly less, but the intramuscular injections cause pronounced soreness. None of the compounds should be given to patients with liver, kidney or heart disease. The clinical efficacy of dimercaprol (BAL) in antimony poisoning is doubtful. The occurrence of both sulfhemoglobinuria and optic neuropathy have been reported in association with organic antimonial administration.

H. W. Brown. The Action and Uses of Anthelmintics. Clin. Pharmacol. & Therap. 1:87, 1960. Use of Gentian Violet in Children Infected with Ascaris Lumbriocoides. J. Pediat. 28:160, 1946. T. S. Bumbalo and L. J. Plummer. Piperazine (Antepar) in the Treatment of Pinworm and Roundworm Infections. M. Clin. North America, p. 575, 1957. B. Combes, A. Damon and E. Gottfried. Piperazine (Antepar) Neurotoxicity. New England J. Med. 254:223, 1956. J. W. Beck, D. Saavedra, G. J. Antell and B. Tejeiro. Treatment of Pinworm Infections in Humans with Pryvinium Chloride and Pryvinium Pamoate. Am. J. Trop. Med. & Hyg. 8:349, 1959. B. Maegraith. Schistosomiasis in China. Lancet 1:208, 1958. Zoheir Farid. Treatment of Multiple Helminthic Infections in Egypt with Dithiazanine. J. Trop. Med. & Hyg. 67:200, 1965. Thomas S. Bumbalo. Single-Dose Regimen in Treatment of Pinworm Infection. New York J. Med. 65:248, Jan. 15, 1965.

"In our area, where the rate of worm infestation is not very high, the new drug thiabendazole (Mintezol) has been introduced for experimental study. Has this agent been tried in an area in which there is a high incidence of infestation throughout the population?"

Reply: Yes, David Botero R. has reported such a study from Colombia, where it is said that over 80% of the population is infested with intestinal helminths and many people suffer severely from such infestations. In a series of 132 ambulatory patients, harboring 284 intestinal worm infestations, he obtained best results with the drug against *Strongyloides stercoralis, Ascaris lumbricoides* and hookworms. Effectiveness was very weak for *Trichuris trichiura*, and there was no effect at all in cases of *Taenia solium* and *T. saginata* infections. In a children's institution in New York, Harry Most's group found the drug highly effective in both strongyloides and enterobius infestations.

David Botero R. Treatment of Human Intestinal Helminthiases with Thiabendazole. Am. Jour. Trop. Med. & Hygiene. 14:618, 1965. Harry Most, Meir Yoeli, William C. Campbell and Ashton C. Cuckler. Treatment of Strongyloides and Enterobius Infections with Thiabendazole. Am. J. Trop. Med. & Hyg. 14:379, 1965.

"With the increasing influx along the East Coast of individuals from regions where filariasis is endemic, we are beginning to be somewhat concerned with the problem of filarial elephantiasis. Is there anything new in this therapy?"

Reply: In India, B. N. Prasad has reported

a study of the use of sodium fluoride. The subjects were patients with limb swelling, history of lymphangitis, lymphadenitis and fever and rigor at frequent intervals. Sodium fluoride, 0.5 mg. twice daily after meals, was given for 27 months and measurements of the elephantiastic limb were made at monthly intervals in 190 patients with known filariasis. Cure was considered to have occurred when the affected limb and the control limb showed equal measurements. It was found that 13.67% of patients were cured, 69.79% improved. It was felt that the drug had its suppressive action on the microfilaria or on the mother filaria and that its presence might inhibit the lymphatic obstructions seen with high calcium levels in filariasis. This was an interesting preliminary study and confirmation has not yet been had, so far as I am aware.

Birendra N. Prasad. Fluoride in Filarial Elephantiasis. Indian J. Dermat. 9:79, 1964.

"In the treatment of schistosomiasis the use of the standard antimony preparations has been difficult because of the high incidence and severity of the reactions. Has any newer antimonial been shown to be equally effective and less toxic?"

Reply: In the Tropical Disease Clinics of the New York City Health Department, Zaki and his associates treated 69 Puerto Rican patients with viable eggs of Schistosoma mansoni in the stools with 10% solution of Astiban in total dosage of 15–20 ml. given during 4 or 5 days, 66 other patients receiving a 6.3% solution of Fuadin in dosage of 60–80 ml. given during 40–50 days. Cure was considered established by 6 negative stools in a follow-up period of 4 months. The cure rate with Astiban was 79.6% and with Fuadin 80.4%. There was vomiting in 45% of the Astiban and 23% of the Fuadin-treated patients; joint or muscle pain in 30 and 51% respectively; rashes in 24 and 3% respectively; anorexia, gastric discomfort or nausea in 44 and 36%, respectively.

Mahfouz H. Zaki, Howard B. Shookhoff, Max Sterman and Stanley de Ramos. Astiban in Schistosomiasis Mansoni: Controlled Therapeutic Trial in a Nonendemic Area. Am. J. Trop. Med. & Hyg. 13:803, 1964.

"I have heard that there is a new drug available for the treatment of trichinosis. What of this?"

Reply: At the University of Texas, Orville Stone's group reported the probable cure of a single case of trichinosis with the new drug thiabendazole (Mintezol), but unfortunately B. H. Kean and Donald Hoskins, in New York, were not able entirely to confirm this experience in their 4 patients, in whom treatment was initiated with the drug in dosage of 25 mg./kg. twice daily for 5–7 days, 31–36 days after infection. Clinical improvement was noted within 48 hours of beginning administration, but the drug did not kill all the larvae. All patients experienced severe nausea, and psychic symptoms developed in 2 of them. There was also transient dermatitis in all and drug fever in 1. The drug certainly needs much more study before one can be certain of its status.

Orville J. Stone, Charles T. Stone, Jr., and J. Fred Mullins. Thiabendazole – Probable Cure for Trichinosis: Report of First Case. J.A.M.A. 187:536, Feb. 15, 1964. B. H. Kean and Donald W. Hoskins. Treatment of Trichinosis with Thiabendazole (Mintezol). J.A.M.A. 190:852, Nov. 30, 1964.

"In my experience dithiazanine (Delvex) has been highly efficacious against Strongyloides infection, but it has been disturbingly toxic. Has pyrvinium pamoate (Povan), which is effective against oxyuriasis, been tried in strongyloidiasis?"

Reply: Yes, in New York, Wang and Galli used this drug in doses from 2.0 to 6.4 mg./kg./day for 7 days in the treatment of 12 confirmed cases of strongyloidiasis, while another 12 patients were treated with conventional dithiazanine iodide enteric-coated tablets in doses of 6.0 mg. to 20.8 mg./kg./day for 7 days as a comparative control group. In the pyrvinium-treated group the stools of 11 patients were consistently negative after the treatment, whereas in the dithiazanine group only the stools of 8 patients were consistently negative after the treatment. There were only mild side effects associated with the pyrvinium treatment but they were severe in association with the dithiazanine therapy.

Chung C. Wang and Gloria A. Galli. Strongyloidiasis Treated with Pyrvinium Pamoate. J.A.M.A. 193:847, Sept. 6, 1965.

"Occasionally I have an adult patient with a tapeworm and usually have difficulty in getting out the scolex in the first treatment. Is there any new departure in this therapy?"

Reply: Several years ago E. L. Lloyd, in Edinburgh, reported the successful treatment of 3 patients by pituitary injection after quinacrine (Atabrine). In a typical case, after purgation on the evening before, the patient was given 1 Gm. of quinacrine orally at 6:00 a.m. and at 7:07 a.m. he was given Pituitrin, 0.5 ml. intramuscularly, and 7 minutes later the worm began to pass. After a cup of tea at 7:25 a.m., 8 ft. of yellow-stained worm with scolex, all in one piece, arrived at 7:30 a.m. The patient had no side effects at all, breakfasted at 8:00 a.m. and returned to active duty after lunch.

Then there is the DeRivas transduodenal intubation method, as modified by Rosen and Kiefer, which seems to be very little known but has the merit of not only being frequently successful but of using no drugs of high potential toxicity. In a typical case, as reported by Robert Lussky and associates (Northwestern University), a Rehfuss tube is passed into the duodenum and, with fluoroscopic control, the tip is placed in the second or third portion of the duodenum. Then in quick succession, 45 ml. of 50% magnesium sulfate, 45 ml. glycerin, 60 ml. of a mixture of equal parts magnesium sulfate and glycerin, and finally 500 ml. physiologic saline at 130° F. are introduced into the tube. Within a very few minutes, usually after only minimal abdominal cramps, there occurs a copious bowel movement containing the entire worm and scolex intact. This form of therapy is based on the fact that protozoan and metazoan intestinal parasites cannot survive more than 10 minutes immersed in either glycerin or saline warmed to 130–140° F.

E. L. Lloyd. Pituitary (Posterior Lobe) for Tardy Tapeworms. Practitioner 185:329, 1960. D. DeRivas. Intestinal Parasites. Am. J. Trop. Med. & Hyg. 12:477, 1952. S. W. Rosen and E. D. Kiefer. Treatment of Tapeworm Infestation. J.A.M.A. 167:2065, 1958. Robert Lussky, John L. Sever and Bernard H. Adelson. Treatment of Beef Tapeworm Infestation by Transduodenal Intubation. Quart. Bull. Northwestern Univ. M. School 33:240, 1959.

XANTHOMATOSIS

"I have a patient with xanthomatosis who has not responded to the usual drugs used in treatment of atherosclerosis, i.e., nicotinic acid, d-thyroxine and cholestyramine resin. What do I do now?"

Reply: In Australia, M. A. Mishkel has reported the somewhat effective use of Atromid, which is described as a mixture of 2.2% w/w androsterone in ethyl (parachlorophenoxy) isobutyrate. The dosage for men was 2.25 Gm. daily initially and for women 1.5 Gm., given in the form of 250 mg. capsules. All patients were then maintained on 6–9 capsules daily for up to 1 year. The mean falls in cholesterol and triglyceride levels after 40 weeks of treatment in the successfully treated cases were 31.9 and 5.7%, respectively, with serum phospholipid levels following closely but no effect on serum uric acid. Best responses were obtained in patients with milky serum. Tendon xanthomata and tuberous xanthomata of long duration were most resistant, and eruptive xanthomata and planar xanthomata of the hands were most amenable. There was usually only slight regression of xanthelasma.

M. A. Mishkel. Treatment of Xanthomatosis with Atromid. M. J. Australia 2:828, Nov. 21, 1964.

YAWS

"What is the preferred drug therapy in yaws?"

Reply: Penicillin. Treat as for syphilis.

YELLOW FEVER

"Those of us who have children of our own or young friends who are in the Peace Corps are concerned about yellow fever. Fred Soper and Austin Kerr and their devoted associates have pretty well cleaned the thing up in the western hemisphere, but there is plenty of it still in Africa. And a lot of the kids are out there. Is there *nothing* that approaches specific therapy?"

Reply: No.

Index